The Psychoanalytic Study of the Child

VOLUME THIRTY

Founding Editors

ANNA FREUD, LL.D., D.SC.
HEINZ HARTMANN, M.D.
ERNST KRIS, PH.D.

Managing Editors

RUTH S. EISSLER, M.D.
ANNA FREUD, LL.D., D.SC.
MARIANNE KRIS, M.D.
ALBERT J. SOLNIT, M.D.

Editorial Board

RUTH S. EISSLER, M.D.
ANNA FREUD, LL.D., D.SC.
PHYLLIS GREENACRE, M.D.
EDITH B. JACKSON, M.D.
MARIANNE KRIS, M.D.
RUDOLPH M. LOEWENSTEIN, M.D.
ALBERT J. SOLNIT, M.D.

Associate Editor

LOTTIE MAURY NEWMAN

The Psychoanalytic Study of the Child

VOLUME THIRTY

New Haven
Yale University Press
1975

Copyright © 1975, Ruth S. Eissler,
Anna Freud, Marianne Kris, and Albert J. Solnit.
All rights reserved. This book may not be
reproduced, in whole or in part, in any form
(except by reviewers for the public press),
without written permission from the publishers.
Library of Congress catalog card number: 45–11304
International standard book number: 0-300-01916-5

Designed by Sally Sullivan
and set in Baskerville type.
Printed in the United States of America by
The Colonial Press Inc., Clinton, Massachusetts.

Contents

Thirty Years Later   xi

PROBLEMS OF DEVELOPMENT

Dorothy Burlingham
   Special Problems of Blind Infants:
   Blind Baby Profile   3
Bertrand Cramer
   Outstanding Developmental Progression
   in Three Boys: A Longitudinal Study   15
Steven L. Dubovsky and Stephen E. Groban
   Congenital Absence of Sensation   49
W. Ernest Freud
   Infant Observation: Its Relevance
   to Psychoanalytic Training   75
Katrina de Hirsch
   Language Deficits in Children
   with Developmental Lags   95
Martin A. Silverman, Katherine Rees,
   and Peter B. Neubauer
   On a Central Psychic Constellation   127

CONTRIBUTIONS TO PSYCHOANALYTIC THEORY

Rose Edgcumbe and Marion Burgner
   The Phallic-Narcissistic Phase:
   A Differentiation between Preoedipal and
   Oedipal Aspects of Phallic Development   161
Irving B. Harrison
   On the Maternal Origins of Awe   181

ALEX HOLDER
Theoretical and Clinical Aspects of Ambivalence   197
PATRICK MAHONY AND RAJENDRA SINGH
The Interpretation of Dreams, Semiology,
and Chomskian Linguistics: A Radical Critique   221
BURNESS E. MOORE
Toward a Clarification of the Concept
of Narcissism   243

CLINICAL CONTRIBUTIONS

MARIA BERGER AND HANSI KENNEDY
Pseudobackwardness in Children: Maternal
Attitudes As an Etiological Factor
Foreword by Anna Freud   279
ROBERT EVANS
"Hysterical Materialization" in the
Analysis of a Latency Girl   307
CHARLES FEIGELSON
The Mirror Dream   341
MAURITS KATAN
Childhood Memories As Contents of
Schizophrenic Hallucinations and Delusions   357
JEROME D. OREMLAND
An Unexpected Result of the Analysis
of a Talented Musician   375
JOSEPH SANDLER, HANSI KENNEDY, AND
ROBERT L. TYSON
Discussions on Transference: The
Treatment Situation and Technique
in Child Psychoanalysis   409
HEIMAN VAN DAM, CHRISTOPH M. HEINICKE,
AND MORTON SHANE
On Termination of Child Analysis   443

APPLICATIONS OF PSYCHOANALYSIS

A. *Clinical Applications*
GILBERT W. KLIMAN
Analyst in the Nursery: Experimental Application

of Child Analytic Techniques in a Therapeutic
Nursery: The Cornerstone Method 477
Moses Laufer
Preventive Intervention in Adolescence 511
William Thomas Moore
The Impact of Surgery on Boys 529
Albert J. Solnit and Beatrice Priel
Psychological Reactions to Facial and
Hand Burns in Young Men: Can I See
Myself Through Your Eyes? 549
Norman E. Zinberg
Addiction and Ego Function 567

B. *Applications to Other Fields*
K. R. Eissler
The Fall of Man 589
Joseph Goldstein
Why Foster Care—For Whom for How Long? 647
Jeanne Lampl-de Groot
Vicissitudes of Narcissism and
Problems of Civilization 663
Leonard Shengold
An Attempt at Soul Murder: Rudyard
Kipling's Early Life and Work 683
Stephen M. Weissman
Frederick Douglass, Portrait of a Black
Militant: A Study in the Family Romance 725

Index 753

Bibliographical Note

S.E. *The Standard Edition of the Complete Psychological Works of Sigmund Freud,* 24 Volumes, translated and edited by James Strachey. London: Hogarth Press and the Institute of Psycho-Analysis, 1953–1974.

Writings *The Writings of Anna Freud,* 7 Volumes. New York: International Universities Press, 1968–1974.

IN MEMORIAM

The Editors regretfully announce the death of Dr. René A. Spitz. This distinguished pioneer psychoanalyst was an original member of our Editorial Board. An appreciation of his work will appear in the next volume.

Thirty Years Later

In 1945, the first volume of *The Psychoanalytic Study of the Child* was introduced by its editors as follows:

> The contribution of psychoanalysis to the study of the child covers many areas. In therapy the range extends from child analysis to child guidance and group work; in theory, from the basic problems of genetic psychology to those concerned with the interrelation of culture and the upbringing of the child. While many psychiatric techniques and many concepts upon which psychologists and educators rely bear the imprint of psychoanalytic thought, contributions to this Annual center on psychoanalytic hypotheses. It is hoped that from this center contacts with neighboring fields will be established.
>
> This Annual is an Anglo-American venture. We hope that in following volumes we may include contributions from other countries.

The "Anglo-American" venture was established by the three editors: Anna Freud, Heinz Hartmann, and Ernst Kris. Ruth S. Eissler joined the editors in 1949, and Marianne Kris in 1957. Lottie M. Newman became associated with the *Study* in 1950. Supported by an editorial board of distinguished analysts, the three managing editors stood for the highest standards in psychoanalysis. This goal is as valid in 1975 as it was in 1945.

In 1945, there were only a few psychoanalytic publications, and these few had during the last years of World War II become more and more interested in psychosomatic medicine, brief psychotherapy, and military psychiatric experiences—understandably enough, since the war emphasized the need for quick and effective therapeutic help. During this period in England, Melanie Klein's school was prominently represented in the English psychoanalytic literature. In other European countries, where psychoanalysis had once prospered, it either was officially abandoned—as in Germany, Austria, and Italy—or could not be openly practiced—as in the Netherlands, France, and Czechoslovakia.

There was one place, though, from which news reached the United States from time to time, news of interesting developments based on Freud's thought. This was the work done at the Hampstead Nurseries, where Anna Freud and Dorothy Burlingham, with a staff of collaborators, took care of infants and young children whose families had been bombed out or killed. For several years we received reports about the activities at Hampstead through the Foster Parents' Organization, and we were thus informed not only of the help that was given these children and their mothers, but also of the scientific work that was carried out at the same time. This experience was described by Anna Freud and Dorothy Burlingham in two books: *Infants Without Families* and *Children in Wartime*.

If the difficulties of psychoanalysis in the years between 1938 and 1945 have a certain similarity to the state of affairs in 1975, we must not overlook that in the 30 years separating us from the end of World War II we have also experienced a tremendous upsurge of interest in psychoanalysis. In particular, as psychoanalytic theory was useful in understanding and treating psychic disorders in the armed forces as well as defining our limitations in curing them, young physicians returning from the armed forces felt a great interest in and need for psychoanalytic training. This was the moment when the first volume of *The Psychoanalytic Study of the Child* made its appearance. It at once filled a great need, and subsequent volumes have continued to do so.

The founding editors promised a continued venture into those areas of psychology which either had been neglected or were not yet accessible to psychoanalytic research. The development of psychoanalytic ego psychology opened up new avenues of investigation: (1) the study of the narcissistic disorders; (2) the development of the early infant-mother relationship, which was largely studied by direct observations; (3) the impact of sensory disturbances, due to deprivation and deficits in the ego, could be pursued after normal development had been understood in terms of the structural theory and the mutual influences of ego and id.

Much of the spadework in these areas had been done by Anna Freud and Dorothy Burlingham at Hampstead, and by Heinz Hartmann and Ernst Kris in this country. From the start, Sybille K. Escalona, Phyllis Greenacre, Margaret S. Mahler, René A. Spitz, Katherine M. Wolf, and many others contributed the results of their research to *The Psychoanalytic Study of the Child*. Berta Bornstein published her classic papers on the technique of child analysis in these volumes.

If one follows the contents of the individual volumes year by year, one obtains a clear view of the history of psychoanalysis during the past 30 years. In 1965, the Monograph Series of *The Psychoanalytic Study of the Child* was added to the annual volumes. These monographs contained the result of research done by individual authors or a group of authors; reports which because of their completeness and length cannot be fitted into the Annual.

The *Study* and the first volumes of the Monograph Series throughout the 30 years contain an impressive record of the psychoanalytic research, clinical and theoretical, done at the Hampstead Child-Therapy Clinic under Anna Freud's leadership. Their papers on the early development of the child, on borderline disturbances, on the specific impact of trauma, on the psychological problems of children in hospitals, on special pathology found in small children who survived in the concentration camps, on problems of adolescence served to enrich the volumes of *The Psychoanalytic Study of the Child*. Dorothy Burlingham's studies of the blind child, direct observations of the small child, Anna Freud's formulation of the Developmental Lines and the Developmental Profile were brought to fruition in the reassessment of developmental difficulties and childhood disturbances, in particular, the infantile neurosis.

This comprehensive work, to a large extent published in the 30 volumes of the *Study*, was done with the stimulation and cross-fertilization of the investigations of authors in the United States. In particular, the theoretical papers by Heinz Hartmann, Ernst Kris, and Rudolph M. Loewenstein were basic to the development of the science of psychoanalysis and the refinement of psychoanalytic concepts. These, in turn, stimulated the interest in normal and abnormal development of the child, and guided the method of direct observation.

To originate and carry out this Anglo-American venture during the last years of World War II was, indeed, a remarkable feat. Communication between the two countries was at best slow, if not at times disrupted. It was certainly not easy to find a publisher willing to launch a new psychoanalytic annual at that time. However, A. S. Kagan of International Universities Press undertook this task, and remained during the following 25 years a loyal and faithful friend of this publication. The editors, authors, and readers of *The Psychoanalytic Study of the Child* owe him warm thanks.

Yet, as it happens with so many creations, the *Study* gradually developed a life of its own; in this case, it grew up and migrated to Yale. This, however, was the final outcome of a particular situation which had existed for many years. Yale had presented during the last 30 years an ever-increasing hospitable and happy climate for psychoanalytic teaching and research. In particular, Anna Freud, Ernst Kris, Marianne Kris, Seymour L. Lustman, and Albert J. Solnit were attached as teachers and researchers to Yale University. Thus, when a few years ago *The Psychoanalytic Study of the Child* was invited by the Yale University Press to become one of its children, the editors accepted this invitation, feeling that their publication has not really emigrated from New York but has returned to Yale, where so many of its contributions had originated.

THE EDITORS

PROBLEMS
OF DEVELOPMENT

Special Problems of Blind Infants

Blind Baby Profile

DOROTHY BURLINGHAM

IN OUR ATTEMPTS TO APPLY THE DEVELOPMENTAL PROFILE (ANNA Freud, 1965) to blind children, we found that special provisions must be made for the fact of blindness. While many of the developmental factors that the Baby Profile (W. E. Freud, 1967, 1971) assesses are the same, others are unique to the blind. In this paper I shall concentrate on the latter. In singling out specific areas for observation and evaluation, I have a double purpose in mind. On the one hand, careful attention to these areas will help in the completion of a Baby Profile for the Blind, which in turn might aid us in deciding some of the unanswered questions concerning the development of the blind. On the other hand, the detailed understanding of the blind baby's specific needs can serve as a practical guide to help mothers of such infants.

All mothers of blind and physically handicapped children need guidance with the tremendous problems they face, but we can help

---

The material used in this paper stems from the author's work with the Study Group for the Blind at the Hampstead Child-Therapy Course and Clinic, London: Annemarie Curson, Alice Goldberger, Anne Hayman, Hansi Kennedy, Elizabeth E. Model, and Doris Wills. The Hampstead Clinic is at present supported by the Field Foundation, Inc., New York; the Foundation for Research in Psychoanalysis, Beverly Hills, Calif.; the Freud Centenary Fund, London; the Anna Freud Foundation, New York; the National Institute for Mental Health, Maryland; the Grant Foundation, New York; the New-Land Foundation, Inc., New York; and a number of private supporters.

them only if we ourselves understand the special requirements of blind babies.

Family Background

In all our contacts with infants we attempt to learn a great deal about the background of the parents, their personal characteristics, their relationship to each other, and their past experiences. With parents of a blind infant it is especially important to determine whether similar abnormalities have occurred on either side of the family. If they have, we should attempt to find out whether the parents have been warned beforehand by either pediatrician or obstetrician that blindness may be transmitted to their child. We have two significant examples where mothers blind from an early age and married to blind husbands ignored all warnings and did not see why they should not claim the right to produce children. This contrasts very sharply with the almost ubiquitous tendency of mothers to blame themselves unreasonably for the child's handicap.

For this reason, when we examine the personal history of a sighted mother, we must pay special attention to the period of her pregnancy because it is of the utmost importance to find out whether she undertook any action which might have played a part in her producing a blind child, whether this was at the time of conception or in the intervening period before she gave birth. Regardless of whether rational or irrational, her belief that some action or behavior on her part is responsible for her baby's blindness will have a profound effect on the mother's sense of guilt and attitude to the infant.

In looking at the period after birth, we need to focus on six aspects that are especially significant for a mother's relationship to a blind infant:

1. The length of time during which the mother regards the baby as normal

2. The actual moment at which either mother or pediatrician recognizes the visual defect

3. The actual manner in which mother, or father, or both are informed of the finding

4. The mother's or parents' (as well as grandparents') manifest and latent reactions to the information and subsequent changes in their attitudes to the baby

5. The length of time during which the mother was estranged from the baby (if she so was) and the duration of her concentration on the handicap

6. The extent of the parents' eventual return to the baby as a person and the manner of recognizing his specific needs.

BODY NEEDS AND FUNCTIONS

SLEEP

It is obvious that blind babies will take longer than normal ones to establish a sleeping pattern with distinction between day and night. Such a delay in the sleeping pattern might even prove significant for the early diagnosis of defective vision.

It is well known that even sighted children may develop the habit of waking in the night, wishing to play, much to the distress of their parents. It is only logical that this happens much more frequently with the blind for whom there is no alternation between light and darkness.

It is worth investigating whether, in contrast to this, it is easier for blind children to fall asleep when they are put to bed because one of the distractions, namely, visual stimulation, is absent from the situation.

On the other hand, the baby's favorite sleeping positions, the specific sleeping arrangements (location, clothes), and the parental attitudes to sleep, though they should be noted, may be expected to be similar to those found in sighted children. Parents of blind infants also want them to sleep at specific times.

FEEDING

In the interaction between mother and blind child during feeding the absence of visual contact is of overriding significance. The observer should note how far the mother replaces this with skin contact or vocal contact, the extent to which the baby listens to the mother's ministrations and seeks communication with her, and the degree to which the mother is able to recognize and respond to these approaches.

Rooting or pleasurable sounds, signs of hunger or thirst—any mother would be pleased to answer to such signs: these areas have nothing to do with vision and a mother concerned about her baby, sighted or blind, would be relieved by such signs. The indications of hunger and thirst, the patterns of food intake, passive or active feeding would be similar for blind and sighted, but other factors are not.

Since the blind baby cannot watch the approach of food to his mouth, it should be noted especially in what manner the mother inserts the nipple, bottle, or spoon into the baby's mouth and whether there is a moment of hesitation on the mother's part in the expectation that the infant will react to the approach of breast or bottle. We should also note any changes in the mother's handling before she is aware of her baby's blindness and after she has this knowledge.

Instead of noting the infant's watching of the feeding operations, the observer must give the same attention to the infant's listening to them.

Special note should be made of mouth movements toward food and body postures since we do not know how far these are occasioned only by the sight of food and how far other sensory avenues, for example, smell, play a part here. Such clues to self-feeding as hand-reaching movements toward the mother and toward food, grasping, will have to be expected to occur later than in the sighted.

We can assume that interruptions of the feeding process are even more unpleasurable to the blind since nipple, bottle, or spoon, when removed from physical contact with the blind infant, disappear completely from his awareness.

Other Needs

PROTECTION AGAINST INAPPROPRIATE STIMULI AND PROVISION OF APPROPRIATE STIMULATION

Although most of the needs listed for sighted children apply equally for the blind, there are some quantitative and qualitative differences for which the Profile will have to make provision. One is that the role of auxiliary ego which every mother has to play is an extended one; the blind child is altogether more vulnerable and needs more protection and assistance. The other concerns the blind infant's extreme need for response and stimulation. This is not easy for the mothers since as sighted individuals they are more alerted to a visual interchange and get discouraged if they receive no response to their efforts of attracting the baby visually. The observer should note here whether this causes the mother to withdraw or whether she is inventive in finding other modes of interaction and stimulation.

STABILITY AND FLEXIBILITY OF ROUTINE ARRANGEMENTS

It may be important to keep in mind here that blind infants profit more than the sighted from the stability of routine arrangements and less from their flexibility. Since they are prone to be frightened of anything new and lack reassurance by the mother's glance, routine as the recurrence of expected events is helpful and gives the infant a feeling of security.

Prestages of Object Relationships

It is obvious that with the blind the anaclitic relationship lasts longer than with sighted children. Security is found in the mother's closeness and in her ministrations. Interruptions of the anaclitic relationship are therefore all the more disastrous for the blind.

The means by which the blind baby recognizes his mother, on the other hand, are far from obvious. It would be very important to know which perceptual modalities the infant uses, whether it takes a longer time for him to know that a different person is feeding him, and whether, on the contrary, he is more sensitive to such changes than sighted children.

Indications of Pleasure and Affects

PLEASURE-UNPLEASURE SIGNS

While the reaction to unpleasure would be the usual ones, such as withdrawal and crying, we cannot expect the blind infant to show the normal manifestations of pleasure since his concentration on listening, even if pleasurable, and the immobility required for listening prevent the visible manifestations of pleasure from appearing. It may well be that observers are misled into thinking that the blind infant is indifferent when in reality he is engaged with pleasurable acoustic impressions (Burlingham, 1972).

All infants derive much pleasure from sucking their fingers. However, in the blind infant, the last phase in finding the hands—looking at them before bringing them to the mouth—is missing. This may make a difference in the important developmental step of hand-mouth coordination and has to be taken into account.

We should also observe carefully whether the blind infant develops other means of gratification.

PLEASURABLE USE OF THE MOUTH FOR APPROACH, GRASPING, PERCEIVING, AND EXPLORING

The use of the mouth should be especially noted and described in even greater detail than normally. For exploration and differentiation, its use can be quite extraordinary. Blind children find the mouth the finest tool for differentiating and for acquiring knowledge of objects (spatial relations, surfaces, texture, shape); therefore it is of importance to know when and how this ability and preference develops, whether the blind's use of the mouth as a tool persists into later stages because it is rewarding, while the sighted give it up at an early age when other methods take its place. In any event, the persistent use of the mouth in the blind, despite its pleasurable elements, should not be interpreted solely as a manifestation of oral gratification, because it substitutes for and serves the purposes of important ego functions.

At a later age, I observed a little girl who in examining a room went along the wall, stopping to feel everything she met and could reach; she felt the floor with her feet and hands and finally with her tongue. Similarly, I know of a blind woman who, when she wanted to examine a fine detail of an object, secretly felt it with her tongue.

AVAILABILITY OR ACCESSIBILITY OF AFFECTS

Just as the pleasure manifestations of the blind infant differ from those of the sighted, his affective responses require special attention.

It is my impression that the blind's affective responses are less strong or wide in range than those of the sighted. This is probably due to lack of response or withdrawal on the part of the mother, as a result of which there may be reduced input of stimulation. But even if the mother is highly inventive in stimulating the infant, the absence of vision greatly reduces the input of the many diverse signs, gestures, and facial expressions by which the sighted recognize and respond to affective expressions.

In contrast, the blind infant's limited understanding of what is going on around him gives rise to specific affects expressing this. Thus we should be alert to look for signs of bewilderment, fear, and confusion, which in the blind occur frequently.

For these reasons, it is especially important not to make hasty judgments concerning the inappropriateness of affects in the blind. So often the observer is unaware of what the infant is reacting to, or why he shows the opposite reaction from the expected one. Very careful study is therefore required to determine not only the nature of the affective response but also its probable source—whether pleasure or distress or lack of affective manifestations occur in response to external or internal stimulations.

Motility and Aggression

AGGRESSION

When we look for signs of aggression in blind infants we should note in particular its lack where aggression would be expected; for instance, distress rather than aggression as a response to frustration. There is great fear of showing aggression when the dependence on the caretaking person is all-important. Only subtle ways of showing aggression are then permissible and tolerable.

MOTILITY

Like the sighted, the blind infant becomes more active and more mobile in relation to the opportunities for pleasurable discharge, which are stimulated by the caretaking person. While the avenues of discharge available to the blind do not differ from those of the sighted, it is very interesting that for the blind the feet seem to play a far more important role than the hands. The blind baby's use of the legs as a means of discharging libidinal and aggressive drives should therefore be explored. Moreover, a possible delay in the use of the hands in general (Fraiberg, 1968; Wills, 1968) should be noted.

The early preponderant use of the legs contrasts with the marked delay in motility, which becomes apparent at a later stage when the child has some awareness of the dangerous consequences of moving into the unknown. When the blind toddler has learned to walk, he will do so, but he will stay in the same place.

Despite the normal maturation of the motor apparatus a certain retardation of motility in the blind is expectable for several reasons. There is for the blind infant no known environment—such as walls, furniture, windows—which on the one hand gives stability and on the other tempts the growing toddler to move toward things or around them. Movement for the blind occurs in a vacuum. Although sound provides a certain amount of orientation, this is not sufficient.

This lack of environmental stimulation is further reinforced by the mother's protective attitude which is designed to guard the child's endangering himself as soon as independent movement is possible. These two influences act together as a delaying force.

State and Function of the Mental Apparatus

It is evident that when vision is absent, one or more of the other senses will be called on to take over some of its functions. In many respects, however, the development of the other senses has to be stimulated and taught. The substitution of sensory modalities brings disorder into the usual sequence of the development of the sensory apparatus as well as the ego functions dependent on them. We must therefore take into account that—

1. Perception and attention are dependent on the use of listening
2. Exploration and recognition rely on touch
3. Reality orientation takes place via sensations called forth by

sound, touch, vibrations, and probably also odor. These need to be integrated with each other before one can expect the blind child to have some awareness, for instance, of space

4. Memory traces are laid down by means of acoustic and other sensory modalities and will therefore differ greatly from visual memory traces.

The diminished sensory input requires a far greater intellectual effort on the part of the blind to arrive at the same degree of understanding that the sighted have of the environment. Special attention needs to be given to whether the infant is helped or hindered in this respect by the parents' efforts.

In this context, I also want to reemphasize that a blind child's apparent withdrawal from the external world need not be a reaction to unpleasure or a sign of lacking interest. Quite the contrary, it is a prerequisite for intensive listening and therefore a normal manifestation.

Forerunners of Fixation Points

There is no doubt that blind children more than others have a notable fixation in the stage of autoerotism. Again, this is partly attributable to the fact that they, much more than others, are "left to their own devices." Lacking perceptual stimulation and frequently also stimulation from the mother (who tends to pay less attention to a quiet baby), the blind infant spends much time in such autoerotic activities as rocking and swaying.

In the blind, the eyes often become a libidinized area, and their investment is significantly increased by examinations of and surgical interventions to the eye, restriction of touch after operations, which are so frequently necessary. Such experiences should be carefully noted.

Altogether blind infants have greater difficulty in progressing from the familiar and known to the unfamiliar and unknown. This in itself may create the semblance of fixation on a particular stage of development.

General Characteristics

In the Profile for sighted children we list general characteristics that have special prognostic relevance for the assessment of their development. These are not applicable to the blind and have to be replaced by others. Frustration tolerance can serve as an example. As with all handicapped children, frustration in the blind is the order of the day and a basic fact of their lives to which the children adapt in some way or other.

Instead I suggest a number of characteristics that might have special prognostic relevance for the blind's normal or abnormal development—
1. The infant's ability to make use of his remaining senses
2. The infant's ability to respond to appropriate stimulation
3. The infant's ability to express needs and wishes
4. With advancing ego development his intellectual ability to use the meager sensory data at his disposal for adequate orientation.

Summary

In selecting certain sections of the Profile for comment, I have tried to underscore two basic considerations in assessing the blind. On the one hand, we need to give special attention to those areas which are most affected by the impact of blindness; on the other, the usual behavioral manifestations we observe may have a different meaning in the blind.

The amendments I propose are a first step toward constructing the Baby Profile for the Blind. As our knowledge of blind babies increases, others will be added.

An early application of the Blind Baby Profile would be very helpful in assessing the normal or abnormal development of the blind, in sorting out the factors that are due to blindness, or to additional brain damage, and those that derive primarily from external sources and therefore can be influenced by appropriate guidance.

BIBLIOGRAPHY

BURLINGHAM, D. (1972), *Psychoanalytic Studies of the Sighted and the Blind.* New York: Int. Univ. Press.

FRAIBERG, S. (1968), Parallel and Divergent Patterns in Blind and Sighted Infants. *This Annual*, 23:264–300.

FREUD, A. (1965), *Normality and Pathology in Childhood.* New York: Int. Univ. Press.

FREUD, W. E. (1967), Assessment of Early Infancy. *This Annual*, 22:216–238.

——— (1971), The Baby Profile. *This Annual*, 26:172–194.

NAGERA, H. & COLONNA, A. B. (1965), Aspects of the Contribution of Sight to Ego and Drive Development. *This Annual*, 20:267–287.

WILLS, D. (1968), Problems of Play and Mastery in the Blind Child. *Brit. J. Med. Psychol.*, 41:213–222.

Outstanding Developmental Progression in Three Boys

A Longitudinal Study

B. CRAMER, M.D.

THIS PAPER REPORTS ON THE DEVELOPMENT OF THREE BOYS WHO WERE followed from the age of 4 up to the onset of puberty. These boys attracted our attention because they showed a very steady developmental progression accompanied by only very scanty symptom formation. These three children were part of a group of forty-five children whom we followed and assessed longitudinally. As we studied all these children and gave them developmental ratings, these three boys stood out from the rest of the children: none of the remaining forty-two children showed the same vigorous, steady, developmental pull, the same apparent ease in coping with conflicts and new adaptational tasks, and the same relative lack of symptomatology.

In concentrating on these three children we hoped to illuminate several issues.

1. We wondered if we could determine the factors (environmental, developmental, dynamic, structural) that could account for their particular "style" of development and functioning or could be correlated with it.

Dr. Cramer was research psychiatrist at the Child Development Center, New York. This study is part of a larger study conducted over the years at the Child Development Center. Dr. Cramer is presently chief of the Geneva University Child Guidance Center. I wish to thank Dr. Peter Neubauer for his suggestions in writing this paper.

2. Following Anna Freud (1965), we consider the unhampered forward movement of development basic to a conceptualization of normality in children. These three children can be viewed as representing one form of normality; or, put differently, their particular form of development and functioning might throw some light on the *clinical* definition of certain aspects of normal functioning.

As most psychoanalytic studies are based on pathological cases, the study of children who show no obvious pathology, or a relative lack of pathology, can be expected to contribute to the understanding of the differences *and* similarities between pathology and normality. This study follows the relatively recent trend of psychoanalytic approaches to so-called normal functioning, which Kris (1951) considered an underdeveloped area in psychoanalysis.

Description of the Study

These data stem from a larger study conducted at the Child Development Center in New York.[1] This research was designed to study the development of a large group of nonclinic children and to classify them in different groups according to developmental criteria (for a detailed description of the study, see Flapan and Neubauer, 1972).

The children were assessed at yearly intervals at the mean age of 4, 5, and 6; they were seen again at age 8½. The three children described in this study were seen again at age 10, and two at age 13. The assessments were based on the following sources of information: interviews with the mother, the teacher, and the child; there were two periods of observation in the classroom, and a battery of psychological tests (Wechsler-Binet, Goodenough, CAT, Rorschach). At age 8½ an interview with the father was added.

Once the totality of the material had been gathered, it was reviewed and each child was placed in one of four groups at each yearly assessment, according to the status of his developmental

[1] The directors of the study were Peter B. Neubauer, M.D. and Dorothy Flapan, Ph.D. Other aspects of this study are reported by Silverman, Rees, and Neubauer in this volume.

progression. Problems of reliability and validity of the clinical judgment passed by several clinicians for each assessment were described in a separate paper (Flapan and Neubauer, 1970). The four groups were:

1. Progression in development has been maintained.
2. Progression in development has been maintained, but with significant accompanying pathological features.
3. Progression in development has been interfered with in significant areas.
4. Progression in development had been interfered with in significant areas, but is again proceeding.

Out of fifty-two children seen initially only forty-five remained available at the third follow-up.

In each of the first three yearly assessments, four fifths or more of the children were judged as belonging in either group 2 or group 3 (Flapan and Neubauer, 1972); *during the same period, only three children were consistently found to belong in group 1.*

It is these three children who were selected for special study. While many group 2 children can be considered normal, certain characteristics differentiated them from group 1 children: group 2 children showed all sorts of symptoms—ego restrictions, affective disturbances, zonal behavior; moreover, some of these symptoms persisted over several assessments, a finding we did not come across in group 1 children to the same extent. In addition, quite a few group 2 children dropped to group 3 in further assessments, thus showing progressive developmental pathology. In the three group 1 children, we saw no such weakening of the developmental progression.

There were other differences between these three boys and the rest of the children. *Reliability* between various sources of information was particularly high in these three boys; parents, teachers, psychiatric observers showed high agreement in describing these children's characteristics; the strength of these children was emphasized by all with the exception of the psychological reports which consistently (in most cases) pointed out more pathology. These three children evoked almost unanimous *praise and admiration* from various sources (adults and peers as well). We became attentive to the fact that this admiration might have played an important role in determining the favorable diagnostic evaluations they received. I shall come back to the relation between a "favorable" diagnosis and the presence of certain value-laden character traits and functions in the discussion. In this respect, it is interesting to note that the only three children who consistently were diagnosed as steadily progressing in their development (group 1) were boys, a finding that may suggest a bias in favor of males or male attributes in our diagnostic assessments (Cramer, 1971).

These boys' behavior, verbal and nonverbal, was generally easy to "read," in contrast to the other children's where the judge felt the need for more information about fantasies and "underlying" dynamics before he was able to assess specific behavior diagnostically. The three boys' behavior was often easy to interpret in terms of adaptative rather than defensive processes.

When the meaning of observations is interpreted without the benefit of validation offered by the psychoanalytic situation, one is often tempted to see many behaviors in defensive terms (for example, activity as reaction formation against passivity, independence as warding off wishes to merge). We frequently found this to be a valid approach when we evaluated the other children; whereas with the three boys we felt that the activity, the independence, and other behaviors were "genuine," age-appropriate acquisitions that served defensive purposes to a minimal degree.

It was often difficult to assess the share of the three psychic structures in a particular type of behavior. In pathology this division is easier to see as regression returns the structures to earlier forms, before structuralization has occurred (Lampl-de Groot, 1962).

The interpretation of observational and interview data is a problem inherent in all observational studies. Moreover, each method of investigation, whether observational, experimental, or reconstructive, makes accessible only certain areas of a person's functioning. While the areas tapped by each method are limited, each in turn tends to highlight certain aspects. "In the case of psychoanalysis," for example, "what its method has made accessible to observation . . . is centered in the sphere of conflict" (Hartmann, 1950, p. 100). Assessments by psychological tests, observations in classrooms, and interviews with parents and teachers, carried out on a yearly basis over a long span of time, might tend to elicit material pertaining primarily to the nonconflictual sphere. It must be stressed, however, that the three boys described in this paper represented a type of "outstanding developmental progression," by comparison with the other forty-two children who were studied by the same method and who thus constituted a control group. The reliance on yearly cross-sections in a longitudinal study of a large number of children yielded a mass of diverse data, some factual, others permitting various levels of inference. While these data illuminate some areas of functioning with much confirmatory material, other areas such as the vicissitudes of affect, unconscious fantasies, and mental representations of objects could not be determined. These could be obtained only through the psychoanalytic process. It is not likely, however, that essentially "healthy" children as those to be described will be subjected to analysis.

Some Characteristics Found in the Three Children

FAMILY BACKGROUND

Ideally, we would need a "developmental profile" of the environment to match the developmental profile of the children, but our research data in this respect are limited. Only a few significant features are singled out. These children belonged to middle-class families, with highly educated and professional parents. Two of the fathers were engineers, one was a writer; one mother was a teacher, one a psychologist, one did not work.

With the exception of one mother, these parents stood out by the firmness of their parental and educational attitudes. The father typically stressed discipline and fostered mature behavior and intellectual pursuits. They showed great devotion to the boys and spent much time with them.

The children attended "progressive" schools which fostered self-expression.

The families did not fit an ideal model: Chris's parents separated, after much marital strain, when he was 15 months old and the father moved away. Jerry's mother was chronically depressed, and was in psychotherapy; she contemplated divorce several times. Jim's mother was a very high-strung person, quite "phallic," very demanding and critical of her colleagues.

EARLY DEVELOPMENTAL HISTORY

We first saw the children at age 4. Our data about their early history are therefore scanty, of a retrospective nature, and must be considered with caution. Two factors stood out, however: there seemed to have been no marked problems around feeding and weaning. The first phases in the process of individuation and separation from the mother seemed gradual and smooth. This relative lack of friction was, however, not present during toilet training, when strong "battles of will" occurred. The other factor we detected was that from infancy on drive discharge of libido and aggression was lusty and assertive.

PHASE PRIMACY

Since we used an optimal capacity for developmental progression as our main yardstick for assessments, it is not surprising that we found a vigorous progressive push in these cases, a feature that can be assessed well only in longitudinal overviews and which suggests something like a "progressive drive" (A. Freud, 1965).

All three children showed clear phase dominance, with well-defined, phase-related characteristics during the phallic, oedipal, latency, and prepuberty phases. All three children clearly established phallic primacy and entered a well-defined oedipal constellation, which was minimally contaminated by oral and anal impulses, a feature that sharply distinguished them from the other children seen in the study. One was hard put to designate in them clear fixation points, again a feature that differentiated these children from the others in the study. This is not to say that their health was maintained by a "split" from past experiences or investments. Over time these children showed—simultaneously with clear phase delineation—consistencies of basic patterns, and their lives were as determined by their past as those of neurotics. But the modalities of the genetic continuum may differ in healthy and pathological states, especially in the degree to which newly emerging patterns are contaminated by early constellations.

The examination of these three children's development suggested that while phase dominance and delineation are to be considered as *relative*, there was a clearer demarcation of phase-related conflicts, functions, and structures in these children than in the rest of the cases studied. A review of the conflicts predominant at each age in Chris's development illustrates definite changes in phase primacy over time.

At age 3;10, we found his need to be independent, strong reaction formations against passive wishes, and a fear of being controlled in the forefront. Anal conflicts were the main motivational forces behind these features; they were exploited by a beginning regression from oedipal conflicts. The departure of his father (who moved to a distant city) created a particular conflict which he attempted to face with an early—perhaps precocious—identification with the "lost object."

At 4;10, typical and intense castration anxiety had developed; it was aggravated by two external events: a head trauma and his mother's engagement. The main defensive maneuvers rested on anal regression and identification with the mother's fiancé.

At 5;9, the main conflict crystallized around oedipal impulses and the fear of retaliation they provoked; the main defensive devices were identification, active mastery of anxiety situations, and attempts at being a "good boy." The anal regression had subsided.

At 8;6, castration anxiety had been "soft-pedaled"; the central conflict was crystallized around the ego ideal and issues of self-esteem: he wished to excel and demanded perfection in performance. The anxiety was linked to narcissistic aspirations, and social pressure had become an important incentive. The defenses were directed mainly against superego anxiety. Chris clearly attempted to make punishment more realistic and ego-syntonic.

At age 10, a regression had occurred with a renewal of the conflict with a pregenitally perceived, phallic mother, very much on the model of the conflict described as typical for prepuberty by Blos (1962). Moral issues were still very active, but were concerned with less personalized, more abstract subjects such as pollution and the Vietnam war.

At age 12;11, with puberty approaching, the oedipal conflict was again in the forefront, as was the attempt to ward off anxieties over his "underdog" position (passivity, inferiority) by an active, fighting stance.

Phase relatedness and dominance of certain conflicts and defenses can thus be documented, although not in as "purified" a form as in textbook descriptions such as Erikson (1950) gives in his timetable of stage-related tasks. It seemed valuable to describe this phase dominance, because the clinician is usually exposed to the *lack* of phase relatedness and the carry-over of characteristics from previous phases in his patients.

CONTINUITY AND CHANGE

The capacity to progress in development automatically implies the capacity to change. Yet side by side with these changes, there was also clear evidence of continuity over the total span of development. The simultaneous presence of persisting features and changing patterns, of continuity within discontinuity, is a most baffling aspect of development, yet the interaction of these two factors greatly influences development. Kris (1950) referred to it as the problem of behavior constancy and anticipated that detailed observations over long periods of time would greatly enhance our knowledge.

This persistence seen in pathological as well as in healthy children suggests the presence of a basic constellation or basic core (Weil, 1970) that colors and determines all the vicissitudes of development.

The conflict over bisexuality, for example, was illustrated very clearly in two of the children by the persistence until age 8;6 of feminine fantasies (fantasies of birth). Although this conflict was mild and relegated to a background position, it remained active over many years. The activity-passivity conflict was particularly marked—and persistent—in these three boys, who exercised a continued, careful vigilance over situations with potentials of enforced passivity.

In the case of Chris, we observed the persistence of a conflict with a stringent superego and of a somewhat exaggerated identification with the adult. We also saw very clearly the persistence of the theme of being the underdog, which in his case became something like a "personal myth."

Our observations certainly demonstrated clearly that conflicts—even intense ones—are an inherent part of *normal* and pathological development.

In these children phase-related conflicts and persisting conflicts existed over the observed span of development. In this respect, these three children do not differ essentially from grossly pathological children (in whom one can also see new conflicts linked to new developmental acquisition). In fact, Freud (1937) made it clear that certain basic conflicts are a continuous challenge inherent in human life. It is interesting to note that he mentioned the conflict over passivity, which we saw consistently in these three children, as basic—and inevitable—in the psychology of men.

Presence of conflict, therefore, is not the relevant issue. Rather, the important questions are: if a persisting conflict does not lead to developmental arrest or to pathology, what are the factors that contribute to this lack of pathogenicity? Is the absence of fixations a necessary requisite of health, or are there "normal" fixations that do not necessarily lead to pathology (Hartmann, 1954); and if so, are there corrective factors? Again, Freud's statement (1937) is pertinent: "even in normal development . . . residues of earlier libidinal fixations may still be retained in the final configuration" (p. 229). Even if a conflict is not phase-related, are there certain factors that safeguard it against chronicity? More generally speaking, what differentiates a normal and a pathological conflict? Certain developmental criteria—the phase appropriateness of the conflict—remain essential in this distinction, but how do we apply criteria of phase relatedness to certain "basic" conflicts that may linger "sotto voce" during long spans of development?

A. Freud's comments (1965) regarding the diagnostic and prognostic significance of regressions might be applicable to these questions. She said, "Unluckily, in our clinical appraisal of regressions as ongoing processes, it is almost impossible to determine whether in a given child's case the dangerous step from temporary to permanent regression has already been taken or whether spontaneous reinstatement of formerly reached levels is still to be expected. Thus far, I know of no criteria for this, even though the entire decision about the child's abnormality may depend on this distinction" (p. 106).

I wish to stress here that *continuous* conflict appears to be part of "normal" development and that it is indeed often impossible to determine the factors that differentiate "normal" and pathogenic conflict.

Certain structural characteristics—mainly general ego reactions—may complement the developmental approach in describing safeguard devices against pathogenic evolutions. It is here that the application of Hartmann's concept of secondary autonomy, and Kris's "optimal distance from conflict" may prove diagnostically helpful.

CONFLICTS, REGRESSIONS, AND EGO REACTIONS

The age span covered by the first two or three assessments corresponds roughly to the period during which these children are in the midst of the infantile neurosis or in the process of disengagement from the oedipal conflict and of entering latency. During this period the nature of conflicts, the defense organization, and the fate of regression play a most decisive role in determining further development. It is therefore particularly enlightening to study an unfolding personality at this "critical" time.

I shall present material illustrating some of the vicissitudes of the infantile neurosis in Jerry. He was a "pushy," independent boy, who generally showed intense reactions. As in the other two boys, there was an intense negativism around the age of 3. At 4;2, he was a typical phallic-oedipal boy: he showed his erections to his mother, competed much with peers, said he wanted to get married; he was quite masculine and strongly identified with his father. The involvement with his mother was intense, with frequent battles of will and occasional hitting of her. He had some mild separation problems; he took stuffed animals to bed. In school, there was some overconcern over aggression. He showed superior skills in intellect and use of words. He needed to succeed. There was no evidence of zonal behavior, no ongoing regression, and no clear-cut fixation.

At the next assessment, at age 5;1, we saw burgeoning manifestations of regressive moves. Jerry's mother was three months pregnant; he knew it, and had asked to taste her milk. He showed clear anal concerns, described the number and shape of bowel movements, and giggled when he used anal talk. His fantasies were concentrated around the pregnancy. He said *he* would have a baby next year and explained to a boy, "You were born in yourself," illustrating his own pregnancy wish. He also showed evidence of an anal birth fantasy when he made such comments as, "You were born in a dirty, stinky place." The negativism, already present during the previous year, was accentuated, as was the battle of wills with his mother.

Side by side with the regressive manifestations, Jerry showed an advance in his libidinal and ego development. His play was typically phallic-oedipal; beside the aggression toward his mother, he was very affectionate with her.

The identification with his father was clear and strong. His self-assertion remained powerful. He refused to be placed in situations of passivity. He tended to treat adults like equals. He accepted to undergo the psychological tests if he was allowed to "take over." He clearly indicated his wish always to be brave and to act maturely. He had progressed in reality-adapted behavior and cognitive development.

In this assessment, manifestations of anal regression and the negative oedipus complex could be seen clearly. The feminine wishes were defended against by reaction formations ("I hate girl stuff," he insisted while playing with planes and trains). He also relied strongly on the identification with his father, whom he imitated in many respects.

The regressive trends that were observable did not involve oral components; they were confined to the anal phase, which he had just pulled out of. Moreover, the regression was limited and partial. It did not prevent simultaneous drive progression, and it did not affect his ego and superego functions, though his object relations, especially with his mother, showed signs of anal regression. Just as regressive and progressive moves existed side by side and balanced each other, passive-feminine and active-masculine aims competed with each other, with the active ones usually gaining the upper hand.

During the next assessment, at age 6, the regression had

deepened and symptoms had occurred. The mother had given birth to a baby boy. By the end of her pregnancy, Jerry's interest in female anatomy and sexual curiosity had tremendously increased. Right after the birth of his brother, Jerry had a few episodes of soiling and bed wetting. He cried often, and was very taunting and controlling with his mother. He exhibited babyish behavior. He regressed to baby talk, wanted to be dressed, to sit on his mother's lap, and showed a renewed interest in his flannel blanket. At that time there were clear oral manifestations: he became fussy about food; he asked to suck at mother's breasts.

Side by side with these regressive trends phallic and oedipal themes were clearly in evidence. They predominated in his play activities, in which he was "all boy." The strong identification with his father had persisted. While Jerry often expressed anger at his mother, he also showed much affection for her. He no longer hit her.

Jerry's need to act maturely had much increased. There was an intense need to refuse help, to be reality-oriented and responsible. He tended to be self-critical; mistakes and criticism upset him much. His sense of values had markedly increased. He showed good controls and frustration tolerance, and his intellectual development progressed well.

The infantile neurosis seemed to be at its peak. His conflicts were intensified by the birth of a sibling. While the regression now involved the oral sphere, it did not prevent *simultaneous progression* in libidinal, ego and superego acquisitions. The conflicts invaded larger portions of the personality. In addition to the oedipal conflict, there were conflicts over feminine and passive wishes, conflicts over anal derivatives and aggressive impulses toward the mother (and the baby), and conflicts over oral impulses.

In terms of Jerry's health, the crucial factor was that the regression was not "wholesale"; it did not involve the totality of libidinal investments and *it allowed for simultaneous progression*. In fact, a reading of the total material showed more evidence of progressive acquisitions than of regressive manifestations. The regression was a partial id regression; ego functions remained relatively uninvolved in the regressive pull. His ego skills, his main defenses, his masculine identification, his relation to reality, his social adaptation in school steadily progressed.

Although Jerry's conflicts increased in intensity, many functions remained intact and kept progressing. In spite of the regression, new structures developed and were strengthened. While Jerry was struggling most with dependency wishes, his ego ideal of mature behavior was reinforced. At age 6, during his deepest regression, he struggled to maintain his independence. This was exemplified when he was asked whether he needed help to go to the bathroom. He replied: "I never need help."

Certain general formulations about the fate of regressions in these children can now be attempted.

Characteristics of Regression

The mutual interactions between regression and progression are central to the appraisal of development. In this appraisal, regression and progression "rates," regression-progression balance, and the defensive use that can be made of progression against the dangers of regressions are important criteria. The extent to which functions and structures are involved in the regression is of foremost diagnostic interest.

In these children, *regressions remain circumscribed.* They do not affect the totality of the drives and they do not suck in the main ego and superego functions.

Controlled Regression

The children tried to contain the regressive flow. Jerry and Chris allowed themselves regressive gratifications, but not without precautionary measures and compensations on a progressive level. When Jerry's mother, aware of his regressive wish, offered to bathe him, he accepted her help, but commented, "I don't know why I let you bathe me, I am a big boy now!" He gave in to the regressive wish, but took a distance from it by naming it and by passing a judgment on it, which revealed that he was aware of his wish being somewhat inappropriate for his age.

Chris, at age 3;10, after his mother went back to work, said, "Babies sure are lucky, because they can have their mommies all the time." He was capable of recognizing in himself and of verbally describing the regressive wish. Moreover, he could express the regressive wish as though he experienced it as something not quite serious, something in the nature of playing. At 3;10, Chris liked playing at being a baby; when his mother went along, offering to feed him with the spoon, he stopped and remarked, "No, I am *really* not a baby," telling her, "It's only for pretend." This example illustrates the child's attempt to *keep regressive gratifications in the realm of fantasy and play.* Taking some distance from it, he judges the situation from a higher level of development. His ego functions, owing to secondary autonomy, can be maintained on a higher level.

While the regressive wishes are indulged in, certain ego functions remain active at higher levels: self-observation, the capacity for verbalization of wishes (rather than merely acting on them), and a watchful stance over what the child accepts as real or as "pretend" in the realm of gratifications. These very sensitive devices are involved in what is best described as "controlled regression" (Kris, 1952).

Regression-Progression Balance

While regressions and progressions coexist side by side, a particular, dynamic interaction between these two currents can also be discerned. It was during the regressions that the strongest mobilization of ego and superego functions toward progressive achievements occurred.

During his deepest regression at age 6 (following his mother's pregnancy), Jerry showed the greatest achievement of independence. He identified with his father's expectations of mature behavior when he announced indignantly: "I never need help." Having internalized his father's demands, he was beginning to shape his ego ideal.

Chris most clearly developed his masculine identification, a somewhat premature adult stance and superego internalization, defenses of an active type, and strengthened reality testing at 3;10, a time when he showed strong regressions.

At first, the progressive move in these children seems hypertrophied (like the exaggerated adultlike behavior) as it was created mainly for defensive purposes. The strong male identification and the marked independence are needed to counteract feminine and passive impulses. But the longitudinal view shows that these progressive moves have been "metabolized," that defensive investments have been lessened, and that the child has made some genuine developmental acquisitions, which have become more autonomous.

The long-term observations of these three children suggest a particular relationship between regression and progression. *Regressions seem to serve as an important incentive for progressions.* It is as if in the face of regressions these children muster their strengths to achieve greater progressive moves. The formula "one step back and two steps forward" is applicable here. The regression acts like a vaccination: a minor insult that mobilizes the organisms reparative progressive forces.

EVENNESS-UNEVENNESS—THE PROBLEM OF PRECOCITY

A. Freud (1965) singled out uneven progression of development as an important factor leading to diverse pathology, depending upon the structures that lag behind or are in advance of the others. It can also be seen, however, that minor and transient unevennesses are ubiquitous. A differentiation between pathogenic and benign unevennesses therefore will have an impact on diagnostic appraisals.

The clearest examples of interstructural unevennesses were seen at the time of regression. In Chris and Jerry, during libidinal regressions to anal and oral aims, we witnessed a forward spurt in ego functioning and in the internalizations leading to superego functions. This created a marked gap between the levels of certain drive gratifications and certain ego and superego functions. In fact, the ego and superego progression suggested precocity in various areas.

There were signs of early internalization of demands. At 3;10, Chris was already quite concerned about right and wrong, without having to rely on the adult's presence. The most pronounced advances were in the area of ego skills. The capacity for verbalization, the use of language, and the fund of information were outstanding. They often spoke in an adultomorphic manner.

At 5;9, Jim indicated properly the complicated names in Latin of a prehistoric animal. Intellectual functioning, especially the capacity for abstraction, was often highly developed.

At 4;10, Jim functioned intellectually like a 6-year-old. His capacity for abstraction was described as sometimes "comparable to that of an adult." The psychologist described Jerry at 5 years as "displaying the rough-and-tough approach of a hard-headed adult." Moreover, these children's consistent insistence on their independence impressed and sometimes intimidated the observers.

When these three boys are compared to all the other children in the study, it is evident that they functioned at an advanced level in so many areas as to suggest precocious development. The precocity is, however, best judged when each child is taken as his own control. Then the existing unevennesses appear less marked, since in each child the essential areas of his personality were not left far behind from the most advanced acquisitions. In a longitudinal overview of each child, one saw that the unevennesses were mostly of a transient nature, and that at the next assessment the child had "caught up." There were exceptions to this. Chris, for example, always remained somewhat too adultlike in his intellectual functioning, his use of verbalization, and his need to treat the adult like a peer (a trait that was seen in all three boys).

In these boys, the advanced ego and superego development could not be equated with the precocities that Hartmann (1950) suggested might lead to obsessional neurosis. In their cases, libidinal development kept the pace of ego development, with rich possibilities of gratification. These boys' precocities rather illustrate and support a suggestion made by Anna Freud (1954), who said, "I believe that precocity is cured, often spontaneously, when the progression of development catches up with it; regressive phenomena profit less from the spontaneous forward moves in the child" (p. 43). In the same article, Anna Freud quotes Kris as stressing that "environmental stimulation belonging to a higher level of development may be an essential factor in spurring on the progressive, forward moving trends toward development" (p. 43). This conception is applicable to the demands of mature behavior made on these boys by their parents, especially by their fathers.

Here again we are confronted with the question: what makes certain precocities pathogenic (leading, for example, to that outstripping of ego achievements over drive gratifications typical of obsessional developments), while others serve as an incentive for progression of the *total* personality? The study of these three children offers only suggestive leads: first, there is the relative absence of the backward pull of strong fixation points; second, there was no evidence that the parents of these children selectively forced precocities of ego functions *while simultaneously encouraging libidinal gratification on regressive levels.* Moreover, the parents tolerated unevenness of development at times of increased anxiety (e.g., the birth of a sibling).

As we realized that the benign nature of the regressions, the lack of developmental distortions that followed them, constituted one of the cornerstones of these children's strengths, we turned to an examination of the ego factors that may have contributed to this happy integration of regressive moves.

CHARACTERISTICS OF EGO FUNCTIONING

Self-Observation, Insight, Verbalization

I described earlier how these children controlled regressions by self-observation and verbalization, allowing for a maintenance of reality testing over the content of regressive wishes which are experienced as being a form of play. It was this type of functioning which allowed Chris, at age 3;10, during a period of intense regression, to state, "No, I am *really* not a baby, it's only *for pretend.*" The regressive activity, viewed as being in the nature of play, was thus "detoxified." Such capacity contributes to the maintenance of adequate frustration tolerance.

These children provided evidence of keen psychological insight and the capacity for self-observation.

At age 5;9, Chris, who was struggling with his disappointment in his mother's recent remarriage, was very intent on trying to sort out realities and fantasies. One of his comments, at this time, was: "Untrue stories always end up happily." This unusual bit of philosophizing showed Chris's attempt to come to terms with the lack of fulfillment of his oedipal wishes. In his statement, he shows his understanding of the wish-fulfilling, magic nature of fantasies ("untrue stories").

At 8½, Chris explained why he had frightening dreams: "I have been watching too much Captain Scarlet and Mysterious," thereby indicating his awareness of the seductive influence of TV shows (but also revealing the defensive use of rationalization, as this statement failed to underline the conflictual, intrapsychic source of nightmares). He also realized that he was not good at football tackling "because I am not the kind who likes to go around fighting at all."

The defensive use of self-observation was revealed clearly by his reaction to an anxiety-provoking situation, the onset of school. On the first day of his new school (at age $8\frac{1}{2}$), he had a stomachache and was carsick. On the way to school, he took his mother's hand, which he never did otherwise, and said, "I know this sounds very funny, but I feel a little scared. You know, what if nobody I know is there?" His eyes filled up with tears, and he asked his mother how long she would stay. "Until you are ready," was her reply. He said, "Tomorrow, I will be running up there with my friends." When the mother announced she would have to go, he said, "Oh, sure!" laying it on.

In this incident, Chris dealt with anxiety by different means. He examined his behavior with some detachment, and commented on the strangeness of his fear ("I know it sounds very funny, but I feel a little scared"). He had some insight into the nature of his anxiety: the fear of having to deal with new unknown objects, in contrast to the security he found in the contact with mother, a tie that was defensively, regressively reinforced. Then, again showing a capacity for detachment and knowledge of himself, he was able to project a pleasurable experience into the future ("Tomorrow, I will be running up there with my friends"). He had the capacity for detaching himself from the immediate, painful situation, evoking the memory of pleasurable past experiences (playing with friends), and used it to make the future more palatable. Most striking was Chris's *capacity to keep self-observation and judgment intact in the face of severe anxiety.* This might well be an illustration of the "optimal distance from conflict" allowed by secure autonomous functioning.

These children also used insight in the mastery of external (social) threats. Jim, at age $8\frac{1}{2}$, complained that his older brother bent Jim's fingers backward, which made him cry; then he explained, "He does that in defense; you see he is very small for his age. All the boys are bigger than he is; he feels very bad about that, but then he feels bad when I punch him in the mouth" (here he identified with the aggressor).

These examples demonstrate that although self-observation and rational explanations of behavior are extensively used for defensive purposes, this does not detract from the adaptive use made of these functions. In fact, it was impressive to note how often *defenses coincided with and contributed to adaptation in these children.* Hartmann (1939) suggested that certain defensive functions may contain an inherent guarantee of reality anchoring, thus simultaneously serving adaptation. (The clinical evaluation of such correlation between defense and adaptation is crucial in determining ego strength.) These functions did not operate at the expense of, or instead of, active involvement (as would be the case in pathological cases of self-observation). They prepared for action and contributed to mastery through understanding.

These children's keen understanding of reality addressed itself not only to external reality, but to inner, psychological reality as well. Moreover, these children were very keen on establishing differences between what is real and what is imaginary, magical.

Reality Orientation and Fantasy-Reality Ratio

Children vary in the regulation of fantasy expression. Some readily verbalize their fantasies, others tend to act on them immediately; still others establish a firmer division between fantasy and action, and tend not to allow fantasies to impinge on reality-directed attitudes.

In Jerry and Chris, and to a lesser extent in Jim, we noticed a keen observance of reality, a constant effort to inject reality into their judgments and actions, a careful weighing of irrational behavior (fantasies, fears, affects) against the norms of the reality principle. Their cognitive functioning revealed an unusual ability to understand the logic of causal relationship. Their interest in how things worked and in factual information was repeatedly illustrated. Their play was characterized as realistic (i.e., not involving much magic) and not artistic; when playing, they often reminded others, "It's only for pretend."

A constant concern with the distinction between real and

imaginary was well illustrated by Chris. At age 6, he often asked what was real; for example, he stated, "Kansas is real, because it's on the map," displaying his ability to recognize an abstract symbol (a name on a map) as representing the reality of a town. He also asked, "Is Dorothy [from the Wizard of Oz] a real person? No, I am not going even to think about that book being real!" Similarly, he said that he wished he could avoid having dreams. Here we see how much he needed to relegate fantasy material to the realm of the unreal; in fact, he wished he could ward off dreams, the main source of irrational thinking.

At 10, he explained that a good dentist was one who explained what was going to happen "because young children are scared. My dentist has all sorts of techniques to make you feel less scared." Chris then proceeded to explain the details of the anesthesia, using precise words like novocaine, muscle relaxation.

When he was asked what he did when he was in a scary situation, he replied, "I don't build up phony courage, I don't pretend I am not scared. I like to face reality! I know the doctor is going to hurt." He also explained, "I used to get scared sick by my dreams, but if you don't think you will get a dream, then it doesn't come" (an illustration of the need for omnipotent control).

When asked if he liked daydreams, he said, "Yes, when I am bored, I daydream; about the free time period, what I will do." He responded to the question, "Do you ever daydream about wild things, like Superman, or other things?" with "No, I am honest. I don't want to dream about these things. I don't want to disappoint myself." But at age 12;11, he revealed that many of his daydreams dealt with grandiose, wish-fulfilling thoughts such as excelling in sports.

The curtailing of fantasies was well illustrated in the course of psychological testing. Both Jerry and Chris gave sparse responses in the projective tests. Jerry, at 6, responded, "A design" to card 1 of the Rorschach; to card 2, he said, "The same, only a little different." At $8\frac{1}{2}$, he refused to respond to the CAT, "The pictures are dumb—my stories would be dumb—the cards are for babies—it would be embarrassing—I hate telling stories!" The sparseness of responses was surprising in view of these boys' high intelligence (Jerry had an IQ of 158 at $8\frac{1}{2}$, and Chris at the same age of 148).

Jim, at 8½, did not care to respond when he was asked what he would wish for if he were granted three magical wishes. Similarly, when asked what he wanted to become, he said he had no idea.

Several factors are responsible for such behavior: a consistent effort to maintain the distinction between fantasy and reality, the use of realistic explanations and judgments in defense against anxiety-provoking situations, an attempt to curtail magical fantasies, a consistent need to observe and test reality. The most important elements in maintaining such reality orientation and control of fantasies turned out to be a superior intellectual endowment; a good capacity for abstraction and conceptualization; an ego ideal of "mature behavior" reinforced by parents who did much to enhance verbalizations and rational explanations; a need to emphasize active measures and identifications. It seemed that these children experienced dreams and fantasies as a powerful influence that would make them passive recipients, threatening their basically alloplastic orientation and active stance.

These were children who wanted to master their environment and to be in control of themselves. They needed to protect themselves against the invasion of unpredictable stimuli and uncontrolled, primary process thinking. The irruption of illogical, uncontrollable thoughts may have been experienced as a narcissistic injury by these boys who had such talents for good cognitive grasp and intellectual mastery.

This particular relationship between reality thinking and fantasy thinking may be described in terms of proportions between secondary and primary process; it may also be seen as a special form of isolation which functions in these boys very much like the type of isolation normally used in intellectual activity where one must temporarily focus on certain aspects of a problem.

The containment of fantasies and general reality orientation were central in these children's defensive, adaptative, and developmental modes. These functions helped in controlling the anxieties inherent in regressive and retaliative fantasies. They contributed to a relative lack of reliance on projection and denial and allowed for defensive devices that were essentially reality-syntonic. Furthermore, the defensive use of containment of fantasies and reality orientation was undistinguishable from the adaptive one. Whatever price was being paid for the upkeep of defenses served simultaneously the purposes of adaptation. (This is in contrast to cases where the major defensive maneuvers interfere with adaptation to external and internal reality.) This particular form of reality allegiance seemed to be a main factor in the ability to control regressions, magical thinking, fears of retaliation. It allowed for that optimal distance from conflicts, which is at the core of these children's functioning.

This type of reality orientation could also be discussed from the point of view of its contribution to pathology. We know that certain forms of "clinging" to reality betray a pathological fear of instinctual manifestations. But in these three boys, we saw no evidence of compromise formations resulting from the upward pressure of large sections of pathologically repressed material, nor did we see a curtailment of drive expression.

THE ROLE OF IDENTIFICATION

Running through the assessments was evidence of an intense "thirst" for identification with the father, a very firm and well-delineated masculine identification, and a particularly clear taking over of the father's attitudes and values. The identification with the father became the central core around which defenses, character traits, and progressive movements were organized.

The vicissitudes of identification were well illustrated in Chris. At age 3;10, Chris seemed excessively adultlike in his manner of speech; he became angry when he was offered help before he was ready; he insisted on independent functioning. When he was frightened, he played at frightening his teddy bear. "I am not scared, my friend is." He was preoccupied with rules and tended to moralize other children, "You should talk, not hit." He had made an intense, even exaggerated identification with the adult: he wanted to take care of himself and had internalized interdictions.

He often played at visiting his father, who lived far away. In fact, his identification was so intense because it was used in a defensive effort to cope with the "loss" of the father. Chris consistently identified with the active party when he was coping with anxiety or regressive dependent wishes. His yearnings for a masculine model were particularly evident when he begged his mother's boyfriends to play with him, while he excluded his mother from the play.

At the time of the next assessment (age 4;10), Chris's mother had become engaged and Chris had regressed and developed symptoms (separation fears, soiling, demandingness). In this situation the curative effects of identification could be observed. Chris's mother, alarmed by his sadness, increased dependency, and separation fears, asked the biological father to send his old clothes to Chris. He then wore his father's hat at night; when he received jockey shorts, he announced, "I feel like a man now." The acute symptoms subsided in a few days.

While this solution involved an essentially magical identification, a form of imitation, displaying mostly defensive determinants, the longitudinal data proved that a real spurt in development also took place. This was fostered primarily by Chris's strong identification with his mother's fiancé, whom he imitated in several respects (driving, shaving).

This example demonstrates the central role of identification with a father figure. It is as if all the strength that can be mustered by the child is concentrated in the process of identification. This identification is a powerful defensive tool covering a wide spectrum of anxieties—castration anxieties and phobic elements (fear of death, of dogs, and nightmares) stirred up by murderous wishes, a host of anal and oral aggressive aims as well as feminine tendencies. The marked economy of means thus achieved indicates how identification is put to use by the synthetic function and becomes a basic ingredient of ego strength and progressive thrusts of development.

When Chris was seen at 5;9 the regressive elements were no longer visible. He was fully in the oedipal phase and strongly identified with his stepfather, with whom he shared many activities. Chris wanted to have his last name changed to his stepfather's name. At the same time the mother's remarriage intensified the oedipal rivalry, which was apparent in Chris's play: as superman he played out many grandiose omnipotent fantasies. Thus identification with the stepfather's real characteristics coexisted with magical modes of identification with qualities of omnipotence.

The new situation also contributed to a new and transient conflict, in which the superego was prominent. Chris showed increased concerns about what was right and wrong, and often seemed confused about the two sets of values and interdictions existing in his two homes (his mother's home and his father's home). He dealt with his conflict by injecting rationality in punishment (in long discussions about what is right, the logics of punishment) and by attempting to identify more with the readily available model, the stepfather with whom he lived.

At $8\frac{1}{2}$, the identification with the stepfather had been further reinforced, but some deflection of goals had taken place: he now wanted to become an athlete.

Throughout Chris's development, he showed a strong need to identify with the adult and with the father, a strong concern with justice, some overcontrol, and demand for mature behavior. These characteristics have contributed both to Chris's best assets and to his difficulties. His tremendous capacity to identify with a new father enabled him to move out of regressions and to fulfill superego and ego-ideal demands by developing ego attitudes and character traits consonant with the father's values. But the pull to identify with the adult was also responsible for his adultomorphic behavior, with the overcontrol of "babyish" tendencies.

The feature that probably accounts for the "normality" of such development is that identification is not limited to the taking over of parental values in the superego and ego ideal, but also implements these values by *actual modifications in the ego.* (This contrasts with cases where introjection of values occurs without the corresponding ego modifications that allow for the fulfillment of superego and ego-ideal demands.)

This was well illustrated by Jerry, who at $8\frac{1}{2}$ said, "I am like my father in almost every way." He also announced that he wanted to be like his father when he grew up. Indeed, throughout his development, he fulfilled, by his independent behavior, his ego ideal of maturity, much on the model of his father's expectations. Jerry was the child who at 6 announced that he intended to become an engineer "and I will not change my mind," as if what he was and what he would become were closely related, betraying a strong sense of identity and confidence that he would realize his projected goals. He was also a child who consistently showed a very masculine stance and a pattern of identification with the *active* party. *He* initiated the questions in the interviews; he was the organizer and "director" of play with children; he "never needed help"; and he became the judging party who pronounced, "*You* are wrong."

Jim, too, was consistently described as very masculine, his own boss, and having a great need to emulate his older brother and his father. He too tended to reverse roles with the adult (he "examined" the examiner, made the tester guess what his drawings meant), and, more than the other two children, identified with the aggressor. Jim acknowledged that he was afraid at night. "I am afraid of the dark . . . because there is a big poster of Frankenstein on my wall." (Why don't you take it off then?) "Because in the day I throw darts at it." (Does that make you feel good?) "Yes, very much so."

In regard to identification, these three children had a tendency to reverse roles and turn passive into active in a way that surprised many observers who felt these boys had the poise of an adult. The identification with the active party was used defensively against passive-regressive wishes and against fear of retaliation. It also resulted in a narcissistic gain, because it helped deny their actual inferiorities as children.

At the height of the oedipal conflict, these boys were strongly drawn to their fathers (it is important to note that the three fathers as well as the stepfather were unusually available and willing to spend time with their boys). This often coincided with increased manifestations of aggression against the mother, in an effort to turn away from her. Each boy actively sought to identify with his father, clearly internalizing his values in his ego ideal. In this process the child gathered progressive momentum, pulled out of regressions, simultaneously expanded ego functioning and reinforced sexual identity.

The keystones of this identification process were the *activity* it implemented in defensive maneuvers and the *progression* it achieved in libidinal, ego and superego development. Moreover, these children's resources enabled them to match the demands of their ego ideal by actual modifications of the ego, thus defending against problems of low self-esteem, which (as will be seen) were nevertheless intense. Inasmuch as identification can be described as *the* main phase-appropriate defensive device of the oedipal phase, this was well documented in our material.

Discussion

PREDICTION AND OUTCOME

These three boys were rated at age 4, 5, and 6 as showing continuous progressive development; follow-ups at 8½, 10, and 13 years indicated that these early assessments had good predictive value. They maintained the developmental progression and retained the relative absence of pregenital fixations.

Such characteristics as developmental style (as seen, for example, in their regression-progression balance), main defenses (for example, the use of active, alloplastic maneuvers, identification, cognitive mastery), dominant conflicts (for example, Chris's concern with the underdog position of the child in the oedipal triad), typical ego functioning (reality orientation, the curtailment of fantasies) were all present early and showed a remarkable consistency over time, a finding that underscores the value of such concepts as a "basic core" of personality functioning.

While these children had ample capacity to move from one developmental issue to another, they simultaneously showed great continuity, a continuity that was basic to their strong sense of identity. This study of basically healthy children invites a comparison with severely disturbed children, whose pathology usually also shows great continuity, but in their case it is the effects of fixation and rigidity that persist. Thus, continuity of pattern can result either in healthy or in abnormal development. It would therefore be of interest to study the interplay of the functions and structures that persist *and* change in their mutual effect.

With regard to predictions, we are better at making them when pathological rather than "healthy" items are concerned. We are fairly certain about the predictive value of marked fixations, ego distortions, and developmental arrests; we are much more insecure when it comes to predicting healthy development. Many colleagues who heard this clinical material kept saying, "You have to wait a few more years before deciding on these children's diagnosis and health"—a remark that denotes a basic skepticism about our ability to detect health.[2] Yet this study indicates that the early assessments were correct in stressing the strengths of these children. I believe that more detailed longitudinal studies of nonpathological children will contribute further *positive* criteria of normality (as normality is still often diagnosed by *exclusion* of pathology).

PATHOLOGICAL AND "NORMAL" CONFLICT

The study of these children's conflicts certainly underscored a point that possibly has not been sufficiently emphasized: namely, that the presence of conflicts, even intense and protracted conflicts, cannot be equated with the presence of pathology. These children were often intensely involved in conflicts (such as conflicts over autonomy and control with the mother during toilet training and again in prepuberty). Yet these conflicts often contributed very significantly to progressive achievements and to the acquisition of new adaptational skills, rather than to pathology.

Similarly, the study of these children impressed on us the usefulness of the concepts of secondary autonomy and conflict-free functioning. These concepts prevent one from adopting a one-sided, reductionistic point of view that would attribute all functions to drive derivatives (Hartmann's [1955] genetic fallacy) or defensive devices. For example, when we were confronted with the clinical finding of these boys' continuous stress on activity and masculinity, we always suspected—according to our basically conflict-oriented epistemology—that this stance was in defense against passive merging and homosexual wishes. While this was partly true, a *longitudinal* view allowed us to see that these traits were solid acquisitions which did not show much lability over time and which we could not explain solely on the basis of defense. (Longitudinal studies can do much in helping us detect more the healthy than the pathological outcomes.) These characteristics had attained a certain degree of autonomy from conflict. The concept of secondary

---

[2] A. Freud (1965) warned that information gathered in evaluations of development does not necessarily provide much understanding of what constitutes normality: "But the indications which emerge are more useful for the diagnosis of pathology and a revelation of the past than they are for deciding issues which concern the normal and the outlook for the future" (p. 55f.).

autonomy can thus be fruitfully applied *clinically* and is an essential tool in the assessment of health and ego strength—a point that was repeatedly stressed by Hartmann (1952).

In studying these cases the question of what constitutes the differences between a "normal" and a pathological conflict was constantly on our mind. While no definite answer can be given, the study of these cases provides some leads. Among the factors that play a vital role are: the remarkable resistivity of the ego in face of regressions; the reliance on reality testing, verbalization, cognitive functioning, and self-observation in controlling impulses, fantasy expressions, and regressions; and the capacity to achieve autonomous functioning under stress. This capacity can also be described as gaining "an optimal distance from conflict" (Kris, 1950). It would be most important to determine what contributes to this optimal degree of secondary autonomy, and which functions promote ego strength and healthy resistivity to regressions. This is obviously a basic problem in psychoanalytic theory, one which has often been stated but not resolved.

Dealing with this question, one is always tempted to explain functioning, normal or pathological, in terms of genetic determinants. Early object relations, especially, are called upon to explain much of later development. Our early developmental data are too scanty to approach the problem from this angle. Yet, our observations indicated that continuing *external* influences played an important role in determining the continuous progressive push in these children. The parents provided many gratifications at higher levels of developments, and they were sufficiently sensitive to allow their children to regress when needed.

Another factor that contributed to these children's strength can be referred to as the organizing function (Hartmann, 1947), which must be regarded as an independent variable and, like other new developmental acquisitions, cannot be explained only by genetic determinants.

One must assume that throughout development, functions and structures influence and stimulate each other, contributing mutually to their maintenance and growth. The conception of development as a spiral rather than a straight line is applicable here. Indeed, we could see how various functions, such as reality orientation, cognitive ability, defensive styles, object relations, kept contributing to each other and to the total picture of ego strength and progressive development. Thus it is useless to single out special items as being the main determinants of the personality, whether in the sense of pathology or normality. The clinical example of these children's particular reality orientation illustrates this point. This was indeed an outstanding feature in these three boys. Yet some colleagues felt that in view of this reality orientation one could not consider these children normal. They saw in it a case of "reality adhesion," a defensive device frequently found in obsessional patients. But one part cannot explain the whole, and our longitudinal observations disclosed a generally healthy, lusty drive discharge in these boys.

Hartmann's (1939) concept of hierarchy of functions, under the guidance of an integrating or organizing function, has to be applied here. Reality orientation is of utmost adaptive importance, but, as Hartmann pointed out, there are times when a functional organization must give way to another one. At times of creative thinking, during orgastic experiences, and while practicing psychoanalysis, one should temporarily and partially be able to abandon reality orientation in favor of other, more primitive modes of functioning. In view of the obvious lack of obsessional pathology in these children, one can only assume that their functioning was dominated by reality orientation at certain times (for example, when they were interviewed), while they must have submitted to more primitive modes of functioning at other times. The *capacity for an optimal timing—according to overall psychic needs—of functional dominance* must be considered an essential characteristic of ego strength and probably also of progressing development.

The particular interplay between regressions and progressions in these children might proceed from a similar dynamism. Progressive moves may find their economic sources in renewed contacts with earlier modes of gratifications and functioning, allowing for a second try at "unfinished business"; thus a "door" must remain open toward primitive functioning, allowing for an enriching recapitulation of regressive modalities before progressive acquisitions can be obtained (the mechanism which Kris described as "regression in the service of the ego"). This door need not be wide open; in fact, these children maintain an alert watchdog function (by specific ego functions) over the regressive moves.

THE INFLUENCE OF NARCISSISTICALLY CHARGED CHARACTERISTICS ON DIAGNOSTIC CRITERIA

The children described here do not correspond to a normative model of normality. They had outstanding intelligence, powerful personalities, leadership qualities, marked successes in adaptation. Typically, they used cognitive mastery when faced with psychological challenges, and they adopted particularly strong, active, alloplastic modes of adaptation. The literature contains a clinical description of a "normal" child which is quite similar to these boys. L. Murphy (1956) characterized Colin as having the ability to go into action to express his needs or assert himself, a strong resistance against any pressure from the adult, strong autonomy and initiative, realism in fantasy life, strong masculine identification, defensive aggression, and quick recovery from emotional disturbances. This boy too had very high intelligence, qualities of "natural" leadership, and a "regal commanding air" with adults. His ego ideal appeared to control his socialization more than his conscience. The similarities with the three boys in this study are obvious.

These boys were the object of praise and admiration from parents, teachers, peers, and the participants in the study. In many ways they had outstanding qualities that might lead them to develop the character structure described by Freud (1916) and Jacobson (1959) as the exceptions. In view of these considerations it is of interest to examine their *narcissistic development*.

At the assessment made in the middle of latency (at 8½ years), all three boys were struggling with self-esteem problems. All three were sensitive to criticism, feared failure, and avoided tasks that they might fail. At 13 years, the mothers of Jim and Chris reported that the boys might not feel sure of themselves. They greatly resented being treated like children or being pushed around. In their adultomorphic demeanor, they denied their smallness and approached adults as equals in a somewhat grandiose way.

At 12;11 years, Chris gave many examples of his concern about being an underdog, his resentment at being treated like a lesser person; he daydreamed of being a sport hero in the center court of the Coliseum, outshining everyone else; he thought he was the smartest of his class (which might well have been true) and that he could get straight A's if he tried.

Naturally, as his mother pointed out, "He has never experienced much failure." These children's "natural" talents protected them against a full realization of their limitations, just as Helen of Troy, because of her extraordinary beauty, was able to neglect the usual social taboos (Jacobson, 1959). Parents of exceptional children also invest them very particularly; such children can easily be used as narcissistic extentions of the parents, and their exceptional characteristics are all the more reinforced when the parents themselves have problems of self-esteem regulation. That this was the case was clearly demonstrated in our last contact with Chris's mother. She described Chris as "sublime" and "wonderful." During the interview, she reported that Chris had his front tooth broken accidentally by his younger brother. At this point, the mother—usually a cheerful person—broke down in tears. "I had such an angry reaction to my younger boy. He damaged my Chris! My *perfect* Chris! It was so upsetting that something permanent, a physical damage was done to my child." Later she acknowledged that she felt much closer to Chris than to his brother and strongly identified with Chris. "Like him, I was the underdog; my father was unloving, he abandoned us; he *broke* my heart." Her child's broken tooth reminded her of her own feeling of castration and of being unloved by her father. Chris had to be perfect to help her defend against her own feelings of unworthiness and castration. This also helped us understand why Chris felt so much like an underdog (he identified with the rejected castrated mother; after all, his father also left him); and like her, he strove to be perfect, thus also identifying with his mother's defensive, narcissistic style.

Tartakoff (1966) described a particular form of narcissistic character disorder, which she called the Nobel Prize Complex. In persons who have known steady success and easy adaptation throughout their development, good adaptation may become an end in itself, which brings considerable narcissistic gratifications, as good performances followed by gratification become an institutionalized method of self-esteem regulation, especially in socially ascending, American families. Tartakoff described that this particular form of narcissistic orientation may contribute to limitations in the depth of object relations and may result in severe disillusionment later in life when the expectation of exceptional performances is not fulfilled. In analysis, these persons—often psychoanalytic candidates—use this form of "normality" as a formidable source of resistance. We may thus study with profit the predisposition to certain forms of pathology that accompanies what we call "normality," especially when normality is linked with outstanding qualities.

Propensities for particular forms of narcissistic development are present in the three boys described in this study. *A particular narcissistic investment of mature, rational behavior may be the price they will pay for functioning in their particular environment.* This could be an example of what Eissler (1960) called the "psychopathology of normality." (However, narcissistic investments are not pathological per se. The role of "healthy narcissism" in normal children was stressed by L. Murphy [1962].)

It is clear that these children's particular reality orientation and cognitive mastery brought them much narcissistic gratification. Hartmann (1956) stressed that with development, a change in the nature of pleasurable experiences occurs. New sources of pleasure derive from "participating in the world of the grownups." Indeed, these children may have felt that they would get much parental love if they renounced prolonged regressive gratification.

Their reluctance to express fantasies also may have stemmed from a fear of narcissistic injury. Fantasies are "for babies," as one of the boys put it. They represented a threat to these boys' need for mastery of their *internal* world.

Indeed, one of the cornerstones of these boys' characterological makeup was their need for active mastery and control of external *and* internal forces. This was clear in their strong investment of intellectual mastery. They showed an omnipotent, at times even grandiose, investment of knowledge and active mastery, *which may correspond to basic values in Western civilization.* We greatly admire qualities that ensure self-reliance, autonomy, and omnipotent control over internal and external events, all qualities that were highly developed and narcissistically invested in these boys.

It seems that our concept of normality is strongly infiltrated by values that stress the above-mentioned qualities, in which case we may tend to see children who do not have them to the same degree as automatically less "normal." This must have influenced our diagnostic assessments of these children, indicating how difficult it is to formulate an operational definition of normality.

It is difficult to predict what price these three children will have to pay for their good and mature functioning and for the narcissistic orientation it may enhance. I can only point to the correlation between their outstanding developmental progression and certain narcissistic gratifications. The question can probably be answered only in the analytic situation.

Summary

In a longitudinal study of forty-five children, three boys showed continuous, unusually vigorous, developmental progression and relative lack of symptomatology. These boys had several characteristics that could account for this particular development. Regressions generally were controlled owing to the maintenance of autonomous functioning of crucial ego functions: verbalization, cognitive mastery, reality testing, containment of fantasies, self-observation. Regressions, acting like a catalyst, were often followed by marked progressive gains with new acquisitions. Identification played a central role in pulling these children out of regressions. These boys had a basic active and alloplastic orientation. Their defenses also served adaptive purposes to a high degree. The maintenance of secondary autonomy of functions allowed for an "optimal distance from conflicts." Good performance and mature behavior were the object of particular narcissistic investments, corresponding to the parents'—and our civilization's—ego ideal. These children's particularly outstanding characteristics in terms of developmental progression and ego functioning were also discussed in terms of their possible correlation with the development of narcissistic character traits.

BIBLIOGRAPHY

BLOS, P. (1962), *On Adolescence.* New York: Free Press of Glencoe.
CRAMER, B. (1971), Sex Differences in Early Childhood. *Child Psychiat. Hum. Develpm.*, 1:133–151.

EISSLER, K. R. (1960), The Efficient Soldier. In: *The Psychoanalytic Study of Society*, 1:39–97. New York: Int. Univ. Press.

ERIKSON, E. H. (1950), *Childhood and Society*. New York: Norton.

FLAPAN, O. & NEUBAUER, P. B. (1970), Issues in Assessing Development. *J. Amer. Acad. Child Psychiat.*, 9:669–687.

——— ——— (1972), Developmental Groupings in Pre-School Children. *Israel Ann. Psychiat. & Rel. Discipl.*, 10:52–70.

FREUD, A. (1954), In: Problems of Infantile Neurosis. *This Annual*, 9:16–71.

——— (1965), *Normality and Pathology in Childhood*. New York: Int. Univ. Press.

FREUD, S. (1916), Some Character-Types Met with in Psycho-Analytic Work. *S.E.*, 14:309–333.

——— (1937), Analysis Terminable and Interminable. *S.E.*, 23:209–253.

HARTMANN, H. (1939a), *Ego Psychology and the Problem of Adaptation*. New York: Int. Univ. Press, 1958.

——— (1939b), Psychoanalysis and the Concept of Health. In: Hartmann (1964), pp. 1–18.

——— (1947), On Rational and Irrational Action. In: Hartmann (1964), pp. 37–68.

——— (1950), Psychoanalysis and Developmental Psychology. In: Hartmann (1964), pp. 99–112.

——— (1952), The Mutual Influences in the Development of Ego and Id. In: Hartmann (1964), pp. 155–181.

——— (1954), Problems of Infantile Neurosis. In: Hartmann (1964), pp. 207–214.

——— (1955), Notes on the Theory of Sublimation. In: Hartmann (1964), pp. 215–240.

——— (1956), Notes on the Reality Principle. In: Hartmann (1964), pp. 241–267.

——— (1964), *Essays in Ego Psychology*. New York: Int. Univ. Press.

JACOBSON, E. (1959), The "Exceptions." *This Annual*, 14:135–154.

KRIS, E. (1950), Notes on the Development and on Some Current Problems of Psychoanalytic Child Psychology. *This Annual*, 5:24–46.

——— (1951), Opening Remarks on Psychoanalytic Child Psychology. *This Annual*, 6:9–17.

——— (1952), *Psychoanalytic Explorations in Art*. New York: Int. Univ. Press.

LAMPL-DE GROOT, J. (1962), Ego Ideal and Superego. *This Annual*, 17:94–106.

MURPHY, L. B. (1956), *Personality in Young Children*: Vol. 2, *Colin—A Normal Child*. New York: Basic Books.

——— (1962), *The Widening World of Childhood*. New York: Basic Books.

TARTAKOFF, H. H. (1966), The Normal Personality in Our Culture and the Nobel Prize Complex. In: *Psychoanalysis—A General Psychology*, ed. R. M. Loewenstein et al. New York: Int. Univ. Press, pp. 222–252.

WEIL, A. P. (1970), The Basic Core. *This Annual*, 25:442–460.

Congenital Absence of Sensation

STEVEN L. DUBOVSKY, M.D.
AND STEPHEN E. GROBAN, M.D.

LITTLE CLINICAL INFORMATION IS AVAILABLE ON THE PROBLEM OF psychological development in the face of severe sensory disturbances. There is, however, widespread agreement on the importance of sensation to development. In the experimental literature, studies of rats (Holloway, 1966; Cragg, 1967), kittens (Pettigrew and Freeman, 1973; Annis and Frost, 1973), and chimpanzees (Reisen, 1961) have confirmed that a certain quantity of sensory input is necessary for continued growth and differentiation of the nervous system. Furthermore, the quality of sensory input in early life has been demonstrated to play a vital role in the later development of affective ties, mothering behavior, and adult heterosexual relationships (Harlow, 1958; Harlow and Zimmerman, 1959; Harlow and Harlow, 1966).

In the literature on human development, the importance of early sensory experience has also been strongly emphasized. Freud (1923) stated, "The ego is first and foremost a bodily ego" (p. 26). Spitz (1965), Fraiberg (1964, 1968), and Call (1964) emphasize the

---

Dr. Dubovsky is Assistant Professor of Psychiatry, University of Colorado School of Medicine, Denver, Colorado. Dr. Groban is Clinical Instructor, Department of Psychiatry, University of California, San Diego, California. We would like to express our gratitude to Dr. Robert N. Emde for his valuable suggestions and contributions to our thinking.

essential role of sensation in early ego formation. For Piaget (Flavell, 1963), infant cognitive development, resulting from the experience of actions with concrete objects, is directly dependent on sensorimotor development. Ongoing sensory input has been said to be the foundation upon which is built a body ego (Call, 1964; Freedman, 1971), the self (Kohut, 1971, 1972; Mahler, 1968; White, 1963), ego strengths (Jessor and Richardson, 1968), reality testing (White, 1963), impulse control (Jessor and Richardson, 1968), affects (Freud, 1920, 1926), and object relations (Spitz, 1965).

Lack of adequate sensory stimulation is said to result in "emotional starvation" (Spitz, 1965) and "irreversible affective and ego deficiencies" (Schneider, 1962; Wilson, 1971). Certainly, our expectation would be that congenital absence of sensation would lead to serious developmental disturbances. Curiously enough, however, the few available case reports emphasize the apparent competence of the individual who is congenitally deprived of sensation (Freedman, 1972; Wilson, 1971). Nowhere is this more evident than in the available studies of congenital absence of tactile and painful sensation. In some reports, no psychological data are provided (McMurray, 1950; Schneider, 1962; Ogden et al., 1959; Sternbach, 1963; Campbell, 1970). In other studies, patients are described as having essentially normal developmental and psychological histories (Cohen et al., 1955; Magee et al., 1961; Winkelmann et al., 1962; Rapoport, 1959; Jewesbury, 1970; Murray, 1973), even when development has been followed over time (Magee et al., 1961; Rapoport, 1959)! Some reports mention only an "exaggerated concern for others" (Cohen et al., 1955; Kane et al., 1968), or "temper tantrums" and occasional self-injury in childhood (Thrush, 1973). The study of how such patients develop in the face of apparently overwhelming congenital handicaps would be of enormous importance because it might highlight some essential factors which we too readily take for granted. It might also give us a better understanding of the adaptability and plasticity of the human organism.

This report concerns a patient with congenital disturbances in surface sensory modalities, enteroception, pain and pleasurable sensations. Unlike other cases reported in the literature, he received an extensive psychological workup and was followed in psychotherapy. We make some preliminary observations regarding his unique development in the interest of stimulating further discussion of our understanding of how such patients and their physiologically normal counterparts adapt and grow.

Case Report

Dan C., an 18-year-old caucasian male, was referred to us by the Orthopedic Service at the request of his mother. She had agreed with him that when he was 18, she would no longer be responsible for his care, and felt that only a long-term institution could provide the care he needed.

The orthopedic staff had experienced considerable difficulty in managing Dan's hospitalizations for chronic osteomyelitis of his right foot. Each time he entered the hospital and was separated from his mother, and preceding each discharge, he seemed to be agitated and combative, often threatening the medical staff. He was discharged several times before maximal healing of the osteomyelitis could occur because his behavior could not be tolerated.

Many neurological diagnoses had been attached to Dan's evident absence of numerous sensations. Dan reported that he could not feel pain, temperature, light touch, deep touch, and vibration below his neck. He could sometimes feel deep touch in the cranial nerve distribution. As a result of the absence of pain, he had incurred numerous burns, lacerations, and other injuries which he noticed only when they were called to his attention by someone else. He never experienced headaches, toothaches, and abdominal pain or cramps. The only physical discomfort he had ever experienced occurred when he was kicked in the groin by a schoolmate. He was able to "shut off" this discomfort when he was kicked a second time by preparing himself prior to the blow. Dan did not know the position of his hands and feet if he was not watching them. He slept with a light on at night because he could not be sure he was lying down without orienting himself visually. He reported a good sense of balance and learned to ride a bicycle at age 16. He enjoyed swimming. Although he said his vision and hearing were keen, he never experienced discomfort with intense light or sound.

Dan had never felt hunger or thirst, but had evolved a regular feeding schedule based on the knowledge that he should eat three meals a day and drink fluids regularly in order to remain healthy. He could not distinguish tastes, but could distinguish odors. He denied ever having felt tired, but slept several hours each night based on his assessment of how active he had been during the day. He also went to sleep when he was anxious.

Dan could sense bowel and bladder distention, although these were not uncomfortable for him. He could not feel the passage of urine or feces. He did not sweat in hot weather, although he did sweat under his arms when anxious.

As striking as the absence of uncomfortable sensation was Dan's report of having experienced virtually no pleasurable sensation. He did not feel pleasure when he was touched, held, or rocked, or with eating, defecating, exposure to sexually provocative material or kissing girls. He had experienced occasional erections, which were unrelated to sexually provocative experiences. Although he had never had intercourse, he had attempted to masturbate while fantasizing about heterosexual intercourse. This had not resulted in ejaculation or any sense of pleasure.

Dan had always given the impression of having superior intelligence. Formal psychological testing showed superior scores in cognitive tests with below-average scores on performance. His overall IQ was 102. Grade-equivalent scores and comprehension were 12.9+, other scores in the Peabody individual achievement test being appropriate to the grade he would be in were he attending school (grade 11).

Physical and neurological examination and special studies confirmed numerous, severe deficits. Dan had many deformities of his extremities due to amputation of most distal phalanges of his fingers and toes, including his left thumb. Several active and smoldering infections were present as well, including cellulitis in his right hand and chronic osteomyelitis of his right foot. Dan walked on crutches to keep weight off this foot. There was an absence of response of blood pressure to standing up, and an erratic response of body temperature to infection and pyrogens.

Motor strength was normal in all extremities. Vestibular and cerebellar functions were intact. Sensory examination showed an absence of appreciation of light touch, deep touch, temperature, joint position sense, vibration, 2-point discrimination, and stereognosis below his neck. Deep touch was appreciated variably in the cranial nerve distribution. Pinprick was not appreciated over his entire trunk. It was variably appreciated on his face, but was not felt as painful. There was no pain sensation in response to sharp pinprick, extreme cold or muscle ischemia. There were no deep tendon, plantar, or abdominal reflexes.

While motor conduction velocities on EMG were normal, sensory conduction velocities could not be obtained. No peripheral sensory nerves could be found on biopsy. A histamine flare test (test of function of sensory nerve axons) was abnormal. All other studies, including EEG, auditory and visual evoked potential, complete blood count, VDRL, BUN, glucose tolerance test, liver function tests, heavy metal screen and chromosone studies were entirely normal. This was compatible with a diffuse peripheral neuropathy said to occur sporadically (congenital sensory neuropathy) with disturbances of surface and enteric sensory reception (painful, pleasurable, and neutral), autonomic dysfunction, disturbance in temperature regulation, and trophic nerve dysfunction. Due in part to confusion in the literature until recently as to how this condition is distinguished from other sensory syndromes (including simple congenital absence of pain), a definitive diagnosis was not made until Dan's most recent hospitalization. His physicians had also been curiously reluctant to investigate his condition, despite its rarity, and had seemed satisfied with a tentative diagnosis of syringobulba.

Because of our wish to evaluate and understand his development and behavior, and in accordance with Mrs. C.'s wishes, Dan was transferred voluntarily to the psychiatric unit.

EARLY DEVELOPMENTAL HISTORY

Dan was the younger of two children. There was no family history of neurological disease. His father had worked in a uranium mine prior to his conception. His mother remembered no instances of exposure to toxins, drugs, radiation, or trauma during gestation. An old hospital note states that he was a breech presentation delivered vaginally at a gestational age of 34 weeks. Poor sucking, difficulty swallowing, and infrequent leg movements were noted in the neonatal and newborn periods.

The mother remembers that Dan cried "from birth" when she was out of sight. She said, "God, I couldn't get away from him." Dan's crying stopped as soon as she was near, so she carried him with her constantly until he began to walk. Because he never cried when he was not fed or when his diaper was wet, his mother evolved a system of regular feedings and diaper changes. Dan usually ate when he was fed from a bottle, but did not demand food.

His mother told us that Dan had always seemed interested in exploring his environment visually. He showed no evidence of stranger distress as long as she was present. Whenever he tried to sit up, he toppled over. He began to crawl at 12 months, first pulled himself up at $3\frac{1}{2}$ years, and walked a few steps at $4\frac{1}{2}$. Development of walking was not complete until he was 8 years old. Dan remembers learning to walk, and told us that he often tripped over his own feet as he did not know where they were if he did not look at them. He said his first words at 11 months and began speaking in sentences at 15 months.

The first injury Mrs. C. could recall occurred when Dan lacerated his finger at $2\frac{1}{2}$ years without crying. At 4 years, while beginning to walk, Dan lacerated his leg on a chair. The resulting infection necessitated hospitalization and a bone transplant. The hospitalization was the first time Dan was away from his mother, and visiting was restricted to once a week because of isolation procedures. Dan remembers a sense of panic at not being able to see his mother and at having his movement restricted by forced bed rest. This resulted in uncontrollable crying and such extreme agitation that he was confined to a straitjacket. His distress subsided immediately when he was reunited with his mother.

Dan and his mother remember that at the age of $4\frac{1}{2}$ years he lacerated his left thumb, with subsequent osteomyelitis which required amputation of the thumb. Hospitalization for this procedure was accompanied by panic and agitation. Subsequent hospitalizations for wounds and infections have taken up more than half of Dan's life. Dan felt helpless, terrified, and angry during the hospitalizations which occurred from age 4½ to 8. Mrs. C. remembers that when he was about 8 years old, she began to feel a sense of relief during her son's hospitalizations. As it became clear that the hospital staff could take over responsibility for his care, she used the time Dan was in the hospital to "rest up." Dan was beginning to think of the hospital as a "second home," and his agitation during hospitalizations diminished as long as his ability to move around the hospital was not restricted. Dan's mother consistently reappeared when he was discharged, and was the only reliable caretaker when Dan was out of the hospital.

Dan started the first grade at age 6. Although his mother does not remember frank school phobia, he fought with the other children because they made fun of his awkward gait. This caused him to be expelled after three months. Other attempts at returning him to school ended in expulsion for fighting. Dan's mother and sister had taught him to read and write by his sixth year. At age 11 he reentered school in the sixth grade. Without the vestibular sensation provided by constant movement, he had to look around constantly to know whether he was standing or sitting. His incessant activity was felt to be a sign that he was uncooperative and he was expelled again. Most of the next three years were spent in the hospital, during which time Dan taught himself history, math, and English. At age 14 he entered the ninth grade and was expelled again because of constant motion and belligerence toward his teachers and peers.

ADOLESCENT DEVELOPMENT

After Dan completed the ninth grade at age 15, the family moved so that the father could pursue a job offer. When their financial situation worsened, Mr. and Mrs. C. began to argue with increasing frequency. Dan remembers fearing that the family would break up and there would be no one to look after him. His injuries began to increase in frequency, and this had the effect of mobilizing his mother to hospitalize him. Hospital notes for the first time began to comment that he seemed to be prolonging his hospitalizations by picking at wounds and infected areas and excessively using injured limbs. Dan recalls feeling that the only thing he could be sure of during these uncertain times was that he had the power to injure himself. Injuring himself also had the effect of attracting his mother's attention when she was around, and of prolonging hospital care when his parents were fighting excessively. Both Dan and Mrs. C. note that by the age of 16, many of his injuries occurred in his mother's presence. For example, while he was soldering a radio kit, Mrs. C. walked into the room and told him to be careful. This made Dan "nervous" and he "accidentally" dropped a piece of hot solder on his hand, which he noticed only when he smelled burning flesh. His mother reacted with anger at his not being more careful, and they began to argue. During this and many subsequent arguments, Dan's mother frequently hit him. Dan did not fight back and was never seriously injured.

DAN'S MOTHER

Mrs. C. told us that she grew up in a large rural family. She felt close to her mother, whom she described as a warm, hardworking housewife. Her father was a miner who drank frequently and slapped her sporadically from the age of 5 to 10. As a result of this experience, she promised herself never to hit her own children. She was confused and upset when she found herself hitting her son.

Mrs. C. described herself as a woman who enjoyed physical contact as a sign of affective warmth. She experienced her son's lack of response to her cuddling as a rejection. In an attempt to elicit a physical response from Dan, she progressed from putting her arm around him to pushing him to get his attention. She had always been convinced that he had a serious physiological disturbance which prevented him from responding. But by the time Dan was 12, she had begun to slap him when he did not respond. The slapping progressed to punching, kicking, and striking him with chairs. She felt increasingly tired and worn out and began to realize that he would never be able to take care of himself. Frustrated by the lack of support from her husband and by seeing Dan's condition gradually worsen, Mrs. C. began to wish that Dan would go away. When Dan was younger, Mrs. C. harbored the thought that he would one day be able to take care of himself and she would be relieved of her burden. The inability of the doctors to make a definitive diagnosis helped prolong her hope that the correct diagnosis would be one with a favorable prognosis. As Dan grew older, however, she became increasingly aware that he would suffer progressive disability and deformity and that whatever the actual diagnosis, he would always need a caretaker.

DAN'S FATHER

Mr. C. worked for many years as a uranium miner and later as an electrician. We were not able to speak with him, although we made many attempts to do so. Mrs. C. felt that her husband was put off by Dan's illness. He seemed to feel that his exposure to uranium was to blame for Dan's condition. His emotional unavailability to Dan was probably related in part to this feeling, as well as to the realization that caring for Dan was a task too enormous for one family to undertake. It seemed that, unable to convince his wife that she was taking on an almost impossible task, he withdrew his support from her, expressing his guilt by outbursts of anger at his wife, and by ridiculing Dan's appearance.

DAN'S SISTER

Betty is 1½ years older than Dan and had a normal prenatal, birth, developmental, and medical history. Mrs. C. reports no physical battles with her. When Betty was 18, she moved into an apartment of her own. This had been planned by the family for some time. She moved back home for six months at 19, and then married and moved to another city. When interviewed together, Betty and Mrs. C. were mutually empathetic and seemed to respect each other's life situations. Betty was working at a job she enjoyed, had definite vocational plans for herself, and seemed to enjoy her relationship with her husband and child. She said that her 6-month-old son was developing normally.

DREAM HISTORY

Dan remembered two dreams in his lifetime. The first occurred when he was very young and was characterized by a frightening sense of "suffocation," having to do with his mother not being with him. At the age of 17, a day before discharge from the orthopedic service, he dreamed he was being strangled by a disembodied hand. He woke up with the conviction that the hand was still strangling him and it took him several minutes to realize that he was awake. This dream made him quite anxious and he woke himself up because he "didn't like" the experience of having an unpleasant dream.

COURSE IN PSYCHOTHERAPY

Following Dan's transfer to our psychiatric facility, one of us (S.G.) assumed responsibility for his ward care. He was also followed in office psychotherapy twice a week by the psychiatrist who first saw him on the orthopedic service (S.D.). We had an immediate sense of admiration for the work done by Mrs. C. in caring for Dan and were convinced it would take many of us to do her job. We felt very protective toward Dan and found ourselves going out of our way to help him. The ward therapist arranged an allowance for him, lent him clothes, and found himself feeling "motherly." Dan slept late, ensuring that the staff would regularly wake him up in time for breakfast. He precipitated minor "accidents" from which the staff rescued him. This increased our watchfulness over him.

Dan's psychotherapist felt aloof and intellectual with him, in response to Dan's "stickiness." Dan prolonged interviews with numerous questions after the time was up, and it was often necessary to lead him out the door. In initial contacts, he tried on the therapist's hat and coat, sat in the therapist's chair, and seemed to have difficulty distinguishing himself from the therapist.

Dan acknowledged with his therapist that when he was frightened, he became agitated and acted angry and provocative to ensure that people would remain in view, if only to fight with him. Most frightening was the thought of losing caretakers, whether it resulted from the possibility of discharge or simply from a change of shift. He was able to control his behavior when he was reminded why he was frightened and encouraged to express in words his need to have someone in sight.

In the presence of his therapist, Dan began to question how much he could do for himself. While discussing his mother's overprotectiveness, he lighted a cigarette and dropped the lighted match on his lap. Continuing to talk, he carefully picked up the match in order to avoid burning himself, remarking in an offhand way that he could not tell how tightly he was holding the match without looking at it. Several minutes later he asked the therapist if he had noticed the match-dropping episode and went on to say that he had been testing the doctor's response. His mother would have hit him and called him an idiot, making him doubt his ability to take any responsibility for his own caretaking. He thought that the therapist was watching him carefully to see if he was capable of avoiding injury, and he was sure that the therapist would have grabbed the match if he had actually been in danger of burning himself. At the end of the session, he asked the therapist to button his coat, remarking that he was not yet ready to be entirely on his own.

As Dan became more skilled at tolerating affects and expressing them in words, he began to speak of what he called a "return" of sensations which he did not remember ever having felt. While soaking his hand under a faucet, he experienced a sense of discomfort which made him withdraw his hand. When he saw that the hot water was turned on, he reasoned that he must have experienced the sensation of "heat." Later he reported a "return" of his ability to distinguish objects placed in his hand and some increase in joint position sense at his ankles and wrists. Several examiners found a consistently improved ability to appreciate temperature, deep touch, stereognosis, and joint position, although there was no change in appreciation of pinprick, painful stimuli, light touch, and vibration. There were no neurophysiological or biochemical changes that could be measured. The patient reported feeling that now that people were taking care of him reliably there was "something to live for" and he expressed an increased interest in "looking after" himself. The number of injuries he experienced diminished rapidly and only a suppurative osteomyelitis of his heel remained.

After three months of hospital treatment the staff felt increasingly "drained," and a curious split in their attitude toward Dan developed. Some staff members felt that he needed long-term hospitalization on another ward, while others thought he should be on his own. We began to look after him less assiduously. In response to our diminished attention, Dan became angry and provoking, threatening to kill the staff and blow up the hospital. He told his therapist that he was feeling "killed" and "blown up" and wanted a more active part in the process. For the first time, seclusion was necessary. Dan remarked that when 10 to 15 staff members gathered to confine him, they were risking injury to look after him. But he was careful to ensure that they were never hurt. Dan's "accidental" injuries increased, and his osteomyelitis worsened.

While interpretation led to an improvement in Dan's behavior, the ward staff felt that working with him was too consuming of time and energy. They complained that they gave Dan a lot and got "nothing in return." After working with Dan for four months, we could empathize with Mrs. C.'s insistence that she did not want Dan to live with her anymore. Dan's ward doctor began to make arrangements for his transfer to an institution geared to long-term inpatient treatment. Dan reacted to the transfer with panic, anger, and sadness. He cried several times, and we felt an empathic sadness with him. Dan said that just as pieces of his body had been "knocked off," his ward therapist was "knocking off" pieces of his mind by transferring him. Soon there would be nothing left. Expressing these thoughts and feelings in words was definitely helpful because further self-destructive behavior did not occur, although Dan was willing to undergo further injuries if it would ensure ongoing care. Because of our guilt over transferring him, we were unable fully to appreciate his need to know that he would have such care. He demonstrated this dramatically.

As part of planning for his transfer, arrangements were made for Dan to sleep outside of the hospital in a boarding home. The next day he broke into a store in front of a policeman. He was arrested and released, and within several hours was arrested again for attempting to steal a car while a policeman was watching. He was then jailed. At first he felt safe, and he remarked that jails seemed more dependable than hospitals in taking care of him. During his second day in jail, he began to feel that his mobility was limited by the cell and that he would not get appropriate medical attention because the police did not understand his illness. He discussed this with his jailers, who called the ward doctor and requested transfer back to our hospital. We were encouraged by the fact that Dan had assessed his situation realistically, expressed feelings and needs in words, and been able to take effective adaptive action. There were no more illegal activities.

On his return to us we reassured Dan that we would continue to "watch over" him. Dan replied that even if his arms and legs were cut off, he would "keep going." After five months in our hospital, Dan will be treated with long-term inpatient care at a nearby institution. He will be followed by us in psychotherapy aimed at examining events that interfere with his ability to use his superior intelligence and capabilities in the service of maximal adaptation.

Discussion

One reason why few reports exist of long-term follow-up of patients with severe sensory deficits may be that few people survive childhood without an intact sensory apparatus. How, then, did Dan manage to survive?

MOTHERING

Most important was his mother's recognition of his need for her constant attention. She was able to assess his continuous need for her to supply sensory input. Her realization that "from birth" he was anxious when she was out of sight led her to prolong an intense relationship with him. Realizing that he was unable to walk, she supplied him with mobility. Mrs. C. rapidly responded to his need to form a functional link between Dan and an environment he could not feel. She was able to adapt her mothering activities to her son's average expectable environment (Hartmann, 1939). As Dan grew, Mrs. C. made the judgment that he could not use visual information sufficiently to keep from injuring himself, and she reminded him when he was in danger and arranged for medical care. Based on her assessment of his capabilities and incapabilities, she allowed him increasing mobility, but aided him with reality testing, impulse control, and intellectual functions.

Mrs. C.'s judgments were for the most part correct and were made without the benefit of a definitive diagnosis or psychiatric consultation! Additional input and support from Dan's physicians might have eased her burden in caring for him. However, hearing early in Dan's life that his capabilities, and even his lifespan, were limited, might well have proved discouraging. Even though she acted in part out of a need to perform a task which seemed impossible, and to obtain gratification from a prolonged symbiotic relationship with her son, Mrs. C.'s persistence seems heroic. When Dan grew to early adolescence, his mother became uncertain of his capabilities. This was reflected in her behavior which fluctuated between extreme attentiveness and insistence that he function autonomously. At this point, consultation with her doctors would definitely have helped to ameliorate her confusion and pain. Lacking sufficient information to be sure in which direction to proceed, tired out by the lack of sensory feedback many mothers need from their children, she sought help from the hospitals with which she had worked.

EGO DEVELOPMENT

It is generally assumed that ego development presupposes a certain measure of perceptual and sensory input. How did Dan acquire his achievements in the face of his severe somatic defects?

If we remember Hartmann's (1939) definition of the ego as "the specific organ of adaptation" (p. 50), it is undeniable that adaptive ego functioning developed. Dan was able to make use of his cognitive abilities to learn new manual (e.g., repairing radios) and intellectual (e.g., reading and writing, diagnosis of infections) skills. He developed creative thought, impulse control, and external reality testing. His capacity to test interpersonal reality allowed him to infer from the actions of others when his inability to separate from them was making them too anxious to function efficiently as caretakers. Having made this observation, he was often able to distance himself until their anxiety diminished sufficiently for them to continue working with him. To the extent that Dan was able to learn to verbalize his needs and affects and increase the observing ego function, the potential for ego growth existed (Blanck and Blanck, 1974).

Defensive functions of the ego that developed were predominantly denial, projection, and reaction formation. Repression, sublimation, and similar mechanisms were not used significantly. Internal regulatory mechanisms also developed. For example, Dan said he would never rob a bank because it was "wrong." He carefully avoided injuring other people during his aggressive outbursts, preferring to injure himself when angry.

Dan's mother served a number of auxiliary ego functions (Spitz, 1965), including interpretation of sensation, mobility, reality testing, impulse control, and intellectual functions. Dan, in turn, developed a continuing ability to mobilize people to serve functions normally carried out by autonomous sectors of the ego. His nurses were auxiliary organs of sensation and motility who arranged day-to-day activities such as eating and sleeping. His ward physician supplied impulse control and arranged continuing hospital care. His psychotherapist was an auxiliary observing ego and an organ of reality testing. It is likely that Dan learned from these people additional means of adaptation, which he could apply to some degree on his own. This may explain his increased ability to control impulses, express internal experiences verbally, and develop observing ego functions.

Another explanation for Dan's development of adaptive ego function in the absence of surface and enteroceptive sensation is that he was able to make use of intact sensory modalities such as hearing, vision, and smell. Blind children to varying degrees are able to make use of auditory and tactile sensation for psychological development (Burlingham, 1965; Fraiberg, 1968; Nagera and Colonna, 1965). Kohut (1971) states that the "auditory modality may . . . take over . . . when there is a defect in the visual area" (p. 118). Freedman et al. (1971) suggest that other sensory pathways are of help to congenitally deaf children in psychological development. Schaffer and Emerson's (1964) "noncuddlers" did not seem to find physical contact rewarding in infancy, apparently on a biological basis. Yet they were able to develop attachment behavior, mediated by vision. Finally, Kohut's (1971) work with adult patients suggests that an infant who does not receive sufficient physical contact uses visual stimulation "to substitute for the failures that . . . [occur] in the realm of physical (oral and tactile) contact" (p. 117). In Dan, it is possible that vestibular sensation, vision (Spitz, 1965; Bronson, 1963), and hearing (Freedman et al., 1971) substituted to a sufficient degree for absent tactile and enteroceptive sensations to provide a perceptual framework for ego development. We do not have enough information to comment on the importance of his sense of smell.

Many organisms can shift to another sensory modality (e.g., touch) when one modality (e.g., vision) is impaired, possibly providing physiological information for adaptation, learning, and development (Bach-y-Rita, 1972; Fraiberg, 1964). It is an interesting speculation that Dan may have made use of "parasensory" neural pathways at a peripheral or central level to provide necessary sensory information. If this occurred, words for such "paratactile" information would not exist as these pathways would not ordinarily be used by people with intact sensory apparatuses.

When Dan's caretaking was assured, he was able to turn some of his attention away from the task of forcing others to care for him. This allowed him to attend to whatever sensory information was available and resulted in more affective and cognitive ties to various body parts. This may have led to the "return" of sensation he noticed.

AFFECTIVE DEVELOPMENT

A striking finding was that Dan developed differentiated affects in the absence of any experience of physical pain or pleasure. Freud (1926) remarked that we commonly treat "the feeling of loss of object as equivalent to physical pain" (p. 171), and our own expectation was that without an obvious sensory substrate, affective development could not occur (Hinde, 1972). However, Freud (1926) goes on to suggest that the *experience* of mental unpleasure depends on mental development, and not on the experience of physical pain. The *expression* of mental pain involves the use of words that are also used to describe physical pain, because "the same state of mental helplessness" (p. 172) prevails when physical and mental pain are experienced. Our experience with this case supports the view that mental unpleasure is not dependent on an intact pain perception system. Dan was quite capable of expressing such affects as anxiety (we were empathetically anxious with him), anger, and sadness (he was able to cry). He did not seem to experience grief (e.g., over loss of an object or body part) or depression (Beck, 1967), possibly because of his failure to differentiate self and object representations.

Dan's unpleasurable affects may have first arisen in the "perceptual unpleasure" that Freud (1926) believed a young child experiences when his mother is out of sight. "Innate recognition mechanisms" (Sackett, 1966), which mature independently of experiential factors, may have further conditioned such affects. We cannot know exactly what Dan meant when he said, "I'm anxious," "I'm sad," or "I'm angry." However, his obvious experience of disturbing affects underscores the fact that unpleasurable affective experiences are the complex endpoint of cortical integration of peripheral sensory, central nervous system (Hebb, 1946), and experiential phenomena, superimposed on a substrate of independently developing innate mechanisms.

Dan's experience of pleasurable affects was even more complex. Proximity to his mother was a soothing experience, and he was calm and relaxed when allowed to remain in view of and interact verbally with an important caretaker. Mastery by active participation (Freud, 1920) later seemed to provide the feeling of being in control, which Dan found very reassuring. An extreme example of this was his marked self-destructive behavior, which seemed to represent an attempt to participate actively in a process that was gradually destroying his body. Dan often remarked that it "felt good" to know that he could actively cause the kind of disfigurement and disability that was going to happen to him anyway. It cannot be said, however, that Dan ever seemed "happy." His sarcastic attempts at humor reflected his derisive view of himself and his future. He also seemed to lack the capacity for empathy, although he was able to note other people's apparent mental state without an affective response of his own unless his caretaking was affected.

DAN'S SENSE OF SELF

The recent understanding of the importance of the self leads us to consider our patient's apparent failure to develop a differentiated, cohesive sense of self. Dan did not seem to experience himself as a separate entity and usually referred to himself in reference to another person. He did not seem to experience people as entities separate from the functional roles they played in his survival, and people who played the same functional roles were virtually interchangeable for him. His conviction that only a "bullet in the brain" could kill him would seem to reflect the unmodified expression of what Kohut (1972) has called the "grandiose-exhibitionistic body-self." (This may also have reflected some awareness of other people's fantasy that he really was indestructible.) Comments such as "Your clothes look nice today. When are you going to give them to me?" may have reflected an unmodified wish to merge with an idealized self-object (Kohut, 1971). When he said, "You look good, how do I look?" he seemed to be stating a need to observe and be observed by us.

Dan's failure to develop a cohesive, autonomous sense of self, while developing other psychological structures, supports the contention that the development of self and adaptive ego function may follow separate lines (Kohut, 1966, 1971, 1972; Levin, 1970). While ego development may occur independently of a number of somatic factors, the self may originate as and remain a "body self" dependent on what Mahler (1968) calls the "sensoriperceptive organ." Freud (1923) seems to suggest that the self[1] "is ultimately derived from bodily sensations, chiefly those springing from the surface of the body. It may thus be regarded as a mental projection of the surface of the body" (p. 26). This view is reinforced by Spiegel (1959): "If we now interpret the word 'self-representation' literally (i.e., as representation of the self), we are obliged to say that the self and body are identical" (p. 86).

It should be remembered that separation-individuation (Mahler,

---

[1] Freud often used "das Ich" to refer to what many authors now call the self, and not the ego (Levin, 1970).

1968) did not occur. "Practicing" would have been impossible, if Dan was to retain the necessary sensory input and protective functions his mother provided. The prolonged mother-child symbiosis was necessary for survival. However, Dan did not have the opportunity to internalize many aspects of his mother, who remained constantly at his side. This resulted in deficits in his ability to regulate chaotic internal experience when his mother was not present. Along with failure to develop differentiated self and object representations, the ongoing, intense mother-child bond with its constant visual focus on Dan's body may have contributed to an excess of what Kohut (1972) calls "unmodified, archaic, exhibitionistic libido" (p. 375). In the absence of events leading to "rapprochement," object constancy did not develop (Mahler, 1968). Dan's fragmented, chaotic sense of self was associated with disorganization of effective ego functioning. This supports Kohut's contention that "the self may serve as an organizer of ego activities. [If] . . . the self is poorly cathected . . . then ego functions may . . . be disconnected one from the other and be lacking in firmness of purpose and integrated cohesion" (Levin, 1970, p. 180). The self may, therefore, serve as a frame of reference against which perceptions of internal and interpersonal states may consistently be judged (Spiegel, 1959). Dan's ability rapidly to categorize other people and use them adaptively, as well as his capacity to judge the degree of danger to his health at any given time, would have been further aided by a cohesive sense of self.

It is difficult to conceptualize Dan's particular object-instinctual line of development. We hope to be able to make some comments about this when we have had more experience with him.

IMPLICATIONS FOR HUMAN DEVELOPMENT:
THE ADAPTIVE APPROACH

In attempting to formulate the salient aspects of Dan's psychological development, it is useful to mention Waddington's (1966) comments, originally made regarding organ development:

> . . . the developing system has an inbuilt tendency to stick to the path, and is quite difficult to divert from it by any influence. . . . Even if the developing system is forcibly made abnormal . . . it still

tends to get itself back onto the canalized pathway and finish up as a normal adult. . . . Developing systems do not always reach the fully normal adult state. The point is that they have a tendency to do so. . . . One can make a mental picture of the situation by thinking of the development . . . as a ball running down a valley. It will, of course, tend to run down to the bottom of the valley, and if something temporarily pushes it up to one side, it will again have a tendency to run down to the bottom and finally finish up in its normal place. If one thinks of all the different parts of the egg, . . . one would have to represent the whole system by a series of different valleys, all starting out from the fertilized egg but gradually diverging and finishing up at a number of different adult organs [p. 48f.].

We may extend this formulation as follows: the human infant is confronted by potential channels of adaptive psychological development (ego, affects, self, object-instinctual), determined in part by his genetic endowment, his neurophysiological equipment, and early mothering experiences. The pressure to develop adaptive psychological structures and mental functions is enormous. Despite temporary alterations, it is extremely difficult to cause an individual to deviate from his potential channels of adaptive development. Should one pathway of adaptive development be blocked, e.g., by deficiencies in physical endowment or early experience, the human organism is flexible enough to shift to other potential developmental channels. Despite our expectation that Dan could not survive, let alone develop competence, in the face of such severe neurophysiological deficits, he developed ego functions, internal regulatory mechanisms, and some differentiated affects. When sensory information useful for development was unavailable, his central nervous system possessed sufficient plasticity to make use of other channels to obtain information. Lacking the sensory equipment and appropriate experience for the development of a cohesive sense of self, Dan was able to make use of others to help organize his own ego activities. His remark that he will continue to "keep trying" is an eloquent testimony to human adaptation in the face of great adversity.

While developmental possibilities open to any individual are in part innate, they are greatly specific to the individual and to his "average expectable environment." Thus, excessive aggressive behavior might be considered symptomatic in a middle-class neighborhood, but would be adaptive in a slum where aggression directed against an individual needs to be met with counteraggression. Behavior which often seemed maladaptive (e.g., "accidental" injuries and Dan's deliberate effort to be jailed when he felt completely abandoned) was adaptive under the circumstances (hospital personnel needed to be reminded that Dan could not be on his own). Lack of separation-individuation can be seen as adaptive given the precondition that early experiences promoting this would have led to death. It is most useful to think of Dan's development as following a path uniquely adaptive for his survival.

THERAPEUTIC IMPLICATIONS

Dan's mother had no way of knowing how to continue to care for a child like Dan, and we took over for her. Our first, most important task was to evaluate, diagnose, and understand Dan's handicap and deficits as well as his capabilities. We next had to assess those factors that facilitated adaptation. These included caretaking and the provision of auxiliary ego functions in a hospital, in doses sufficient to ensure survival. Our initial psychotherapy involved empathetically reflecting back to him ego states that were related to utilization or lack of utilization of his adaptive potential. This included teaching him to develop words for intrapsychic events. During this time, structured hospital care also served the purpose of helping him to increase his ability to tolerate anxiety and to keep him from converting affects into action. When he was anxious, Dan reacted in the only way he knew: by provoking fights and getting himself injured. When we controlled his behavior and reflected his anxiety back to him, he was able to discuss the affect in words. Dan called this "getting in touch with his feelings." He could then add information himself. For example, he interpreted an increase in privileges as a sign that he would soon be on his own. He was also able to apply additional information from the past. When he burned himself while soldering in his mother's presence, he interpreted her warning to "be careful" as meaning that he should *not* be capable of being careful when he was in her presence. To

Dan, being careful when she was around meant losing her protective functions entirely.

We next asked Dan if there was some different way such situations could be handled. This was the beginning of our mutual investigation of those functions he could begin to carry out on his own. As his sense of connection to various body parts increased, he was more able to ask appropriately for and obtain efficient caretaking. Our progress in working with him can be measured in part by his increased ability to heal many wounds, the diminished incidence of self-destructive behavior, and his increasing use of language instead of action as a tool of communication. We have not yet had sufficient experience with Dan to agree with Freedman (1971, 1972) and Wilson (1971) that early serious somatic deficits set limits on new psychological structure that can develop. We suspect, however, that the limits of his psychological growth are beyond our expectations.

Summary

This fascinating and complex patient had a congenital absence of most surface and many enteroceptive sensations including touch, pain, temperature, vibration, joint position sense, stereognosis, and visceral sensation. Sensations arising from the oral, anal, and genital regions were absent, and pleasure was not experienced with surface pressure, cuddling, eating, defecating, urinating, and erections. He had disturbances in blood pressure and body temperature regulation, as well as in wound healing. Despite impaired development of a sense of self, identifications, object constancy, and empathy, he developed competence in many spheres. Adaptive and defensive functions of the ego as well as mechanisms of internal control and differentiated affects developed despite our expectation that this could not have occurred. The roles of empathetic mothering, auxiliary egos, and plasticity of the human organism in development are discussed. The importance of considering each individual as proceeding along developmental lines uniquely adaptive for him is given renewed emphasis. Further evidence is provided to support the concept of a separate developmental line for the sense of self, probably more directly tied to somatic experience than to ego development. The usefulness of a psychotherapeutic approach which emphasizes a knowledge of the patient's adaptive potential as well as his deficiencies is underscored.

BIBLIOGRAPHY

ANNIS, R. C. & FROST, B. (1973), Human Visual Ecology and Orientation Anisotropies in Acuity. *Science*, 182:729–731.
BACH-Y-RITA, P. (1972), *Brain Mechanisms in Sensory Substitution*. New York: Academic Press.
BECK, A. T. (1967), *Depression*. New York: Hoeber.
BLANCK, G. & BLANCK, R. (1974), *Ego Psychology*. New York: Columbia Univ. Press.
BRONSON, G. (1963), A Neurological Perspective on Ego Development in Infancy. *J. Amer. Psychoanal. Assn.*, 11:55–65.
BURLINGHAM, D. (1965), Some Problems of Ego Development in Blind Children. *This Annual*, 20:194–208.
CALL, J. D. (1964), Newborn Approach Behaviour and Early Ego Development. *Int. J. Psycho-Anal.*, 45:286–294.
CAMPBELL, A. M. G. (1970), Hereditary Sensory Neuropathy. In: *Handbook of Clinical Neurology*, ed. P. J. Vinken & G. W. Brayn. Amsterdam: North Holland Publishing Co., 8:180–186.
COHEN, L. D., KIPNIS, D., KUNKLE, F. C., & KUBZANSKY, P. E. (1955), Observations of a Person with Congenital Insensitivity to Pain. *J. Abnorm. Soc. Psychol.*, 51:333–338.
CRAGG, B. G. (1967), Changes in Visual Cortex on First Exposure of Rats to Light. *Nature*, 215:251–253.
FLAVELL, J. H. (1963), *The Developmental Psychology of Jean Piaget*. Princeton, N.J.: Van Nostrand.
FRAIBERG, S. (1968), Parallel and Divergent Patterns in Blind and Sighted Infants. *This Annual*, 23:264–300.
——— & FREEDMAN, D. A. (1964), Studies in the Ego Development of the Congenitally Blind Child. *This Annual*, 19:113–169.
FREEDMAN, D. A. (1971), Congenital and Perinatal Sensory Deprivation. *Amer. J. Psychiat.*, 127:1539–1545.
——— (1972), On the Limits of the Effectiveness of Psychoanalysis. *Int. J. Psycho-Anal.*, 53:363-370.
——— CANNADAY, C., & ROBINSON, J. S. (1971), Speech and Psychic Structure. *J. Amer. Psychoanal. Assn.*, 19.765 770.
FREUD, S. (1920), Beyond the Pleasure Principle. *S.E.*, 18:1–64.
——— (1923), The Ego and the Id. *S.E.*, 19:3–66.
——— (1926), Inhibitions, Symptoms and Anxiety. *S.E.*, 20:75–175.
HARLOW, H. F. (1958), The Nature of Love. *Amer. Psychologist*, 13:673–685.
——— & HARLOW, M. (1966), Learning to Love. *Amer. Scientist*, 54:244–272.

——— & Zimmerman, R. R. (1959), Affectional Responses in the Infant Monkey. *Science*, 130:421–432.
Hartmann, H. (1939), *Ego Psychology and the Problem of Adaptation*. New York: Int. Univ. Press, 1958.
Hebb, D. O. (1946), On the Nature of Fear. *Psychol. Rev.*, 53:259–276.
Hinde, R. A. (1972), Concepts of Emotion. In: *Physiology, Emotion and Psychosomatic Illness*. Amsterdam: Associated Scientific Publishers, pp. 3–13.
Holloway, R. (1966), Dendritic Branching. *Brain Research*, 2:393–396.
Jessor, R. & Richardson, S. (1968), Psychosocial Deprivation and Personality Development. In: *Perspectives on Human Deprivation*. Washington, D.C.: National Institute of Child Health and Human Development (USDHEW), pp. 1–87.
Jewesbury, E. (1970), Congenital Indifference to Pain. In: *Handbook of Clinical Neurology*, ed. P. J. Vinken & G. W. Brayn. Amsterdam: North Holland Publishing Co., 8:187–204.
Kane, F. J., Downie, A. W., Marcotte, D. W., & Perez-Reyes, M. (1968), A Case of Congenital Indifference to Pain. *Dis. Nerv. Syst.*, 29:409–412.
Kohut, H. (1966), Forms and Transformations of Narcissism. *J. Amer. Psychoanal. Assn.*, 14:243–272.
——— (1971), *The Analysis of the Self*. New York: Int. Univ. Press.
——— (1972), Thoughts on Narcissism and Narcissistic Rage. *This Annual*, 27:360–400.
Korner, A. F. & Grobstein, R. (1966), Visual Alertness As Related to Soothing in Neonates. *Child Develpm.*, 37:867–876.
Levin, D. C. (1970), The Self. *Int. J. Psycho-Anal.*, 51:175–181.
McMurray, G. A. (1950), Experimental Study of a Case of Insensitivity to Pain. *Arch. Neurol. Psychiat.*, 64:650–667.
Magee, K. R., Schneider, S. F., & Rosenzweig, N. (1961), Congenital Indifference to Pain. *J. Nerv. Ment. Dis.*, 132:249–259.
Mahler, M. S. (1968), *On Human Symbiosis and the Vicissitudes of Individuation*. New York: Int. Univ. Press, pp. 7–31.
Murray, T. J. (1973), Congenital Sensory Neuropathy. *Brain*, 96:387–394.
Nagera, H. (1968), The Concept of Ego Apparatus in Psychoanalysis. *This Annual*, 23:224–242.
——— & Colonna, A. (1965), Aspects of the Contribution of Sight to Ego and Drive Development. *This Annual*, 20:267–287.
Ogden, T. E., Robert, F., & Carmichael, E. A. (1959), Some Sensory Syndromes in Children. *J. Neurol. Neurosurg. Psychiat.*, 22:267–276.
Pettigrew, J. D. & Freeman, R. D. (1973), Visual Experience Without Lines. *Science*, 182:599–601.
Rapoport, J. L. (1959), A Case of Congenital Sensory Neuropathy Diagnosed in Infancy. *J. Child Psychol. Psychiat.*, 10:63–68.
Reisen, A. H. (1961), Stimulation As a Requirement for Growth and Function. In: *Functions of Varied Experience*, ed. D. W. Fiske. Homewood, Ill.: Dorsey Press, pp. 68–71.

SACKETT, G. P. (1966), Monkeys Reared in Isolation with Pictures As Visual Input. *Science*, 154:1468–1473.
SCHAFFER, H. R. & EMERSON, P. E. (1964), Patterns of Response to Physical Contact in Early Human Development. *J. Child Psychol. Psychiat.*, 5:1–13.
SCHNEIDER, S. F. (1962), A Psychological Basis for Indifference to Pain. *Psychosom. Med.*, 24:119–132.
SPIEGEL, L. A. (1959), The Self, the Sense of Pain, and Perception. *This Annual*, 14:81–109.
SPITZ, R. A. (1950), Psychiatric Therapy in Infancy. *Amer. J. Orthopsychiat.*, 20:623–633.
——— (1965), *The First Year of Life*. New York: Int. Univ. Press.
STERNBACH, R. (1963), Congenital Insensitivity to Pain. *Psychol. Bull.*, 60:252–264.
THRUSH, D. C. (1973), Congenital Insensitivity to Pain. *Brain*, 96:369–386.
WADDINGTON, C. H. (1966), *Principles of Differentiation and Development*. New York: Macmillan.
WHITE, R. W. (1963), *Ego and Reality in Psychoanalytic Theory*. New York: Int. Univ. Press.
WILSON, C. P. (1971), On the Limits of Effectiveness of Psychoanalysis. *J. Amer. Psychoanal. Assn.*, 19:552–564.
WINKELMANN, R. K., LAMBERT, E. H., & Hayles, A. B. (1962), Congenital Absence of Pain. *Arch. Derm.*, 85:325–339.

Infant Observation

Its Relevance to Psychoanalytic Training
W. ERNEST FREUD

THE PSYCHOANALYTIC TEACHING PROGRAMS THAT ADDED INFANT observation[1] to their curricula usually did so in order to acquaint the student with "the solid knowledge of child development" (A. Freud, 1970) and to enable him to get the "feel" of the baby, the mother, and the family (Bick, 1964). Such experience was thought essential for understanding and helping child and adult patients and invaluable as an aid to reconstruction in analysis (Freud, 1937; E. Kris, 1956; A. Freud, 1966; Kennedy, 1971). However, the specific bearing that infant observation has on the actual work of the analyst would seem to need further elucidation.

I shall leave aside the question of how one can be a good enough

---

The author, a research psychoanalyst at the Hampstead Child-Therapy Clinic, draws on experience with students of the Clinic and with students of the London Institute of Psycho-Analysis who are training for adult analysis. I am indebted to Dr. J. Stross, pediatrician at the Well-Baby Clinic of the Hampstead Child-Therapy Clinic, who furthered my own baby observations, and to the dedicated student observers without whose inspired cooperation this venture would not have been possible.

The Hampstead Child-Therapy Clinic is at present supported by the Field Foundation, Inc., New York; the Foundation for Research in Psychoanalysis, Beverly Hills, Calif.; the Freud Centenary Fund, London; the Anna Freud Foundation, New York; the National Institute of Mental Health, Bethesda, Maryland; the Grant Foundation, New York; the New-Land Foundation, Inc., New York, and a number of private supporters.

[1] The term "infant observation" is used to denote observation of the infant, the mother, and the mother-infant interaction.

analyst (Mitscherlich-Nielsen, 1970) without experience in infant observation—or for that matter without training in child analysis—and also steer clear of such problems as feasibility, implementation, staffing (Beiser, 1973), and student evaluation. Instead, I shall look at what is involved in observing a family in its natural habitat.[2] In London the three psychoanalytically orientated teaching centers (the Institute of Psycho-Analysis, the Hampstead Child-Therapy Clinic, and the Tavistock Centre) developed and use basically similar kinds of infant observation, though the setups vary in detail. At the Institute and at Hampstead the student is required to follow the development of a newborn baby through visiting a family for one hour once a week during the first academic year. Often there is a sibling of toddler age present too, so that the student can learn "to observe and understand the unfolding interaction between mother, infant and the whole family" (Training Prospectus of the Institute, 1973/74). After the visit the student writes a report on his observations. It is circulated and discussed in weekly seminars under the guidance of a seminar leader, who ideally should be at home in both adult analysis and child analysis and have had some experience of pediatrics. The optimal number of students for a group seems to be four, especially if they are evenly matched as to gender and (at the Institute) medical and nonmedical background. In this way each student will learn not only about the family he observes but about three other families as well.

On the whole, first year students are psychoanalytically inexperienced. They are in the early stages of their own training analysis, are starting attendance at formal lectures, and usually have to wait a year before they are entrusted with a supervised training case. Naturally they long for clinical experience and responsibility.

[2] We are aware of the intrusive nature of such an enterprise, but it should not be overlooked that many house-bound mothers welcome a sympathetic listener whose presence may be a great support, quite apart from the prestige value that is sometimes in certain circles attached to such an interesting "possession." One of our mothers tried to provide herself (for various reasons) with an additional observer from another institution.

At Yale a free Well-Baby Clinic service is offered to mothers who volunteer for research. The Hampstead Well-Baby Clinic also offers a free service, but does not take for granted the right to impose observers on the families.

Infant observation offers a first "case load" (mother, infant, and the rest of the family) that provides relevant and meaningful experience.

At the Institute a preliminary meeting between seminar leaders and students is arranged before the summer holidays, to give more time for finding families in which a baby is expected around October, when courses start. Most of the Hampstead students arrive from abroad in the fall; they are usually assigned to a baby from the Well-Baby Clinic (where they also observe), and care is taken to match observer and family.

Briefing

The best introduction to the student's activities is through the briefing, which in many ways parallels Freud's recommendations on technique (1912, 1913). The student is instructed to use his free-floating ("evenly suspended") attention,[3] and is not allowed to take notes in the family's home. Although this may initially lead to free-floating anxiety, the instructions are firm. The procedure serves as an excellent preparation for the next stage of training when the student will have to listen to his patients and write reports for his supervisors after sessions.

Observers are not supposed to moralize or adopt a critical attitude to the way a mother handles her infant, and they must not attempt "wild analysis" (Freud, 1910). As with patients, it is advisable not to tell the mother much about oneself, but at the same time the observer should feel free to satisfy the family's curiosity about his "credentials." He should feel equally free to turn questions back (as in analysis). It is always easier to be truthful than to invent a lie. In any case, he is advised to make a mental note of those occasions when questions appear to be in the service of a latent, inappropriate need rather than in the service of a manifest and appropriate one. He will refrain from "interviewing" the

---

[3] See also A. Freud's description (1951) of the Hampstead War Nurseries: "The observational work itself was not governed by a prearranged plan. Emulating the analyst's attitude when observing his patient during the analytic hour, attention was kept free-floating and the material was followed up wherever it led" (p. 20).

family, but in keeping with analytic tradition he will gradually build up a picture from what is volunteered—and from what is conspicuous by its absence, which may well be significant.[4] He is encouraged to build up a working alliance by enlisting the mother's interest in his wish to learn as much as possible through her about the baby's development and her interaction with the baby. The mother is with the baby nearly all the time and therefore "knows best." She will function optimally when her mothering is attuned to her personal needs, and we stress that each mother (like each baby) has her own style of functioning, just as the observer is likely to be at his best when he can let himself be himself. We tell him: "If in doubt, be yourself, be natural, and use your common sense!"

During observation time nothing should be left out. For example, if the mother discreetly goes upstairs with the baby to change his nappies, the observer might well pluck up courage and ask whether he could follow her. When such incidents are taken up in the seminar, we refer to the "fundamental rule" (Freud, 1913) and explain why analysts are dependent on getting as much consciously known information from the patient as possible and how easily one omission begets another. However, if the mother, in spite of her original willingness, later does not want a stranger (especially a male observer) present during breast feedings, this must always be respected. If the choice of family for observation appears to be in most other respects a good one, and if the observer can cope with his disappointment, he is encouraged to continue visiting. Some of the students who were deprived of observing breast feeding (for whatever reason) nevertheless became first-rate observers and succeeded in maintaining excellent relations with the mother.

The Role of the Observer

Observers are usually concerned about the role they are supposed to play, and the more guidance we can give them the easier will be their task. Many applicants for analytic training come from the medical profession, which generally requires an actively helpful,

---

[4] The procedure adopted by the well-baby clinics at Yale and at Hampstead has previously been described (W. E. Freud, 1967, p. 218).

supportive, and often authoritative role (not least in psychiatry), while those coming from academic psychology may have relied greatly on their "scientifically objective" orientation. Either extreme may well be a handicap in assuming the role of "participant" observer. While this is the general expectation, the student should feel free to decline or oppose anything he really dislikes or thinks he cannot cope with. Participation may extend to anything a member of the family may ask him to do, short of becoming emotionally involved. It may range from bringing in the milk bottles on arrival to holding, feeding, bathing, or changing the baby; from reading to, or playing with, an older sibling, or taking him to the toilet; from collecting with mother another child from nursery school to going shopping with mother and infant at the supermarket. Each situation will be instructive and may provide unexpected opportunities for learning more about the family. Advice, guidance, and reassurance should on the whole be avoided, on the same grounds as they are in analysis. The student is encouraged to think in what ways and for what reasons his role resembles or differs from that of the analyst.

Direct Observation and Observation in the Analytic Situation

Although the student has been given many recommendations derived from analytic technique, we stress that his objective, and therefore the way in which he is expected to use these recommendations, is very different. The analyst has access to preconscious and unconscious material by dealing with the patient's major transference and resistance manifestations. Free association in the adult, or extended observation of the child patient's play and other reactions, puts the analyst in the unique position of being able to trace, illuminate, and reconstruct the origins of the patient's pathology. He communicates his findings whenever indicated, with a view to bringing about changes and reintegrations in the patient's personality.

By comparison, the sphere of the student observer's activities is rather restricted. In his relationship with the infant's *mother,* he is dependent on what she chooses to tell him and on his observations of her behavior. Its meaning can be understood with the help of what is reliably known about the connections between surface behavior and underlying unconscious elements (A. Freud, 1957). In addition, the character of a family can often be inferred from the individuality of their home; from their attitude to food, pets, cleanliness; and from their display of possessions. These usually tell something about the relative emphasis put on orality, anality, and phallic-exhibitionistic competitiveness. A baby girl's name may be a pointer to the parent's wish for a boy. Religious orthodoxy may curtail a family's range of preferred activities. Yet it would be rash, without deeper material, to pinpoint determinants of a parent's choice of occupation, as one may occasionally be tempted to do. In one of the families we observed the father became a milkman at the time of the baby's birth.

Altogether, all conclusions the observer may draw have to be tentative and have to be treated with the utmost caution. The emphasis on not jumping to premature conclusions serves as a good *preparation* for the understanding of psychoanalytic observation, which is, after all, the aim of the course.

With the *baby* the observer is, in the absence of verbal communication during the first year of life, even more restricted to direct observation of what shows through manifest behavior (Spitz, 1950). Notwithstanding this limitation, I have tried to show in earlier publications (1967, 1971) how, by focusing on various areas, a comprehensive picture of an infant's "personality" is gained. To the wide range of topics new ones can be added.

With the Baby Profile in mind, we can in turn look at the baby's body needs and functions—sleep-waking patterns; feeding (with special attention to the mother-infant interaction during feeding); pleasure-unpleasure indications and drive development (libido and aggression). We scrutinize progression of ego development (sensorimotor), and especially the state and functioning of the mental apparatus. We look for forerunners of defenses and identification, and we gauge the infant's affective states and responses. We are on the lookout for forerunners of fixation points, tendencies to regression and conflicts (clashes between competing needs). We think that some general characteristics have special prognostic relevance for future pathological and normal development (W. E. Freud, 1971).

Technique of Observation

Observation is, as we know, anything but objective (Anthony, 1968). The student is alerted to such hazards as personal blind spots, scotomization, interference by his own problems and preoccupations, or distortions through prevailing interests.

The observer's written reports on each visit to the family are the *recorded data* (however selected), invaluable not only for discussion and enlightenment in the seminars, but also for scrutiny in later research work and longitudinal studies. They will in any case be needed in connection with making predictions (M. Kris, 1957).

The *understanding of the data* can become a crucial issue, for observer and analyst alike. In both situations it is essential to distinguish clearly between observational material and the observer's understanding of it. As a safeguard against "the neglect of environmental influences and reality" (Greenson, 1974) we aim in our teaching to instill a healthy respect for the difference between "fact" and opinion, or speculation. In the analytic process the patient's free associations provide not only facts but also many links between them. They speak for themselves, and there is usually nothing so convincing to the patient as when one can quote to him the very phrases he used, or in slips of the tongue lets him repeat what he just said.

We stress that many factors are usually involved in any one situation and that comprehension of what has been observed may well remain fragmentary, if not incomplete. We show how easy it is to read into an observation what need not be there. A baby's crying, e.g., may be due to any number of circumstances—hunger, tiredness, pain, heat or cold, or other internal and external discomforts that may remain unrecognized by the observer.[5] Adultomorphizing should always be exposed. A favorite example is that of the mother who proudly told the observer that her 3¾-month-old baby had said her first words, "Daddy is coming," which in Hebrew sounds roughly like "Ababa." The observer

---

[5] It is least likely to be due to feeling "depressed," as has been said in a Kleinian infant observation seminar.

commented: "As far as I could tell Mary was babbling and gurgling and blowing bubbles between her lips, which seemed to give her pleasure."

Another example is that of a father who was convinced that his 3½-month-old daughter looked at him with contempt. Of course, not only parents but observers too may misinterpret what is going on.

While analysts can take their bearings from several directions, e.g., from the continuity of the patient's themes, the contiguity of associations, and the context in which they occur, the observer will have to rely mainly on context as an aid to understanding. More likely than not he will find himself without many vital pieces of information. However, issues can often be decided by turning to the mother for enlightenment (see W. E. Freud, 1971, p. 187f.). How easily even the experts can be baffled is shown by the following example. During a well-baby clinic visit Erna (age 4;9) played "doctor," wearing the toy stethoscope. Each time she put it on she trampled with her feet. One of the staff members asked why a doctor had to "dance." The mother at once explained that Erna was imitating the doctor rushing up the stairs to see another patient.

Desirable Attitudes

A major part of our work, often unobtrusive, is directed toward fostering desirable attitudes in the student, especially those thought to be assets in the later use of analytic technique. Some of them, like refraining from moralizing, criticizing, advice, or guidance, have already been mentioned; others have been touched on in connection with the hazards of interpreting observational data.

We help students who have in previous nonanalytic work with clients developed a zest for "rushing in where angels fear to tread" to become attuned to the slower pace of interaction required in analysis. Analysts are expected to be patient and bide their time. Mother-infant observation can be made a good training ground for this. The seminar discussions of the observers' experiences with mother and baby provide opportunities for consolidating a thoughtful and cautious approach. For example, there usually is a baby that feels decidedly uncuddly when held. The student learns that there just are uncuddly babies and that it would be rash to assume that their development will for this reason be unhealthy. (For other examples, see W. E. Freud and I. Freud, 1974.)

Subtly and almost imperceptibly we try to encourage those attitudes that "should not need to be taught" (Greenson, 1972), i.e., humility and respect for the integrity of the person in our care—here primarily the mother.

Another area in which the seminar can be of help is that of language. The use of scientific and psychoanalytic jargon (sometimes popular with beginners and often inappropriately applied) should be firmly discouraged. On the other hand the student is helped to express difficult terms in everyday language—a process which is in part dependent on a better understanding of the meaning of concepts. The student's cooperation is enlisted by referring to the analytic situation, where the patient's use of jargon or big words alerts us to his camouflaging something else. We point out that the patient gains if his analyst can clearly and concisely communicate with him, especially when it comes to elucidating associative material and to phrasing interpretations. The observational setup itself, in which the student is alone with one other person (counting the breast-feeding mother and baby as one symbiotic unit), is a good preparation for the intimacy of the analytic situation. No opportunity need be missed to relate the observer's activities with those of his future analytic work.

Widening of Awareness

The student will become attuned to "listening with the third ear" (Reik, 1948) to the undertones and overtones of what the mother, or other members of the family, might say or do. The Baby Profile's sections on the Auxiliary Ego (W. E. Freud, 1967, pp. 228–236), which deal with "Assessment of the Mother's *Manifest* Responses to the Baby" and with "Assessment of the Mother's *Latent* Attitudes," exemplify what I have in mind. After a short time the student can work out this Profile section. It clarifies his impressions and deepens his positive cathexis of mother and infant.

Anything in the material that lends itself to illustrating preconscious and unconscious processes can be used as an introduction to psychoanalytic thinking. The student will experience for himself the mother's "forgetting" of visiting times and other parapraxes.

By comparing observations of different babies, he will become aware of the wide range of individual variations and the normality of differing rates of emotional development. Moreover, by observing individual children over a period of time, he will learn about the variations in the infants' behavior constancy and regression rate (E. Kris, 1950).

If the observer can discern a particular pattern in the mother's interaction with her offspring, he may well expect traces of similar reactions to appear in her relationship with himself. For example, Mrs. A. stated that "she did not feel it necessary to adjust her whole life to fit in with a baby's needs" (age 11 weeks). One week later she said in a somewhat resigned and frustrated tone of voice that the baby was very unpredictable—"he sleeps from seven to thirteen hours at night and takes his feeds in a variable manner as well." This mother, who disliked feeling pinned down, had gone out shopping on the observer's first visit, and had taken the baby "for a walk" and let the observer wait for 15 minutes on the third visit.

When different impressions are compared, it soon becomes obvious that the relationship between an individual mother and her observer is unique, just as the relationship between an individual mother and her baby is unique. Similarly, we point out, each analyst's relationship with any one patient will differ from that with any other.

We try to broaden the student's outlook in yet another direction by trying to make him aware of the child's view of the world, which differs through being limited by phase-adequate understanding (Freud, 1908). For example, Judy (13 weeks) had cried and struggled when fed with the spoon. "Twice when she was yelling, Katie (her 1-year-10-months-old sister) came and inspected her anxiously. The mother's opinion was that Katie was bothered by Judy's messiness." It was a time when the older girl was already using the pot and had achieved some control of her own messiness. She may have thought the baby was crying out of distress over having been messy. Equally age-adequately, she may have wondered what the mother was aggressively doing to Judy to make her cry.

Concepts

It would be interesting to know how many concepts commonly used in child development are also used in psychoanalysis. Observations of mother, infant, and sibling seem to provide, inter alia, most of what is needed in psychoanalytic theory, practice, and research. The question is to what extent concepts should be taught systematically, e.g., from the writings of Freud (Nagera, 1969a, 1969b, 1970a, 1970b), or developmentally, say, around the developmental lines (A. Freud, 1963a), in connection with diagnostic conferences (A. Freud, 1962), or ad hoc from clinical material as it presents itself in infant observation.

We found it most rewarding to clarify concepts as they presented themselves through the students' observations, taking into account their special interests, with the seminar leader at the helm to direct attention to anything of special relevance. The early physiological manifestations will facilitate introduction to specific topics, e.g., *somatic channels of tension discharge*, from which we can proceed to the developmental line "from physical to mental pathways of discharge"; *somatic compliance*, when later use is made of somatic channels for psychosomatic and conversion phenomena (A. Freud, 1974). Related topics are *spread of excitation* and *equipotentiality of intake channels*, e.g., looking, grasping, feeding (W. E. Freud and Nagera, 1968).

The following example illustrates *body memory:* "When she sucks her thumb, Nancy (1;10) strokes her upper lip with one of her fingers of the same hand." This was understood as a body memory, whereby she re-created the early comfort of the feeding situation when the areola of her mother's breast touched her lips. The meaning of the gesture probably was: It was so nice to be a baby. (What a pity the analyst cannot see what exactly a patient's hand is doing when it is near his mouth.)

When mouth-hand-ego integration and activity related to the development of the body ego (e.g., long alternating sequences of touching the body and touching the side of the cot) are observed, we refer to Hoffer's papers (1949, 1950). Comments on the *affective climate* may lead to discussion of the *coenesthetic* mode of functioning (Spitz, 1945)—"Any animal knows as a matter of course when somebody is afraid of him, and acts without hesitation on this knowledge" (Spitz, 1965, p. 136f.)—and thence to *empathy*. As an example of a mother's empathy, I cite the following observation: "As last week, the mother makes mouth movements unconsciously while spoon-feeding solids to her 3-month-old baby boy." The next example illustrates mutual empathy between mother and child. "Mrs. T., who seems very identified with her baby daughter and who is known to have separation problems herself, found that the baby's sleep pattern was disturbed whenever she left the house in a prearranged manner. When, by contrast, she followed the infant's rhythm, made no plans, and went out on the spur of the moment, then the baby did not become upset." (While such examples may well be regarded as inconclusive, they nevertheless point in a certain direction.)

Observations of an older sibling are often most rewarding. For example, "Without asking if she wanted to use the potty, the mother presented Emmy (nearly 2;4) with the potty and put her on it. Emmy sat on the potty at the end of the room far from the television. The news was on and Emmy demanded that the station be changed. Mrs. D. changed the station. Then Emmy said that the volume should be lowered. Mrs. D. lowered the volume. Emmy peed in the potty and when Mrs. D. asked her if she was finished, she said, 'No.' Mrs. D. replied that she really thought Emmy had nothing more to do. Emmy continued to dictate orders from her seat on the potty." No one who has witnessed such scenes and discussed their implications is likely to doubt that struggles over *control* have their strongest roots in the *anal phase*. We are entitled to skepticism when, in connection with diagnostic inquiries, a mother tells us that "Toilet training was uneventful."

Some of the concepts are introduced most strikingly via the mother, e.g., *ambivalence* (the mother who confesses to the observer that when she left the pram outside the store, it had also occurred to her that someone might snatch the baby). *Conflicts,* especially over weaning or going back to work, are commonplace. Infant observation graphically illustrates not only the ebb and flow of ongoing development (e.g., the inevitable *regression* of an older sibling in connection with the existence of the baby—A. Freud, 1963b) but also well-established concepts, like *sibling rivalry* and openly expressed *aggression* to the baby, especially when the latter is fed by the mother in the sibling's presence. Sometimes an older girl's *penis envy* of the baby brother can be observed.

The importance of actually experiencing what is taught probably makes itself felt more in the area of learning concepts than elsewhere. It is in line with the value many analytic authors put on the "experiential" (Fleming and Benedek, 1966), and we share the view that education is the accumulation of experience, rather than facts (Welbourn, 1966).

Defenses

Among the concepts, the defenses (A. Freud, 1936) have a special place in our esteem, not least because we would like to contradict the widely held belief that they are signs of abnormality and have (like warts) to be removed—in this case by analysis. Our main task is to show how indispensable they are for normal development and maintenance of mental functioning.

At any one time our observational setup may offer the student a three-tier opportunity to become conversant with defenses:

1. In the baby he can discern the first "primitive reactions to unpleasure" (incidentally, still the best operational definition) which "suggest or foreshadow the kind of defense he is likely to adopt in the future" in terms of protest, avoidance, withdrawal, regression, somatization (W. E. Freud, 1971, p. 189). Whenever we are dealing with forerunners, there is always the possibility of new discoveries[6] and from then on the student's enthusiasm leads to spotting more defenses as they abound on the other two levels.

2. In the slightly older sibling a preponderance of primitive archaic defenses can be seen: those closer to positive ego consolida

---

[6] The whole question of chronology of defenses received new impetus from Anna Freud's (1974) suggestion to look closer at their connection with the developmental lines.

tion, like imitation, introjection, and identification, as well as others, like projection and denial. Children often deny what is unpleasant by creeping under the bedclothes and stuffing their fingers into their ears (A. Freud and Burlingham, 1939–1945, p. 320). Others may avoid unpleasure by withdrawal into sleep. As ego building proceeds, so does sophistication of defenses.

As long as our orientation is anchored around the *pleasure principle* and the mechanisms are seen in terms of defensive maneuvers against *unpleasure*, it should be easy to understand how, in the process of coping with anxieties, more and more aspects of ego activity can become involved in defensive activity. Freud's (1920) vivid example of *passive into active* (the game of the 1½-year-old boy who made his mother disappear and return), and the eagerness with which young infants enter into peekaboo games around the time of weaning (or initiate them) bear this out.

3. In the adult members of the family the student may guess at some defenses almost from the start. For example, on his second visit the (American) observer met the father and "though we got along well, he perhaps exposed some of his feelings about observers when he stated that American foreign policy sticks its nose in the business of the other countries of the world. This comment was made during a brief discussion of President Nixon." (This suggests displacement.)

Of special interest to us are those childhood theories that mothers invent, as *rationalizations*, in order to cope better with conflicts over weaning, going back to work, or gaining greater independence. For example, "Mrs. K. noted that Tom (7 months) did not like her to go out of the room and leave him alone. She said he did not need the physical contact with her, but just likes 'having me around.' She does not seem too pleased about this, but will nevertheless stay with him." Two weeks later she commented on a friend who had gone away for a fortnight, leaving her 6-month-old child in the care of a nanny. When the mother came back the child smiled in recognition, but when she later went out on an errand the baby wept inconsolably. "Mrs. K. was surprised because she would not have expected such a young child to know the difference between the mother and other adults. Her next remark was to tell me that Tom will now let her leave the room and will play happily on his own for quite a long while." (For another example, see W. E. Freud, 1967, p. 224.)

It is instructive to clarify, whenever possible, what kind of unpleasure is defended against and to ponder about the extent to which defenses are dependent on the object world or, corresponding to the state of superego development, independent of it. Though fortuitous, some acquaintance with defenses nevertheless provides an introduction to what will later be encountered in analytic technique, where the "resistances are repetitions of all the defensive operations that the patient has used in his past life" (Greenson, 1967, p. 36).

Technique

The interaction between observer and observed is basically different from that between analyst and patient. Although similarities exist, they are approximations and no more than foreshadow technique. We can prepare the student observer in several ways:

1. As already mentioned in the briefing, the observer has to be sparing in giving information about himself, even if he need not aspire, like the analyst, to "be opaque to his patients and, like a mirror, . . . show them nothing but what is shown to him" (Freud, 1912, p. 118). If he introduces foreign matter into the situation, he will "muddy the water" and unnecessarily complicate his task.

2. He is taught to expect—either in the mother, or in the material—reactions to any moves on his part, like being early or late, cancellations of visits, or interruptions during holidays. As in analysis, he is advised to prepare the mother for any changes in advance, especially for the final separation.

3. The advantages of waiting can be recommended by illustrating the disadvantages of inept intervention, i.e., when an observation is unwittingly aborted. "The mother went to get a cup of tea. The baby (3 weeks), who had been lying quietly in his cot, started whimpering; so I picked him up and rubbed his back. He quietened down and I put him back after the mother came back with the tea." We pointed out that the situation was not an emergency, and that it might have been instructive to wait for the mother's reaction to the infant's signals of discomfort.

Although it has been said that *countertransference* manifestations can be discerned in the observer, we feel that problems of countertransference are best left within the province of the student's personal analysis, where, after all, most of the work toward preparing him will have to be done.

Conclusion

1. If infant observation is such a versatile, meaningful, and directly relevant teaching tool, why do many training centers not use it at all? Why was it not made a requirement for all training courses long ago? Our impression is that, apart from those directly concerned, few are aware of what is involved. One purpose of this paper was to show what it is all about.

2. Is it possible in the available teaching time to do justice to the students' observations, reports, the knowledge of child development, the links with analysis and the relevant literature? The amount of attention given to each will vary with the seminar leader's predilections, but within the framework of psychoanalytic training the overriding objective and commitment are to initiate the student into the world of analysis. This orientation will have to be reflected on all levels, from the briefing onward, so that perforce we will often find ourselves discussing analysis rather than infant development. Clinical aspects have priority over theoretical ones; as in analysis, it may therefore be best to follow the main theme as it develops, branching out whenever required. The literature can often no more than be touched upon and the student directed to sources. Additionally, seminar leader and students contribute from their own specialized knowledge and reading.

3. When and how do observations end? The student's cathexis of the family and of his observational activities increases as the baby develops and as his acquaintance with analytic implications deepens. All along he is encouraged to formulate and record his impressions through making retrospective and prospective evaluations and predictions. This activity serves to impress on him how difficult it is to predict with accuracy in early infancy, while on the other hand it bolsters his confidence in what he has, from prognostic pointers, intuitively grasped. Yet, no sooner has he acquired a taste

for the longitudinal view than his observations come to an end with the end of the first academic year. Family and observer have to decathect each other, and the small student group in which he began his training is absorbed into bigger ones. Other areas of the curriculum become more important, little time is left for follow-up visits, and further pursuit of observations lacks support and incentive. Are we not throwing away unique opportunities by letting this kind of clinical experience lapse too soon? We suggest that it is as essential to acquire experience of normal development against which later analytic reconstructions can be checked (A. Freud, 1951), as it is to acquire experience of childhood disturbances that may facilitate neuroses.

On the theoretical side infant observation has, in the widest sense, made a major contribution by adding the developmental point of view, which permits us to look at processes in their forward move to learn more about how each step in the infant's experiences serves as a foothold and basis for the following ones. It is the indispensable complement to the genetic point of view, by which phenomena are pursued back to their origins. Only by using the two together can we hope to improve our understanding of normal and abnormal manifestations (A. Freud, 1965).

Since more extensive and intensive observation is clearly needed, I cannot help wondering whether the time has not come for a radical reappraisal of existing teaching programs.

It should not be beyond the ingenuity of training committees to design a psychoanalytic curriculum that is based on longitudinal clinical experience at the center, with theoretical teaching built around it. The student would then follow a baby's development from the antenatal clinic to latency, or beyond (through follow-ups). Apart from his observations in the family's home, he would spend time observing in a maternity hospital, well-baby clinic, mother-toddler group, nursery school, and perhaps school. The program would be integrated with experience of adolescents, participation in a diagnostic unit, and the training in child and adult analysis. It would make for a more cohesive and rounded-off learning experience.

Whoever thinks that it would take an unduly long time should reflect that at present (at least for graduates of the Hampstead

Child-Therapy Course) a combined child-adult training also takes six years.

SUMMARY

Mother-infant observation is presented as a meaningful and versatile tool directly relevant to the teaching of psychoanalysis. It serves to prepare the candidate for successive stages of his psychoanalytic training. Some of the differences, as well as parallels, between direct observation and observation in the analytic situation are pointed out and discussed.

The question is posed whether the time has not come for a radical reappraisal of existing curricula: most institutes provide a genetic view of infantile life, based on analytic reconstruction through following mental processes back to their origins. Observing ongoing progressive development would seem the ideal complement. It is suggested that training be organized around a central experience of intensive longitudinal studies of the first four to six years of the child's life.

BIBLIOGRAPHY

ANTHONY, E. J. (1968), On Observing Children. In: *Foundations of Child Psychiatry*, ed. E. Miller. Oxford: Pergamon Press, pp. 71–123.
BEISER, H. R. (1973), Can the Psychology of Childhood Be Taught to Students of Psychoanalysis? *J. Amer. Psychoanal. Assn.*, 21:727–744.
BICK, E. (1964), Notes on Infant Observation in Psycho-Analytic Training, *Int. J. Psycho-Anal.*, 45:558–566.
BRITISH PSYCHO-ANALYTICAL SOCIETY AND INSTITUTE OF PSYCHO-ANALYSIS (Session 1973/74), *Training Prospectus*. London: 63, New Cavendish Street, W1M 7RD.
FLEMING, J. & BENEDEK, T. (1966), *Psychoanalytic Supervision*. New York & London: Grune & Stratton, pp. 20–34.
FREUD, A. (1936), *The Ego and the Mechanisms of Defence*. London: Hogarth Press, 1968.
——— (1951), Observations on Child Development. *This Annual*, 6:18–30.
——— (1957), The Contribution of Direct Child Observation to Psychoanalysis. *Writings*, 5:95–101.
——— (1962), Assessment of Childhood Disturbances. *This Annual*, 17:149–158.
——— (1963a), The Concept of Developmental Lines. *This Annual*, 18:245–265.
——— (1963b), The Role of Regression in Mental Development. *Writings*, 5:407–418.

——— (1965), *Normality and Pathology in Childhood*. New York: Int. Univ. Press.
——— (1966), The Ideal Psychoanalytic Institute. *Writings*, 7:73–93.
——— (1970), Child Analysis As a Subspecialty of Psychoanalysis. *Writings*, 7:204–219.
——— (1974), A Psychoanalytic View of Developmental Psychopathology. *J. Philadelphia Assn. Psychoanal.*, 1:7–17.
——— & BURLINGHAM, D. (1939–1945), Infants Without Families: Reports on the Hampstead Nurseries. *Writings*, 3.
FREUD, S. (1908), On the Sexual Theories of Children. *S.E.*, 9:205–226.
——— (1910), 'Wild' Psycho-Analysis. *S.E.*, 11:219–227.
——— (1912), Recommendations to Physicians Practising Psycho-Analysis. *S.E.*, 12:109–120.
——— (1913), On Beginning the Treatment. *S.E.*, 12:121–144.
——— (1920), Beyond the Pleasure Principle, *S.E.*, 18:7–64.
——— (1937), Constructions in Analysis. *S.E.*, 23:255–269.
FREUD, W. E. (1967), Assessment of Early Infancy. *This Annual*, 22:216–238.
——— (1971), The Baby Profile. *This Annual*, 26:172–194.
——— & FREUD, I. (1974), Die Well-Baby Klinik. In: *Jahrbuch der Psychohygiene*, ed. G. Biermann. München/Basel: Ernst Reinhardt Verlag, Vol. 2, pp. 119–137.
——— & NAGERA, H. (1968), Range of Ego Modalities in a Case of Overeating (unpublished).
GREENSON, R. R. (1967), *The Technique and Practice of Psychoanalysis*, New York: Int. Univ. Press.
——— (1972), Beyond Transference and Interpretation. *Int. J. Psycho-Anal.*, 53:213–217.
——— (1974), Transference: Freud or Klein. *Int. J. Psycho-Anal.*, 55:37–48.
HOFFER, W. (1949), Mouth, Hand and Ego-Integration. *This Annual*, 3/4:49–56.
——— (1950), Development of the Body Ego. *This Annual*, 5:18–23.
KENNEDY, H. (1971), Problems in Reconstruction in Child Analysis. *This Annual*, 26:386–402.
KRIS, E. (1950), Notes on the Development and on Some Current Problems of Psychoanalytic Child Psychology. *This Annual*, 5:24–46.
——— (1956), The Recovery of Childhood Memories in Psychoanalysis. *This Annual*, 11:54–88.
KRIS, M. (1957), The Use of Prediction in a Longitudinal Study. *This Annual*, 12:175–189.
MITSCHERLICH-NIELSEN, M. (1970), Was macht einen guten Analytiker aus? *Psyche*, 24:577–599.
NAGERA, H., Editor (1969a), *Basic Psychoanalytic Concepts on the Libido Theory*. London: Allen & Unwin.
——— (1969b), *Basic Psychoanalytic Concepts on the Theory of Dreams*. London: Allen & Unwin.
——— (1970a), *Basic Psychoanalytic Concepts on the Theory of Instincts*. London; Allen & Unwin.

——— (1970b), *Basic Psychoanalytic Concepts on Metapsychology, Conflicts, Anxiety and Other Subjects*. London: Allen & Unwin.

REIK, T. (1948), *Listening with the Third Ear*. New York: Farrar, Straus.

SPITZ, R. A. (1945), Diacritic and Coenesthetic Organizations. *Psychoanal. Rev.*, 32:146–162.

——— (1950), Relevancy of Direct Infant Observation. *This Annual*, 5:66–73.

——— (1965), *The First Year of Life*. New York: Int. Univ. Press.

WELBOURN, R. B. (1966), The Training and Education of a Surgeon. *Proc. Roy. Soc. Med.*, 59:934–936.

Language Deficits in Children with Developmental Lags

KATRINA DE HIRSCH, F.C.S.T.

AS REMEDIAL THERAPISTS WORKING WITH CHILDREN WHO PRESENT difficulties with spoken, printed, and written language we are in an ambiguous position. We are not in the usual sense educators. We certainly are not psychotherapists. The children referred for language and learning difficulties frequently come with a file of reports from specialists which lend themselves to very different interpretations.

Consider the reports from the teacher, the neurologist, and the psychiatrist on a fifth grade boy referred to us for remediation. The teacher states that the boy reads two and a half years below the class average, that his spelling is bizarre, and that he absolutely refuses to write a composition. His marks in math are not impressive either. She describes the boy as an underachiever in terms of his high intellectual potential. His performance is curiously uneven. By now he is so discouraged that he can hardly bear to try. Perhaps he is just lazy.

The neurologist writes that this boy's prenatal, natal, and postnatal history is ambiguous. He was a little late passing developmental milestones. He did not use phrases until the age of 33 months. He has always been moderately hyperactive. The EEG is negative, as is the classical neurological examination, except for mild cerebellar signs which might or might not be significant. At

---

Consultant in Language Disorders, N.Y. State Psychiatric Institute; Consultant to the Robinson Reading Clinic, Columbia Presbyterian Medical Center, New York.

any rate, his coordination is poor, not so much for large muscle activities as for graphomotor skills, to wit, his atrocious handwriting. He appears to suffer from a learning disability (which is the reason he was referred in the first place) probably on the basis of minimal brain injury.

The psychiatrist believes that as a result of neurotic conflict the boy presents an arrest in ego development and has insufficient psychic energy available for academic requirements. Punitive handling has complicated the situation.

The parents are confused, angry, and guilty. The child's failure is experienced by them as a severe narcissistic blow.

All of these diagnostic labels—underachievement, learning disability, minimal brain injury, arrested ego development—have some essential validity. None of them, however, takes into account the complex interactions between physiological and psychological aspects of functioning, interactions which in turn are crucially affected by the emotional climate of the child's home.

I shall attempt in the following pages to discuss some of the characteristics of a number of children referred to clinics and offices with a variety of dysfunctions that escape precise classification. Many of these youngsters present atypical developmental patterns that are reflected not only in perceptuomotor deficits but above all in failure to master receptive and expressive aspects of language that require a high level of central integration. Among such children I have singled out two groups whose maturational delays and imbalances are fairly striking.

In view of the reciprocal relationship between language and developing ego functions, the question is raised what linguistic deficits mean in terms of children's psychic structure.

The problem of labeling and its implication for referral and therapy is taken up. Two cases are briefly discussed because in spite of similar physiological deficits, they did well with different kinds of management.

Description of the Children

The children whom I shall describe, rather than discuss in terms of labels, range from 2 to 18 years. The severity of their dysfunction extends from mild to severe. Some are in need of assistance at the preschool level. The difficulties of others do not become evident until they are faced with academic demands. Their difficulties are recognized relatively late because the children did not appear to be atypical, at least at first glance.

Nevertheless, these children *are* different. They present varying degrees of perceptuomotor deficits, uneven development, inconsistency of response, lability of affect, and little resistance to the normal stress and strain of growing up. They are vulnerable children. They exhibit symptoms singly or in a variety of combinations: irritability, poorly established early sleep and feeding rhythm, the disorganized and global motility typical for younger subjects, occasionally severe disorders of body schema and praxis, motor clumsiness, primitive perceptual and visuomotor experiences, fluctuations in attention, and a lowered threshold for anxiety. They have trouble with organizing and integrating experiences into cohesive wholes. The management and patterning of all kinds of information—perceptual, linguistic, and conceptual—present difficulties.

These children show no evidence of a circumscribed cerebral insult of the kind found in individuals who have suffered the loss of a previously established function. They do not present positive signs on the classical neurological examinations and the EEG. Nor do they suffer from significant sensory deficits or marked intellectual impairment.[1] Their difficulties are less gross. Ajurriaguerra (1966) points out that the effects of even subtle interference with central integrative processes are less drastic but far more global in younger than in older individuals. The less differentiated and the more plastic the organism, the more diffuse and more generalized are the symptoms (and at the same time the greater is the potential for compensatory adjustments). Whatever may have happened to the central nervous system of these children (and I specifically exclude children with verifiable brain injury, for example, epileptic children, etc.) happened to a system in the process of formation and can be assumed to have interfered with maturation and integration in

---

[1] These children are often called "organic." The concept, according to Clements (1973), has been broadened of late to include a wide spectrum of dysfunctions, sometimes based on genetic variations.

many areas and on many levels of physiological and psychological functioning.

The more complex a function the more vulnerable it is. Language is a highly differentiated function; it is thus not surprising that we find linguistic deficits frequently in conjunction with other disturbances. Early linguistic difficulties are red flags in terms of subsequent academic failure. Even more significantly, they interfere from the very earliest age with developing ego functions that are essential for learning and for the child's total adaptation to his world.

Language comprehension requires ability to process intricately patterned inputs. Our children have difficulty breaking up the totality of a pattern and to synthesize parts into wholes. Their perceptual organization is diffuse. How do these babies, who have trouble analyzing and structuring patterns, make sense out of the buzzing confusion in which they are embedded? How do they detect the inherent regularities in the swiftly flowing stream of speech? [2]

Normal babies begin very early to respond selectively to many linguistic events (Friedlander, 1970). Seemingly passive infants apparently do an enormous amount of discriminative listening.

Lewis (1963) describes how children learn to understand language. They first respond to the intonational features which carry the emotional load of communication and are an integral part of the mother's affectively colored caretaking activities. Very slowly, phonemic patterns become intertwined with situational and intonational features until, very gradually, as further differentiation takes place, phonemic patterns become dominant relatively independent of the situation.

The mother's ongoing vocal and verbal exchange with her baby differs from her communication with older children and with adults in rate, rhythm, and dynamic accent. It provides the matrix from which spring early communicative attitudes as well as the enjoyment in verbal give-and-take, which is essential for language acquisition and later learning. The mother caresses the baby with

---

[2] The discussion of the crucially important communicative, interpersonal aspect of language is beyond the scope of this paper.

her voice; she tailors her own utterances to his specific developmental needs; she endlessly repeats sounds, words, and phrases, thus providing him with the data that allow him to detect and to organize the recurring intonational and phonemic signals into more or less stable categories. Wyatt (1969) describes this interaction as a mutual feedback based on unconscious identification. Piaget (1923) calls it "contagion verbale."

Language develops in the matrix of a close mother-child bond. There are mothers who do not "tune in," who either fail to provide carefully dosed stimulation and feedback or who swamp the baby with their verbalizations, thus failing to make him aware of the crucial features of input.

The children I am discussing may fail to take advantage of the cues provided by the mother. They may not stimulate her to engage in vocal and verbal play. As a result, those children who need stimulation most usually get least. Some of them may not even separate out speech from the background of noise. They may experience speech as a diffuse undifferentiated flow. At 18 months when normal children begin to discover phoneme and word boundaries, these children are bathed in a sea of sounds and do not grasp the underlying schemata.

By the age of 3 or 4, normal children are quite familiar with the small connective words, the number, space and time markers that provide a net of relations and are the framework for the organization of experience. The child who lacks understanding of such words lives in a confusing universe—and this confusion may in turn interfere with the organization of his inner and outer cosmos. He is limited to the Here and Now. His world has few shades and few signposts.

The child who is unable to deduce from the incoming messages the phonemic and syntactical rules underlying the surface structure of language tends to tune out. He has learned *not to listen*. Difficulties with processing input and withdrawal into fantasies interact. Missing the more subtle aspects of communication, the child finds the pull of fantasies more compelling, and invests less and less in listening except when the message is highly cathected and verbalizations are relatively short.

Kagan et al. (1960) point out that certain children fail to acquire the set of symbols that would allow them to conceptualize important aspects of their experience. The acquisition of these symbols, however, depends on adequate interpretation, and in order to conceptualize experience the child must understand the grammatical structures that provide him with linguistic options.

Both receptive and expressive language represent intricate structures. It is precisely with the structuring of perceptuomotor, affective, linguistic, and conceptual configurations that our children have the greatest difficulty. Such difficulty with structuring is typical for delayed or disordered development. Development, according to Werner (1957), proceeds from relative globality and lack of differentiation in the direction of increasing articulation and hierarchic organization. Successive stages of development are characterized by the emergence of new forms of organization and novel structures of increasing complexity. The performance of the children we work with could therefore be expected to be more primitive, more global, and less differentiated than that of children whose developmental course runs more smoothly.

Among the numerous children who present maturational delays I have picked out two subgroups—prematurely born and educationally unready children—because their maturational lags and imbalances in all areas of functioning appeared to be striking.

PREMATURELY BORN CHILDREN

In the course of a reading prediction study (de Hirsch et al., 1966a, 1966b) we had an opportunity to investigate 53 children born before term with birthweights ranging from 2,240 grams to 980 grams. By comparing these children with a control group, we hoped to learn something about maturational deficits. Children born before term are by definition immature at birth, and there is some evidence that some of this immaturity may persist for varying periods of time.

We excluded those children who had been diagnosed as brain-injured, whose IQs fell a standard deviation below or above the norm, who showed sensory deficits, and who, on psychiatric evaluation, presented symptoms of psychopathology.

We saw the children two or three times between the ages of $5\frac{1}{2}$

and 8. While there were considerable differences among them, I could, without prior information, distinguish most of the prematurely born from those born at term—which suggests that the prematures had certain characteristics in common. I would say that I recognized them because they somehow looked "unfinished" and "immersed."

With regard to those features that were treated statistically; one aspect measured was motility patterning. The prematurely born children hopped across the room—if indeed they were able to hop—like 4-year-olds. Their entire body was involved. Differences in motility patterning between prematures and controls were statistically significant in the direction of greater globality in the case of the prematures. Some of them were hypoactive and tended to slump. Most others were entirely at the mercy of a thousand environmental stimuli.

Their visuomotor gestalts were both primitive and fluid and only rough approximations of the designs to be copied. They flowed into each other and were rotated in space. In the visuomotor area differences between prematures and controls also reached statistical significance. The children's ability to imitate tapped-out patterns—to respond to auditory gestalts—and to reproduce them was inferior.

As a group the prematurely born brought to mind Bender's observations on "primitive plasticity" (1966).[3] One could say that their maturational status resembled that of younger children. At kindergarten age those born at term surpassed the prematures in 36 out of 37 tasks. On 15 tasks the differences were significant statistically. Among the 15, 11 were verbal tasks. Recognition of words heard, language comprehension, word-finding, story organization, and ability to categorize were all significantly poorer in the prematures than in controls. It is of interest that in no single oral language dimension were the prematures superior. Differences in favor of controls were overwhelming on the so-called prereading tasks.

---

[3] Bender uses the term "plasticity" the way embryologists use it: "as yet unformed but capable of being formed"; and she uses it primarily for schizophrenic children. See also de Hirsch (1965).

Twenty-eight months later, the performance of the prematurely born children in reading, writing, and spelling—all of which require a high level of neurological integration—was poorer than that of controls.[4] Statistically treated aspects of this study thus demonstrated that, at least at kindergarten age, many of the prematurely born children represented a "high risk" group in terms of subsequent academic achievement.

Notes added to the children's protocols and an inspection of their individual profiles conveyed a clinical impression of each child's style as a learner. They showed that certain features were common to virtually all the prematurely born children. Clinically, they struck us as disoriented in time and space and as if they did not know how they fitted into the scheme of things. It is of interest that the 16 prematurely born children in Caplan's study (1963) showed identical problems with spatial and temporal categories.

The human figure drawings of our group were bizarre only in a few instances. However, they were crude—stick figures mostly—and they did not look as if they were anchored down. Many were slanted on the page and others seemed to float in space. The premature likewise had trouble remembering the dates of their birthdays, identifying the times of day, recalling past events.

Disorientation in space and time is characteristically found in

[4] In a study of the interplay of prematurity, intrafamily dynamics, and "idiogenic" cognitive organization, Caplan et al. (1963) found a preponderance of cognitive disorders in the prematures as compared to controls. In their sample of 16 subjects the differences between the two groups were even greater at ages 11 to 12 than they had been between the ages of 6 and 7.

The discussion of the relationship between cognitive and linguistic dimensions has gone on for generations and cannot possibly be reviewed here. It is well known that language stabilizes perception and also serves as a mediator for nonverbal performances (Luria, 1961). Verbal children talk themselves through a puzzle (this is how subjects with good linguistic endowment compensate for perceptual deficits). Language makes possible operations such as categorization and serializing. It allows the individual to determine the common property of things and to group them into larger entities, thereby facilitating the shift from associative to cognitive levels of operations. Thus, what Caplan calls "cognitive disorders" in his premature population may be closely related to linguistic deficits especially at higher age levels when the two tend to fuse (Vygotsky, 1962). See also Scholnick and Adams (1973).

children presenting disorders of spoken and printed language. Difficulty with sequencing and serial-order manipulations are frequently seen in dyslexic youngsters.

Disorientation in time has, however, other important implications. The pleasure principle operates *now*. The reality principle demands submission to time. Children have difficulty relinquishing immediate gratification until they have acquired some comprehension of the linguistic structures that denote temporal relationships. In dysphasic children, one observes that their capacity to wait grows with their increasing understanding of linguistic forms that represent the future. Their anxiety decreases. Pain does not last forever, mother will return *soon*. Time concepts and academic performance are closely related. Work requires postponing of gratification in the service of a distant goal.[5]

The prematures' approach to the examiner and the testing situation differed from that of the children born at term. Separation was much harder for the prematures. "Infantile" was the most frequently mentioned term in their protocols. Some had to be taken on the examiner's lap to enable them to get through the testing. They needed massive support and demonstrated little autonomy. Their need for oral gratification was enormous; they devoured masses of candy during testing sessions.

The premature children's ego organization appeared to be loose and fragmented. We were impressed with the ebb and flow of their attention. More than full-term children, they moved in and out of focus. The level of their performance fluctuated. This variability may have resulted from the children's difficulties sustaining psychic energy for longer periods of time, but one also felt that smooth managing of inputs presented difficulties, that some of the children's basic perceptual experiences were unstable, and that their frame of reference tended to shift from one moment to the next.

Their anxiety—Greenacre (1941) described its organic stamp—

---

[5] Leshan (1952) found time orientation to vary with social class, perhaps because so many deprived individuals have no future, literally or figuratively. There is little incentive to work for uncertain rewards. Goal orientation and a stake in achievement are closely linked to the ordering of life in terms of sequencing. Some groups do not experience life in these terms.

appeared to be diffuse and amorphous. One cannot but feel that their poorly patterned, primitive, perceptual experiences were contributory factors (see also Kurlander and Colodny, 1965).

Many of the prematures impressed one as dependent, passive, and shadowy. They appeared to be immersed in fantasies to a point where they were unable to invest in age-appropriate tasks. I do not want to give the impression that all of our prematures were handicapped; there were some vigorous and lively children among them, who had considerable ego strength,[6] but they stood out in the group. And they did not necessarily do well on testing. They were still wedded to the pleasure principle and unable to mobilize their plentiful energy in the service of tasks that were unrelated to their drives. And among the 53 prematures there were, of course, a few who managed very adequately and did not present a significant developmental delay.

It would be a gross simplification to ascribe the relatively poor performance of the prematurely born children solely to the factors just described—to their deficits in the primary ego apparatus, their trouble with early homeostasis, and their lack of power over their bodies and the environment. Surely, the profound anxiety and sometimes despair aroused in mothers by premature birth, the prohibition against the handling and fondling of these babies, the worry over their slow early development (Kaplan and Mason, 1960), the guilt feelings because such children are often unwanted, must of necessity have interfered with the mothers' handling of their infants. Psychiatric help enabled some mothers to respond both to the children's legitimate needs for protracted infantilization and to their emerging readiness for autonomy. The prematures' difficulties were inextricably bound up with their mothers' anxiety, which flowed over to these children, thus constituting a configuration in which it was difficult to tease apart crucial environmental, physiological, and psychological determinants.

It is therefore of interest to look at a second subgroup of children whose history is not burdened by their mothers' intense anxiety but who nevertheless show a similar clinical picture.

---

[6] Ratings of ego strength were based on the independent judgment of three observers. We found statistically significant differences between the prematurely born children and controls in favor of the latter.

EDUCATIONALLY UNREADY CHILDREN

Large numbers of 5½- to 7-year-old children are referred to us because of questionable readiness for first grade entrance. This is, of course, a preselected group. However, in the course of a second predictive investigation (Jansky and de Hirsch, 1972) we found among 400 randomly selected kindergarten pupils a fairly well circumscribed group whose test performance reflected a high risk of failure in the elementary grades. These children came from a variety of socioeconomic backgrounds; their IQs ranged from high to low.

The early development of educationally unready children does not necessarily present marked deviations. The majority are boys, and many of them are small in size. Bentzen (1963) believes that learning problems in boys may be the response of the immature organism to the demands of a society that fails to make appropriate provision for the biological age difference between boys and girls. Tanner (1961) found that around the age of 6, males lag 12 months behind females in skeletal age. Some are very bright; Ilg and Ames (1965) call them the "superior immatures." They retain some of the global responses previously described as characteristic of prematurely born children. They frequently turn the whole head, for instance, when asked to flex the tongue. They have an inordinate need for motor outlets. They are distractable and cannot stick to a task for longer than 10 minutes at a time. Their frustration threshold is low.

Laterality is often ambiguous.[7] Auditory perceptions are not

---

[7] In neither of the two predictive studies (1966 and 1972) was ill-defined laterality at this early age predictive for subsequent reading disorders. Identical symptoms mean different things at different ages. A 10-year-old who switches hands during writing would be suspected of central nervous system irregularity because by this age certain functions should be locked into place. McFie's research (1952) suggests that in children with reading disabilities, the neurological organization corresponding to dominance is not normally established in either hemisphere. Subirana (1961) has found that the EEGs of strongly lateralized children are more mature than those of others. This does not exclude the significance of genetic factors.

sharply defined.[8] They are poor listeners.[9] They do not follow the line of a simple story; they do not suggest alternate solutions. Some appear to be so preoccupied with the psychosexual conflicts typical of this particular age that they cannot listen to directions. Others simply have trouble interpreting all but the most primitive grammatical constructions. They cannot sort out, for instance, the difference between "the dog chases the boy" and "the boy chases the dog," or the difference between "mother's cats" and "mother cat." Their kindergarten teacher may complain about their trouble following directions. Visual verbal forms also are unstable. Letters such as *p* and *q* appear to pivot. Directionality continues to be an arbitrary matter. "Tap" and "pat" look more or less alike. Indeed, in some cases, ground and figure are not sharply differentiated. When presented with the word-matching section of the Gates Reading Readiness Test, one 6-year-old told me angrily: "It's just a jumble, it looks like ants crawling around the page." While this was, of course, a phobic response, it also reflected the child's inability to structure and organize the printed configurations on the page into some kind of pattern.

Some of these children learn to compensate for their earlier plasticity. With the help of conceptual and contextual clues they become good readers. (Ability to compensate depends largely on cognitive endowment, ego strength, and environmental support.) The overwhelming majority, however, are "stuck" with often severe spelling disorders. They do not remember the overall gestalt of the word, or its internal design. They have little "physiognomic" ability. Words never become familiar or stable enough for recall. The children may do relatively well on a spelling list, but fail to reproduce correctly the identical words when they are embedded in a sentence. They are unable to maintain a linguistic gestalt

---

[8] In speaking of auditory and visual perceptions in this context, I mean *verbal* auditory and visual perceptions. Many of the children described here have no trouble distinguishing between shades of sounds in the environment and do very well with discrimination among shapes and forms.

[9] During the course of development children become sensitive to successively different aspects of their environment. At age 4 and 5 the "critical" time for learning to listen may have passed.

(French, 1953) even when ego functions are relatively unimpaired.

Dysnomia (word-finding difficulty) is frequently seen among educationally unready children. They can match colors, but cannot name them. They forget the names of favorite characters on their TV programs. These are the same youngsters who a few years later have trouble retrieving the names or the sounds of the alphabet. Picture naming was a powerful predictor of reading failure in Jansky's kindergarten screening battery (1972).

Despite high intelligence in many cases—as evidenced by their problem-solving ability and their often superior performance on psychometric tests—one finds a delay in physiological maturation and a lag in ego development which appear to go hand in hand. These children continue to move their bodies globally; their reflex behavior, tonus, and posture belong to a chronologically younger age. Their outstanding trait is impulsivity. They cannot wait; they cannot postpone gratification; and, as Anna Freud (1965) puts it, they cannot "carry out preconceived plans with a minimum regard for the lack of immediate pleasure yield, intervening frustration, and the maximum regard for the pleasure of the ultimate outcome" (p. 82).

Drive control constitutes a central problem.[10] Aggression is primitive and expressed through action rather than verbally. The amorphous nature of the stimuli on the Rorschach plates tends to arouse disorganized and chaotic responses and makes it difficult for such youngsters to reject aggressive and fairly primitive fantasies. The stories they tell in response to pictures are filled with references to food and longings for early instinctual gratification. The material clearly shows that the children have not begun to move out from a fairly egocentric universe and are preoccupied with conflicts belonging to an earlier psychosexual phase. Wish-fulfilling and magic solutions are ready at hand. Anna Freud's statement (1965) that a measure of advance in ego development and drive control is

---

[10] Lack of control over drives is, of course, not related solely to linguistic deficits. In some cases it appears to be one aspect of the child's biological dysfunction, the "organic drivenness" syndrome. The forces that propel the children appear to be related to their difficulty in organizing their inner and outer cosmos. Secondary conflicts are, of course, the rule rather than the exception.

a necessary forerunner of the ability to work is strikingly demonstrated in the case of these children. They are not ready for formal education. At older ages some of them develop compulsive-obsessivelike mechanisms. At age 8 a youngster's Bender copies may be scattered all over the page, while at age 13 the same youngster might encase each single copy to anchor it down on the page, as it were. These defenses appear to be directed not so much against forbidden impulses as against fears of disintegration (Kurlander and Colodny, 1965). Whatever their origin, these mechanisms constitute one more barrier to learning. An important avenue for research would be the choice and the structure of defenses used by these particular children.

Language and Psychic Organization

If one looks at both prematurely born and educationally unready children, the question arises whether lags in ego development and delay in patterning perceptuomotor and linguistic stimuli should be regarded as two separate phenomena or rather as manifestations of a pervasive organismic immaturity[11] that invades all sectors of the personality and interferes with the orderly organization of experience.

In the prematurely born children, maturational deficits are in all probability related to the original physiological lag and one might ask, as Weil (1961) does, whether the organism's inherent tendency to structuralization and the capacity for integration are weaker in these children than in others.

In the educationally "unready" children, one might hypothesize a physiological variant. Orton (1930) and his pupils, most Scandinavian researchers (Herman, 1959; Hallgren, 1950), and Owen et al. (1971), who tested the parents and siblings of dyslexic children, maintain that reading and spelling difficulties are found in given

[11] The concept of maturation as put forward by Bender (1958) is based on the theory of functional areas in the brain and the personality which develop longitudinally according to a recognizable pattern. A maturational lag, then, could be defined as a retention of primitive experiences in perceptuomotor gestalts, body imagery, and conceptualization of time and space.

families. This is borne out by the large number of family files piling up in our clinics and offices. That severe immaturity may be genetically determined was postulated by Zangwill (1962). It is possible (though I have no way to prove it) that it is not the reading and spelling disorder per se which is genetically determined, but rather the underlying maturational defect that is reflected both in deficits of spoken and printed language and perhaps also in delays in the structuralization of the ego.

It may be worth while to trace in greater detail the specific and intricate meshings of lags in both the linguistic and the psychic organization—what Edelheit (1968) calls the deeply rooted reciprocity between language and ego development.

Linguists are primarily concerned with the formal properties of language. The main interest of academic psychologists centers around the role of language in cognition. Both disciplines have largely neglected to probe the part language plays in the child's growing ability to define himself, to gain control over drives, and to cope with reality demands. It is to the psychoanalytic literature that one must turn for more penetrating insights into the relationship between linguistic and psychic structure (Atkin, 1969; Edelheit, 1968, 1969; Rosen, 1967; Peller, 1966; Katan, 1961; Waelder, 1960; Balkanyi, 1964; Kolansky, 1967; Frank, 1969).

Rappaport (1961) speaks about the repercussion of the organic dysfunction on the epigenesis of the ego. This implies, however, a cause-and-effect relationship, and does not take into account the *interactions* between the two. While a severe lisp, for instance, may interfere with the child's social relationships, it should not be overlooked that a need for oral gratification may enter into lisping and in turn reflect attitudes which might be unacceptable to the group in the first place.[12]

Rappaport ignores the fundamental fact that the development of language is a major determinant in the differentiation and growth

---

[12] To assume, as does Rousey (1969), that other specific sound substitutions, such as *f* for *th,* reflect highly specific emotional constellations—in this case, a disturbance in the early and significant relationship with the father—seems to be a gross simplification. Among other things, it neglects to take into account the inherent laws of phonemic development.

of the ego itself. Indeed, Edelheit (1969) considers the ego as a language-determining and language-determined structure.

Verbal signs heavily reinforced by intonations reassure the child that the mother will return even if she is gone for a while, and they thus contribute to object constancy. In the children discussed here, the very perceptual experience of the mother is probably more fragmented and more diffuse than that of others. Being unable to stabilize their experience by means of language, they are doubly handicapped. It would be of interest to explore the possibility of a delay in development of object constancy in "organic" children and to investigate what such delay—if any—means in terms of the children's adaptation to and trust in the world.

The appearance of the ego as a psychic structure and the emergence of verbalizations occur more or less simultaneously during the last two phases of the separation-individuation process (Mahler, 1971). Rosen (1967) states that the symbolic use of words is the most crucial step in the process of individuation. Since individuation itself seems to be a prerequisite for the development of language, it is clear that these processes are reciprocal and that disturbance in one will be reflected in the other.

Children probably have some sensorimotor schemata that give rise to a vague and fleeting sense of self before they use words. It is quite true that without a fairly well developed sense of self, of being separate, verbal dialogue cannot take place. On the other hand, the distinction between the "me" and the "not me" is enormously strengthened when the child understands and uses concepts such as "mine" and "I" (Peller, 1966). One sees this clearly in schizophrenic children. Their unstable ego boundaries are mirrored in their severe communicative deficits. Their idiosyncratic use of language reveals the dominance of archaic and primitive affects and drives. Words for these children are not necessarily tools for adaptation to reality or for communication.[13] As in dreams, words

---

[13] This becomes very clear when one compares the language deficits of dysphasic and schizophrenic children. The language of the latter may reflect the displacements and condensations of the primary process, while in the former, verbalizations, no matter how primitive, serve mainly the secondary process (de Hirsch, 1967).

are played with, condensed, truncated (Werner and Kaplan, 1963); they tend to express instinctual needs. For 8-year-old Ted, who refused to learn the name of the letter *K* because "he has too many spikes," numbers and letters were not referents, but the things themselves: they expressed inner states, in Ted's case, archaic fears of aggression and retaliation.

In young children one can observe the many ways language fluctuates depending on its use for the primary or the secondary process. "Baby talk" is an example of the use of language in the service of regression. Syntactical constructions change into more primitive ones, word-order rules no longer hold, phonemic profiles flatten out, iterations of sounds and words become more frequent, sentence melody changes in the direction of nursery rhymes, and singsongs often accompany rhythmic movements. Pitch rises, and the oral gratification function of language moves into the foreground. A little later, the child's language changes back into more age-adequate linguistic forms and the cognitive and communicative functions of language reassert themselves.

Listening to a 4-year-old talk to himself while he plays with his train, one may notice initially that his verbalizations are in the service of mastery. As the play changes and the train comes to stand for power and potency, syntax dissolves, novel words are invented, meanings are used idiosyncratically, pitch fluctuates. In other words, as the child slips back and forth between the different levels of organization, the formal features of language reflect these changes.[14]

Katan (1961) describes how the externalization of magical and omnipotent fantasies by means of words renders these fantasies less dangerous and contributes heavily to reality testing, one of the crucial functions of the ego. Dysphasic children take much longer

---

[14] Vygotsky (1962) distinguished between the "meaning" of a word and its "sense." Sense, he says, contains all the private and perceptual associations of the word. He talks, of course, about inner speech which, he maintains, is saturated with "sense." It seems to me that in the egocentric speech of young children (Piaget, 1923), which accompanies their fantasies during play, we find the same saturation with the "sense" of words—verbalizations drenched with affect rather than related to thought processes.

than others to emerge from their magic universe. Lacking verbal concepts, they have far fewer opportunities to test their fantasies against reality, which is one of the reasons why the differential diagnosis between autistic and dysphasic children is often difficult to arrive at.

Inner processes enter consciousness by being associated with their verbal representation (Frank, 1969). Verbalizations help establish control and reduce acting out. Many years ago we worked with a 4-year-old who had been referred by an analyst because of a moderately severe receptive-expressive aphasia and who could not be retained in his nursery school because of severe hyperkinesis and uncontrolled aggressiveness. Thomas did not strike us as a particularly hostile youngster. His aggression was somehow different from that of neurotic children; it had a quality which has been described as "organic drivenness." Since the boy was unable to reconcile his behavior with the demands of the environment, there were many secondary conflicts. Moreover, he suffered from feelings of guilt about being "bad," as do many such children. Some two years later, when he had acquired reasonably effective, if primitive, verbal tools, I heard him say upon entering the room, "This is one of my days, take the junk [toys] away—it sets me off." The fact that this youngster had learned to label his behavior and the underlying feeling states meant that he was no longer entirely delivered to the forces that drove him.

Anna Freud (1936) wrote,

> The association of affects and instinctual processes with word representations is stated to be the first and the most important step in the direction of the mastery of instinct which has to be taken as the individual develops. Thinking is described in these writings as an "experimental kind of acting, accompanied by displacement of relatively small quantities of cathexis together with less expenditure (discharge) of them" (Freud, 1911, p. 221). This intellectualization of instinctual life, the attempt to lay hold on the instinctual processes by connecting them with ideas which can be dealt with in consciousness, is one of the most general, earliest, and most necessary acquirements of the human ego. We regard it not as an activity of the ego but as one of its indispensable components [p. 162f.].

The ontogenesis of language cannot be separated from consciousness, which, according to Edelheit (1968), confers meaning and structure on the world and which includes an awareness of self, an awareness that is an essential condition of superego development. Waelder (1960) felt that a prerequisite of superego formation is the capacity for introspection and the ability to stand back and regard the self from an imaginary vantage point.[15] It implies the capacity to abstract, which in turn is intimately bound up with language.

It was fascinating to watch the parallel emergence of superego precursors and linguistic forms in another dysphasic boy who was started on a language-stimulation program at the age of 30 months. As his speech improved, he was able to talk about his difficulties with self-control, and after a particularly stormy session, he stood himself in front of the mirror and said: "Brian, you are a horrid little boy."

Piaget (1932) says that cognitive development must have reached a certain stage to enable the child to internalize moral values. While this is undoubtedly true, one might raise the question whether the internalization of moral demands does not also require the ability to use certain linguistic options. Conscience implies a choice. "I would like to swipe the candy, but *if* I did, I would feel badly." The nonverbal child might or might not swipe the candy. If he did, he might anticipate punishment, but in the absence of linguistic options his chances to internalize moral values would be limited.

If linguistic development were in some ways related to superego formation, one would expect deaf individuals to be delayed in this respect. There is a great deal of new research directed toward the relationship between cognitive and linguistic dimensions in deaf children (Furth, 1974), but very little work has been done on the ego and superego development in youngsters who have profound hearing losses. Lesser and Easser (1972) say that the deaf show a relative lack of the self-observing ego, a conscience formation different from that to be expected, and they add that deaf children

---

[15] It should be added that this also includes an awareness of the tool of language itself as revealed in the linguistic jokes most 7- and 8-year-olds delight in: "Did you ever see a butter fly?" (Gleitman, 1973).

regress easily to primary process thinking. The few deaf individuals I have observed closely appeared to follow very rigid rules of behavior (which does not necessarily mean that they had internalized a value system). It was evident that they dealt in absolute categories. Things or people were either black or white; there were few shades because these children did not have at their disposal sophisticated and differentiated linguistic tools.

It is, of course, essential to stress that in innumerable cases, physiological lags and neurotic conflicts resulting in arrested ego development or regression to an earlier psychosexual phase may have independent roots, but nevertheless interact. The 7-year-old who has failed to solve conflicts belonging to the oedipal situation, and who does not catch on to reading in the first and second grade because of a constitutional weakness in the language area, will look on his failure as a conclusive confirmation of the grave doubts he has about himself. His failure intensifies feelings of helplessness and impotence, which in turn prevent him from using his compensatory resources. We encounter this kind of interaction day in and day out in the children referred for language and learning disabilities. Specific weaknesses provide a convenient focal point for phobic responses.

The Implications of Labeling for the Choice of Therapy

Calling our children "brain-injured," no matter whether or not we add the word "minimal," is unjustified in the absence of positive signs on the classical neurological examination and a conclusive history of cerebral insult (Birch, 1964). This label, furthermore, does not account for genetic variations. It is an inferential diagnosis, conveying to the parents and to the environment, including the children themselves, that they are physically and mentally crippled. Saying that they suffer from minimal cerebral dysfunction also constitutes an inferential diagnosis, but it has at least the advantage that the term refers to processes rather than to structure.

If one were to describe these children rather than label them, one might say that their experiences in a number of areas are less stable, more fragmented, cruder, and above all far less under the control of the ego than those of other children. To say that their experiences resemble those of younger subjects is valid, but the fact that they are actually older—and thus encounter a different environment and expectations—results in significant developmental imbalances[16] as well as in a different structuring of their defenses.

Bender (1955) feels that a maturational lag reflected clinically in primitive patterning is precisely what constitutes nonfocal brain injury.

Conrad (1948) in his work on adult aphasia speaks of the phenomenon of "dedifferentiation." We observe in our children simplified organizational schemata and what is probably a defect in differentiation of more complex gestalts.

Starting with early sensorimotor experiences and continuing all the way up to higher psychic functions, our children appear to have difficulties responding to and integrating gestalts—a difficulty which may be reflected in delayed development of the integrative function of the ego. Evidence of problems with gestalts is seen clearly in the lack of flow in the children's handwriting, in the absence of sentence melody when they read aloud. Pick (1931) called it "Sprachgefühl"—feel for language.[17] One also sees it when after months of painstaking work, the dyslexic youngster suddenly integrates subskills, "takes off" and reads. Watching the process, one feels that it does not consist of adding one skill to another, but rather that the gestalt suddenly "jumps out" (de Hirsch, 1954).

It would be fascinating to inquire whether the tendency to fragmentation, the difficulty in grasping wholes, and the instability of the gestalt experience influence the formation of the very easiest object relationships. Perhaps these children are slower than others in linking need gratification with the percept of the person who provides it.

Unfortunately, the problem of labeling is not an academic one,

---

[16] The problem of "critical" periods comes up in this context; the time (and it clearly varies for different functions) in which basic organizations and structures are laid down (Connelly, 1972).

[17] Many years ago Pick (1931) said that the processes of language do not consist of a collection of elements, rather they are from the very beginning patterned structures ("gestaltete Strukturen").

since in a large number of cases the label determines the choice of therapy. The child who is said to present minimal brain dysfunction may receive appropriate medication. However, he may miss out on the psychological support from the psychotherapist who lends him his own ego attributes—interest in mastery, pride in achievement, and willingness to push through. He has nobody to turn to if he needs help with the secondary conflicts arising from his situation. On the other hand, the youngster who has been correctly diagnosed as suffering from lag in ego development may be exposed to years of interpretative therapy to the neglect of his educational needs, which tend to snowball and result in additional problems and conflicts (A. Freud, 1974).

In my experience, the preschoolers who have significant linguistic deficits and lags in readiness skills do best with an intensive relationship therapy. This can be done either by a psychotherapist who can simultaneously carry out a careful language-stimulation program in the framework of his own approach and who can work with the mother; or by a language therapist who has some idea of the psychological implications of the child's behavior, who has learned to listen to what the child is trying to say even on a nonverbal level.

Weil (1973) suggests educational therapy for such children before latency, in preparation for analysis. The educator, on the other hand, must be alert to signs which point to the necessity for psychiatric intervention.

In many cases, the contribution of specific handicaps is slight and the child's educational difficulties are directly related to neurosis. While the decision in such cases is relatively clear-cut, it is not always easy to convince the parents. They often come to us precisely because we are *not* psychiatrists. Consulting an educator seems to be less threatening. Furthermore, the parents may previously have been told that the child's problem is "developmental," "organic," or "familial," and it may be difficult for them to understand that such conditions do not exempt the child from conflict but are, rather, precipitating factors.

There are other children whose significant neurophysiological lags are closely intertwined with their psychological problems.

Some of them are so preoccupied with intruding fantasies that they are unavailable for remediation and have no psychic energy available for academic requirements.

Tonia is an example. She was a small, dainty, little girl with a tiny face and masses of very dark hair. The child looked anxious and somewhat distraught. There was a frantic, worried air about her.

She had been rejected for the second time by every private girl's school in town, which had been a blow to her parents. She was currently in the third grade of one of the more acceptable public schools in the silk-stocking district in Manhattan. She managed in math, but she was nevertheless at the bottom of her class in reading, writing, and spelling, although she scored an IQ of 125 on the verbal and one of 112 on the performance section of the WISC. She hated school, she had no friends, and her mother said she was totally unable to concentrate.

There were no doubts as to Tonia's specific deficits. At this late date she reversed the letters in her own name and signed her drawing: "Msi Tonai" (for Mis Tonia). She transposed sounds in words and scrambled words in sentences even in speaking. Her verbalizations were rushed, indistinct, and poorly organized. She told endless stories in which people went to and fro, but it never became clear what they were doing and why they were there.

Tonia's responses to the CAT pictures raised more questions than they answered, but they pointed to sexual preoccupations. The bathroom picture, above all, elicited a good deal of excitement.

Tonia's mother told me that the child's early development had been uneventful, except for speech which had been late to emerge. Tonia had nightmares during which she twitched all over. She did not easily talk about her feelings, the mother added. Apart from her failure at school, the main complaint was "stubbornness." It was only when I specifically asked about toilet training that I got the full story. Tonia had stopped wetting early. Bowel training, on the other hand, had been a traumatic affair. The child was afraid of the toilet, she refused to perform, and suffered from extreme constipation. The nurse became terribly upset, as did the mother, with the result that the child held on to her stools for as long as 10 days. Suppositories and enemas were not particularly helpful and produced endless scenes. The power struggle lasted for nearly two years, but things straightened out when the nurse left.

I suggested that the parents discuss Tonia's problems with an analyst. Nothing came of it, however, because they could not bring themselves to go any further.

In the meantime the child had settled down in the office,[18] and although she would much rather have played and often looked longingly at the dollhouse, she did try to apply herself to the educational task. The returns were woefully limited. Tonia's many spatial and linguistic difficulties continued to plague her. Above all, she was unable to stay with any one activity. "Things run around my head like squirrels," she said. She asked innumerable questions, not taking the time to listen for the answers. She became more and more restless swaying in her chair and complaining about her peers: "They think I'm crazy and dumb, but I'm not, am I?"

Over the next few months it became increasingly evident that Tonia was intensely preoccupied with sexual fantasies in which beatings played a predominant role. None of these fantasies was elicited; they would spill over against her wish—she appeared to have no way of defending herself against them. Not only did they make Tonia feel terribly guilty, but they played havoc with learning. No wonder she was drawn to the dollhouse—play would have given her some outlet for her fantasies.

Since nothing solid was being accomplished, I made another urgent appeal to the parents, who finally agreed to send the child into analysis while continuing with remedial work. The analyst was a man, which initially eliminated some of the transference problems that might otherwise have been troublesome. The remedial therapist was quite capable of dealing with the vicissitudes of the analytic process as it intruded into the educational situation. Tonia soon understood which kinds of material belonged to the remedial setting and which to the analyst's office. Above all, the analyst and the therapist were in close contact.

There were no very sudden changes; but when one looked at the

---

[18] Dr. Jeannette Jansky was the therapist who worked with both of the children described here. She also did the psychological work-ups.

child two years later, she was a different girl. What had apparently happened was a developmental spurt that was reflected in both the physiological and the psychological segments of the personality. One might ask whether such a spurt would by itself have worked the changes we observed. I do not think so. I believe that the analytic process, by relieving the child of preoccupations belonging to an earlier psychosexual phase, enabled her to respond to teaching and to compensate for her specific deficits.

The stubbornness that had so upset the mother was now in the service of autonomy and adaptation. Her academic work improved considerably because Tonia could bend her energies to the task at hand.

She was accepted in a private school. Her spelling still was quite poor; her compositions were vivid but not exactly elegantly formulated, and she still had trouble with punctuation. She read with pleasure and she now had a few friends.

In Tonia's case remedial work and analysis were carried out simultaneously. She would have fallen too far behind if remedial help had been postponed. Without analysis, on the other hand, she would not have been accessible to remediation.

Nick's case is different. His specific difficulties were, if anything, more massive than Tonia's. To begin with, the family history of language difficulties was heavily positive. In the past we had worked with two other members of the father's family, and we had seen three others in consultation because of delayed speech development and various disorders of printed and written language.

Nick immediately impressed us as strikingly immature physiologically. Although he is in the fourth grade, his second teeth are just coming in. He was a slight, blond boy with a charming face, but when we first saw him more than three years ago he looked as if he had not quite jelled. Nick was incredibly hyperactive, as a result of which his family found it difficult to cope with him. His kindergarten teacher had called him a "buzz-bomb." Sitting still was a major problem. For the past two years he had been on Ritalin which helped in the learning situation. His drawing of a human figure was quite primitive, his Bender copies those of a much younger child. He had a terrible time managing the pencil and his hand tended to shake because he had to press so hard to control it. Nick's oral language was quite immature. He had not incorporated basic syntactical rules and would cheerfully say: "I dag clams" because he had the vague feeling that the past tense of "dig" is irregular. He would tell one excitedly that they had a "firebrush" close to the house when he meant a "brushfire." Nick was (and up to a point still is) a clutterer and appears to lack anticipatory schemata—his verbal formulations are quite poor. Nick had a dysnomia of gigantic proportions—he could not recall color names until he was 7 years old.

It is easy to see the implications of these deficits for learning the letters of the alphabet or, for that matter, their sound equivalents—Nick had to tie the shape of the letter and its name to some concrete clue in order to remember it. His retention of whole words was terribly poor as well. It took him forever to learn to recognize the printed word "kitten": he was apt to lose it when he saw it in different contexts. He simply could not hold on to the verbal visual gestalt. If only he had had a feel for the flow of a sentence, it would have been easier for him to compensate for his perceptual instability by guessing from the surrounding syntactical and contextual configurations what the options were. Unfortunately, he had no feel for it. It was the combination of perceptual instability and linguistic deficits that accounted for his massive reading disability.

Psychologically, Nick was a solid boy. He had the age-appropriate conflicts which he handled rather well. He had his difficulties; his boiling point was low, and he was very easily frustrated (in his case there were good reasons for it). Yet, he never gave up, even when he was occasionally close to tears. He was fiercely jealous of his younger brother, but nowadays he is occasionally amused by him. He treats him the way he treats his animals—Nick lives surrounded by lizards, two dogs, three cats, and a much beloved snake—roughly but good naturedly.

Nick is bright. He does well in math, and he is a collector of facts. He is a vivid, entertaining boy with a delicious sense of humor, and he has many friends.

He more or less owns the office. He has been coming for over three years, which means that his unusually devoted mother had to drive him four times a week from one of the Connecticut suburbs to Manhattan.

For the first time this year Nick is beginning to look like a latency boy. He is much less hyperactive, but during lessons he wriggles in his chair. In spite of intensive efforts his handwriting still is atrocious and his spelling remains quite poor, though it is less bizarre than it had been. However, he is developing a feel for the flow of a sentence. It makes all the difference because it helps him guessing from context and to compensate up to a point for his continuing perceptual instability. To everyone's amazement he is now reading at the mid-third-grade level, and the other day he wrote a composition half a page long. For Nick this is a tremendous achievement. The next year will probably show further physiological changes and we expect considerable gains.

Nick illustrates the gross physiological immaturity described earlier in this paper. In his case one would be entitled to speak of a maturational defect rather than a lag. While his deficits will become less obvious with ongoing development, I believe that one will find residuals in later years. I feel sure, nevertheless, that Nick will in the last instance do well. He is determined to be an explorer, an excellent illustration of his ability to sublimate his hyperkinesis and to use his passion for animals.

What enabled this grossly immature youngster to cope? In contrast to many other physiologically immature children, he has a great deal of ego strength. His capacity to relate is impressive. He uses his therapist constructively. It is this relationship that enabled the boy to mobilize the more than normal quantities of energy he needed in order to benefit from remedial measures. I feel (though it would be difficult to prove) that in some of these children a very close identification with the remedial worker is a powerful factor in neurophysiological maturation.[19] Another asset in his ability to

---

[19] This statement is of course debatable since maturation has been defined as the organism's inherent tendency to evolve new structures relatively independent of environmental influences. Koffka (1935) stated that any perceived gestalt is the product of inner organization *and* training. Schilder (1964) felt that training and stimulation play a significant part even in those functions in which maturation of the central nervous system is of primary importance. This is true, above all, during transitional states.

work. In contrast to many other immature children, he has made the shift from the pleasure to the reality principle. Finally, he had the full support of his family.

Remedial therapists confronted with sometimes conflicting reports from a variety of specialists need some awareness of the complexity of the presenting symptoms. They must realize that an identical configuration of deficits may or may not result in failure, depending on the child's inherent strength and the kind of support he can draw upon to compensate for his deficits. Without such awareness, they will not be in a position to make appropriate referrals, nor will they be able to map out adequate remedial strategies. No matter which specific techniques are employed, the therapist will have to work with the child's affects in order to mobilize the energy he needs to compensate for early adaptive failure.

Summary

This paper attempts to describe a group of atypical children whose sometimes severe physiological deficits represent one aspect of a pervasive organismic immaturity that is reflected in difficulties with integration on all levels—perceptuomotor, linguistic, cognitive, and in terms of the ego's organization. The specific constellation varies from child to child. The impact on the child's functioning depends on his ability to mobilize his adaptational resources. The child's genetic endowment, including his greater or lesser vulnerability to stress; his prenatal, natal, and postnatal history; the emotional climate in which he is raised; the social scene of which he is part—all interact in complex ways.

The crucial role of the home and, more specifically, of the nature of the mother-child bond has not even been touched upon and is beyond the scope of this paper. Suffice it to say that at the very earliest ages the characteristics of the children discussed here tend to alter the normal response patterns of the mother (Thomas et al., 1963; Weil, 1970a), which in turn modify the child's perception of self and contribute to his pathology. I refer here to what Weil (1970a) calls the "multifaceted complimentary series of interactions."

The premium our society places on success is another factor that enters the situation in the case of learning-disabled children. It is against the background of the mother-child communication—nonverbal and verbal—and the demands of the larger society that these children's difficulties have to be assessed.

BIBLIOGRAPHY

AJURRIAGUERRA, J. DE (1966) Speech Disorders in Childhood. In: *Brain Function*, ed. E. C. Carterette. Berkeley: Univ. California Press, 3:117–140.
ATKIN, S. (1969), Psychoanalytic Considerations of Language and Thought. *Psychoanal. Quart.*, 38:549–582.
BALKANYI, C. (1964), On Verbalization. *Int. J. Psycho-Anal.*, 45:64–74.
BENDER, L. (1955), *Psychopathology of Children with Organic Brain Disorders*. Springfield, Ill.: Thomas.
——— (1958), Problems in Conceptualization and Communication in Children with Developmental Alexia. In: *Psychopathology of Communication*, ed. P. H. Hoch & J. Zubin. New York: Grune & Stratton, pp. 155–176.
——— (1966), The Concept of Plasticity in Childhood Schizophrenia. In: *Psychopathology of Schizophrenia*, ed. P. H. Hoch & J. Zubin. New York: Grune & Stratton, pp. 354–365.
BENTZEN, F. (1963), Sex Ratios in Learning and Behavior Disorders. *Amer. J. Orthopsychiat.*, 33:92–98.
BIRCH, H. G. (1964), *Brain Damage in Children*. Baltimore: Williams & Wilkins.
CAPLAN, H., BIBACE, R., & RABINOVITCH, M. S. (1963), Paranatal Stress, Cognitive Organization and Ego Function. *J. Amer. Acad. Child Psychiat.*, 2:434–450.
CLEMENTS, S. D. (1973), Minimal Brain Dysfunction. In: *Children With Learning Problems*, ed. S. Sapir & A. C. Nitzburg. New York: Brunner/Mazel, pp. 159–172.
CONNELLY, K. (1972), Learning and the Concept of Critical Periods in Infancy. *Develpm. Med. & Child Neurol.*, 14:705–714.
CONRAD, K. (1948), Beitrag zum Problem der parietalen Alexie. *Arch. Psychiat. Nervenkr.*, 181:398–420.
DE HIRSCH, K. (1954), Gestalt Psychology As Applied to Language Disturbances. *J. Nerv. Ment. Dis.*, 120:257–261.
——— (1965), The Concept of Plasticity and Language Disabilities. *Speech Pathol. & Ther.*, 8:12–17.
——— (1967), Differential Diagnosis Between Aphasic and Schizophrenic Language in Children. *J. Speech & Hear. Dis.*, 32:3–10.
——— JANSKY, J., & LANGFORD, W. S. (1966a), Comparisons between Prematurely and Maturely Born Children at Three Age Levels. *Amer. J. Orthopsychiat.*, 36:616–628.

——— ——— ——— (1966b), *Predicting Reading Failure.* New York: Harper & Row.

EDELHEIT, H. (1968), Panel Report: Language and Ego Development. *J. Amer. Psychoanal. Assn.*, 16:113-122.

——— (1969), Speech and Psychic Structure. *J. Amer. Psychoanal. Assn.*, 17:381-412.

EKSTEIN, R. (1965), Historical Notes Concerning Psychoanalysis and Early Language Development. *J. Amer. Psychoanal. Assn.*, 13:707-730.

FRANK, A. (1969), The Unrememberable and the Unforgettable. *This Annual*, 24:48-77.

FRENCH, S. L. (1953), Psychological Factors in Cases of Reading Difficulties. Presented at the 27th Annual Conference of the Secondary Education Board, New York.

FREUD, A. (1936), *The Ego and the Mechanisms of Defense.* New York: Int. Univ. Press, rev. ed., 1966.

——— (1965), *Normality and Pathology in Childhood.* New York: Int. Univ. Press.

——— (1974), A Psychoanalytic View of Developmental Psychopathology. *J. Philadelphia Assn. Psychoanal.*, 1:7-17.

FREUD, S. (1911), Formulations on the Two Principles of Mental Functioning. *S.E.*, 12:215-226.

FRIEDLANDER, B. Z. (1970), Receptive Language Development in Infancy. *Merrill-Palmer Quart.*, 16:7-52.

——— (1973), Receptive Language Anomaly and Language/Reading Dysfunction in "Normal" Primary School Children. *Psychol. in the Schools*, 10:12-18.

FURTH, H. G. (1974), The Concept of the "School for Thinking." In: *The Learning Disability Child* [Proceedings of a Symposium on Current Operation, Remediation and Evaluation]. Dallas: Univ. Texas Health Science Center.

GLEITMAN, L. (1973), Metalinguistic Capacity. Position paper presented at the meeting of the Language Panel on Head Start. Sponsored by the Rand Corporation, Washington, D.C.

GOODMAN, K. (1972), Reading: The Key Is in Children's Language. *Read. Teacher*, 25:505-508.

GREENACRE, P. (1941), The Predisposition to Anxiety. *Trauma, Growth and Personality.* New York: Int. Univ. Press, 1952, pp. 27-82.

HALLGREN, B. (1950), Specific Dyslexia (Congenital Word-Blindness). *Acta Psychiat. Neurol.* (supp. 65), 1-287.

HERMAN, K. (1959), *Reading Disability.* Springfield, Ill.: Thomas.

ILG, F. L. & AMES, L. B. (1965), *School Readiness.* New York: Harper & Row.

JANSKY, J. & DE HIRSCH, K. (1972), *Preventing Reading Failure.* New York: Harper & Row.

KAGAN, J., MOSS, H. A., & SIGEL, I. E. (1960), Conceptual Style and the Use of Affect Labels. *Merrill-Palmer Quart.*, 6:261-276.

KAPLAN, D. M. & MASON, E. A. (1960), Maternal Reactions to Premature Birth Viewed As an Acute Emotional Disorder. *Amer. J. Orthopsychiat.*, 30:539-552.

KATAN, A. (1961), Some Thoughts About the Role of Verbalization in Early Childhood. *This Annual*, 16:184–188.
KOFFKA, K. (1935), *Principles of Gestalt Psychology*. New York: Harcourt, Brace.
KOLANSKY, H. (1967), Some Psychoanalytic Considerations on Speech in Normal Development and Psychopathology. *This Annual*, 22:274–295.
KURLANDER, L. F. & COLODNY, D. (1965), "Pseudoneurosis" in the Neurologically Handicapped Child. *Amer. J. Orthopsychiat.*, 35:733–738.
LESHAN, L. (1952), Time Orientation and Social Class. *J. Abnorm. Soc. Psychol.*, 47:589–592.
LESSER, S. R. & EASSER, R. B. (1972), Personality Differences in the Perceptually Handicapped. *J. Amer. Acad. Child Psychiat.*, 11:458–466.
LEWIS, M. M. (1963), *Language, Thought and Personality in Infancy and Childhood*. New York: Basic Books.
LURIA, A. R. (1961), *The Role of Speech in the Regulation of Normal and Abnormal Behavior*, ed. J. Tizard. New York: Liveright.
MAHLER, M. S. (1971), A Study of the Separation-Individuation Process. *This Annual*, 26:403–424.
McFIE, J. (1952), Cerebral Dominance in Cases of Reading Disability. *J. Neurol., Neurosurg., & Psychiat.*, 15:194–199.
ORTON, S. T. (1930), Familial Occurrence of Disorders in Acquisition of Language. *Eugenics*, 3(4):140–147.
OWEN, F. W., ADAMS, P. A., FORREST, T., ET AL. (1971), Learning Disorders in Children. *Monogr. Soc. Res. Child Develpm.*, 36:1–77.
PELLER, L. E. (1965), Language and Development. In: *Concepts of Development in Early Childhood Education*, ed. P. B. Neubauer, Springfield, Ill.: Thomas, pp. 53–83.
——— (1966), Freud's Contribution to Language Theory. *This Annual*, 21:448–467.
PIAGET, J. (1923), *Language and Thought of the Child*. London: Routledge, 1932.
——— (1932), *The Moral Judgment of the Child*. New York: Free Press, 1965.
PICK, A. (1931), *Aphasia*. Springfield, Ill.: Thomas, 1973.
RAPPAPORT, S. R. (1961), Behavior Disorder and Ego Development in a Brain-Injured Child. *This Annual*, 16:423–450.
——— (1964), Childhood Aphasia. *Pathway School Symposium*. M.I.T. Research Lab of Electronics, Cambridge, Mass.
ROSEN, V. H. (1966), Disturbances of Representation and Reference in Ego Deviations. In: *Psychoanalysis—A General Psychology*, ed. R. M. Loewenstein et al. New York: Int. Univ. Press, pp. 634–654.
——— (1967), Disorders of Communication in Psychoanalysis. *J. Amer. Psychoanal. Assn.*, 15:167–190.
ROUSEY, C. L. (1969), A Theory of Speech. Presented at the Annual Meeting of the American Association of Psychiatric Clinics for Children, and at the Winter Meeting of the American Psychoanalytic Association, 1970.
SCHILDER, P. (1964), *Contributions to Developmental Neuropsychiatry*, ed. L. Bender. New York: Int. Univ. Press.

SCHOLNICK, F. K. & ADAMS, M. J. (1973), Relationships Between Language and Cognitive Skills. *Child Develpm.*, 44:741–746.
SUBIRANA, A. (1961), The Problem of Cerebral Dominance. *Logos*, 4:67–85.
TANNER, J. M. (1961), *Education and Physical Growth*. London: Univ. London Press.
THOMAS, A. ET AL. (1963), *Behavioral Individuality in Early Childhood*. New York: New York Univ. Press.
VYGOTSKY, L. S. (1962), *Thought and Language*. Cambridge: M.I.T. Press.
WAELDER, R. (1960), *Basic Theory of Psychoanalysis*. New York: Int. Univ. Press.
WEIL, A. P. (1961), Psychopathic Personality and Organic Behavior Disorders. *Comprehens. Psychiat.*, 2:83–95.
―――― (1970a), The Basic Core. *This Annual*, 25:442–460.
―――― (1970b), Children with Minimal Brain Dysfunction. *Psychosocial Process* [J. Jewish Board of Guardians]. 1:80–97.
―――― (1973), Ego Strengthening Prior to Analysis. *This Annual*, 28:287–301.
WERNER, H. (1957), The Concept of Development from a Comparative and Organismic Point of View. In: *The Concept of Development*, ed. D. B. Harris. Minneapolis: Univ. Minnesota Press, pp. 125–148.
―――― & KAPLAN, B. (1963), *Symbol Formation*. New York: Wiley.
WYATT, G. L. (1969), *Language, Learning and Communications Disorders in Childhood*. New York: Free Press.
ZANGWILL, O. L. (1962), Dyslexia in Relation to Cerebral Dominance. In: *Reading Disability, Progress and Research Needs in Dyslexia*, ed. J. Money. Baltimore: Johns Hopkins Press, pp. 103–114.

On a Central Psychic Constellation

MARTIN A. SILVERMAN, M.D., KATHERINE REES, AND PETER B. NEUBAUER, M.D.

IN THIS PAPER, WE SHALL DESCRIBE THE EMERGENCE OF A CENTRAL psychic constellation which is observable during the preoedipal period. Our observations were made in the course of a longitudinal study in which we utilized observational techniques, supplemented by therapeutic material, to investigate the course of development and fate of the conflicts and structures associated with the prelatency period. We shall try to demonstrate that this central constellation emerges by the age of 3 or 4 out of the coordination of certain key variables into a relatively stable, cohesive, psychic organization which persists as an influential factor and which seems to play an important role in codetermining the pattern of further development, including the form and early outcome of the struggles of the oedipal period. The constellation's stability derives from the organization of its constituent elements into a dynamic equilibrium which persists despite changes in the elements themselves as development proceeds.

Dr. Silverman is Senior Psychiatrist, Child Development Center of the Jewish Board of Guardians; Clinical Instructor, Division of Psychoanalytic Education, Department of Psychiatry, State University of New York, Downstate Medical Center. Miss Rees is Child Therapist, Child Development Center of the Jewish Board of Guardians. Dr. Neubauer is Director, Child Development Center of the Jewish Board of Guardians, New York City; Professor, Division of Psychoanalytic Education, Department of Psychiatry, State University of New York, Downstate Medical Center, New York City.

Ever since Freud's momentous discovery of the role of the oedipus complex in human mental life, psychoanalysts have centered their attention upon oedipal conflicts and the ego's efforts to resolve them. Advances in ego psychology and research into the events of the preoedipal period have greatly broadened our perspective of development, but the knowledge thus gained has not yet been fully integrated into the mainstream of psychoanalytic theory and practice. There have been many contributions to our understanding of the preoedipal and oedipal periods and of the organization and functioning of the ego. This may be the time for psychoanalytic investigators to pull together the large quantity of information about early development that has been gathered over the years and to make use of it to enhance and refine our understanding of the origins, structure, and fate of the oedipus complex and further development. We hope in this communication to contribute to such an integration by describing what may be a significant aspect of the transition from preoedipal psychic organization to the developmental currents of the oedipal and latency periods.

In 1966, we embarked upon a long-range longitudinal study of eight children who at that time were between 3 and 3½ years of age. We set out to study the patterns of developmental change and evolution which were taking place. We were especially interested in the modifiability of early neurotic patterns and the ultimate fate of early patterns of conflict and conflict resolution.

We drew up a detailed Developmental Profile, derived from the outline devised by Anna Freud (1965), on each child twice yearly for three years and yearly thereafter. Our Profiles were based upon data obtained from multiple sources. In addition to the full clinical records available to us, we observed the children extensively in the classroom, paying attention to their relationships with the teachers and the other children, the fantasies expressed in their play and in their verbal communications, their physical activities and intellectual interests, and their involvement with the various people in their lives (including the investigators). The teachers kept a daily log on each child and met with us regularly to share their observations and impressions. The children and each of their parents were interviewed by one or more of the investigators and each child underwent a battery of psychological tests prior to each Profile. The study is still in progress.[1]

For the first Profile, a detailed account of each child's personal and family history was compiled. In addition to our own research, we also had access to the data gathered in a lengthy study of each child before his acceptance to the nursery school. The majority of the children had older siblings who also had attended the Center nursery school, which provided an additional rich source of information about the family. Some of the older siblings also had been in treatment at the Center. A staff member regularly saw at least one of each child's parents during the first three years of the study. One of the children had been a subject of a detailed infant study, the raw data of which were made available to us. It is significant that the main patterns of family interaction observed for each child at the beginning of the study seemed to have remained quite stable throughout the course of the investigation.

THE CENTRAL CONSTELLATION

Although at the time of the first Profile, the children's development was marked by considerable fluidity and change, certain observations stood out quite clearly. There were plentiful derivatives from prephallic levels of libidinal organization, with wide variation from child to child. All the children showed evidence of having reached the phallic phase of libidinal development, but not all were firmly engaged in it. In most of the children there was little evidence of involvement in oedipal fantasies and conflicts at the time of the first Profile.

As we followed the children through the "oedipal period" and on into latency, we were increasingly impressed that in our initial Profiles we had described a constellation of central characteristics which had become organized in such a way as to have reached relative stability, so that it was bound to exert an important impact upon further development. There were wide individual variations in the relative significance of each of the constituent elements of the

---

[1] Dr. Bertrand Cramer, who was a member of the research team during the first three years of the study, describes other aspects of our study in this volume.

constellation. In general, however, the components could be grouped into four overall areas, the assessment of which provided a key to each child's readiness at 3 or 3½ to move in certain directions.

The areas which we have come to view as particularly significant are: the pattern of phase progression, drive balance and discharge patterns, the impact of early variations in ego equipment and organization, the self and object representations, and the modes of regulating self-esteem with which the latter are associated. When we watched the children progress into late latency, we were increasingly impressed by the finding that what had been basic in each of these areas at the beginning of the phallic-oedipal period continued to be observable, despite all the changes which took place thereafter.

By the time the children entered the phallic and oedipal period, the inherent tendency to consolidation and integration underlying the increasing efficiency of operation of the developing psychic apparatus seemed to have coordinated and organized these psychic components into a remarkably stable constellation of forces. As we followed the children into latency, we found that this central constellation played a highly significant role, in interaction with the effects of ongoing maturational and experiential influences, as a codeterminant of the form and content of the children's oedipal conflicts, the options available for their resolution (or failure thereof), and the personality organization observable in latency.

We do not view the constellation as constituting a binding together either of pathological components exclusively or only of components arising out of normal developmental sequences. We would rather describe the process as a binding together of "core" variables in which conflictual and nonconflictual elements combine to form a characteristic psychic organization.

The Components of the Central Constellation

The variables which we shall describe emerged from the assessment data as significant areas which seemed to be coordinated with one another into a developmentally meaningful, dynamic, interaction system. These variables are an expression of the developmental forces, drive expressions, ego functions, and patterns of object and self regulation which have crystallized by the fourth year of life.

PHASE PROGRESSION

When we correlated current observations with the historical data on each child, it became apparent that each child had his own style of developmental progression. There were individual variations in the pattern of progressive and regressive movements, including variations in intensity of conflict engagement, strength of the progressive pull, ease of regression, range of movement to and fro, degree of fluidity and overlap, and the extent to which various modalities were affected by regressive shifts (Silverman and Neubauer, 1971).

There was evidence of advance to the phallic level, but each child had his own particular combination of prephallic and phallic elements. The impact of conflict at earlier levels upon the course of the phallic phase varied from one child to another. The range included fixations which impeded advance to higher levels, fixations which served as potential attraction points for regression in some areas without greatly interfering with general progression, and contamination of phallic interests and activities by derivatives of earlier conflicts. A few children seemed to shift fluidly back and forth between oral and phallic or anal and phallic interests without dominance at either level of libidinal organization.

It is not possible to speak of drive progression without describing the ego attitudes which are correlated with drive organization. In addition to responding to the specific tasks imposed in each new psychosexual phase, the ego had developed a characteristic attitude toward libidinal or aggressive drive pressure in general, regardless of its phase-specific form. Historical data seemed to point to three sources of this ego attitude: the relative strength of the drives, the child's perception of the reliability of his environmental objects, and his capacity to tolerate drive tension and secure object gratification. In other words, by $3\frac{1}{2}$, the ego of each child had developed a characteristic way of responding to the intensity of the drive demands imposed upon it, of assessing the availability of suitable environmental resources with which they might be satisfied, and of pursuing, capturing, and utilizing those resources.

DRIVE BALANCE AND DISCHARGE PATTERNS

Our data suggested that by the time they had reached the age of 3½, our children had reached a point of relative stability in the balance between libidinal and aggressive drive expression. The interplay between variations in drive endowment (Alpert et al., 1956) and crucial experiences during the first few years seemed to have determined the way in which libidinal and aggressive drive components had developed, intertwined, and fused with one another during the first three years in each child. The way in which each child's ego had experienced and executed drive demands during the first year or two seemed to have determined the pattern with which the ego sought and experienced pleasure thereafter. The form of aggressive drive expression and ambivalence conflicts seemed to have acquired relative stability as a result of passage through the oral and anal phases. The effect of defense systems, of course, played an important role.

Each child had experienced the onset of the capacity for independent assertion and execution of libidinal and aggressive drive demands differently during the toddler phase. These differences had greatly influenced his view of his ability both to assert himself independently and to move into and enjoy the focused, assertive, independent, competitive explorations and activities of the phallic phase. We saw that the children had come through the prephallic period with various quantities of aggressivity which had to be controlled. The degree to which aggressive drives had been tamed and neutralized (as well as the mechanisms employed for that purpose) also varied from one child to another at the beginning of the phallic phase.

We have seen that inability to mobilize aggressive energies in the pursuit of drive satisfaction in the prephallic period can be the harbinger of a restricted ability to be assertive and competitive during the phallic-oedipal period (an example will be described later on). Another child, Mark, possessed a strong, innate or congenital aggressivity, which enabled him vigorously to pursue libidinal objects during his second and third years despite the repeated loss of important objects. In the phallic phase, however, he was unable to restrain his aggressivity enough to hold on to his objects (and preserve his object representations against sadistic attack) once he had pursued and captured them. He was so terrified of driving off or destroying his objects, or of incurring terrible, punitive reprisal, that he was forced to abandon oedipal, rivalrous strivings and to turn to previously treasured inanimate objects onto which he could safely divert his aggressive attacks. He could not sufficiently engage himself in oedipal struggles to resolve them and move into latency. He was very intelligent and perceptive, but had little interest in learning for its own sake. He used his skills rather to charm and manipulate people, as well as to defeat and hurt them. In grade school, he used his intellectual abilities in the service of narcissistic withdrawal rather than employing them in the pursuit of knowledge.

THE DEVELOPMENTAL EFFECT OF EARLY VARIATIONS IN EGO EQUIPMENT AND ORGANIZATION

In each child we followed, a unique way of perceiving and responding to life situations and adaptational pressures had developed by the time of the first Profile. Although we did not directly study the children's development during the first three years, our data strongly suggested that these individual patterns derived in part from innate dispositions and equipmental variations which had been evident very early in their lives. The historical information we received (one child had also taken part in a thorough infant study, conducted by Annemarie Weil and Anneliese Riess) indicated that from the beginning each child had shown innate preferences for using certain modalities rather than others for relating to and interacting with the outside world. There was evidence of intrinsic variations in tension tolerance and in thresholds of response to external stimulation. The children differed in their perceptual sensitivities as well as in their patterns of assessing and integrating information. Motor activity patterns varied from one child to another and there were significant variations in motor control and in the rudiments of cognitive control apparatuses.

In each case, these variations were observed in early infancy and their impact upon behavior and personality characteristics was readily apparent during the first three years. However vague or unclear they may have been about other matters, nearly all the parents were unequivocally certain about these particular early observations. As we followed the children during the course of the study we were impressed with the ongoing consistency with which these individual characteristics remained observable and with the significant impact which they seemed to exert upon the developmental process.

The observation that variations in endowment, in interplay with environmental experience, contribute significantly to ongoing development is not a new one (Escalona, 1963, 1968; Korner, 1964; Thomas et al., 1963; Weil, 1956, 1970). It is difficult to predict from infant studies alone what will be the eventual developmental impact of early variations (Escalona and Heider, 1959). Longitudinal study beyond the period of infancy is necessary before the meaning of congenital traits and characteristics can be appreciated (Ritvo et al., 1963). By the fourth year, enough structuralization and organization seem to have taken place to indicate which factors have been developmentally significant and to permit reasonable predictions about the fate of the structural and organizational elements to whose evolution they have contributed. Our own findings indicate that by the age of $3\frac{1}{2}$, they have become organized into a relatively stable, central constellation which exerts an important influence upon psychic development thereafter. We do not mean to imply that no change occurs in the individual elements with further development. *The stability to which we refer is that of a dynamic interaction of interrelated factors within an organized, integrated, dynamic grouping or constellation which remains relatively stable despite changes in the constituent elements.*

An example may help to clarify this point. One child as an infant had been relatively inactive motorically but very alert and active perceptually, with precocious discriminative powers. Possessing a high degree of visual and tactile sensitivity, Karen had related to people largely through those modalities, quietly savoring contact in favorable circumstances, but closing her eyes and withdrawing into sleep when conditions were unsatisfactory. By the age of 3, she had developed a pattern of motor restriction, underaggressivity, vigilant avoidance of excessive stimulation, and defensive scotomization, coupled with exquisite perceptual sensitivity and a rich and active fantasy life. As we followed her development further, we were impressed both with the stability of this pattern and with the important role it played in her overall development.

In another of our children, Jack, we saw how from infancy, an unusual capacity to tolerate tension was combined with a particular perceptual style of slow, thorough observation and assessment of his objects and environment. Such attributes significantly influenced his ongoing development and contributed to the evolution of a psychic constellation which included low-keyed, measured interaction with objects, steady drive progression and integration, much problem-solving activity in the realm of fantasy, and a highly developed use of his intellect for careful observation, empathic understanding, the working over of drive demands, and scientific explorations. These individual variations in ego function became an important factor in his ongoing development.

SELF AND OBJECT REPRESENTATIONS AND
THE REGULATION OF SELF-ESTEEM

In the process of passage through the normal autistic, symbiotic, and separation-individuation phases (Mahler, 1968), each child in the study appeared to have developed a unique set of self and object representations and a related group of mechanisms for preserving self-esteem and narcissistic well-being that greatly influenced his current and ongoing perception of himself and of the object world in general.

One aspect of this involved self-object differentiation (Jacobson, 1964). Disturbances in this area could be traced to regressions, the impact of endowment, the effect of certain conflicts, or environmental interferences. A second facet involved the nature of the self and object representations. We saw that the way in which the children viewed themselves and their main objects, consciously and unconsciously, affected the way they approached the tasks of the phallic-oedipal period in important ways.

A third aspect was the economic one. By the time a child had reached the age of 3 there might already have been a significant depletion in the narcissistic cathexis of the self representation, an overidealization of his objects, or a pattern of narcissistic grandiosity, excessive self-preoccupation and withdrawal from objects. In such instances, the disturbances were carried over into the phallic and oedipal struggles, coloring their form and contents and imposing limitations upon their outcome. At the time of the first Profile, we already could see which aspects of the self representation received special narcissistic cathexis and we could discern certain aspects of the evolving ego ideals, including whether they contained demands which were excessively high or low.

Another item of importance involved the maintenance of self-esteem. It was significant whether or not self-esteem regulation was based upon realistic self and object representations and actual achievements. In some instances the ego had acquired confidence in its ability to maintain control over tension states, achieve independent mastery, and secure affection and approval from its objects. In others, for various reasons, self-esteem was dependent to a significant extent upon the provision of certain external supplies.

We could offer many examples of the significance of this developmental dimension. Mark, for example, who had difficulty regulating the expression of his aggressivity, had suffered a number of object losses (including that of his father) early in his life. His image of himself as dangerously destructive to his objects and of men as weak, disappointing, and helplessly vulnerable to illness and death contributed in an important way to his need hastily to give up his rivalrous oedipal ambitions and to the weakness of his striving toward a masculine identity.

Jeanette's alertness, superior intellectual endowment, high tension tolerance, adaptability, and unusual capacity for self-control and delay were quickly recognized by her dependent and ambitious but unsuccessful parents. In their eagerness to realize their ambitions vicariously through her, they actively reinforced her high self-expectations and fostered the development of a lofty ideal self to which she aspired. The central constellation observable in her fourth year was organized about the need to maintain this idealized self representation. She easily advanced into a phallic libidinal organization, in which her fantasies included an all-powerful, illusory phallus. Yet, the need to be in continual command of an adulatory environment and her inability to risk defeat severely compromised Jeanette's ability to engage herself in oedipal, rivalrous struggles, and she entered latency as a haughty, lonely girl who was incapable of intense social relationships and hampered by the burden of unresolved oedipal and preoedipal conflicts.

A Clinical Illustration of the Central Constellation

We have chosen a child in whom all four component areas of the central constellation are well defined and in whom the contribution of the constellation to oedipal and early latency development is particularly clear. The psychological makeup of this child also afforded us an unusually good view of her fantasy life and intellectual processes; she has received no psychological treatment to complicate the developmental process.

KAREN AT THE BEGINNING OF NURSERY SCHOOL

Karen was just 3 years old when she started in our nursery school. She stood out not only for her delicate prettiness, but even more for her sober demeanor and quiet aloofness. She keenly observed all the activities, but held back for a long time from direct participation. Although she obviously yearned for attention from the teachers, her overtures were so meek and tentative that they often went unanswered. She was happy when they responded in a friendly but low-keyed manner, but had to pull away when they were effusive with her. When her overtures were ignored, she was dejected and withdrew temporarily into a solitary reverie, accompanied at times by autoerotic activity.

Karen could more easily accept the friendly approaches of the other children, and gradually reached out for friendship with them, but she tended to withdraw whenever there was more than one other child in the play. She occupied herself mainly with simple, solitary activities that afforded her a good vantage point for observing the others. She alternated in her play between competitively making the tallest towers and constructing carefully tended buildings and enclosures, which she populated with people and animals.

In her individual interview with a male observer, Karen appeared to be very interested in him, but froze after she had taken two steps into the room. She stood there during the interview and poured out a stream of anxious, loosely organized chatter, the content of which concerned feelings of helplessness, conflicts over eating and biting, yearning for her father, who had just gone on a plane trip, fear of being overexcited sexually the way she had been at times with her father and brother, and guilt over masturbation and sex play with her brother. At home, Karen continued to compete actively with her brother for her mother's attention. She indicated repeatedly that she felt cheated (of attention, oral supplies, her father, and a phallus), but was unable to maintain an angry attack upon her mother without soon making up to her.

EARLY HISTORY

Karen had been conceived in the hope of saving a crumbling marriage. Her mother characteristically staved off anxiety and depression via flamboyant bravado, seductiveness, a stream of chatter, and immersion in a kaleidoscopic sea of sensation. Her father was charismatic, creative, and unpredictable. During Karen's infancy, her mother became increasingly anxious and depressed as the inevitability of a divorce became obvious. The father left the home when Karen was 8 months old, but he continued seeing the children three times a week until the divorce, when Karen was 2½, after which he temporarily left the state. Although his contact with the children was irregular thereafter, with absences of many months at a time, Karen remained loyally attached to him.

Karen was so motorically inactive during the first few days after her birth that her mother worried about her. She developed colic, which lasted for four months. She was noted from the very beginning to be unusually alert, perceptive, and visually observant. Like her older brother, Karen very early discriminated between men and women. She showed a clear preference for men, and made an early attachment to her father.

Blocked tear ducts had to be pressed out each day by her mother during her first year. They were finally probed free by the doctor when Karen was 12 months old. Teething, which took place quickly, was associated with a moderate amount of discomfort.

Karen's mother tended to offer the breast to her frequently as a universal panacea. When weaning was attempted at 6 months, Karen resolutely refused to accept a cup, and continued at the breast until it was abruptly removed at 10 months. She refused milk in any form for the next year and a half. Mrs. K. was intermittently depressed and anxious during Karen's first year. Most of the time, she responded appropriately to Karen's needs, but there were times when she was less available. At other times, apparently in response to her own needs, Mrs. K. picked Karen up to cuddle and feed her when she actually had been quietly asleep. Rather than protesting these ill-timed, intrusive stimulations, Karen responded by closing her eyes and "falling asleep."

Toilet training was begun at 2 years of age and took about a year to complete. On the toilet Karen showed anxiety that began with fear of falling in; the flushing also disturbed her. She made no protest against the toilet-training demands and did well for a while, but when her parents were divorced and her father moved away, a general ego regression took place, during which she wet herself intermittently day and night, and she tended periodically to retain her stool. Her father returned when she was 3 years old; she responded by recovering from her regressive episode and attaining complete control of toilet functions.

When she was about 2½ years old, she began to masturbate and was seduced by her 4½-year-old brother into mutual genital explorations, which continued intermittently thereafter with the mother's tacit approval. Karen's brother, the only sibling, was good looking, aggressive, and talented, and Mrs. K. scarcely concealed her preference for him.

DEVELOPMENTAL ASSESSMENT AT 3 YEARS

Phase Progression

At 3 years, Karen showed intense libidinal wishes and longings, with an adherent attachment to her aims and objects and intense fear both of overstimulation and of loss. Despite intermittent temporary flight and emotional withdrawal, she maintained cathexis of her objects via vivid fantasy relationships to them even when they actually were absent or unavailable. Her persistent longings and her efforts to seek out new possibilities of finding the gratifying relationships for which she yearned encouraged continual psychosexual progression.

A fluid libidinal organization seemed to have emerged, in which persistent oral yearnings had become interwoven with powerful longings to receive a penis. These unified longings contributed to the yearning for a man as a rescuer and provider, although inability to risk the loss of her mother prevented Karen from pushing away from her. There was a capacity for fluid, progressive-regressive shifts within her drive organization, without firm closure and with only relative phallic primacy. There had been a weakness in her anal level engagement and in her ability to control and dominate her objects. The early sexual play with her brother seemed nevertheless to have promoted early vaginal awareness and fantasies (e.g., a lollypop was found in her vagina when she was 2½ years old) which, combined with her observations of her mother's coquettish interest in men and her early attachment to her father, had stimulated movement into phallic and oedipal interests.

Drive Balance and Discharge Patterns

Karen showed intense libidinal cathexis of object representations, accompanied by a relative inability to mobilize aggressive energies either to assert and secure possession of her objects or to do battle with them. The genetic roots seemed to include both innate and experiential factors.

Karen had been relatively inactive motorically as an infant, relating to the world largely via perceptual (especially visual and tactile) channels. She had possessed a considerable need for sensual contact from infancy on, enjoying the contact when it was presented in a comfortable fashion and withdrawing from it by tuning out and turning off contact when it was intensive or hyperstimulating. From the combination of innate inclinations and the effect of repeated experiences with objects who were inconsistent, often overstimulating, and difficult to control or influence, she had developed a pattern of pursuing objects by studying them, learning to anticipate their behavior, and adapting her own behavior to make herself pleasing to them, rather than aggressively demanding from them what she needed or complaining when they failed her.

The Developmental Effect of Early Variations in Ego Equipment and Organization

From earliest infancy, Karen had presented a striking combination of relative motor inactivity and a high degree of visual alertness and perceptual activity. She had tended to use tactile sensitivity and visual pursuit as her favored modalities for relating to the world around her. She also had tended from very early on to withdraw from ill-timed intrusions and experiences of overstimulation by closing her eyes and retreating into a sleeplike state. These early characteristics seemed to have developed from her particular endowment, reinforced by ongoing experiences (the pattern of feeding and maternal handling, the lacrymal duct probing, uncomfortable teething, maternal depression and anxiety, and her father's departures), especially during the first year.

An early tendency to employ a defensive style centering about flight, avoidance, and withdrawal, rather than mobilizing aggressive energies to demand gratification and fight off unwelcome intrusions, had persisted as a basic, ongoing characteristic. Karen had become particularly sensitive, empathic, and observant, but was continually on guard against the possibility of being overwhelmed by excessive stimulation. Associated with this was an ego attitude toward her own aggressive and libidinal impulses in which vivid, relatively undisguised fantasies could be tolerated, but their direct motor expression was prohibited. The ego avoided the possibility of their enactment, at the expense at times of an extensive restriction of ego activity in general.

Karen's learning capacity was enhanced by acute powers of observation, a ready capacity to absorb rote information, a vivid memory, and a fine sense of color and form. It was hindered, on the other hand, by her tendency to turn away from painful or disturbing stimuli, avoid the new and unknown, and reduce impinging stimuli by scotomizing the field of attention. Avoidance of competition and an inclination to hold on to what was already possessed, but not seek after more, completed the picture observable at 3 years.

Self and Object Representations and the Regulation of Self-Esteem

Karen's self and object representations centered about vivid images of idealized, loving, and protective objects whom she yearned to possess in reality, although she had little confidence that she might actually succeed in doing so. Although her past experiences had led her to view her objects as potential sources of pleasurable gratification, they also had led her to perceive them as unreliable, frequently elusive or unavailable, and often painfully overstimulating. Correspondingly, she viewed herself as being not quite desirable enough to attract her objects or as strong enough to catch, hold onto, and control them.

Karen's self representation had received insufficient narcissistic investment and she lacked the capacity to mobilize enough aggression to achieve full individuation from her objects. Since her self-esteem was still largely dependent upon the objects' response to her, she was cautious lest she alienate them. She suppressed angry, complaining feelings and made an effort to be good and pleasing to win their favor. Since her defensive style was organized about flight, avoidance, and restriction of activity, she was hindered in her ability to utilize reality experiences to modify either her fears or the contents of her self and object representations. This served to reinforce the tendency to withdraw from interaction with actual, new objects and to turn to her highly cathected, idealized, fantasy objects. She always returned, however, to an interest in the outside world, where she sought objects who might approximate the idealized object representations which she held so dear. This indicated to us that she did not give up hope, but maintained her object cathexis at times of disappointment and injury. It was possible, therefore, that if she were fortunate enough to find the right people, she would be capable of achieving meaningful change as a result of her interaction with these new objects.

THE CENTRAL CONSTELLATION AT 3 YEARS

The initial Profile contained evidence of the coordination of the key developmental factors we have described above into an internally coordinated constellation possessing a high degree of stability. As we have followed Karen's development, we have become increasingly convinced that this constellation has been an influence upon her ongoing development. A strong innate progressive push, reinforced by the forward pull exerted by a sexually stimulating environment, more than counteracted the retarding effects of oral fixations. Since her ego organization permitted wide progressive-regressive fluctuation and an unusual degree of fluidity and overlap, early fixations did not prevent developmental advance, but were carried along and woven into the higher levels of organization which progressively evolved.

Karen's relative inability to mobilize aggression interfered with her ability to take control of and possess her objects and interfered with certain aspects of individuation, but it also contributed to the preservation of her object cathexes at times of disappointment and narcissistic injury. This very sensual little girl's tendency to establish intense, discriminative cathexes and her ability to maintain her object cathexes in fantasy, even in the prolonged absence of her cathected object, helped preserve the availability of constant, positive object representations. Although her self-esteem remained dependent upon positive responses from her more or less idealized objects, she was able to seek out such responses and to use them in the service of developmental progression.

The ability to make restitutive use of fantasy at times of actual frustration and failure enabled her to retreat temporarily when confronted by overwhelming stress. Stemming partly from intrinsic variations in ego endowment and partly from the impact of early experiences of overstimulation and ego inadequacy, she seemed to have developed a well-organized defense system built around avoidance, temporary introversion and withdrawal, flight, and ego restriction. It served to control anxiety, although at the price of reduced ego flexibility and freedom of action, so that developmental progression could proceed. An important aspect of Karen's central constellation was the ability to make good use of environmental resources to facilitate developmental progression.

THE PHALLIC-OEDIPAL PHASE

There was steady movement forward between 3 and 6 years into increasing phallic and oedipal interests. Although phallic organization was attained, her libidinal organization remained fluid, with a plentiful admixture of oral fantasy and conflict and an ease of progressive-regressive alternation. Karen persistently wooed her father, who had returned to the city with his new wife, and there was evidence of intense genital excitement in his presence, associated with wishes to abandon herself to him. She was frightened by her excitement, however, particularly at times of natural regression, and was unable to spend the night at her father's apartment. She maintained an intense, visual, idealizing interest in him as well as vivid fantasies about him when she was not with him, but her activity was restricted in his presence and she had difficulty expressing appropriate anger at him.

There was evidence of intense anger at her mother and of attempts to push away from her, but Karen was inhibited in her expressions of resentment and hostility, which she was unable to sustain for long. There were indications of intermittent longing for closeness with her mother (which at times had to be warded off anxiously) and of inability to give her up as a source of narcissistic reinforcement and libidinal satisfaction. Karen was a fussy eater at school as well as at home and developed a number of transient food intolerances.

At school, Karen was increasingly assertive and capable of a certain amount of verbal aggression and sarcasm, but she continued to be relatively restricted, inhibited, and somewhat phobic. She became increasingly able to woo the attention of her favorite teachers, but remained quite cautious and overly sensitive to rebuff. Her learning and her peer relations progressed, but she was limited to a significant extent by her cautiousness, reluctance to explore the unknown, tendency to scotomize, and relative inability to be competitive. She grew increasingly interested in the male investigator who was following her progress, and gradually acquired the courage to approach him in the classroom and woo his attentions in competition with the other girls. When she finally dared to make physical contact with him, she reacted with excitement that necessitated prompt removal of herself from his presence. In her semiannual interviews with him, she initially showed a wistful yearning for him to be a prince charming who would like her, care for her, and provide her with the feeding breast she had lost and the phallus of which she had been cheated. This fantasy gradually faded and was replaced by increasingly exciting images of being taken for wild roller-coaster rides, being thrown down and run over, and being attacked and torn apart. Castration themes alternated with restitution themes in these fantasies. Retreat to peaceful scenes of mutual feeding became less and less prominent with each set of interviews until it finally disappeared.

THE LATENCY PERIOD

Karen moved into latency via resigned acceptance that she could not obtain from her parents all that she wanted from them. Her mother was absorbed increasingly in pursuing a career and social activities, with less and less time and energy available for the children. Her father remarried when Karen was $5\frac{1}{2}$, and a year later had a son. This half brother aroused in Karen wistful envy of the lovingly fed baby and the fantasy of herself becoming father's bride.

Karen gradually shifted from her parents to her teachers as objects to be wooed and won. She was fortunate in that each year from 5 to 9 her teacher was a perceptive young woman who liked and appreciated Karen and was alert to her need for low-keyed interest, warmth, and approval. Their descriptions of Karen bore a striking resemblance to our original observation of her. They depicted her as a perceptive observer, sensitive to the responses of others, averse to exploring the unfamiliar, and reluctant to take the initiative, although she responded well to gentle encouragement.

Karen became excited but anxious in the presence of men. With familiar men, including her father, she was provocative and seductive, but she shunned direct physical contact (even at 9, she did not like to be kissed by her father). Her reaction to new men in her life was largely one of avoidance. The wildness of the boys and the excitement they aroused in her discomfited her. Her intense wish to be liked, her efforts to please, and her empathetic response to their needs made her very popular with her peers. Although her academic achievements and popularity did much to raise her self-esteem, she continued to feel uncertain of her successes and to worry about losing her place in her friends' affections, even when she was past the age of 9 years. She gradually became able to express anger and to register complaints against her mother (and brother), but she could do so only timidly. She developed a rather typical feminine superego organization, although with more dependence upon external approbation and fear of loss of approval and admiration than the average.

The Theoretical Significance of the Central Constellation

We have described the emergence by the age of 3 or 4 years of a relatively stable, organized, central psychic constellation which persists thereafter as an influential factor. Our conclusions are related to two fundamental propositions regarding human development. One is the notion that development proceeds via a process of sequential organization and reorganization in which new systems of psychic functioning periodically evolve to supersede previously existing systems as dominant, organizational configurations. The other is the proposal that increasing differentiation and hierarchy formation are accompanied in the developmental process by a tendency to internal coordination and cohesion which leads to stability and systemic integrity. To state the latter proposition another way, there is an intrinsic tendency toward synthesis and self-regulation which leads to a "bonding between the interacting components" (Sander, 1973).

The work of a number of investigators suggests that in the course of development there are certain nodal points at which critical reorganizations can be identified. Freud (1905), for example, reconstructed the existence of successive waves of libidinal reorganization in childhood, each of which centers about a particular erotogenic zone. Abraham (1925) defined the epigenetic nature of this sequence of libidinal reorganization. Erikson (1950) later expanded this point of view to include the psychosocial aspects of development and extended its application to the entire life cycle from birth to death.

Spitz (1959, 1965), Ritvo et al. (1963), and others have demonstrated that a sequence of progressive reorganizations can be observed in the first two years in which psychic elements periodically regroup themselves into a new, relatively stable, superordinate organization which supplants the previous one as the current *modus operandi* of adaptation. Each new organizational system has its own way of perceiving, processing, and responding to environmental stimuli and drive demands. The periodic regroupings, leading to new levels of psychic equilibrium, derive only partly from the appearance of new ego structures. In part, they derive from shifts in the coordination or patterning of already existing structures.

Piaget has shown that cognitive development proceeds by means of a complex, epigenetic sequence in which each developmental stage is derived from and represents the outer limit of equilibrium of the previous stage (Silverman, 1971). He has demonstrated that the process of reorganization in each stage leads to the crystallization of an end point of organizational patterning in which firm internal bonding provides relative stability. Cognitive development may be particularly well suited, in fact, to demonstrate the interplay of epigenetic reorganization and synthesis or interaction of constituent elements into stable, dynamic systems within the developmental process. George Klein, for example, has described the evolution during early childhood of an organized system of multiple, cognitive controls which together constitute a lifelong, cognitive style that is unique in each individual. He concluded that in the course of progressive restructuring of psychic mechanisms there evolves a stable, regulating organization which represents an equilibrial balance among individual variations in intrinsic ego equipment, response to the pressure of drive demands, and the necessity of accommodating to environmental restrictions (Klein, 1954, 1958; Santostefano, 1969).

It is our impression that the age of 3 years may be a nodal point at which a crucial, developmental reorganization reaches stability. The child's style of progressive-regressive movement usually cannot be adequately appreciated until he has gone through enough of the total range of his libidinal development at least to have entered the phallic phase. Except in extreme instances, it is also not until then that the developmental impact of prephallic fixations can be gauged. Often enough, the relative balance between libidinal and aggressive drive pressures does not reach a stable enough form for it to be identified accurately before the move forward from anal ambivalence conflicts to phallic phase interests. By the age of 3, the child's ego capacities have had time to unfold and develop, and the impact of his innate endowment has had a chance to demonstrate itself. By then, there has been enough time for him to utilize his resources in interaction with an expanding object world, with its various adaptational demands and its provision of a range of stimuli and opportunities for exercise of the child's mental and emotional machinery. Three years is also the age cited by Mahler (1968) as the time when the separation-individuation process has proceeded sufficiently for relative object constancy and relatively stable self and object representations to have been attained. These various dimensions seem gradually to become organized with one another, under the direction of the integrative function (Hartmann, 1939).

The observation that certain developmental characteristics coalesce early in life into stable, dynamic groupings exerting influence upon further development is not a new one. In addition to Spitz (1959, 1965), Sander (1962, 1970), Escalona (1963), and others have made extensive investigations into the evolution of patterned modes of functioning out of the coordination of the innate rhythms and executive tendencies of the infant with the modifying influence of the mother's responses to him.

Anna Freud (1971) has described an early "psychosomatic matrix," deriving from this interaction, which sets the scene for the development of certain aspects of the pleasure-unpleasure balance, the form and strength of object attachment, certain ego strengths and weaknesses, and the pathway to somatic compliance. These form a matrix, according to Anna Freud, out of which later id and ego structures, conflicts involving the emerging component drives, and the infantile neurosis ultimately develop.

Annemarie Weil (1970) has formulated in rich detail how the interaction between the infant's equipment and early experiences leads to the emergence of a "basic core" of fundamental trends which accompanies the infant as he enters the symbiotic phase. Since the basic core influences and intertwines with later psychological developments, it continues to be evident, according to Weil, as a more or less discrete, psychic organization within the personality as it develops further.

Our own observation of a developmentally influential central constellation in the fourth year dovetails closely with the concepts of the "psychosomatic matrix" and the "basic core." What we have described in this paper appears to be a manifestation of the tendency within the developing psychic apparatus toward periodic regrouping of central tendencies and characteristics into a new, central organization which incorporates the previous one into it as it supersedes it as a central, guiding, developmental constellation. Anna Freud's concept of multiple, converging and diverging, developmental lines (1965) is pertinent in this regard. Periodically, certain key lines of development intersect in such a way that they become mutually coordinated and organized into a relatively stable constellation of forces, which then plays a central role in the developmental process. The central constellation observable in the fourth year would seem to grow out of earlier organizational constellations as they interact with new structures and with the deformations imposed upon the psychic apparatus by new developmental requirements.

We have been tracing the fate of the central constellation itself in the course of further development. What we have seen so far has indicated that it persists with sufficient stability to stamp itself upon the organization of the personality during the oedipal and latency periods. Besides affecting the form and content of oedipal conflicts and the options available for their resolution, it influences character structure, intellectual and cognitive styles, and sublimative potential, at least during the period in which we have followed the children. To understand the degree to which the constellation itself changes in the course of development through childhood and into adulthood will require further longitudinal study, correlated with study and review of the analyses of children and adults. We are not yet in a position to assess this adequately, but we hope to continue our study until the children have reached early adulthood. We are especially interested in seeing what will be the effect of the major shifts and reorganizations that can be expected to take place during adolescence.

It is our impression that our observations fit in with a current tendency in child psychoanalysis to evolve a theoretical formulation which fits the oedipus complex into the mainstream of development at the same time that it recognizes its central role in the organization of the neuroses. We are referring to a shift in emphasis from a formulation which depicts the oedipus complex as *the cause of the neurosis* to one which would consider the oedipus complex as a *dynamically central feature* of a developmental process which may or may not predispose to neurotic solutions of developmental tasks. In this formulation, unresolved oedipal conflicts would appear as a central part of the neurotic process rather than as its source. Anna Freud (1971) stated:

> There is a world of difference between . . . the past and the present scene. What we are pursuing at present are not evaluations undertaken from the viewpoint of any later mental disorder but an elaborate map of infantile mental difficulties as such, or, to express it more succinctly, an enumeration, description, and explanation of any interference with optimal mental growth and development. On the basis of our knowledge of developmental phases, as established by reconstruction from adult analysis, by child analysis, by direct observation of infants and young children, we attempt to do this from birth onward, with the phallic-oedipal phase placed not at the lower but at the upper end of our investigation. . . . It appears almost as a by-product that, while doing so, we also assemble those developmental aspects which, in due course, will lend themselves to the production of conflicts and may even determine beforehand which among the available defense mechanisms the individual's ego will choose to employ and, accordingly, which forms of compromise and symptom formation will be open to him [p. 82].

This is not to say that all neurotic manifestations arise out of processes that begin in the earliest years. A developmental process that is proceeding adequately can be altered at any point, particularly by events occurring in such critical periods as the oedipal stage. An initially adequate developmental process can be transformed in this manner into a deviant one. But even in such a case, it would seem to us that organizational predispositions must also play an important role, along with and in interaction with traumatic experiences, in determining the final outcome.

Psychoanalysis has demonstrated that neurotic disorders consist of unsuccessful attempts to obtain relief from insoluble, unconscious conflict. It has been recognized that the main conflicts underlying the infantile neurosis crystallize during the oedipal period. Advances in ego psychology, investigations into the psychoses and narcissistic disorders, and the opportunity to carry out longitudinal observations of infants and young children, however, have called our attention to the enormous importance of preoedipal development in neurosogenesis. It has even led some investigators to question whether the principal determinant of emotional health or neurosis is the oedipal conflict and its resolution or whether matters are already decided in the period before the emergence of the oedipal conflict. Our study suggests to us that the issue may not be whether the earlier period or the oedipal conflicts are more significant, but how the earlier developments contribute to the content and form of the oedipal conflicts and the means employed to resolve them.

The psychoanalytic view of the developmental process emphasizes the significance of fixation points which impede developmental progression and predispose the individual to regressive flight to escape from the tensions and anxieties created by insoluble conflict at higher levels. The regression, of course, only leads to new conflicts and anxieties at earlier levels of psychic organization. We believe the understanding of neurotic functioning would be broadened by supplementing this genetic point of view, with its emphasis upon fixation and regression, with one which looks upon the developmental process prospectively as a steadily evolving and reorganizing dynamic interplay of psychic forces.

This might help clarify the individual differences among children as they progress through the various developmental phases. Employing the concept of the early crystallization of a central constellation has provided us with an extra vantage point from which to consider a number of questions. One of these concerns the ability of some children to relinquish or modify their maternal attachments relatively easily during the course of their oedipal struggles, while others cling tenaciously to them at all costs. A second involves the factors determining the choice of fantasy or action as the preferred channel of discharge and the impact of this choice upon the oedipal outcome. Other questions which seem to be elucidated concern the choice by different children of different sets of defense mechanisms with which they struggle with their oedipal conflicts, the degree to which oedipal conflicts are object-oriented or narcissistic in orientation, the tendency to employ predominantly positive or negative oedipal solutions, and certain aspects of the structure of the ego ideal and the superego's methods of enforcing its prohibitions.

The value of coordinating the genetic point of view with a developmental one emphasizes the importance of the principles of epigenesis, synthesis, progressive organization and reorganization, and change of function. When the early stages of development are reconstructed in the course of a therapeutic analysis, they may appear to be relatively discrete, well-demarcated, and discontinuous in nature. When one follows children prospectively, however, one sees a great deal of overlap, fluctuation to and fro, and a gradual, shifting metamorphosis in which old mechanisms acquire new functions and old patterns are rearranged and more or less modified in the interest of adaptation to new tasks and new requirements.

Nunberg's emphasis upon the importance of the synthetic function has been very helpful to us. He pointed out that underlying the increasing efficiency of the evolving psychic apparatus is an inherent tendency to integration and consolidation: "The tendency to simplify and generalize, to integrate and the like, reveals that the synthetic function of the ego is subject to an economic principle, which induces the ego to economize expenditure of effort. . . . Synthesis thus brings about not only unity of the whole personality but also simplification and economy in the ego's mode of operation" (1932, p. 153). The concept of a synthetic (Nunberg, 1930) or integrative (Hartmann, 1939) function operative within the developmental process has enabled us to study the ways in which developing structures and functions are fitted together and coordinated into operational systems and subsystems in the course of development.

The Clinical Implications of the Central Constellation

The data emerging from our studies are clinically relevant. The diagnostic evaluation of children is complex and arduous. Symptoms and developmental disturbances, as Anna Freud (1965, 1974) repeatedly has stressed, are significant only insofar as they reflect the existence of meaningful disturbances of overall developmental progression or of key elements within it. Assessment of the pattern of developmental progression is particularly difficult with the prelatency child, for whom the diagnostic task is largely predictive in nature.

In a previous paper (Silverman and Neubauer, 1971), we stated our opinion that with prelatency children a series of cross-sectional Profiles was required to obtain the longitudinal dimension that would permit an assessment of *the developmental significance* of temporary disturbances, symptoms, or imbalances. It is our impression at this point, however, that delineation of the central constellation identifiable by $3\frac{1}{2}$ years can be an alternative means of determining the directions in which overall development is proceeding. It describes the paths being taken by important developmental lines and the ways in which they are knitting together and becoming mutually organized. It has helped us to see the degree to which various patterns and structures are open to change and the directions in which they can be expected to steer developmental responses to the phase-specific experiences and conflicts of the oedipal and latency periods. Since the constellation contains important indications of the basic fabric of the personality organization, it is a key to understanding the way in which the child will deal with the issues which have to be resolved in the years ahead.

If it turns out that treatment is indicated, the central constellation can help the clinician decide which forms of intervention are most likely to be effective. The choice is especially wide with preschoolers, since important areas of the personality are still plastic and are highly vulnerable to outside influence. Mapping out the central constellation can help the clinician to pinpoint the precise target areas toward which therapy should be directed. It may be possible, for example, by strengthening a specific ego function to alter a child's self representation in important ways and to bring about necessary changes in his or her defensive system. Recourse to the central constellation also can help distinguish between those areas which are rigidly locked into a pattern of maldevelopment and those in which longitudinal, developmental pressures are likely to bring about sufficient, fortuitous growth and reorganization that the decision whether or not to intervene in the developmental process can be postponed to a later time. The grasp of the basic personality fabric which the central constellation provides can help the clinician to achieve precision in his choice among the various therapeutic procedures available by pinpointing the impact of each at any point in time. It can help him to decide whether the best therapeutic approach will be a specific educational program, efforts to effect changes in parental handling, the provision of new object relationships, one or another psychotherapeutic approach, or a carefully planned sequence of more than one of these modalities.

We believe that our observations are of significance to the psychoanalyst whether he is working with children or with adults. The psychoanalytic task consists in undoing fixations and facilitating the resolution of repressed conflicts. The method we have been employing for this has been principally genetic and dynamic in its approach, but these points of view have been coordinated more and more over the years with structural and developmental viewpoints. The psychoanalytic method concentrated at first upon reconstructing the emergence of insoluble unconscious conflicts between drive pressures, ego and superego attitudes, and environmental demands. This has been supplemented increasingly by an interest in studying the structural organization within which the conflicts emerge and are perpetuated and in exploring the shifts and changes which take place at successive developmental levels.

It is here that our observations become relevant. We have seen that by the age of $3\frac{1}{2}$, a number of influential developmental factors have coalesced into a relatively stable balance of forces within the personality organization and that this constellation helps to regulate the way in which experiences are perceived and dealt with from that point on. It would seem to us that reconstruction of the emergence of this central psychic constellation out of its constituent components and of its developmental impact (as well as of the internal changes forced upon it by developmental progression) at each level thereafter would enhance the psychoanalyst's understanding of his analysands, whatever their age. It would add to our grasp of the interplay of forces operating within them and, therefore, to the origins of their characterological and neurotic structural formations. It would place us in a better position to define the limits within which we might expect change to take place in our patients and to map out the specific strategy by means of which we might facilitate the attainment of such changes.

Summary

In this report we called attention to a central psychic constellation which is observable by the age of 3 or 3½ and which appears to play an important role as a codeterminant of the form and early outcome of the struggles and conflicts of prelatency and latency. Our findings stem from a longitudinal study of the developmental process in which data emerging from regular observations and interviews have been correlated wherever possible with therapeutic insights.

We attempted to demonstrate that the central constellation arises out of the coordination during the first three years of life of certain key, preoedipal, developmental variables into a psychic organization possessing sufficient cohesion and stability to maintain a significant impact upon the course of further development. Clinical material was adduced to illustrate the constellation and its components. We described certain variables that are particularly significant in the formation of this constellation.

We considered some of the clinical and theoretical implications of our findings. Psychoanalytic investigators have been attempting to integrate the increasingly vast body of data about the preoedipal period with the assumptions concerning the central role of the oedipus complex in human psychic functioning. We hope that our work, which focuses upon the transition between the preoedipal and ocdipal periods, will facilitate the successful completion of this complex and difficult task.

BIBLIOGRAPHY

ABRAHAM, K. (1925), Character-Formation on the Genital Level of the Libido. *Selected Papers on Psycho-Analysis.* London: Hogarth Press, 1927, pp. 407–417.

ALPERT, A., NEUBAUER, P. B., & WEIL, A. P. (1956), Unusual Variations in Drive Endowment. *This Annual*, 11:125-163.

ERIKSON, E. H. (1950), Growth and Crises of the Healthy Personality. In: *Identity and the Life Cycle* [*Psychological Issues*, Monogr. 1]. New York: Int. Univ. Press, 1959, pp. 50-100.

ESCALONA, S. K. (1963), Patterns of Infantile Experience and the Developmental Process, *This Annual*, 18:197-244.

—— (1968), *The Roots of Individuality*. Chicago: Aldine Publishing.

—— & HEIDER, G. (1959), *Prediction and Outcome*. New York: Basic Books.

FREUD, A. (1965), *Normality and Pathology in Childhood*. New York: Int. Univ. Press.

—— (1971), The Infantile Neurosis. *This Annual*, 26:79-90.

—— (1974), A Psychoanalytic View of Developmental Psychopathology. *J. Philadelphia Assn. Psychoanal.*, 1:7-17.

FREUD, S. (1905), Three Essays on the Theory of Sexuality. *S.E.*, 7:125-243.

HARTMANN, H. (1939), *Ego Psychology and the Problem of Adaptation*. New York: Int. Univ. Press, 1958.

JACOBSON, E. (1964), *The Self and the Object World*. New York: Int. Univ. Press.

KLEIN, G. S. (1954), Need and Regulation. In: *Nebraska Symposium on Motivation*, ed. M. R. Jones. Lincoln: Univ. Nebraska Press, pp. 224-274.

—— (1958), Cognitive Control and Motivation. In: *Assessment of Human Motives*, ed. G. Lindzey. New York: Rinehart, pp. 87-118.

KORNER, A. F. (1964), Some Hypotheses Regarding the Significance of Individual Differences at Birth for Later Development. *This Annual*, 19:58-72.

MAHLER, M. S. (1968), *On Human Symbiosis and the Vicissitudes of Individuation*. New York: Int. Univ. Press.

NUNBERG, H. (1930), The Synthetic Function of the Ego. In: *Practice and Theory of Psychoanalysis*, 1:120-136. New York: Int. Univ. Press, 1955.

—— (1932), *Principles of Psychoanalysis*. New York: Int. Univ. Press, 1955.

RITVO, S., MCCOLLOM, A. T., OMWAKE, E., PROVENCE, S. A., & SOLNIT, A. J. (1963), Some Relations of Constitution, Environment, and Personality As Observed in a Longitudinal Study of Child Development. In: *Modern Perspectives in Child Development*, ed. A. J. Solnit & S. A. Provence. New York: Int. Univ. Press, pp. 107-143.

SANDER, L. W. (1962), Issues in Early Mother-Child Interaction. *J. Amer. Acad. Child Psychiat.*, 1:141-166.

—— (1973), Infant and Caretaking Environment (unpublished manuscript).

—— STECHLER, G., BURNS, P., & JULIA, H. (1970), Early Mother-Infant Interaction and 24-Hour Patterns of Activity and Sleep. *J. Amer. Acad. Child Psychiat.*, 9:103-123.

SANTOSTEFANO, S. (1969), Cognitive Controls versus Cognitive Styles. *Seminars in Psychiatry*, 1:291-317.

SILVERMAN, M. A. (1971), The Growth of Logical Thinking. *Psychoanal. Quart.*, 40:317-341.

—— & NEUBAUER, P. B. (1971), Use of the Developmental Profile for the

Prelatency Child. In: *The Unconscious Today,* ed. M. Kanzer. New York: Int. Univ. Press, pp. 363–380.

SPITZ, R. A. (1959), *A Genetic Field Theory of Ego Formation.* New York: Int. Univ. Press.

——— (1965), *The First Year of Life.* New York: Int. Univ. Press.

THOMAS, A., CHESS, S., BIRCH, H. G., HERTZIG, M., & KORN, S. (1963), *Behavioral Individuality in Early Childhood.* New York: New York Univ. Press.

WEIL, A. P. (1956), Some Evidences of Deviational Development in Infancy and Early Childhood. *This Annual,* 11:292–299.

——— (1970), The Basic Core. *This Annual,* 25:442–460.

CONTRIBUTIONS TO PSYCHOANALYTIC THEORY

The Phallic-Narcissistic Phase

A Differentiation between Preoedipal and Oedipal Aspects of Phallic Development

ROSE EDGCUMBE, B.A., M.S. AND
MARION BURGNER, B.A.

OUR PREVIOUS WORK ON EARLY OBJECT RELATIONSHIPS (1972) LED US toward the understanding of development from the viewpoint of object relatedness as well as from the more classical viewpoint of the drives. The *psychological* capacity for object relatedness progresses through levels of maturity, developing out of the infant's biological and self-preservative needs for the libidinal object into gradually more complex relationships. We view these developments as *levels* of object relationships and distinguish them from the *phases* of drive development, though in optimal conditions the two proceed in parallel lines, smoothly and congruently.

The authors are child psychotherapists and research workers at the Hampstead Child-Therapy Course and Clinic, London, which is at present supported by the Field Foundation, Inc., New York; the Foundation for Research in Psychoanalysis, Beverly Hills, California; the Freud Centenary Fund, London; the Anna Freud Foundation, New York; the National Institute of Mental Health, Bethesda, Maryland; the Grant Foundation, New York; the New-Land Foundation, Inc., New York, and a number of private supporters.

This paper forms part of a Research Project entitled "Childhood Pathology: Impact on Later Mental Health." The Project is financed by the National Institute of Mental Health, Washington, D.C., Grant No. MH-5683-09. The paper also forms part of the work carried out by the Hampstead Index Committee, Chairman, Dr. J. Sandler. Our thanks are due to Renate Putzel and Trevor Hartnup for their participation in this study.

In our consideration of later phases of development from this dual viewpoint of object relatedness and drives, of particular interest to us was the phallic-oedipal phase of development. Our examination of the literature disclosed a tendency to assume that entry into the phallic phase is accompanied by the *simultaneous development* of oedipal relationships, so that the terms phallic, oedipal, and phallic-oedipal are often used synonymously. *Yet close scrutiny of clinical and observational material reveals distinct differences in the forms of drive derivatives and in the nature of the child's relationships in the preoedipal phallic phase as compared with the phallic-oedipal phase.* In the preoedipal phallic phase, exhibitionism and scoptophilia are the most pronounced drive components. In the child's object relationships, correspondingly, the real or fantasied use of the genital serves primarily exhibitionistic and narcissistic purposes, to gain the admiration of the object. In the preoedipal phallic phase, the one-to-one relationship is still dominant, since the rivalry of triangular oedipal relationships has not yet developed.

Many authors have described the changes in drive aims and relationships involved in the move into the oedipal phase, as well as the stages and vicissitudes within that phase (Freud, 1923, 1924, 1925, 1931; Lampl-de Groot, 1928, 1952; Brunswick, 1940; Deutsch, 1930). The assumption that a phallic child is also an oedipal child is in part a legacy from the historical growth of psychoanalytic theory. The concept of the oedipus complex was formulated by Freud as early as 1897, several years before his first formulations of the drive theory (1905) and the even later formulations of phase development which Freud added to the *Three Essays on Sexuality* in 1915. In fact, Freud did not differentiate between the phallic and the oedipal phases; for instance, in 1924 he wrote that the phallic phase, in which he saw the male genital organ as taking the leading role, "is contemporaneous with the Oedipus complex, does not develop further to the definitive genital organization, but is submerged, and is succeeded by the latency period" (p. 174).

In his more general formulations of object choice, Freud described the anaclitic nature of the early development of libidinal drives in relation to the object who satisfies the child's earliest self-preservative needs. Since at that time his primary emphasis was on drive development, he did not explore all aspects of the development of relationships through all developmental phases. Thus, he examined the object mainly from the viewpoints of finding an object for drive gratification and the changing expressions of drives toward the object. It is of interest to note that in his description of the oedipus complex he spelled out in more detail than in other phases the various relationships involved.

In order to clarify the development of relationships to self and objects during the early part of the phallic phase, we think it helpful to separate out the preoedipal phallic phase from the oedipal phase proper, since such a separation will enable us to examine in detail the development of object relatedness and drive development in these two phases. Further, we consider it appropriate to trace in more detail both the development of the body representation as an integral part of the developing self representation and the processes of identification affecting these representations. This development of self and body representations and of identifications makes a crucial contribution to the establishment of a differentiated sexual identity, to the narcissistic valuation of the sexually differentiated body, to the development from a two-person relationship to the triangular relationship of the oedipal phase, and to the organization of phallic drive aims in regard to the objects concerned.

THE PHALLIC-NARCISSISTIC PHASE

THE MAIN TASKS

We shall refer to the early, preoedipal part of the phallic phase as the *phallic-narcissistic phase*,[1] and reserve the term *oedipal phase* for the later part of the phallic phase when triangular oedipal relationships are established.

Psychic organization in the phallic-narcissistic phase is complicated by the presence of two factors not encountered in the oral and anal phases: first, the child has to attempt to come to terms with the differences between the sexes in the physical formation of the

---

[1] We are indebted to Anna Freud for this term.

genitals, the dominant erotogenic zone of the phallic phase; second, the child is faced with the task of recognizing and accepting the immaturity of his or her own genital apparatus and functioning. Normal development in the phallic-narcissistic and oedipal phases therefore requires a gradual divergence, in boys and girls, of drive derivatives, fantasies, sexual identifications, and modes of relating to the object, as well as a difference in the sex of the object to be chosen for the oedipal relationship. Every child has the task of consolidating his or her sexually differentiated body image, renouncing the sexual role not appropriate to his or her own sex, and accepting, relative though such an acceptance may be, the indefinite postponement of full adult genital functioning.

THE DEVELOPMENT OF THE BODY REPRESENTATION AND OF IDENTIFICATIONS

The establishment of the body representation has to be traced back to its starting point in the first weeks of life when diffuse, experiential awareness of polarities of feeling gradually differentiates into localized sensory perceptions belonging to specific parts of the body. When the infant starts to distinguish between what is external and what is internal, what belongs to his own body and what is given or taken in from the outside, the body representation has begun to be structured. Such localization of body parts, a process which may be seen as beginning at approximately 3 months with mouth-hand integration, serves to build up and establish the mental structure of a body image (Hoffer, 1950). In the second year of life, with the rapid development of cognitive and affective responses, this body representation becomes firmly integrated with the self representation, and we may surmise that the same mental structure serves both the body and the self representations; subsequently, these representations remain as an established and integral structure (Sandler and Rosenblatt, 1962). It is this representation of body and self which receives the narcissistic investment of the child, an investment which is in part determined by the objects' attitudes toward him (Joffe and Sandler, 1967). The child is aware of sexual differences prior to the phallic phase, but the narcissistic investment of sexually differentiated aspects of the body assumes particular importance with entry into the phallic phase, and with the consolidation of a sexual identity.

The process of acquiring a differentiated sexual identity rests largely on the child's capacity to identify with the parents of the same sex. We understand the process of identification as a modification of the self representation with the aim of acquiring some attributes of the object representation (Sandler and Rosenblatt, 1962; Sandler et al., 1963). And we define the acquiring of a sense of sexual identity as a process starting during the child's second year, continuing through the anal phase, and reaching its peak within the phallic phase.

We choose to restrict the term identity[2] quite particularly to one aspect of the child's self representation—the child's growing awareness of his or her sexual identity, an awareness which is intimately linked with the identifications with the parent of the same sex, as well as with the upsurge of phallic sexual drives with the entry into the phallic-narcissistic phase. Thus we see in the boy the precursors of his oedipal masculine attitudes toward the mother, while the girl[3] similarly manifests precursors of feminine oedipal attitudes toward the father.

Mahler (1958) describes "two crucial phases of identity formation: (1) the separation-individuation phase; (2) the phase of resolution of bisexual identification" (p. 136). With regard to the latter, she is reported to have said:

> The second crucial period of integration of feelings of identity extends from three years to latency, most significantly during the phallic phase with its massive concentration of libido in the sexual parts of the body image. Body-image representations now emerge from pregenital libidinal positions and bisexual identifications to firm establishment of sexual identity. Here not only successful integration of prior pregenital phases, but successful identification with the parent of the same sex and the emotional attitudes of both

---

[2] The concept of identity is a problematic one; it is sometimes used interchangeably with the concept of self representation, for instance, by Erikson (1950, 1956) who describes in careful detail the genetic sequence involved.

[3] While it is misleading to use the term "phallic" for the girl, at present we are at a loss for a more satisfactory one.

parents to the child's sexual identity are of paramount importance. Thus, the distinct feeling of self-identity hinges on solution of the oedipal conflict [p. 138].

We differ with Mahler in regard to timing, because we attach great importance to the phallic-narcissistic (preoedipal) phase as the time in which the child may be expected to acquire and to shape his own sexual identity; having done this, the child is then better able to enter the oedipal phase of development.

SEXUAL ACTIVITY AND FANTASIES

When the genital area first becomes a source of erotic pleasure, there is little difference between boys and girls in the way this pleasure is achieved; both stimulate themselves autoerotically by rubbing or squeezing their genitals; and if sexual pleasure is sought from the object, the child envisages it as taking the same form. Examples of this abound in the literature, starting with Freud's accounts (1909) of Little Hans who, at the age of 4¼ years, asked his mother to touch his penis because, "It's great fun"; and of a 3½-year-old girl who, while her mother was testing the fit of some new drawers, closed her thighs on her mother's hand, saying, "Oh, Mummy, *do* leave your hand there. It feels so lovely" (p. 19). This kind of masturbatory activity indicates only that the child has reached or is entering the phallic phase of drive development. It cannot be taken by itself as an indication that the child has attained the level of oedipal relationships: this can be determined only by the nature of the accompanying fantasies about and attitudes toward the object.

If at this early stage the child engages the object in some form of game indicating a wish for mutual sexual activity, there is little role differentiation between self and object. For example, early in treatment, Derek, a 3-year-old boy, wanted his therapist (a woman) and himself to have toy cars, which were made to chase, bump, touch, and drive over each other as well as their owners. Derek was visibly excited and his game was a thinly disguised form of a masturbatory wish to touch and to be touched. But at this time there was no clear differentiation between the roles of the two participants. Although Derek was already acutely aware of and anxious about bodily differences between the sexes, these had not yet assumed importance for him in terms of *differing sexual roles,* so that it was not yet possible to discern a fantasy of the penis penetrating the woman.

Intercourse fantasies during the phallic-narcissistic phase show a similar lack of differentiation of sexual roles: characteristically they are expressed in terms of activities belonging to earlier drive phases, e.g., oral impregnation and anal birth, or the mixing of urine or feces produced by two people, but with no clear differentiation between the activities of the partners.

For example, Jane, aged $3\frac{1}{2}$, made use of her therapist in the transference situation to reenact her infantile sexual theories of impregnation and birth; one such reenactment concerned her wish to urinate and defecate in the therapist's company so that they could make a baby together. There was, however, no clear indication in the treatment material that this activity involved the displacement of a rival, or that the partners had differing sexual roles.

It is characteristic of the child's relationships in the phallic-narcissistic phase that sexual wishes and fantasies toward an object are expressed within what is still essentially a one-to-one relationship. The third person may be seen as an unwelcome intruder in this exclusive relationship, as in earlier prephallic phases of the mother-child relationship, but this intruder has not yet been awarded by the child the full status of the oedipal rival.

The distinction between phallic-narcissistic and oedipal phases applies equally to normal and neurotic children, from whose clinical material we shall give examples. Our observation of such normal children in the nursery school [4] and family settings suggests, however, that their consolidation of oedipal relationships is achieved more quickly and decisively as compared with neurotic children, whose conflicts interfere with the transition between the two phases.

For example, in the treatment of Stella, who began analysis at about 5 years, there was a long period when phallic drive derivatives were sufficiently abundant to indicate phallic domi-

---

[4] The Hampstead Clinic Nursery School; Mrs. M. Friedmann, Head Teacher.

nance, while her relationships remained essentially on a preoedipal, need-satisfying level. Play with dolls which at first sight appeared to be indicative of oedipal fantasies turned out to be only an expression of her own longing to be well-mothered. A reported early attachment to her father, at about 2½ years, proved to have been part of her search for a substitute for her disappointing preoedipal mother, rather than a turn toward an oedipal father. Although Stella was preoccupied with sex differences and penis envy, her concurrent relationships continued to center on her intense wish to be mothered until the end of the first year of treatment; then there appeared some indications of negative oedipal attitudes toward her mother. Only toward the end of the second year of treatment, when Stella was nearly 7, did full-fledged positive oedipal attitudes and wishes toward her father become firmly established.

EXHIBITIONISM AND SCOPTOPHILIA

We have found from observations of children in the nursery school and in analysis that during the phallic-narcissistic phase the most noticeable component drive wishes are exhibitionism and scoptophilia; either parent (and other people) may be the object of these wishes. Exhibitionistic trends in the anal phase are particularly characterized by the child's demands for his body products to be admired. The move into the phallic-narcissistic phase is, in contrast, characterized by the child's demands that his objects admire his entire body self. The demand, "Look at what I've done" changes into "Look at what I am and look at what I'm able to do." The admiration demanded of and given by the object for the child's body and physical prowess is an important source of narcissistic gratification; the gratification received from the object is subsequently internalized.

The child's curiosity develops as an aspect of ego functioning in the prephallic phases and usually includes interest in sexual matters among the many situations in the world that the small child seeks to understand. With the entry into the phallic-narcissistic phase, however, curiosity becomes sharply focused, under the pressure of phallic drives, on questions of sexual differences and sexual activities; the wish to look now has the urgency of a drive derivative, which distinguishes scoptophilia as a sexual activity from more general curiosity. It is well known that this is an important period of development for the child's future learning capacity; in favorable circumstances the scoptophilic drive component can boost the child's ego functioning, increasing his wish and capacity to learn; whereas unduly severe conflicts over scoptophilia can result in generalized inhibition of curiosity and can later in development drastically reduce his learning capacity.

Castration anxiety occurs during the phallic-narcissistic phase, but it is of a different order from the oedipal castration anxiety. In boys whose castration anxiety and conflicts over competing in the phallic phase are not too severe, the exhibitionistic component normally remains quite marked through the oedipal phase, when it becomes part of the boy's masculine pursuit of his mother. It also continues into latency, though the derivatives normally become further removed from the object, the emphasis shifting to such pursuits as physical prowess in organized games, skill in handicrafts, achievements in intellectual activities.

In girls, normal development is less smooth since they have to contend with a much greater blow to their narcissism than boys. Exhibitionistic and scoptophilic activities make the boy aware of the small size of his penis, whereas the girl is made aware of her complete lack of a penis; and unlike the boy, she must abandon the idea that it will grow. Our observations suggest that the phase of indiscriminate exhibitionistic and scoptophilic activity directed toward objects of either sex is shorter in girls than boys, since girls are so quickly plunged into the problems of penis envy.

Differences Between Phallic-Narcissistic and Oedipal Manifestations

BOYS

A brief clinical example may serve to illustrate the differences between the phallic-narcissistic and oedipal phases of development. These differences can be seen in the levels of relationship to self and object, in drive activity, and in the content of castration fears.

At the beginning of treatment Derek (mentioned above) was 3;1

and Peter was 3;10. Both boys had reached the phallic-narcissistic phase, and in both analyses there was for a long time a central preoccupation with the penis and castration fears before the appearance of triangular oedipal relationships (either in or outside the transference). Both boys were envious of the man's big penis and anxiously aware of the woman's lack of one. Both had fantasies of stealing the man's penis and of having stolen the woman's penis. Each boy consequently feared both the father's anger and the deprived mother's envy; castration was thus feared at the hands of male and female objects. In each boy's analysis there was a phase in which the central theme was the wish to gain the object's admiration through the exhibitionistic demonstration of the penis and its possession, and the protection of the penis against loss by castration or theft. During this phase women were experienced as frighteningly envious and castrating objects. Only in a subsequent phase of treatment did mother (or her substitute) become the desired sexual object whom the boys wished to possess, impress, dominate, and care for in a masculine way. Concomitantly, male objects became rivals for possession of the female, not merely for possession of the penis. Fear of castration by the female grew less, sympathetic concern for her lack of a penis appeared, and a wish to impress and excite her sexually with his own penis was seen in each boy, with a concomitant shift in the intercourse fantasies.

This material shows that as the boy moves from the phallic-narcissistic to the oedipal level, changes occur in all areas: following the consolidation of his sexual identity, he experiences the full intensity of the triangular relationship of the oedipal level, with concomitant changes in the content of castration anxiety and in the aim of the phallic drive. At the phallic-narcissistic level the boy's penis becomes a highly valued body part, his main source of narcissistic and autoerotic gratification, and the focus of his phallic exhibitionistic wishes. He may fear its loss, or wish to be a girl, thus defensively anticipating its loss. Such responses may indicate his expectation of envious attempts by females to take away his penis or of talion punishment from father, or fear of having damaged his penis himself through masturbation. Fears of father's retaliation at the phallic-narcissistic level differ from those at the oedipal level both in content and intensity; at the oedipal level, the boy anticipates punishment for his wishes to castrate and banish father in order to take his place as mother's sexual partner.

This schematic outline of processes during the phallic-narcissistic and oedipal levels tends to obscure an important ongoing process, namely, the boy's developing positive identifications with and his love and admiration for his father.[5] These positive aspects of the relationship with father are maintained and developed alongside the oedipal rivalry; they are not to be confused with the negative oedipal relationship to the father, which may alternate with the positive oedipal relationship to the mother.

As the boy's sexual identification at the phallic-narcissistic level proceeds, he may at times defensively deny his awareness of sexual differences in objects; such defensive maneuvers may result from a valuing, or even overvaluing, of the phallus, with a consequent fear of its loss and a defensive bid to generalize such a prized attribute onto others. In the oedipal phase these defensive maneuvers must be distinguished from the fear of retaliatory castration by father. This denial and confusion must also be distinguished from those manifestations belonging to prephallic phases when he has not yet fully discovered the important differentiating sexual characteristics of his objects and integrated them into his self and object representations. At this earlier stage the child does not defensively deny sexual differences, but merely generalizes from his experiences of his own body and assumes that other people have similar bodies. In the prephallic phase many children are curious about the

---

[5] It is worth commenting that apparent regression during the phallic phase to earlier modes of relating may not be indicative of regression in either drives or relationships. Rather, it may be due to distortion of identification with specific sexual aspects of the parents who themselves have marked prephallic fixations. Derek, for example, showed a marked persistence of oral modes of drive expression: phallic excitement was often expressed in his mealtime behavior. Analysis showed that one of the determinants of this behavior was identification with his parents, especially the father, who used demands and complaints about food to get his wife's attention. Both parents used to get up in the middle of the night to eat. Derek clearly showed a wish for a continuation of the overindulgence he had experienced from his mother in the oral phase. But when, in the phallic phase, he began to identify with the phallic, sexual aspects of his father and father's sexual activity, this identification also reflected the father's own oral fixation and mode of relating to the mother.

differences between the genitals of boys and girls, without this necessarily being an indication of castration anxiety. While the penis seems to become a valued object when the boy is still in the anal phase of development, his interest in the penis is allied to a general curiosity about bodies, their functioning and their differences.

For example, John became interested in whether or not adults possessed a penis when he was about $2\frac{1}{4}$ years old, and firmly in the anal phase. He repeatedly asked his father and mother whether they had a penis, and then his interest spread to other adults whom he began to differentiate according to their possession or lack of a penis. At this time he appeared quite able to accept his parents' explanations about such bodily differences. In the course of toilet training John occasionally evidenced some fear that his penis, like his feces, might be lost, but he was able to reassure himself by means of observing the reality and by reasoning. By the time he was 3 years old, entering the phallic-narcissistic phase, and establishing a sexual identity, however, the increasing importance of his penis made it necessary for him to resort to defensive denial of his mother's lack of penis. At this time, he asked increasingly sophisticated questions about conception, pregnancy, and birth. He was given simple answers, but was now unable to accept his parents' explanations as readily as he had done previously. Instead, he maintained in conversation with his mother: "When I was born I came out of your penis." At the same time, he made active attempts to master his castration anxiety; e.g., he wanted to be allowed to use the breadknife. The prohibition of this activity, as well as of others, enhanced his awareness of being little, and made him long to be "a big man" like father.

Such examples demonstrate that during the anal phase the boy does not yet regard his penis as a confirmation of his masculinity. This confirmation takes place with the move into the phallic-narcissistic phase and consequent drive investment in the genital organs. It is in this phase too, or even earlier, that the boy may envy mother's possession of breasts and her capacity to have babies, but these feelings are partially counteracted by his growing masculine identifications.

GIRLS

While most authors are prepared to conjecture, or to extrapolate from later analytic material, about the formation of the body representation and identifications in boys, they are far less forthcoming about similar processes in girls. To our understanding, the process of establishing a constant representation of the body self follows exactly the same pattern in girls and has the same time sequence as that of the boy prior to the phallic-narcissistic phase. Only after a well-defined self representation has been attained, can the girl, by virtue of her developing ego capacities, begin to make comparisons between her own body and the body of the male. As Ruth Mack Brunswick (1940) puts it: "The active wish for a penis of the little girl arises with the observation of the difference between the sexes and the determination to have what the boy has. This original basis is narcissistic" (p. 276).

The girl experiences feelings and fears of castration different in nature and in complexity from those of the boy. She has to come to terms with the differences between her body and that of the boy; depending upon her narcissistic organization, level of ego development, and interaction with the important objects in her environment, she begins to a greater or lesser degree to accept her female body, a process which is not completed until the end of adolescence, if at all. Unlike the boy, the girl has no external organs to indicate to her the future capacity for achieving female adult functioning; such a prospect has to be realized principally by the adaptive process of identification with the mother and the later positive oedipal fantasies and wishes toward the father.

In examining the course of the girl's development in the phallic-narcissistic phase, we have to consider that envy in the girl may start prior to this phase (Joffe, 1969) and that the wish for a penis may then be on a par with the wish for other objects that she does not possess. It is in the phallic-narcissistic phase itself that specific penis envy occurs and may well denote a rivalry with boys, castration wishes, and a general dissatisfaction with her body. But the observable lack of well-being and lowered self-esteem may include other elements deriving from prephallic phases, such as early oral deprivation, inadequate mothering, sibling rivalry, and feelings of feminine inadequacy compared with mother. Both prephallic and phallic-narcissistic feelings of envy, with their concomitant lowering of self-esteem, may interfere with the development of feminine sexual identification.

Helene Deutsch (1944) emphasizes that feelings of envy are the prerogative of every child, particularly so in relation to a new sibling, and that the "anatomic difference becomes significant only in that phase of the girl's development in which her genitals (that is to say, her clitoris) assume functional importance" (p. 236). Moreover, she carefully distinguishes between the "primary genital trauma" and "penis envy," viewing the former as representing an awareness of genital inadequacy and deficiency which becomes generalized. She writes:

> In the psychologic material gathered from the analyses of adult women, particularly neurotic ones, we find repeated expressions of the lack of an organ, feelings of inferiority, etc. According to my present view, the assumption that these complaints result from the lack of a penis is one-sided. Their real origin is the fact that during a period of biologic development in which the inadequacy of an organ leads to a constitutionally predetermined transformation of the active tendencies into passive ones, no ready organ exists for the latter—in other words, the little girl continues to be organless in a functional sense. Her genital trauma, with its numerous consequent manifestations, lies between the Scylla of having no penis and the Charybdis of lacking the responsiveness of the vagina [p. 230].

Examination of our clinical material and the literature suggests that the development of sexual drive activity and fantasies during the phallic-narcissistic and oedipal phases is less well understood in girls than in boys, and is a subject which deserves further study. We may, however, offer some comments on the observable changes in the girl's relationships during these two phases. It is commonly accepted that for the girl normal development involves dealing with her penis envy by substituting for the missing penis her whole body and its appearance as a source of narcissistic-exhibitionistic gratification. The wish to be admired for her attractive, feminine appearance then becomes part of her positive oedipal approach to father. We have found it necessary, however, to distinguish between this form of feminine exhibitionism as a sign of a wish to be loved on an oedipal level and other forms which are signs of fixation to the phallic-narcissistic phase, or even to earlier preoedipal phases.

Margareta, for example, a nursery school child not in treatment, occasioned much discussion among the staff as to her status in phallic-narcissistic and oedipal development. She was a pretty, dainty, beautifully dressed child, who appeared feminine and self-satisfied. She knew well how to make an entrance and become the center of attention, and soon became known as "the little princess." She had an apparently flirtatious relationship with her father, which was occasionally extended to male observers in the nursery school. When she began nursery school at age 3, it seemed reasonable to suppose that she was entering the oedipal phase. But during her two years in the nursery school it became increasingly apparent that her relationships were superficial; she approached adults briefly in order to be admired, and retreated again once this aim had been achieved. If at times she became more involved, it was only to reveal clearly (at home as well as in school) the obstinate behavior more appropriate to the relationships of a toddler in the anal phase. Throughout the two years she remained aloof from the other children, never making any lasting friendship. Margareta had a younger brother, of whom she had at one time been overtly and intensely envious. This overt envy had subsequently disappeared. The superficiality and lack of development in Margareta's relationships eventually led the staff to conclude that her feminine exhibitionism was not a sign of true oedipal development, but was rather a defense against intense, unresolved penis envy, which had apparently prevented her from moving satisfactorily into the oedipal phase. Since low self-esteem and feelings of deprivation in girls often become organized around penis envy, the prephallic determinants in Margareta's personality must also be taken into account.

Fixation in the phallic-narcissistic phase is more easily ascertainable in girls who do not show Margareta's deceptively feminine development. Alice, for example, was a 3-year-old who did not appear at all feminine to the nursery school staff and observers. She had an older brother who was favored by the mother because of his more amenable and compliant behavior. Alice was preoccupied with "being big," and her conversation made it clear that she equated this with being a boy. She was intensely competitive with boys and interested only in activities and possessions which had some phallic significance. All her relationships, however, remained on the level of a negativistic toddler in the anal-sadistic phase. There were no signs of feminine attitudes toward her father and other male objects. Alice's difficulties were so marked that the nursery school staff soon concluded from the observations of her that although she was clearly in the phallic phase of drive development, she was quite unable, because of her conflicts, to make the move to oedipal relationships. This conclusion was confirmed when Alice entered analytic treatment.

In contrast to these two girls, Jane (whose infantile sexual theories were mentioned earlier) gradually brought material which was unmistakably oedipal in content, in that the triad of oedipal relationships predominated. For instance, after some months of treatment, Jane frequently cast her mother at home in the role either of a witch or a bad wolf, who had then to be appeased and placated with sweets. Then, in an analytic session, Jane brought the following sequence of fantasy material: while looking out of the window, she maintained, as she often did, that the therapist lived at another Clinic house across the road, that Dr. A. (who had conducted the diagnostic interviews with her in that house) was the therapist's "father" (i.e., husband). Jane next remarked upon a log in the garden opposite and fantasied that a daddy bear and a baby bear were sitting on it together, only hastily to amend this to include the mother bear as well. Two days later Jane instructed her therapist to be father, changing this to Santa Claus, who was to bring her presents while she slept. There had obviously been allied material during this time, and it was thus considered appropriate to interpret to Jane that she wanted her father to give her a very special present, a baby. Some four months later, Jane spontaneously asked the therapist whether she remembered her story of the daddy and baby bears sitting on the log together. This question came within the context of Jane having shared the parents' bedroom on a holiday and having been very much aware of parental intercourse. When the therapist, at one point, put it to Jane that when she grew up, she too could have a "daddy" all to herself and play such "love games" with him, Jane first looked extremely pleased, but then soberly remarked that it was a very long time to wait.

In Jane's material we see some of the paradoxes that the girl has to negotiate in the oedipal relationship. She continues to be dependent on her mother to meet her basic needs, and she wishes too to preserve a positive identificatory relationship with her and yet she also has to face her ambivalence toward her mother and her envy of her, as well as the pressures of her sexual fantasies toward father. It is therefore hardly surprising that many psychoanalysts, including ourselves, have found it so difficult to disentangle the different wishes, fantasies, and affects that make up adult female sexuality.

Effects of Fixation at the Phallic-Narcissistic Level on Later Development

In the treatment of adolescents and adults who have a strong fixation at the phallic-narcissistic level, we often find that they have failed to consolidate their oedipal relationships in childhood, with the consequence that their later relationships are deficient in truly oedipal characteristics.

The role of phallic-narcissistic fixation in the disturbances of adolescence and adulthood requires a separate study; on the basis of the cases examined so far, we briefly mention a few points. It was often possible to reconstruct that regression from a brief and imperfectly resolved oedipal level of relationships to the phallic-narcissistic level had occurred in childhood. Regression had at that time served as an adaptive attempt to cope with such problems as loss of self-esteem following the object's rejection of oedipal overtures, doubts about the oedipal object's acceptance of the patient's femininity or masculinity, and continuing difficulties in establishing a firm sexual identity due to conflicts. Regression to the phallic-narcissistic level was also used to cope with discrepancies between the ideal and the real self representations; such discrepancies often had roots in prephallic levels, but were heightened by disappointments and conflicts at the phallic-narcissistic and oedipal levels. While as adults these patients were often able to have heterosexual intercourse (thus indicating the relative intactness of their drive development), their relationships to their objects were frequently characterized by interactions on a phallic-narcissistic level; for example, an inability to achieve a reciprocal relationship in which the object's real qualities and characteristics are recognized and valued, and in which the needs and demands of the object are accepted; a tendency to use the object solely as a source of admiration or condemnation, as a substitute for internalized approval or sanctions; an emphasis on exhibitionistic and voyeuristic behavior in relation to the object; an incessantly phallic-competitive interaction with the object. Indeed, we were struck, as we examined the level of object relationships of these patients, how many of them could also be described as *hysterical characters,* and we would further suggest that in the hysteric the phallic-narcissistic level rather than the oedipal one is the nodal point of the regressive behavior. Much of what is often described as oral-demanding behavior in hysterics is perhaps better understood as a manifestation of phallic-narcissistic demands for admiration and narcissistic supplies from the object.

The cases we have referred to, both child and adult, demonstrate that development may be held up in the phallic phase, not so much with regard to drive development but more so in the appropriate relatedness to self and objects, so that the normal move into oedipal relationships does not adequately take place. This does not imply that fixation and conflict are found only at this level. Indeed, all these cases had major conflicts on prephallic levels which were at least partially responsible for their difficulties in the phallic-narcissistic and oedipal phases, and this also applies to other cases we have studied. We have concentrated particularly on phallic material in these cases because they show in exaggerated form the normal processes of phallic phase development in regard to both drive development and object relationships.

Summary

We have differentiated between the phallic-narcissistic and oedipal phases of development. While both are under the same dominant drive organization, they differ radically with regard to relationships to self and objects and drive and ego manifestations.

Within the phallic-narcissistic phase we have specifically examined the building up of the body self representations, the processes of identification and the acquisition of a sexual identity, the contributions made by the scoptophilic and exhibitionistic component wishes, and the differences between phallic and oedipal manifestations in these processes in boys and girls. Pseudooedipal relationships, i.e., phallic-narcissistic relationships, have been differentiated from oedipal relationships proper, with regard to the child's mode of relating to self and objects.

BIBLIOGRAPHY

BRUNSWICK, R. M. (1940), The Preoedipal Phase of the Libido Development. In: *The Psychoanalytic Reader*, ed. R. Fliess. London: Hogarth Press, 1950, pp. 261–283.

BURGNER, M. & EDGCUMBE, R. (1972), Some Problems in the Conceptualization of Early Object Relationships: Part II. *This Annual*, 27:315–333.

DEUTSCH, H. (1930), The Significance of Masochism in the Mental Life of Women. In: *The Psychoanalytic Reader*, ed. R. Fliess. London: Hogarth Press, 1950, pp. 223–236.

——— (1944), *The Psychology of Women*. New York: Grune & Stratton.

EDGCUMBE, R. & BURGNER, M. (1972), Some Problems in the Conceptualization of Early Object Relationships: Part I. *This Annual*, 27:283–314.

ERIKSON, E. H. (1950), *Childhood and Society*. New York: Norton.

——— (1956), The Problem of Ego Identity. *J. Amer. Psychoanal. Assn.*, 4:56–121.

FREUD, S. (1897), Letter 71. In: Extracts from the Fliess Papers. *S.E.*, 1:388–391.

——— (1905), Three Essays on the Theory of Sexuality. *S.E.*, 7:125–243.

——— (1909), Analysis of a Phobia in a Five-Year-Old Boy. *S.E.*, 10:3–149.

——— (1923), The Infantile Genital Organization, *S.E.*, 19:141–145.

——— (1924), The Dissolution of the Oedipus Complex. *S.E.*, 19:173–179.

——— (1925), Some Psychical Consequences of the Anatomical Distinction between the Sexes. *S.E.*, 19:243–258.

——— (1931), Female Sexuality. *S.E.*, 21:225–243.

HOFFER, W. (1950), Development of the Body Ego. *This Annual*, 5:18–23.

JOFFE, W. G. (1969), A Critical Review of the Status of the Envy Concept. *Int. J. Psycho-Anal.*, 50:533–545.

——— & SANDLER, J. (1967), Some Conceptual Problems Involved in the Consideration of Disorders of Narcissism. *J. Child Psychother.*, 2:56–66.

LAMPL-DE GROOT, J. (1928), The Evolution of the Oedipus Complex in Women. In: *The Psychoanalytic Reader*, ed. R. Fliess. London: Hogarth Press, 1950, pp. 207–222.

——— (1952), Re-evaluation of the Role of the Oedipus Complex. *Int. J. Psychoanal.*, 33:335–342.

MAHLER, M. S. (1958), In Panel: Problems of Identity, rep. D. Rubinfine. *J. Amer. Psychoanal. Assn.*, 6:131–142.

SANDLER, J. & ROSENBLATT, B. (1962), The Concept of the Representational World. *This Annual*, 17:128–145.

——— HOLDER, A., & MEERS, D. (1963), The Ego Ideal and the Ideal Self. *This Annual*, 18:139–158.

On the Maternal Origins of Awe

IRVING B. HARRISON, M.D.

PHYLLIS GREENACRE'S STUDIES ON AWE HAVE FIRMLY ESTABLISHED THE concept of phallic awe in the psychoanalytic literature. Her account of the developmental phase at which it is first experienced, its metapsychology and clinical manifestations, its characteristic quality, the circumstances responsible for its arousal, and its impact on the lives of gifted persons stand unchallenged.

Greenacre's definition of awe, derived from the Oxford Dictionary, emphasizes *reverential dread.* A second signification in that dictionary centers upon the experience of *wonder,* the implications of which seem to me to enrich the full understanding of awe phenomena. Therefore I shall cite both significations and note some special features of the word.

I

The word *awe* first appeared in the English language, according to the Oxford Dictionary (1933), in 855 A.D.; it has been in continuous use throughout the centuries. Its original, now obsolete, usage was descriptive of the subjective emotion of fear, terror, or dread. Two current significations exist. First: examples from 950 A.D. illustrate that "From its usage in reference to the Divine Being, this passes gradually into: dread mingled with veneration, reverential or respectful fear; the attitude of mind subdued to profound reverence in the presence of supreme authority, moral

---

Faculty member and training analyst, New York Psychoanalytic Institute. Based on a paper presented at the American Psychoanalytic Association, December 1974.

greatness or sublimity or mysterious sacredness." Second: "The feeling of solemn and reverential wonder tinged with latent fear, inspired by what is terribly solemn and majestic in nature, e.g. thunder, a storm at sea." It is noted that Ruskin wrote in 1851: "It is possible to conceive of terribleness without being in a position obnoxious to the danger of it, and so without fear; and the feeling arising from this contemplation of dreadfulness, ourselves being in safety, as of a stormy sea from the shore, is properly called *awe*."

Awe includes a range of related feeling states. At one extreme are feelings of reverence; at the other, those of wonder. Within this range are feelings which have an element of the uncanny, surpassing beauty, or mystery; tremulous feelings, as of the marvelous, and religious feelings, sometimes considered ineffable. Besides the range of feeling states from reverential to wondrous, there are degrees of fear, from states almost devoid of it to those in which dread or terror predominate.

Ecstasy has manifold expressions, some of which are undoubtedly variants of awe. Feelings of wonder or of ecstasy may be aroused in aesthetes in situations which fail to elicit a like response in others. Sometimes awe arises with no perceptible stimulus. Sensitive individuals describe a sense of mysterious specialness of the moment or of the scene. *Déjà* phenomena may resemble these in their affective quality. Some persons apparently live in a state of subdued awe much of the time, and may consider this as evidence of their contact with the Godhead.[1] It is of far-reaching importance, as will be shown, that the psychoanalytic understanding of awe has centered upon the impact of the phallus, and that the religious feelings linked to awe have been explained psychoanalytically almost exclusively in terms of the child's need for and fear of the father.

Although phallic awe is well known, I shall present some simple examples because what appears to be phallic awe, as described by adolescents and adults, can in analysis sometimes be related to elements pertaining primarily to nonphallic attributes of the mother's body.

Greenacre reported her observations of awe in 1947, 1953, and

[1] The related oceanic feeling will be discussed in another paper.

1956. Only selected observations which relate to the present effort will be noted here. She states that awe experiences in childhood are invariably colored by earlier events, especially those causing physiological distress and early infantile fright. In this context she mentions the "prehensile" quality of vision and the intensity of visual cathexis which in some children occurs as early as 6 months. In contrast to early ego experiences of "narcissistic mortification," which fall within the period of infantile amnesia (Freud, 1939, p. 74), awe can be experienced "only after a child is sufficiently developed to realize himself fairly well as a separately functioning being, no longer confused between the I and the other" (Greenacre, 1956, p. 9).

According to Greenacre, the firm establishment of body-ego boundaries, and thus the sense of separateness of the self from the other, generally occurs in the latter half of the second year. In the awe experience, however, there is always a degree of regressive loss of ego boundaries. She notes that the severity of the effect of witnessing the adult's erect penis depends very much on the character of the narcissistic elements in the ego at the time. Witnessing the mother's body may also arouse awe. She refers to observations of parturition and pregnancy as having the same impact, and relates a dream that calls to mind the Isakower phenomenon, as well as one of a machine representing the act of coitus. She subsumes a wide range of stimuli under the heading of collective alternates. In general, it may be said that Greenacre's work on awe lies within the realm limited by Freud's emphasis on the role of the father in early development.

As far as I could ascertain, Freud (1913, 1939) made only two explicit references to awe. In 1913, he came startlingly close to one dictionary description of awe. Explaining the original connotation of taboo, he stated that it was "wholly and solely 'objectified fear'. That fear has not yet split up into the two forms into which it later develops: veneration and horror" (p. 25). ". . . 'holy dread' would often coincide in meaning with taboo" (p. 18).

"Veneration" and "horror" and "holy dread" describe affective experiences, which thus lend themselves to clinical and introspective study. "Taboo," which is as foreign to German as to English, leads to considerations both exotic and behavioristic. Freud followed the theme of taboo to speculations on the prehistory of culture and thus away from clinical considerations. The prohibition against touching observed in the behavior of obsessive patients was linked to certain primitive ceremonials. Psychological ontogeny came to be considered, to some extent, as a recapitulation of the archaic heritage; in this approach, the developmental role of the mother receded in importance. As one pursues themes associated with awe in Freud's writings, one discovers many pertinent items under the headings of the uncanny and of religious feelings (1919, 1927, 1930) and, in a very different vein, of the occult, mystic experiences, poltergeists, and the "double." Freud placed uncanny feelings in the realm of aesthetics—"understood to mean not merely the theory of beauty but the theory of the qualities of feeling" (1919, p. 217)—and therefore somewhat foreign to psychoanalysis. As Lewin (1961) relates, however, Freud himself devised a method for the investigation of feelings such as anxiety and depression, which had previously been considered elemental.

In *Moses and Monotheism* (1939), Freud acknowledged that religious emotion attains a greater sublimity, profundity, and majesty than any other human emotion. Describing the reemergence of the primal father in the establishment of monotheism, Freud also observed: "Admiration, awe and thankfulness for having found grace in his eyes—the religion of Moses knew none but these positive feelings towards the father-god" (p. 133). He amplified that statement with another which contains a summation of his otherwise unexpressed views on awe, although he placed this once again in the context of cultural evolution. Such "feelings only become fully intelligible when they are transposed into the primitive and infantile setting. A child's emotional impulses are intensely and inexhaustibly deep to a degree quite other than those of an adult; only religious ecstasy can bring them back. A rapture of devotion to God was thus the first reaction to the return of the great father" (p. 134). Religious feelings are here seen to arise from awe feelings in childhood; only in the historical sweep of the Moses opus, however, does Freud deal with the importance of the latter, and there he bases them exclusively on the child's relation to the father and considers them in a neo-Lamarckian context. For example, he wrote, "what seems to us so grandiose about ethics, so mysterious and, in a mystical fashion, so self-evident, owes these characteristics to its connection with religion, its origin from the will of the father" (p. 122).

II

When the implications of the second Oxford definition of awe, which pertains to wonder, are considered, clinical, personal, and literary examples readily come to mind. Thus, Robert Plank (1957) quotes an autobiographical account by Jane Austen, who had an experience of wonder when she was a girl of 5 or 6. In this vignette, elements suggestive of the momentary loss of self-object boundaries —reminiscent of the infant's regression after nursing—are evident; it also reveals connections between awe, wonder, and religious feelings: "Quite suddenly, after a moment of quietness there, earth and sky and tree and wind-blown grass and the child in the midst of them came alive together with a pulsing light of consciousness. There was a wild foxglove at the child's feet and a bee dozing about it, and to this day I can recall the swift, inclusive awareness of each for the whole—I in them and they in me, and all of us enclosed in a warm lucent bubble of livingness." The child is described as having looked for the source of this "happy wonder," and having concluded that it must be God, "because it was the only awesome word she knew" (p. 385). As we have learned from Greenacre, awe is first experienced only after self-object differentiation has been accomplished, and it always—even in early childhood—involves regression. The early experiences to which this child regressed must have involved her infantile relationship with her mother; I regard this description ("all of us enclosed in a warm lucent bubble") as confirmatory.[2]

Clinical accounts of wondrous awe experiences are not uncommon during the course of some analyses, and these often prove to be quite complex. In the following two examples, the patients experi-

---

[2] The bee's penetration of the flower has been used poetically as a thinly veiled sexual symbolism. Bradley (1973), who notes that fact, adds interesting evidence that the bee and its honey have rich symbolic connections with the nipple and breast and its product.

enced awe during a dream; in the first, she also experienced awe in relation to its manifest content during the next analytic session. The patient reported the dream on the first visit after an overnight hospitalization for a breast biopsy which was negative. The night before the procedure, she dreamed: "The whole dream was just this magnificent tree, like a Christmas tree, with its branches *laden* with wonderful gifts! They seemed to reach out toward me, and bow down as if heavy with them. But my feeling was—of something— just *beyond* real gifts—so splendid—marvelous!"

This patient had entered analysis with unusually intense penis envy, alternately vilifying her husband for his "softness" and berating herself for being so unfair. She was driven to glorify her children, especially to deny their slightest departure from superiority. An early memory was of seeing her father in bed, with his hair tousled and standing up, and looking like a clown. She never completely worked through the feeling of being deprived and cheated, nor her conviction that if the analyst were a *real* man, and if she were worthy of the slightest self-respect as a woman, he would find her irresistible and disregard taboos. Behind these phallic phase problems was an intense oral problem, which centered on a remembered experience at age 2: the patient's mother, who had been away for some time, returned home, in an atmosphere of excitement, with a present. It was around the time of the patient's birthday, and close to Christmas, and this particular present turned out to be a sibling. The patient could recall her disappointment. She never thereafter liked her younger sibling or her mother. She felt slapped in the face by her father's attention to other girls or women.

The tree in the dream was, she supposed, a phallic symbol. It seemed mysterious. It must have had to do with the feared surgery—a castration threat. Speculations about the gifts were unmistakably oral. I felt that the dream probably included the symbolic representation of witnessing the erect penis of her father. She could not date "the clown" experience, but believed, as I do, that it was after her disappointing "gift" at 2. I also concluded that the gifts on the tree alluded to all the longed-for oral gifts emanating from her mother, which would include a phallus. Her mother was in fact unable to provide genuine and full maternal warmth, as a result of which the patient had suffered considerable oral deprivation. The tree, drooping with oral gifts, was a primitive, bisexual (phallic breast) symbol, containing a representation of the mother's breast, which, at last, she would have for herself as (dream) compensation for her own terrible loss. Under the stress of an anticipated mutilation, she regressively revived an awe-arousing observation of her mother's breast which she had originally made in infancy, perhaps while envying her nursing sibling.

The second example is from a 40-year-old writer, who early in his analysis had a classic dream of his body as phallus. In a large office where he had worked, he was gliding back and forth, inclining his body in space merely by willing it, and thereby changing his direction in order to go into a corridor. This occurred before the fascinated gaze of a secretary. He alluded spontaneously to a feeling of mixed astonishment and pleasure in the dream, but, he said, there was something more, indefinable, mysterious! He recalled how large the building seemed. His account indicated that the phallic element was associated with voyeuristic and other fantasies about his mother's body. The associations will not be recounted in full. The following details support the impression of an awe experience relating to the mother. After a depressing quarrel with his wife the night before, he had experienced a "sensual itch" which disturbed the "global peacefulness" of the bath to which he had retired. He masturbated, but not to orgasm. His initial feeling was of being rocked in the ocean. In the dream, the element of wonder combined with phallic exhibitionism, just as, in the preceding evening, his genital arousal occurred in a deeply regressive context suggestive of fantasies of being in his mother's body.

It is significant that both these patients were vulnerable to depression when disappointed. Other patients with marked orality and more severe depression also related dreams that revealed deeply regressive wishes such as being in the womb, attended at times by intense feelings of wondrous awe.

III

All awe experiences contain some measure of fear. In many, the fear element is all but imperceptible, and awe is indicated only by a special quality, sometimes considered ineffable. The child's initial experiences of wonder have in general the same developmental requirements as those of phallic awe, but they are aroused, usually a little earlier, by a particular incident involving awareness of the mother's breast or some other attribute of her body. The infant's recognition of mother's breast as a separate object is established earlier than that of the father's phallus. The repeated experiences with the mother's breast and body facilitate such self-object differentiation. Thus the recognition of the breast as a separate object may come to have, under optimal developmental conditions, a gentler impact than that of the relatively foreign paternal phallus.[3] With respect to the infant's object representations, I also distinguish between the infant's awareness of mother's body as claustrum and an earlier, less well-differentiated awareness. Presumably the infant's earliest fluctuating awareness of his own cold, wet, or hungry self alternates with a loss of self when a symbiotic merging occurs. Thus a complex situation normally evolves. During the developmental phase of the nursling, a gradual differentiation between self and breast regularly alternates with the loss of boundaries as the infant sinks into contented sleep, paradigmatically at the mother's breast. With good mothering and other fortunate circumstances, the infant's needs do not rise to the point of trauma during this process. Later, usually in the early oedipal phase, the mother's body gains object meaning as potential receptacle or womb. I suggest that the initial recognition of mother's breast and, later, of her body customarily gives rise to wondrous awe.

This basic state of affairs, i.e., the development of wondrous and of phallic awe, tends to be obscured by two factors—by very early trauma occurring well before self-object differentiation, and by other premature startling observations made by the infant or young child. Both, in my opinion, tend to skew the awe experience in the direction of anxiety or fear. The most severe distortions seem to be caused by very early trauma occurring well before the arousal of

---

[3] Loewald (1951) cites the danger of a regressive pull toward engulfment by the mother, with loss of the self. I believe that this is more likely when there has been early trauma.

phallic awe. As a result of such distortions, later responses to awe-arousing stimuli are attended by horror, terror, or dread. The analysis of examples of presumably phallic reverential dread in which fear is extreme may reveal a symbolic core related to a maternal element—e.g., smothering or engulfment—rather than to the paternal phallus.

Although Greenacre does not draw the same conclusions as I do, her work clearly establishes that startling observations for which the preoedipal or even early phallic phase child is unprepared have an immense impact on the immature child. Among such observations are witnessing parental intercourse, the genitalia of either parent, menstruation or childbirth, bodily deformation, or a death in the family. A highly unusual and intense affect exhibited by the parent (e.g., pain, fear, grief or rage) may, by giving rise to bewilderment, alter the child's later awe experiences. The impact of such experiences depends on their frequency and the child's stage of development. When they occur too early, the subsequent awe is markedly colored by anxiety or dread, which often reveals itself in response to a symbolic representation of the mother's body. Awed fear of whirlpools, pits, and of caverns is not, in my clinical experience, a vicissitude reflecting exclusively the genital phase, but rather is the expression of distortion by pregenital or "too early" phallic phase trauma. In such a context, phallic symbols, e.g., the pendulum, are usually traceable to the fantasy of the mother's destructiveness, represented as a concealed and dangerous phallus. A readiness for superstition and belief in magic and miracle may be one of the later consequences of such traumatic overexposure.

In cases revealing narcissistic symptomatology wondrous awe often becomes an eery dread, as is well illustrated in the short stories of Edgar Allan Poe. Somewhat suggestive of such a change is the account of a young analysand whose castration anxiety had prevented manual masturbation throughout his adolescence. During his entire infancy and early childhood his bitter and often depressed mother was pregnant almost continuously. She remained phallic in his unconscious. The day after his girlfriend persuaded him to let her masturbate him, he described his "overwhelming" orgasm as "dynamite!" He was clearly awed by the experience. He went on to use the metaphor of riding a surfboard along a great roller. Then he paused and concluded, "But then this enormous wave flips you and comes crashing down on you. Phew, it was scary." I learned that his sexual experience was followed by a nightmare and profound anxiety.

In 1966, I described a patient's uncanny feeling on entering the aqueduct of the Pont du Gard. Viewing his experience as an identity disturbance, I attributed it to a revival of awe and envy of his father's greater urinary stream. But the interior of the mother's body was also symbolized: a review of the data provides an account of a search on a hillside for the source of the original water supply for a village.

As a boy of 10, this patient had been present when his maternal grandfather, in terminal coma, ceased to breathe. As the assembled family was acknowledging that the old man had just died, the boy's mother called out, "Papa!" and breathing resumed briefly. The event became a screen memory for seductive and frightening experiences to which he had been subjected by his mother in early childhood. The boy had never outgrown the awe of a mother who possessed such power; he retained a striking tendency to revere impressive women as well as to seek wondrous awe experiences in nature.

Slochower (1970) attributed Freud's disturbance on the Acropolis to *mater nudam* as symbolically represented by the Parthenon, and claimed that my 1966 paper was predominantly concerned with the conflict with the father. I had, however, made explicit mention of the significance of the temple sacred to the goddess, and was struck by the specific element of awe as stimulated, at least in part, by the mother's body symbolically represented. Moreover, I referred explicitly to awe in relation to such stimuli. In fact, the present study is in part an attempt to pursue the questions which my 1966 paper evoked. Kanzer's (1969) analysis of Freud's account emphasizes the role of the brother, in an oedipal context distorted by conflict over death wishes toward a sibling.[4]

---

[4] Freud's own account of his experience, when studied in the context of his correspondence with Rolland (Cornubert, 1966), and of his comments in *The Future of an Illusion* (1927), is suggestive of awe of the mother as a result of early trauma—a topic that will be taken up in a separate paper.

I now turn to clinical indications of how very early infantile trauma may alter later awe experiences. Borderline patients sometimes experience acute states of depersonalization and related disturbances when awe is aroused in them in adolescence and adult life. Archaic ego states are then evident, and early vicissitudes of narcissism involving confusion between the self and the other again are prominent; grandiosity and terror may coexist or alternate. The fluidity of boundaries can be glimpsed in the analysis of such awe experiences in which it is difficult to untangle the web of dread and rage, humiliation and triumph, megalomania and devastation. Here we are dealing with the vicissitudes of aggression. Freud's views on related issues are touched upon in Strachey's Introduction to *Civilization and Its Discontents* (1930).[5]

An etymological study of awe reveals a definite linguistic link to the primal distress of suffocation. Freud dealt repeatedly (1916/17, 1933) with the respiratory distress of birth as a primary source of anxiety. It is to such primal fear and to the subsequent reexperience of such feelings that I refer. They seem to arise during states of physiological distress in infancy and early childhood and, I believe, later in response to certain psychological stresses in susceptible persons.

With respect to the word *Angst*, and the idea that it, like awe, relates to early respiratory distress, it is, of course, presently beyond the bounds of psychology to date the dawn of psychic activity. Nevertheless, objections to Freud's concept of birth trauma based on the incomplete maturation of the cerebral cortex at birth seem unwarranted, at least in the present consideration. Patterns of physiological discharge which subsequently contribute to characteristic affective complexes, and hence to basic self-feelings, originate demonstrably in response to the earliest stresses, and vary among infants in the intensity, duration, and frequency of such discharge (see Stone, 1971; Walsh, 1968, 1971). Obviously such experiences contribute to memory in its broadest sense.

---

[5] In *Civilization and Its Discontents*, Freud traced the origins of religious feelings to the earliest events in self-object differentiation. He concluded, however, that the relationship with the father ousts the oceanic feeling from a place in the foreground.

This is consistent with Mahler's (1968) account of the gradually evolving and extremely complex earliest development, although these data must be taken as no more than a guide to the correlation of material obtained in adult analysis, in which only inferential impressions about early mental events can be made. The latter can be tested only indirectly through observation of infants and children, child analysis, and data derived from other fields such as linguistics, religion, and mythology.

In the distortion of awe which can occasionally be seen during the analysis of borderline patients, the essential psychic experience is of overwhelming power *(mana)*, which is totally ambiguous with respect to its locus because of regression toward a state in which there are no boundaries or limits. Hence this primary undifferentiated force cannot be discriminated. It is at one and the same time an expanding megalomanic outrage and the horror of dissolution or annihilation of the psyche. Momentarily the afflicted individual relives an instant of total disorientation, with a sense of awfulness which cannot at that moment be discriminated in terms of whether it is impinging or exploding. Such an incident may occur instead of awe, as the following example illustrates.

In the analysis of a 20-year-old borderline student, I made a mistake in interpreting a dream element. It was not a premature interpretation in the sense that it lacked the basis of earlier analytic work; rather, it was injudicious and overwhelming because the patient was at that moment not prepared for it. She began to shriek, her face contorted with rage and horror, and tears began to flow as she gasped and sobbed. In her first coherent sentence she cursed me for knowing what was in her brain when she herself did not. It was, she said, *awful*. I believe that a primitive distorted awe experience had occurred. Awe was aroused by the omniscient interpretation. Her rage was an exaggerated, but understandable response to my mistake; she had detected my narcissistic gratification in being able to provide a remarkable interpretation and bring about a startling insight. At the moment of raging the patient may have been psychotic, but a few seconds later she was able to describe lucidly her traumatic awe experience, as I have delineated. Many other clinical incidents, fortunately less dramatic, have convinced me that momentary episodes—sometimes expressed as loss of equilibrium or time sense (i.e., *déjà* phenomena)—have the same or similar determinants (Kohut, 1971).

Greenacre's observation (1953) that aggression is aroused in the awe experience can be extended somewhat. For instance, an aggressive or destructive element has been noted in many situations in which the infant or young child acknowledges the separateness of an object, e.g., the mother or a part of her body, or even an inanimate object (Winnicott, 1969; Galenson and Roiphe, 1973). This is but another way of referring to self-object differentiation and the establishment of new object representations in the ego. Freud (1923) commented on the release of aggression in the process of identification which leads to the formation of the superego. The latter is, I believe, a specific instance of a general principle: in the process of identification there is a recapitulation of a sequence of events. These begin with regressive efforts to get closer to the object, i.e., to become more like it. The regressive route leads in the direction of loss of boundaries and fusion. Along with other possible factors, the health and maturation of the ego stand in the way of this process, however, and the next step is therefore the full recognition of the separateness and autonomy of that element which the child wishes to make part of himself. Such recognition is, however, a narcissistic wound, a loss of what was experienced as part of the self and must now be given up in order to become a part of the ego. Thus it is in preparation for identification that the release of aggression occurs. Awe involves superego identification. Maenchen (1946), Jacobson (1964), and Reich (1954) trace the superego precursors back to early infancy. Jacobson (1971) refers specifically to the fantasy of being one with the object: "Of course, unconscious, short-lived, partial identifications of this early preoedipal type . . . [are] an important element in our social and love relationships." She directs attention to "idealized images of the parents blended with archaic, aggrandized images of the self" (p. 246), but she does not describe the terrifyingly threatening images of the parents which often coexist with the idealized images.

In certain awe experiences of adults, such identifications are reemphasized by the aesthetic—often architectural—qualities of the stimuli. As I noted elsewhere (1966), many cultural shrines and comparable stimuli to awe are remarkable in that they have an impact upon the individual as a member of a group and at the same time revivify the early awe-arousing experiences which they symbolize. In the healthy awe response to symbolic stimuli, aggression is mastered. Moreover, as if through a tacit preconscious understanding of having shared a class of early experiences, the affected members of the group often share a sense of humility which protects them from the possible humiliation of the overpowering stimulus.

Summary

Evidence has been adduced to support the contention that awe arises in relation to the mother. Normally, such awe is experienced as wonder, or as akin to that feeling. It lacks the terror or dread typically associated with phallic awe. Distortions of both types of awe, as a result of the traumatic impact of earlier experiences, were noted by Greenacre with respect to phallic awe. In this paper they were considered in relation to the mother, and clinical evidence has been offered in support of these propositions. The presentation is intended as a basis for examining Freud's views on religious and oceanic feelings, and for an investigation of current social issues.

BIBLIOGRAPHY

BRADLEY, N. (1973), Notes on Theory-Making, on Scotoma of the Nipples and on the Bee as Nipple. *Int. J. Psycho-Anal.*, 54:301–314.
CORNUBERT, C. (1966), *Freud et Romain Rolland.* These #453, pour le Doctorat en Médicine, Paris.
FREUD, S. (1913), Totem and Taboo. *S.E.,* 13:1–161.
——— (1916/17), Introductory Lectures on Psycho-Analysis. *S.E.,* 15 & 16.
——— (1919), The 'Uncanny.' *S.E.,* 17:217–256.
——— (1923), The Ego and the Id. *S.E.,* 19:3–66.
——— (1927), The Future of an Illusion. *S.E.,* 21:3–56.
——— (1930), Civilization and Its Discontents. *S.E.,* 21:59–145.
——— (1933), New Introductory Lectures on Psycho-Analysis. *S.E.,* 22:3–182.
——— (1936), A Disturbance of Memory on the Acropolis. *S.E.,* 22:239–248.
——— (1939), Moses and Monotheism. *S.E.,* 23:3–137.
GALENSON, E. & ROIPHE, H. (1973), Unpublished manuscript.
GREENACRE, P. (1947), Vision, Headache, and the Halo. *Psychoanal. Quart.,* 16:177–194.

―― (1953), Penis Awe and Its Relation to Penis Envy. In: *Drives, Affects, Behavior,* ed. R. Loewenstein. New York: Int. Univ. Press, pp. 176–190.
―― (1956), Experiences of Awe in Childhood. *This Annual,* 11:9–30.
HARRISON, I. B. (1966), A Reconsideration of Freud's "A Disturbance of Memory on the Acropolis" in Relation to Identity Disturbance. *J. Amer. Psychoanal. Assn.,* 14:518–527.
JACOBSON, E. (1964), *The Self and the Object World.* New York: Int. Univ. Press.
―― (1971), *Depression.* New York: Int. Univ. Press.
KANZER, M. (1969), Sigmund and Alexander Freud on the Acropolis. *Amer. Imago,* 26:324–353.
KOHUT, H. (1971), *The Analysis of the Self.* New York: Int. Univ. Press.
LEWIN, B. D. (1961), Reflections on Depression. *This Annual,* 16:321–331.
LOEWALD, H. W. (1951), Ego and Reality. *Int. J. Psycho-Anal.,* 32:10–18.
MAENCHEN, A. (1946), A Case of Superego Disintegration. *This Annual,* 2:257–262.
MAHLER, M. S. (1968), *On Human Symbiosis and the Vicissitudes of Individuation.* New York: Int. Univ. Press.
PLANK, R. (1957), On "Seeing the Salamander." *This Annual,* 12:379–398.
REICH, A. (1954), Early Identification As Archaic Elements in the Superego. *J. Amer. Psychoanal. Assn.,* 2:218–238.
SLOCHOWER, H. (1970), Freud's *Déjà Vu* on the Acropolis. *Psychoanal. Quart.,* 39:90–102.
STONE, L. (1971), Reflections on the Psychoanalytic Concept of Aggression. *Psychoanal. Quart.,* 40:195–244.
WALSH, M. N. (1968), Explosives and Spirants. *Psychoanal. Quart.,* 37:199–211.
―― (1971), Ordinal Language and Superego Genesis. *Int. J. Psycho-Anal.,* 52:115–125.
WINNICOTT, D. W. (1969), The Use of the Object. *Int. J. Psycho-Anal.,* 50:711–716.

Theoretical and Clinical Aspects of Ambivalence

ALEX HOLDER, PH.D.

The Historical Context

FOR EVERY PSYCHOANALYST, AMBIVALENCE IS PART OF HIS EVERYDAY vocabulary and is perhaps one of the most frequently used (and misused) psychoanalytic terms. It may therefore come as a surprise to find that the term is listed only in the supplement to the Oxford English Dictionary, even though it was coined and introduced into psychoanalytic literature well over half a century ago. The term is there defined as "having either, or both, of two contrary values or qualities." It was Eugen Bleuler who used the term for the first time in a lecture on the subject in 1910.[1] In it, he differentiated between three types of ambivalence—voluntary, intellectual, and emotional ambivalence.

This paper forms part of a Research Project entitled "Childhood Pathology: Impact on Later Mental Health," which is conducted at the Hampstead Child-Therapy Course and Clinic, London, where the author is a child psychotherapist and research associate. The Clinic is at present supported by the Field Foundation, Inc., New York; the Foundation for Research in Psychoanalysis, Beverly Hills, Calif.; The Freud Centenary Fund, London; the Anna Freud Foundation, New York; the National Institute for Mental Health, Bethesda, Maryland; the Grant Foundation, New York; the New-Land Foundation, Inc., New York; and a number of private supporters. The paper is the outcome of research conducted in the Index Department of the Hampstead Child-Therapy Clinic.

[1] According to Grinstein (1956) a paper entitled "Die Ambivalenz" by Bleuler was published in 1914 in the *Festgabe der medizinischen Fakultät* in Zürich.

In the original German version of his lecture, Bleuler used the term *Ambitendenz* with reference to the ambivalence of the will. This ambitendency essentially refers to conscious conflicts over doing or not doing something or over doing one thing as against doing another: to eat or not to eat; to attend a meeting or stay at home; to work or play. Intellectual ambivalence has reference to a high level of ego functioning in the realm of secondary process thinking and reasoning. It is concerned with the condensation of opposites in a single word (e.g., *altus* meaning both high and low) or the simultaneous interpretation of phenomena in a positive and a negative way. Both forms of ambivalence are not primarily related to any other object and any feelings about or toward such an object. Rather, they refer to preconscious and conscious mental processes and to the kind of nonneurotic conflict which we all have to face in our daily lives.

The third form of ambivalence singled out by Bleuler—the emotional or affective ambivalence—became the focus of Freud's formulations on the topic. Bleuler had pointed out that the three forms of ambivalence described by him were interrelated and that it was therefore impossible to draw sharp dividing lines between them. At the same time he recognized that the investment of the same object representation with feelings of love and hate was the most pathogenic form of ambivalence and therefore the most relevant for the understanding of mental illness, dreams, and mythology.

FREUD'S FORMULATIONS DURING THE SECOND PHASE

Freud's correspondence with Fliess [1892–1899] shows that he recognized the importance of the phenomenon of ambivalence in mental disorders from the very beginning of his clinical work. He alludes to the phenomenon again in the case history of Little Hans (1909a) and notably in his case presentation of the Rat Man (1909b), where he elucidates its crucial contribution to the genesis of obsessional neuroses. He points out that a "battle between love and hate was raging in the lover's breast, and the object of both these feelings was one and the same person. The battle was represented in a plastic form by his compulsive and symbolic act of removing the stone from the road along which she was to drive, and then of undoing this deed of love by replacing the stone where it had lain, so that her carriage might come to grief against it and she herself be hurt." (p. 191). He concludes that in considering a number of analyses of obsessional neurotics "we shall find it impossible to escape the impression that a relation between love and hatred such as we have found in our present patient is among the most frequent, the most marked, and probably, therefore, the most important characteristics of obsessional neurosis" (p. 239).

In these earliest discussions of ambivalence, Freud already spells out what is, for him, the hallmark of "emotional ambivalence in the proper sense of the term," namely, "the simultaneous existence of love and hate towards the same object" (1913, p. 157), and as it is reflected in the transference relationship in the oscillations between positive and negative transferences (1912). As he points out in his 1912 paper, in which he uses the term "ambivalence" for the first time, ambivalence of feelings of this kind is a normal phenomenon, "but a high degree of it is certainly a special peculiarity of neurotic people" (p. 106f.).

With the exception of a few instances (1915, 1918) where Freud uses ambivalence to describe the simultaneous existence of active and passive instinctual aims, his extensive discussions of the phenomenon are all concerned with emotional or affective reactions of an incompatible nature which arise in relation to one and the same object. His views about the *genesis* of ambivalence underwent changes in accordance with his modifications in instinctual drive theory and have to be understood in that context.

Thus, during the second phase of psychoanalysis and up to the introduction of the primary dualism between life and death instincts in 1920, the understanding of emotional ambivalence was related to the dualism between the sexual drives on the one hand and the ego instincts (or self-preservative instincts) on the other. Feelings of love were regarded as an expression of underlying sexual drive wishes toward an object, whereas the opposing feelings of hatred were seen as deriving from the self-preservative tendencies and their response to threats and mental pain, initially experienced as inflicted from outside. In 1915, Freud notes,

> Hate, as a relation to objects, is older than love. It derives from the narcissistic ego's primordial repudiation of the external world with

its outpouring of stimuli. As an expression of the reaction of unpleasure evoked by objects, it always remains in an intimate relation with the self-preservative instincts; so that sexual and ego-instincts can readily develop an antithesis which repeats that of love and hate. When the ego-instincts dominate the sexual function, as is the case at the stage of the sadistic-anal organization, they impart the qualities of hate to the instinctual aim as well [p. 139].

There appear to be some inconsistencies in Freud's formulations about the genesis and nature of ambivalence. On the one hand, we find statements which place ambivalence within the context of the relation of the total self to an object and, at the same time, link its emergence with the synthesis of the component instincts under the dominance of genital primacy. On the other hand, Freud refers to oral-incorporative aims and sadistic-anal strivings as ambivalent. How are we to reconcile such apparently contradictory statements?

In the first place, it seems crucial to realize that Freud is looking at the same phenomena from two different points of view, on the one hand, in terms of subjective experience, i.e., the individual's psychic reality; and, on the other, from a descriptive point of view, i.e., as the same phenomena appear to an observer. The confusion of these two points of view is a frequent source of misguided interpretations of mental phenomena and of the development of theories based upon them to which Hartmann has called attention with his notion of the "genetic fallacy." To illustrate my point I cite a brief passage in which Freud (1915) discusses the development of love:

> Preliminary stages of love emerge as provisional sexual aims while the sexual instincts are passing through their complicated development. As the first of these aims we recognize the phase of incorporation or devouring—a type of love which is consistent with abolishing the object's separate existence and which may therefore be described as ambivalent. At the higher stage of the pregenital sadistic-anal organization, the striving for the object appears in the form of an urge for mastery, to which injury or annihilation of the object is a matter of indifference. Love in this form and at this preliminary stage is hardly to be distinguished from hate in its attitude towards the object. Not until the genital organization is established does love become the opposite of hate [p. 138f.].

It is important to bear in mind that Freud here describes oral-incorporative and sadistic-anal phenomena within the context of various stages in the development of object love. In terms of the infant's psychic experience, there is no question of any ambivalence, let alone a conflict over feelings of ambivalence toward an object. The infant's instinctual aim is not one of destroying the object but rather of making it part of the self in order to ensure the permanence of need satisfaction during the oral-incorporative phase of development, and the same aim is achieved during the anal phase by means of the actualization of omnipotent fantasies.

Descriptively and from the point of view of an outside observer, such infantile modes of relating to a specific object fit the definition of ambivalence in a phenomenological sense. But it is erroneous to assume, as it is in the case of symptoms, that a particular surface manifestation is always due to the same causative factors. The understanding of an adult patient's behavior of sucking and biting his wife's breasts during sexual foreplay has to be substantially different from the understanding of the same behavior in a 9-month-old infant.

In 1915, Freud added a paragraph on ambivalence to his *Three Essays on Sexuality* (1905), which throws further light on the apparent contradictions in some of his formulations about ambivalence. Referring to anal sadism, he writes:

> This form of sexual organization can persist throughout life and can permanently attract a large portion of sexual activity to itself. The predominance in it of sadism and the cloacal part played by the anal zone give it a quite peculiarly archaic colouring. It is further characterized by the fact that in it the opposing pairs of instincts are developed to an approximately equal extent, a state of affairs described by Bleuler's happily chosen term 'ambivalence' [p. 199].

Freud is using the term ambivalence here in a wider context, i.e., as referring to any opposing pairs of instinctual tendencies. The context suggests that he was thinking of such polarities as activity and passivity, masculinity and femininity, sadism and masochism. He regarded such innate polarities as facilitating factors in the development of emotional ambivalence toward objects. But he also seems to imply that there is a persistence, in psychic development and life, of certain polarities and conflicts between them, which manifest themselves with particular intensity during certain pregenital phases of development. Thus the anal phase is characterized by the appearance or exacerbation of conflicts between activity and passivity, expulsion and retention, control and submission. Such conflicts and polarities can be seen as providing the blueprint or paradigm for the later emergence of the polarity of ambivalence between love and hate.

If, as Freud suggests, love and hate can hardly be distinguished from each other during the pregenital phases of development and love becomes the opposite of hate only when the genital level has been reached, how do we explain conflicts over ambivalence which we know from clinical experience to exist in children long before they reach the genital level of instinctual drive development? Here we come to a point which, I feel, has not been given sufficient emphasis either in theoretical or clinical formulations. This may be partly due to Freud's own emphasis on the juxtaposition between love and hate in his conceptualization of ambivalence. At the same time, there seems to be an implicit suggestion, in many of his formulations during the second phase of theory formation, of a developmental continuum from the infant's *need*[2] for and dependence on objects to his later love of objects, a link which is perhaps

---

[2] The term *need* is used very widely, and often indiscriminately, in psychoanalytic writings. We speak of sexual needs, emotional needs, instinctual needs, biological needs, and so forth. It would seem appropriate to differentiate between two basic categories of needs: (a) those related to the preservation of life, which might be designated as "biological needs"; and (b) those related to the maintenance of mental health, which constitute "psychological needs." We need to eat and drink as much as we need to dream, but for different reasons: if we are deprived of food and drink, we shall die; if we are deprived of dreaming, we shall go insane. Freud used the term *need* mainly—though not exclusively—with reference to biological needs, arising from the self-preservative instincts. When we consider sexual or aggressive drive wishes and their satisfaction in either direct or sublimated forms, we realize at once the considerable overlap between the biological and psychological aspects of certain needs. In this paper, the term *need* is used to cover both the biological and psychological aspects, although in the context of early individual development the emphasis is on the satisfaction of biological needs which serve self-preservation.

reflected in the German saying "Liebe geht durch den Magen" (love proceeds via the stomach).

Following this line of thought, I would suggest that the child's initial conflict in relation to the mother on whom he is dependent (for the satisfaction of his biological needs and of his emotional needs for love, safety, admiration) is between his *need* of her and his hatred of her insofar as she is experienced as a source of frustration and unpleasure. Freud seems to allude to something like this when he states in 1915: "We do not say of objects which serve the interests of self-preservation that we *love* them; we emphasize the fact that we *need* them, and perhaps express an additional, different kind of relation to them by using words that denote a much reduced degree of love" (p. 137). In the same context he points out that the terms "love and hate cannot be made use of for the relations of *instincts* to their objects, but are reserved for the relations of the *total ego* to objects." He further notes that the affect of hatred arises as a reaction to frustrations of both sexual satisfactions and satisfaction of self-preservative needs. From a developmental point of view, hatred and related feelings of lesser intensity are therefore to be considered as a relatively early affective response to frustrating objects. The term love, on the other hand "can only begin to be applied in this relation after there has been a synthesis of all the component instincts of sexuality under the primacy of the genitals and in the service of the reproductive function" (p. 138). When this stage of development has been reached, the dependence on a particular object for need satisfaction has usually receded very much into the background.

The point I wish to underscore is that the young child simply cannot afford to reject or abandon the object on whose love and ministrations he is dependent for survival. This dependence remains long after the child has reached and passed the point of emotional object constancy, even though it lessens as a consequence of maturation and development. To some extent, we all remain dependent on other objects for survival as well as for the satisfaction of instinctual drive wishes throughout our lives, and for most of us the need for objects persists, even though the quality and content of these needs undergo changes and may lose much of the imperative quality of early childhood and be considerably less in terms of direct instinctual gratification. (These points will be discussed further in relation to clinical examples.)

In the historical context, it is important to bear in mind that the transition from the second to the third phase of psychoanalysis, or from the topographic to the structural frame of reference, had significant repercussions on Freud's conceptualization of the genesis of emotional ambivalence. As indicated, during the second phase he regarded loving feelings as derivatives or expressions of sexual drive impulses. As such they emanated from the system Unconscious. Feelings of hate, on the other hand, were eventually seen as deriving from the so-called "ego instincts"[3] whose aims become basically different from those of the sexual instincts from an early point in development onward. Their chief aim is the preservation of life under the dominance of the reality principle, as opposed to the blind gratification of instinctual drive wishes in accordance with the pleasure principle. In terms of mental topography, then, these self-preservative or ego instincts have to be regarded as a reflection of the functioning of the systems Preconscious and Conscious. Thus, within the topographic frame of reference, feelings of love and hate are seen as deriving from structurally and functionally different parts of the mental apparatus.

FREUD'S FORMULATIONS DURING THE THIRD PHASE

When Freud introduced his concepts of life and death instincts (1920), he came to regard the polarity between love and hate as a direct consequence and expression of the hypothesized opposition between the instincts of life and death. In contrast to his earlier view, both love and hate were then seen as deriving from the same mental structure, the id, the one being a derivative of sexual drive wishes, the other an expression of aggressive drive impulses. Furthermore, Freud put forward the view that the appearance and persistence of ambivalent feelings was due to an insufficient degree of fusion (or integration, as we might say) between the two hypothesized primal instincts. He points out (1923) that ambiva-

---

[3] For a fuller account of Freud's changing views of the place of aggression in his instinctual drive theory, see Edgcumbe (1970).

lence "is such a fundamental phenomenon that it more probably represents an instinctual fusion that has not been completed" (p. 42), rather than being the result of a defusion. This conceptual shift placed more emphasis on the constitutional elements in the predisposition to neurotic conflicts about ambivalent feelings toward an object, a predisposition which was further reinforced by another constitutional given—bisexuality. It also placed more emphasis on the ego's task of integrating and synthesizing these diametrically opposite impulses and feelings toward one and the same object. In the words of Hartmann, Kris, and Loewenstein (1949), "During the oral, anal and phallic phases of libidinal development integration of the drives remains incomplete. It is only the development of the object relation during latency and prepuberty and the maturation of the new modes of discharge provided by the genital organization that allow for what might be considered as optimal integration of the discharge of both drives (Freud). This integration then leads to a diminished proclivity toward ambivalence" (p. 33f.).

Freud's extensive discussions of ambivalence in the father-son relationship in *Totem and Taboo* (1913) and in *Moses and Monotheism* (1939) give the impression that his emphasis on the constitutional elements in ambivalence is derived from such studies. At the same time, he never underestimated the experiential contributions to ambivalence conflicts. He placed both possibilities side by side in a discussion of ambivalence in the mother-child relationship (1933):

> It might be thought indeed that this first love-relation of the child's is doomed to dissolution for the very reason that it is the first, for these early object-cathexes are regularly ambivalent to a high degree. A powerful tendency to aggressiveness is always present beside a powerful love, and the more passionately a child loves its object the more sensitive does it become to disappointments and frustrations from that object; and in the end the love must succumb to the accumulated hostility. Or the idea that there is an original ambivalence such as this in erotic cathexes may be rejected, and it may be pointed out that it is the special nature of the mother-child relation that leads, with equal inevitability, to the destruction of the child's love; for even the mildest upbringing cannot avoid using compulsion and introducing restrictions, and any such intervention

in the child's liberty must provoke as a reaction an inclination to rebelliousness and aggressiveness [p. 124].

This passage leads up to a discussion of the castration complex in girls who hold their mothers responsible for their lack of a penis. This line of thought would suggest that experiential factors play a more crucial part in the ambivalent feelings of girls to their mothers than in that of boys. It would be interesting to know whether this suggestion can be confirmed by comparing the qualities of the mother transference in boys and girls or men and women.

ABRAHAM'S VIEWS

Abraham regarded the first period of life (corresponding to the oral-sucking stage) as preambivalent, the period up to puberty as being characterized by ambivalence toward the object, followed by a period during which, ideally, the individual overcomes his attitude of ambivalence, and love and hate toward the same object can be tolerated without mutual interference. His developmental scheme (1924) undoubtedly relates ambivalence to the objects of component instincts (e.g., oral-sucking and oral-incorporative, anal-retentive and anal-expulsive), which is at variance with Freud's view that the concept of ambivalence should be restricted to the relationship of the total self to an object. Furthermore, Abraham's classification seems to be based on an observer's point of view rather than being a reflection of the infant's psychic experience. This becomes clear in the following passage:

> Within the first—the oral—period, the child exchanges its pre-ambivalent libidinal attitude, which is free from conflict, for one which is ambivalent and preponderantly hostile towards the object. Within the second—the anal-sadistic—period, the transition from the earlier to the later stage means that the individual has begun to spare his object from destruction. Finally, within the third—the genital—period, he overcomes his ambivalent attitude and his libido attains to its full capacity both from a sexual and a social point of view [p. 453].

The attribution of a destructive aim to an infant during his first year of life seems highly questionable. As I pointed out when I discussed some of Freud's formulations relating to the oral and anal phases of development, what may look like a destructive aim from a descriptive point of view is probably more in the nature of a wish for permanent possession of the pleasure-giving object from an experiential point of view. It is a form of "aggressive love," as Anna Freud (1949) has called it.

The views of Melanie Klein and her followers are, to a significant extent, based on some of Abraham's. Ambivalence is a central concept in Kleinian theory, regarded not only as an inherent characteristic of instincts themselves but also of the object which, as a consequence, has to be split into good and bad.

THE EXTENSION OF THE MEANING OF AMBIVALENCE IN THE POST-FREUDIAN LITERATURE

The preceding historical account suggests that, in the majority of his formulations, Freud gave ambivalence a very precise meaning in terms of the simultaneous existence of loving and hating feelings toward one and the same object. Bleuler's much wider view of ambivalence may be one of the historical reasons why in the current psychoanalytic literature the concept is often used with reference to phenomena which are completely unrelated to object-directed feelings of a contradictory quality. Like a number of other psychoanalytic concepts (for instance, those of transference and acting out), the concept of ambivalence has suffered the same fate of having been blurred in its original and precise meaning. It is now often used as a synonym for conflict in general, irrespective of the nature of such a conflict. Laplanche and Pontalis (1973) have summarized this state of affairs very well when they write that psychoanalysis "has often used 'ambivalence' in a very broad sense. The term has thus come at times to mean the actions and feelings resulting from a defensive conflict in which incompatible motives are involved; considering that in such cases what is pleasurable for one agency is unpleasurable for another, one might categorise every 'compromise-formation' as ambivalent. The danger of such a procedure is that the concept may come, in a vague way, to connote all kinds of conflict-ridden attitudes" (p. 28).

An illustration of this indiscriminate use of the term ambivalent can be found in a clinical description which refers to a child's conflict about having some of her secrets revealed to the therapist. The therapist writes that the child, "however, had ambivalent feelings about wanting me to know and not wanting me to know." Such descriptions, which are not uncommon, have nothing to do with ambivalence in the strict sense of the term. It might be more appropriate to speak in this and similar instances about "mixed feelings," leaving it open whether these arise from a conflict between different ego attitudes, between the ego and instinctual drive wishes, or between the ego and the external world (Sandler, 1974).

What needs emphasizing is that although ambivalent feelings can be the cause of severe conflicts and pathology, not all conflict is due to ambivalence. This seems almost too obvious to need saying. Yet the present-day tendency—perhaps more pronounced in clinical discussions than in the literature—of using the term "ambivalent" with reference to any conflict or indecision about a course of action to be taken blurs the issue in three ways. In the first place, it widens the notion of ambivalence to a point where it becomes virtually meaningless. Secondly, it entails the loss of the crucial distinction between conflicts which are specifically and primarily object-related and others which are not at all or only secondarily related to internal or external objects. Thirdly, and perhaps most importantly, it implicitly equates ambivalence with conflict. The existence of ambivalence in an object relationship is in itself no indication of pathology. Freud considered it to be a normal and expectable aspect of every relationship after a certain point in development has been reached. It is the rule rather than the exception that we value and admire certain characteristics in a person, while, at the same time, we dislike, loathe, or despise other attributes of that person. In spite of such opposite feelings, our loyalty and constancy to that object remains, without any tangible signs of conflict between the two sides.

Clinical Applications

It is of some clinical importance to distinguish between those individuals who are capable of tolerating the coexistence of ambivalent feelings without being neurotically conflicted about them and those individuals who do experience conflict over their ambivalent feelings and are capable only of finding pathological solutions to it. It is a distinction which roughly parallels that between normality and pathology. Freud held that neurotic ambivalence conflicts are due either to the intensity of the feelings involved, or to the fact that love and hate are of equal strength, and that in many cases there is evidence of a combination of these two factors. It might be a useful diagnostic pointer to assess not only a child's frustration tolerance but also his ambivalence tolerance.

While I have maintained that the indiscriminate use of the term "ambivalence" for any kind of conflict or mixed feelings serves no useful purpose, it may also be argued that the restriction of the concept to the coexistence of feelings of *love* and *hate* in an object relationship excludes a host of phenomena which undoubtedly bear the hallmark of ambivalence insofar as they reflect the simultaneous existence of opposite feelings toward one and the same object. Perhaps it is only a question of semantics if we accept that we tend to use the term "love" as a generic one to cover a vast range of different feelings of a positive quality toward an object rather than restricting it to those mature relationships where affection and sensuality have become united. In this sense we speak of parental love to include care, concern, admiration, pride, delight, fondness, and affection. We seem to be much more reluctant to use "hate" in a similarly global fashion, indicating that it has retained its meaning as a specific affect along a continuum from dislike, anger, to rage.

Following this line of thought, we might speak either of precursors or derivatives of the love-hate polarity. To such derivatives, in adults, would belong the coexistence of feelings of envy and gratitude in the transference relationship; or the simultaneous activation of wishes to praise or idealize on the one hand and to condemn or devalue on the other. Furthermore, the frequent coexistence of admiration for and fear of one and the same object belongs here, especially if the analysis reveals the fear to be the result of a projection of hostile wishes.

TYPES OF AMBIVALENCE IN CHILDREN

The precursors can be observed in the analysis of children. Especially in very young children, opposite feelings toward one and the same object coexist side by side, without any indications of conflict: a child will kiss his mother's hand one moment and hit it the next; or a child will embrace his younger sibling with such ardor as to nearly suffocate him. These two examples characterize two types of ambivalent manifestations, the first one showing the successive expression of the two sides of the ambivalence; the second, the condensation of the two into one action. This difference is again apparent in the child who wrote to her therapist: "Der (lieben) Frau Doktor—soll der Schlag treffen" ("To the (dear) Frau Doktor—may you be struck down")[4] and the child who referred to his younger sibling as being "nicety," an endearment which is a beautiful condensation of "nice" and "nasty." [5]

Most of the clinical examples in the Index under the heading of ambivalent object relationships describe, in fact, the expression of the two sides of the ambivalence in succession, as the following typical example illustrates.

> The intensity of ambivalence in Amy's object relationships contributes to her pervasive difficulty in handling ambivalent conflicts. In treatment, her ambivalence has been demonstrated most strikingly in relation to her brother. In a game Amy [5 years old] talked about a sister who was "happy" to have a little brother, and then about a boy who had to hide from his sister who wanted to kill him. After six months of treatment, Amy tried to resolve this conflict in games, with the therapist in the role of the sibling, saying, "Sometimes we play together, and sometimes not, and sometimes we can fight."

This mode of expressing the ambivalent feelings toward one and the same object in succession might be referred to as a "temporal splitting of the ambivalence," to distinguish it from the defensive splitting of the ambivalence where one side of the ambivalence is displaced from one object to another.

---

[4] I am indebted to Anna Freud for this example.
[5] I am indebted to Trevor Hartnup for this example.

Ambivalence

The next illustration shows a mixture of the temporal splitting of the ambivalance and indications of a beginning compromise formation between the two sides of the ambivalence in a somewhat older child, a girl aged 7.

> There was heightened ambivalence in Emma toward all her objects: family, friends, therapist. Emma said that she sometimes calls mummy and daddy big fat elephants and muck, adding, "One day I like them and one day I hate them." She said about a friend: "Angela likes her mother one day and hates her another day; just as you teach it here." One day she wrote down what she felt about her therapist and began, "Love, hate, adore, like, nice, horrible," adding, "You see, there are more loves than hates." Later she said to the therapist, "Coming here is my best and my worst." Still later she said about her mother: "I can think mummy is nice and also a pig."

This example suggests Emma's growing awareness and tolerance of the coexistence of both positive and negative feelings toward the same object and a capacity to maintain a positive relationship to such an object in spite of the presence of hostile feelings. More generally, this development seems to be dependent on the consolidation of emotional object constancy as well as on the ego's capacity for integration. The attainment of object constancy would appear to be a precondition for conflicts over ambivalent feelings to arise, followed by a fairly prolonged developmental process in the direction of tolerating ambivalent feelings without mutual interference.

It is clear that love and hatred in a narrow sense refer to very complex feeling states which cannot occur before a considerable degree of psychic development has taken place and a relatively advanced level of object relatedness has been achieved. This would be in line with Freud's view that ambivalence does not belong in the realm of component instincts and their objects but is rather an expression of feelings experienced by the self in relation to another object as a whole. For this reason it is questionable whether one ought to speak of ambivalence in an infant before he has reached a point in development when he is fully aware that the frustrating object toward whom he experiences anger is the same person who gratifies his needs at other times.

Of the two types of ambivalent expression illustrated above, that of the separate activation of the two sides, seems to be—from a developmental point of view—the earlier one since it contains no signs of any attempts at synthesis or integration on the part of the ego. The second type of example, which contains a condensation of or compromise between the two sides of the ambivalence, already shows indications of such integration. In children, this ego capacity for integration and synthesis of contradictory or incompatible ideas or affects is not yet fully developed. Yet, as development proceeds, the ego becomes increasingly intolerant of the simultaneous presence of such incompatible wishes, ideas, or feelings in relation to an object. At this point a conflict situation arises which necessitates the instigation of defensive measures.

DEFENSES AGAINST AMBIVALENCE

Two specific modes of defense seem to be particularly associated with ambivalence conflicts. One of these is the so-called "splitting of the ambivalence," frequently seen in children but not uncommon in adults either. In the past, this mode of defense must have been greatly facilitated by the presence of nurses and nannies in the household. The following Index example from the treatment of a 5-year-old boy illustrates this defensive mechanism:

> Cyril's relationship to his mother is mainly of an ambivalent nature. The therapist has observed that he seems to split this ambivalence, expressing the hate only to his mother, while the expression of love is directed toward his father. He sees his father as all good, his mother as all bad. Later in treatment it seemed that he split this ambivalence toward his mother between the therapist and his mother, seeing the therapist as his good mummy and his own as the bad.

This example reflects the influence of this boy's phallic-oedipal development in determining the displacement of the loving feelings from the mother representation onto another object (father, therapist). One expects that younger children will more frequently show a tendency to preserve the need-satisfying object (the mother) as the good and loved one and to displace the hostile feelings from her onto another suitable object such as a relative, teacher, father, sibling, an animal, or even inanimate objects.

The second mode of defense commonly found in connection with attempts to resolve ambivalence conflicts consists of the repression of one component of the polarity and the reactive reinforcement of the other component, frequently showing itself in an overconcern for the safety and well-being of the loved person. We are familiar with this phenomenon from the analysis of obsessionals. It is also frequently found in children who are trying to come to terms with their intense death wishes against the parent (usually the mother) on whom they are dependent and whose love and care they can ill afford to lose. Clinging behavior and difficulties in separating from the omnipotently threatened object are often associated with this reactive concern, which is well illustrated in the following example of a 6-year-old girl.

> One of Jane's main referral symptoms was her difficulties in separating from her mother. She usually made a big fuss when she had to let her mother go at school, and ever since entering primary school she had insisted on being fetched home for lunch every day. In treatment, she initially became very anxious when she was away from her mother and frequently had to run out of sessions in order to ensure that her mother was still in the waiting room. For many months she could not tolerate the idea of her mother leaving the Clinic while she had her session. What emerged initially in treatment was her tremendous concern for her mother. Apart from a general provocativeness at home and a sadomasochistic quality in her relationship with her mother, there were no tangible signs of hostile feelings toward her. These emerged only after a prolonged period of intensive work on her obsessional defense organization and when the mother transference became the focus of the analysis. This brought to the surface the most intense death wishes against her mother, at first in displaced and distanced forms (e.g., sending away and killing the nasty and bad stepmother, fantasies about destroying the therapist anally), but gradually directly related to her mother who had confronted her with a brother when Jane was 2, who was felt to have deprived her of a penis, and who was now also experienced as a rival as far as Jane's oedipal wishes toward her father were concerned.

Clinically, it is not always easy to make a clear distinction between these two defenses of splitting and repression. With both of them, the link of one side of the ambivalence to a particular object has disappeared, in one case due to displacement, in the other as a consequence of repression. The reactive intensification of the feelings of love or hate toward a particular person usually serves as a pointer to the type of defense which is in operation. On the other hand, it is quite easy to mistake the expressed hatred toward a certain object as the split-off part of the ambivalence belonging to another object when, in fact, the former object may be hated in its own right. Yet this distinction is of considerable clinical importance with regard to the understanding and interpretation of phallic-oedipal material as it emerges in the transference relationship.

PARAPRAXES

Certain forms of behavior and particularly slips of the tongue give indications of strong ambivalent feelings which the patient is trying to hide from conscious awareness for a variety of reasons. What finds expression is then often in the nature of a compromise between the loving and hating feelings. For a beautiful example of this, I am again indebted to Anna Freud who recalled an obsessional child who flung herself at her, embraced her lovingly, and said: "I want to kill you—I mean kiss you." In both children and adults we often find a marked discrepancy between the content of what they are saying and the significance of what they are doing at the same time. Thus a patient talked about the goodness of his mother and about his fondness of her, while at the same time he violently kicked the table leg with his foot. Another patient gave verbal expression to her immense gratitude toward me, quite oblivious of the fact that, at the same time, she was pounding a cushion on the side of the couch with her fist.

Lateness for sessions, misunderstandings about session times, errors in connection with the payment of analytic fees may all be indications of ambivalent feelings, although this is not invariably so. Without exploring each such incident in depth, all we can say is that such behavior is a reflection of a conflict, but it need not necessarily center around ambivalent feelings.

With slips of the tongue it is usually easier to ascertain immediately whether they are derived from a conflict over ambivalent feelings. For instance, a patient who meant to tell me how gentle he could be to his wife when they were in bed together said instead, "And I can be so jealous toward her when we are in bed," revealing the underlying ambivalent feelings toward her. The same patient told me how he got up very early one morning in order to get on with some work which he was anxious to complete. As he got up he heard his wife say to him: "Do you want me to make light?" He mumbled something about seeing enough and followed his intention to work. He realized later that his wife had, in fact, asked him whether he wanted to make love. This "slip of the ear," as we might call it, was therefore not due to an ambivalent conflict; rather, his anxiety-driven need to work left no room for the possibility of obtaining sexual gratification.

Freud's *Psychopathology of Everyday Life* (1901) contains many examples of bungled actions, errors, and other parapraxes which indicate an underlying conflict over ambivalence. Perhaps one of the most impressive examples is that of a father (Freud's patient) who once almost struck his favorite child's head against a heavy gas chandelier. The analysis revealed that this action was an expression of a repressed wish for the death of this now consciously beloved child which originated during the child's earliest infancy when the father wanted to be free and get a divorce from his wife from whom he got little satisfaction (p. 188).

NEED VERSUS LOVE FOR AN OBJECT

In some of his second phase formulations, Freud emphasized the point that a child above all *needs* an object in order to survive. To begin with, the infant is totally dependent on such a mothering object in every respect, i.e., for the satisfaction of bodily needs (food, warmth, hygiene) as well as emotional needs (to be loved, cuddled, smiled at, held). As he develops, he will at first return his mother's love and attention to the extent to which she satisfies his needs. At the same time, he will experience hostile feelings toward her insofar as he perceives her as frustrating, restricting, and uninvolved with him. We know from observations and analyses of blind children how much more prolonged and exclusive this dependence on a caring object is on account of their sensory deficiency. Adults at least have the option to reject and abandon those objects which do not meet their needs—whatever they are—and replace them by others which promise to be more suitable and satisfactory. No such option is open to a child for a great many years. When we therefore speak of a child's ambivalence toward a parental figure—in particular toward his mother—are we right in always conceptualizing it in terms of a juxtaposition between love and hate? Or would it not sometimes be more appropriate to think of it in terms of a conflict between the need for and dependence on the mother on the one hand and a wish to reject her on the other?

Some of the clinical examples in the Index suggest that the child's need to make reparation because of a fear of losing the needed object is often mistaken for an expression of primarily loving feelings (in contrast to a placating or propitiating sort of love). A clinical example will highlight this problem. It comes from a girl who started treatment around the age of 9. The material, classified in the section on "Object Relationships" under "Characteristics: Ambivalent," describes this girl's "deeply ambivalent feelings toward the object" and her increased ability to tolerate the coexistence of loving and hostile feelings toward one and the same object, without being overwhelmed with anxieties of either destroying or seducing the object. The example shows how this ambivalence manifested itself in the transference relationship:

> Whenever Nelly experienced sexual feelings, she became angry with the therapist. She then threw away her toys and her locker key, complained that treatment kept her from important pleasures, and then experienced intense anxiety, panic, hunger, and made the attempt to hold on to the therapist at the very last moment. When the Christmas holidays approached, Nelly was very unwilling to show and bring out the suspicions and anger she felt, still fearful that this would destroy the now very positive relationship in the transference.

Such an example raises the question to what extent the positive feelings in the transference are determined by intense anxieties about the possibility of being rejected by and losing the object on whom the child has become dependent, and whom she feared having offended irreparably. Nelly's efforts to hold on to her therapist after her outbursts of hostile feelings seem to be in the nature of a reparative effort, triggered off by her fears of losing the object's love and based on her need for and dependence on that love. This would mean that we are here dealing not with a conflict between love and hate but rather with one between need and hate.

A similar problem arises in connection with a much younger child, whose *need* for the object to provide her with emotional supplies was much more pronounced. Karen needed to feel loved in order to maintain her self-regard. She was nearly 4 years old when she started treatment. Her clinical material also was classified under "Object Relationships: Characteristics: Ambivalent."

> Karen desperately wanted the love and attention of other people. This much was evident in her incessant demands as well as in her hurt expression when she felt rejected or unappreciated. The anger as well as the self-hatred that resulted from this sense of rejection prompted Karen to increase her demands for attention. The resulting behavior was a clear indication of her ambivalence. Sometimes Karen's demands were a straightforward expression of her affection and need for love. At other times they were colored by a sense of reproach and biting discontent with the people who did not, in her estimation, love her enough.

The greedy demands and overriding need to get something from an object raise the question whether what appears to be affection for the object is not more in the nature of placating the object in order to get from the object what Karen wants for herself. The object seems to be loved not for what it *is* but for what it provides. In this sense, we would not be justified to speak of ambivalence in this instance. Nelly's example is reminiscent of those young children who assure a person of their love in the hope of eliciting what they want (need) for themselves. It is a form of cupboard love; and in conjunction with the anger over the frustration of their wishes, it has very little to do with ambivalence between love and hate.

This distinction between the need of an object and the love of an object is clinically relevant in the treatment not only of children but also of adults. It parallels Freud's distinction, within the positive transference, between affectionate and more directly sexual aspects. In this sense the need of and dependence on the analyst form an essential ingredient of the developing treatment alliance which enables the patient to persevere with the analysis in the face of resistances and at times when negative transference feelings predominate. The patients' awareness, conscious or unconscious, that they *need* the analyst for the resolution of their problems is thus a powerful ally in our therapeutic endeavors. Where it is absent, the likelihood of treatment being broken off prematurely is greatly increased. We are very familiar with this phenomenon from the treatment of adolescents.

"HATE OBJECT"

In a discussion concerned with the simultaneous existence of loving and hateful feelings toward one and the same object, it is pertinent to wonder about the reasons why the object of the aggressive drive impulses apparently shows less stability than that of the sexual drives, and why we generally do not speak of a "hate object" as we do of a "love object."

Some of Freud's formulations referred to previously suggest that, at the beginning of psychic development, the external world is equated with the source of all unpleasure and therefore cathected with aggression. This stage parallels the narcissistic split between the self as pleasurable and the object world outside as unpleasurable. From a developmental point of view, the appearance of ambivalence in an object relationship goes hand in hand with the infant's reluctant acceptance of the fact that the objects in his external world on whom he is dependent are a source of both pleasure and unpleasure, satisfactions and frustrations. At the same time—and in line with the magic-omnipotent mode of his thought processes—he has to cope with the fear that his unmitigated hatred of the needed object might omnipotently destroy it. The growing awareness of the need for the object provides the stimulus for the deflection of the hostility away from the need-satisfying object in order to protect and preserve it. Either the ambivalence is split, or the hostile component undergoes repression. In the former case, the hostility is displaced to any suitable object and we see frequent shifts from one object to another.

I am not sure whether this is a sufficient explanation for the undoubted fact that the link between loving feelings and a particular object is much more stable and persisting than that between hateful feelings and a specific object. While one might be inclined to have recourse to the "adhesiveness of the libido" (Freud, 1937), it would be more appropriate to speak of the mobility of aggressive investments. We reserve our love and admiration for special people, but we are much more indiscriminate in our choice of the victims of our hostility. For some people, this may provide a safeguard against experiencing an intolerable degree of ambivalence in a valued and meaningful relationship. Others again may have reached a point at which their egos have become successful in sufficiently integrating the two sides of the ambivalence so that mutual interference between love and hate is absent, with a concomitant mitigation of hate by love and of love by hate. The prognosis seems worst for those who have to initiate pathogenic defenses against conflicts over ambivalence at an early age, before their egos have attained the full capacity for synthesis and integration.

BIBLIOGRAPHY

ABRAHAM, K. (1924), A Short Study of the Development of the Libido. *Selected Papers on Psycho-Analysis.* London: Hogarth Press, 1927, pp. 418–501.

BLEULER, E. (1910), Lecture on ambivalence, reported in *Zbl. Psychoanal.*, 1:266, 1911.

EDGCUMBE, R. (1970), The Development of Freud's Instinct Theory, 1894–1939. In: *Basic Psychoanalytic Concepts on the Theory of Instincts,* ed. H. Nagera. London: Allen & Unwin, pp. 23–49.

FREUD, A. (1949), Aggression in Relation to Emotional Development. *This Annual,* 3/4:37–48.

FREUD, S. (1901), The Psychopathology of Everyday Life. *S.E.,* 6.

——— (1905), Three Essays on the Theory of Sexuality. *S.E.,* 7:125–243.

——— (1909a), Analysis of a Phobia in a Five-Year-Old Boy. *S.E.,* 10:3–149.

——— (1909b), Notes upon a Case of Obsessional Neurosis. *S.E.,* 10:153–320.

——— (1912), The Dynamics of Transference. *S.E.,* 12:97–108.

——— (1913), Totem and Taboo. *S.E.,* 13:1–161.

——— (1915), Instincts and Their Vicissitudes. *S.E.,* 14:111–140.

——— (1918), From the History of an Infantile Neurosis. *S.E.,* 17:3–123.

——— (1920), Beyond the Pleasure Principle. *S.E.,* 18:3–64.

——— (1923), The Ego and the Id. *S.E.,* 19:3–66.

——— (1933), New Introductory Lectures on Psycho-Analysis. *S.E.,* 22:3–182.

——— (1937), Analysis Terminable and Interminable. *S.E.*, 23:209–253.
——— (1939), Moses and Monotheism. *S.E.*, 23:3–137.
——— (1950), Extracts from the Fliess Papers. *S.E.*, 1:175–280.
GRINSTEIN, A. (1956), *The Index of Psychoanalytic Writings*, 1. New York: Int. Univ. Press.
HARTMANN, H. (1955), Notes on the Theory of Sublimation. *This Annual*, 10:9–29.
——— KRIS, E., & LOEWENSTEIN, R. M. (1949), Notes on the Theory of Aggression. *This Annual*, 3/4:9–36.
LAPLANCHE, J. & PONTALIS, J.-B. (1973), *The Language of Psycho-Analysis*. London: Hogarth Press.
SANDLER, J. (1974), Psychological Conflict and the Structural Model. *Int. J. Psycho-Anal.*, 55:53–62.

The Interpretation of Dreams, Semiology, and Chomskian Linguistics

A Radical Critique

PATRICK MAHONY, PH.D.
AND RAJENDRA SINGH, PH.D.

IN HIS VERITABLE PIONEERING MONOGRAPH MARSHALL EDELSON (1973) rightly sees Freud the dream theorist as the forerunner of modern semiology.[1] Accordingly, Edelson specifies that when "Freud describes the dream as a kind of rebus, he is clearly concerned, and perhaps the first semiologist to state the problem so explicitly, with the translation of the symbolic forms of one symbolic system into those of another symbolic system" (p. 252), i.e., the translation of the verbosymbolic latent dream into the predominant visuality of the manifest dream. Edelson's own guiding interest is to harmonize Freudian and Chomskian tenets, to establish an isomorphism between linguistic deep and surface structures and the dual structure of oneiric activity. Hence, "the semantically interpreted

---

Patrick Mahony is Associate Professor teaching English and comparative literature at the Université de Montréal; he is also in training at the Canadian Institute of Psychoanalysis. Rajendra Singh is Assistant Professor in linguistics at the same university.

[1] In this new vast field dealing specifically with semiology, two other works deserve special mention: Ernesto Liendo (1967) applies a semiology inspired by Luis Prieto to a noticeably Kleinian conception of object relations; the other is by David Liberman (1970).

deep structures underlying dreams are identical with those underlying linguistic forms generated in waking consciousness" (p. 234). All in all, Edelson's own text merits close attention insofar as it makes a daring attempt in semiological innovation, incorporates a sensitive reading of *The Interpretation of Dreams*, and recurrently offers stimulating questions for further speculation and research.

Granted the merits of Edelson's efforts, however, three major objections, each of which will be taken up in detail in separate sections, may be brought against his approach. First and ironically enough, in spite of Edelson's very enchantment with semiology, he neglects to explore the area in dream analysis where Freud made his most striking semiological observations! Secondly, the identifications posited between Chomskian and Freudian concepts are, unwittingly, metaphorical and analogical mentations on Edelson's part. Thirdly, his semiological penchant wrongly induces him to challenge the essential existence of censorship, whose function would putatively be subsumed by the factor of representability; Edelson's contention nonetheless solves nothing, creates problems, and indeed militates against the law of parsimony that he so cherishes and invokes.

I

One could semiologically describe some of Freud's efforts in dream theory as an attempt to establish a comparative grammar of interior media. Semiology of course is used somewhat loosely here as a word, for in the strict sense semiology cannot be extended to mental operations since codes exist only for external phenomena and there are no codes for our thoughts. Nevertheless, for example, what may be called the interior visual media of fantasies may be to some extent considered in relation with external media of a visual nature, such as cinema and television. With admirable effort, Freud strove to trace the translation of the syntactic laws of the latent dream or verbosymbolic mode into the manifest dream or predominantly visual mode. Necessarily, however, as Emile Benveniste (1969) suggested about external communicative systems, there is an inevitable relative distortion of a message put in different media: "There is no 'synonymy' between semiotic systems; one cannot 'say the same thing' in words and in music. . . . Man does not dispose of several distinct systems for the same relation of meaning" (p. 9).

Thus the individuating features of a medium, sensorial and otherwise, change that which is communicated. Now if we bear in mind that fantasies, somatic symptoms, and latent dreams are intrapsychic phenomena or media with visual, kinesthetic, and verbal bases, the "same message" should be somewhat altered in each of the three systems. It follows that a modification of this kind occurs in dreams. The verbosymbolic latent dream is rooted in a wish, or grammatically, in the optative mood; yet sheer visuality (and hence the manifest dream) can directly express only the indicative. The hallucinatory dramatization of that indicative mood is ipso facto enacted in the present tense, and defined by it. In this sense Freud (1916/17) declares:

> . . . a dream does not simply give expression to a thought, but represents the wish fulfilled as a hallucinatory experience. '*I should like to go on the lake*' is the wish that instigates the dream. The content of the dream itself is: '*I am going on the lake.*' Thus even in these simple children's dreams a difference remains between the latent and the manifest dream, there is a distortion of the latent dream-thought: *the transformation of a thought into an experience.* In the process of interpreting a dream this alteration must first be undone. If this turns out to be the most universal characteristic of dreams, the fragment of dream which I reported to you earlier 'I saw my brother in a box' is not to be translated 'my brother is restricting himself' but 'I should like my brother to restrict himself: *my brother must restrict himself* [p. 129].[2]

Freud went on to spell out in some detail the grammar of articulation between the latent and manifest dream; as he insisted, one must discover the "characters and syntactic laws" of the manifest dream by comparing it with the original (1900, p. 277). The semiological value of this grammar is undeniable, as it directly

---

[2] See also Freud (1905): "The dream-work . . . submits the thought-material, which is brought forward in the optative mood, to a most strange revision" (p. 162) and "Thus dreams make use of the present tense in the same manner and by the same right as day-dreams. The present tense is the one in which wishes are represented as fulfilled" (1900, p. 535).

grapples with the problem of representability, of translating elusive points of lexicality and verbal syntax into oneiric pictures. In this way—one not examined by Edelson—Freud anticipated the contemporary semiological challenge of translating the literary form of, say, a novel into the cinematic medium, or par excellence a short story into a silent movie. Laboring under the same difficulties as the plastic arts of painting and sculpture, dreams generally disregard all conjunctions and the relations between the subject matter of dream thoughts (1900, p. 313). Yet dreams do represent logical relationship, which is revealed mainly in their form.[3] Specifically, it is the dreamwork which does "succeed in expressing some of the content of the latent dream-thoughts by peculiarities in the *form* of the manifest dream—by its clarity or obscurity, by its division into several pieces, and so on. . . . Thus the form of dreams is far from being without significance and itself calls for interpretation" (1916/17, p. 177).

In actuality, then, the form of a manifest dream has a dual importance: it may refer to the semantics or the syntax of the latent dream. Semantically, the varying clarity of either whole dreams or their sections may be highly revelatory. Given the fact that *"The form of a dream or the form in which it is dreamt is used with quite surprising frequency for representing its concealed subject-matter"* (1900, p. 332), a hazy dream, for example, may express the female dreamer's confusion about the father of her child, or a dream of absolute clarity might represent the sleeper's wish that a theoretical problem be flawlessly solved. And in another case, a great part of the impression of a dream's absurdity "was brought about by running together sentences from different parts of the dream-thoughts without any transition" (1900, p. 437).

Syntactically as well, Freud's various oneiric translations are worthy of the closest semiological attention:

Either—Or. Though in the great majority of cases, this double conjunction does not succeed in being expressed, occasionally the

---

[3] In effect, visual expression cannot directly contain relations, which characterize thoughts. Both phylogenetically and ontogenetically it is older than thinking in words and is in some ways even nearer to unconscious processes (Freud, 1923, p. 21).

idea of mutual exclusion is represented in a dream by two equal parts (1900, p. 316ff.).

If. Sometimes *if* in a dependent conditional clause is represented by a minor dream episode interrupting the main dream scene which has persisted for some time; this minor scene seems describable in these words: "But then it was as though at the same time it was another place, and there such and such a thing happened." This spectacular case incorporates a multiple translation: the *if* of the latent dream becoming a sequent visual scene; the sequentiality nevertheless is *verbally* describable as *when, at the same time,* which in turn is to be verbally translated as *if* (1900, p. 335).

Because. Though in the preponderant number of instances causality is lost, it may be expressed by the transformation of an image of a person or thing into another, before our very eyes, or by the division of the dream itself into two unequal parts; extra caution is needed here, for the two unequal parts may otherwise indicate two different points of view (1900, p. 315f.). Concerning the transformation of one image into another, and its semiological applications to cinema, a passage from Jakobson's essay on the two types of aphasia is especially pertinent:

> Ever since the productions of D. W. Griffith, the art of the cinema, with its highly developed capacity for changing the angle, perspective and focus of "shots", has broken with the tradition of the theater and ranged an unprecedented variety of synecdochic "close-ups" and metonymic "set-ups" in general. In such pictures as those of Charlie Chaplin and Eisenstein these devices in turn were overlayed by a novel, metaphoric "montage" with its "lap dissolves"—the filmic similes [1971, p. 256].

A promising area of fruitful semiological investigation lies in the evaluation of Freud's and Jakobson's divergent positions. For Freud, the transformation of one image into another may mean causality, which in itself expresses a metonymy, a syntagmatic relationship between two events. Jakobson on the other hand sees image transformation as metaphorical and paradigmatic, thus contrasting with a cinematic metonymic style.

Elsewhere Freud (1905, p. 172) summarily asserts that dreams replace internal associations (similarity, causality) by external associations (simultaneity in time, contiguity in space, similarity in sound), the very components of infantile causality. In this regard, it is by means of scattered remarks in *Totem and Taboo* (1913, pp. 5f., 27, 61, 81ff., 85, 87f.) that we may construct the most insightful synthesis. Contact is the most comprehensive term for the two essential ways of association: similarity or metaphorical contact (characterizing imitative or homeopathic magic, where a similarity exists between the act performed and the result expected) and contiguity or literal contact (characterizing contagious magic, in which the contiguity may be spatial or imagined). One may note here, however, a terminological difficulty insofar as imagined contiguity is not easily differentiated from similarity or metaphorical contact. At any event, parallel to the two kinds of contact postulated by Freud, there are two types of displacement: the displacement operative in obsessional neurosis, where prohibitions glide from one object to another, and displacement operative in the taboo-infected individual, who contaminates those coming in contact with him; hence, perhaps since obsessional neurotics displace, they follow the laws of similarity, substitution, and imitation.

Just As. This is the only logical relation that is highly favored by visuality itself, through the dream mechanism of condensation. More precisely, two entities linked by a common element may be represented by a composite reality, or merely by either of the two entities (1900, p. 319f.).

Logical Connection. Such connections are reproduced by simultaneity in time, like Raphael who in his School of Athens established a conceptual unity between all the poets and philosophers by assembling them all at one time in the same place. For details, dreams express connections by juxtaposing or collocating scenes (1900, p. 314), i.e., by propinquity in time (p. 247).

Independent and Dependent Clauses. With respect to this larger grammatical framework, Freud's suggestions are most provoking:

> The number of part-dreams into which a dream is divided usually corresponds to the number of main topics or groups of thoughts in the latent dream. A short introductory dream will often stand in the relation of a prelude to a following, more detailed, main dream

or may give the motive for it; a subordinate clause in the dream-thoughts will be replaced by the interpolation of a change of scene into the manifest dream, and so on [1916/17, p. 177].

By contrast, in the more localized and specific area of syntactical expression, exemplified in at least three instances, Freudian hermeneutics are too readily venturesome:

1. A dependent temporal clause is represented by an introductory or terminal minor dream, the more extensive part of a dream always corresponding to a principal clause (1900, p. 314f.).

2. "A short introductory dream and a longer main dream following it often stand in the relation of protasis and apodosis [conditional and consequential clauses]" (1933, p. 26). Freud, on the other hand, cites one instance of a screen character adequately representing a conditional sentence. In one of his dreams the substitution of his father for Meynert did not lie in any analogy between them but rather translated "a conditional sentence in the dream-thoughts, which ran in full: 'If only I had been the second generation, the son of a professor or Hofrat, I should certainly have got on faster' " (1900, p. 438).

3. "A dream which is described by the dreamer as 'somehow interpolated' will actually correspond to a dependent clause in the dream-thought" (1933, p. 26f.). Similarly, secondary elaborations, not being especially vivid, are frequently introduced by an "as though" in postoneiric description (1900, p. 489). At any event, to this postulated correspondence between dream segments and grammatical dependence or independence, one may offer two caveats. First, grammar does not necessarily conform to logic. As the linguist Francis Christensen discovered, contemporary American expository prose is characterized by the most important matter being found in *dependent* grammatical structures; likewise, Baroque prose in seventeenth-century England often had the same trait (see Rooney, 1962). Secondly, just as dream condensation and censorship operate on a semantic basis, they may also do syntactically and, for purposes of disguise and screening, devote the longer oneiric scene to a minor issue.

In sum, the formal traits of a dream that Freud hermeneutically invokes include the length of its parts, the placement of a shorter dream episode (either initially, terminally, or as a medial interpolation), juxtaposition, condensation, metamorphosis of one element into another, and obscurity or distinctness of whole or sections of dreams. Or in other words, the form of a dream ranges from its sheerly external aspects (length) to internal ones (haziness and transformation).

With reference to these findings, much more research must be devoted to the formal aspects of the manifest dream, the results of which should be particularly promising for dream interpretation. There is a pressing need for a comparative syntax of the sensorial dream. How does a tactile imagination, for example, represent syntax? On another score, Robert Blank (1958) reported that "The congenitally blind do not have visual dreams." [4] Blank also finds that in the congenitally blind, hearing is the foremost sensory dream element; tactile or kinesthetic next, whereas the gustatory and olfactory are rare. Certainly, the analysis of a dream's form is rendered very difficult by its ephemeral nature. Nevertheless a phenomenological reflection on the nature of dreams—and one is absolutely necessary—should be guided by two essential principles of semiological investigation: the specification of the basic units of a system, and the rules of their combination. To this end, one might explore some of the semiological criteria applied by René Passeron (1962) to painting and by Marcel Martin (1968) and Christian Metz (1968, 1971) to the cinema. Cinematic semiology could be directed to the field of psychoanalytic symbolism, e.g., the Wolf Man's primal scene. Though the scene occurred when he was 1½ years old and was only later put into words, it was singled out among other visual incidents; though preverbal, it was given a signifié, a signified. Could it be that such traumatic visual phenomena (fantasied or real) might be displaced and deformed into various configurational patterns, much as heavily charged

---

[4] Blank says that his finding "will surprise only those who believe in a racial unconsciousness, hereditary transmission of memories, or other Lamarckian concepts" (p. 159). He adds that if a person is blinded before 7, there is little chance of his having visual memories or dreams later on, for the period between 5 and 7 is critical for cerebral structural maturation, the development of the visual center, and the completion of early ego growth.

words are both phonologically and orthographically? These configurational patterns may be assigned, then, to objects or shapes far different from those proper to the primal scene. Thus, on a markedly *visual* basis, some object very dissimilar in shape from a breast may be symbolized for it. It remains to determine the practicality and practicability of determining the symbolic vicissitudes of a transformed visuality. On a simple plane, a straight line may be transformed into a circle, a crooked line, etc. It may be that the plethora of metamorphic possibilities discards any practical application. Yet the retention of the viability of such a concept in mind may afford a correcting alternative to restricting symbolism solely to archetypal, verbal, and other considerations.[5]

A second great need in what may be called comparative oneirics is a study of mass media's influence on the form of dreams. Hence one may ask, Is the form of a dream different in an oral-history society as opposed to a literary and print-oriented society? Does the transformation of one dream image into another take place predominantly in a "movie" culture? To what degree do mass media, each of which has its own syntax, influence the form of the manifest dream? Alongside the very express messages of symbols, the oedipus complex, infantile wishes, etc., syntax itself in dreams is meaning, message. To this extent one may posit some relevance of McLuhan's theories to dreams.

Thirdly, if hypotaxis[6] is to some degree in the formal nature of

---

[5] At any rate, there would be a great use for a grammar of visual deformation and displacement that could do on a visual basis what Jones (1916), for example, did with Punchinello as a verbal symbol, tracing its contaminations and so on. Moreover, such a grammar would help to undercut Jones's contention that "linguistic connections between the symbol and the idea symbolised" (p. 140) are one of the six aspects of true symbolism. The manifold nature of childhood symbolism is even further complicated by the cross-sensory and intermodal possibilities underlined by Howard Gardner (1973). Recent studies indicate more and more that the child, seizing on the modal properties of behavior, may well open his mouth as a response to seeing an open hand. Gardner concludes: "The sensitivity to modal/vectoral properties (which cut across sensory modalities and are manifest in both perceptual and the motoric realm) is, I would suggest further, a necessary antecedent for the use and comprehension of symbols, and remains fundamental to our cognition in the adult years" (p. 206f.).

[6] I.e., sentence structure characterized by subordinate structure and hierarchical organization, exemplified par excellence by the Ciceronian periodic sentence. On

the manifest dream, to that degree the dreams of people whose language is marked by hypotactic structure should be different from those whose language (and basis of their latent dreams) is paratactic. Thus the Whorfian hypothesis concerning language as a determinant of culture could be either somewhat shaken or confirmed by dream evidence.

II

In this section, we shall examine the linguistic aspects of Edelson's proposals. Since he is apparently interested in developing an explicit, generative theory of "dream language" (a cover term we shall use to designate the terminal units in which dreams are represented and various kinds of rules that must necessarily relate these units in a determinable way), some of our comments will necessarily be concerned with his understanding of the generative theory of language, deliberately chosen by him as his model. His larger aim of contributing something to a general theory of what he calls "symbolic function" will also be taken up.

Edelson is interested in developing propositions about "the relation between dreams and language," the outlines of a possible generative theory of dream language, and in examining "the possible status" of the generative theories of language and dream language in relation to a "more general theory of semiology or symbolic function." More specifically, he is concerned with "the determinacy of the meaning of dreams—what aspects of their mode of construction make their meaning determinable" and with "the value of using the linguistic distinction between deep and surface structures for appreciating the consequences of the operations of the dreamwork" (p. 209f.).

Edelson's attempt to provide plausible outlines of a possible generative theory of dream language constitutes a major effort since it could, if it is not devoid of empirical content, have some far-reaching consequences. Chiefly, if his preliminary demonstra-

---

the other hand, in parataxis there are no conjunctions (as in a telegram), or if subordinating and coordinating conjunctions be present, they tend to be deprived of their logical force (as in Biblical style).

tion succeeds, it would show that there are indeed domains of symbolic function other than language that are characterized by a richness and complexity that most generative grammarians believe is restricted to human language.

Since the parameters of the context within which Edelson's proposals must be examined are overwhelming, it may not be entirely out of place to identify some of them rather clearly. Edelson's hopes provide an optimistic counterpoint to Chomsky's pessimism regarding the problem of "extending concepts of linguistic structure to other cognitive systems," which, to Chomsky (1972), does not seem to be in "too promising a state" (p. 75). The study of other languagelike structures has not turned up with anything "even roughly comparable to language in these domains" (p. 74). Chomsky adds:

> Are there other areas of human competence where one might hope to develop a fruitful theory, analogous to generative theory? Although this is a very important question, there is very little that can be said about it today. One might, for example, consider the problem of how a person comes to acquire a certain concept of three-dimensional space, or an implicit theory of "human action" in similar terms. Such a study would begin with the attempt to characterize the implicit theory that underlies actual performance and would then turn to the question how this theory develops under the given conditions of time and access to data—that is, in what way the resulting system of beliefs is determined by the interplay of available data, "heuristic procedures," and the innate mechanism that restricts and conditions the form of the acquired system [p. 73f.].

It is important to note the reasons for Chomsky's pessimism. He believes that although various systems have been shown to be rich and complex, their richness and complexity have never been shown to be of that specific kind that generative grammarians attribute to language systems. He believes that there is "not the slightest reason to believe" that there are other symbolic systems that have specific properties of generative grammars of human languages—say "the distinction of deep and surface structure, the specific properties of grammatical transformations and phonological rules, the principles of rule ordering, and so on" (p. 175). There is "little useful analogy between the schema of universal grammar [generative theory of human language] that we must, I believe, assign to the mind as an innate character, and any other known system of mental organization" (p. 90).[7]

If any other system of mental organization can be shown to have the specific properties of generative grammars, Chomsky would be willing to give up his pessimism. It is, he admits, "quite possible that the lack of analogy testifies to our ignorance of other aspects of mental function, rather than to the absolute uniqueness of linguistic structure" (p. 90). Such a demonstration would also provide an answer to the larger question regarding the number of faculties of the mind. If the theories of the various domains of symbolic functioning were shown to have the specific properties of generative grammars, we would have reason to believe that there is, as Edelson apparently thinks, just one faculty, "the symbolic function," of the mind, not, as advocated by Putnam (1967), for example, several.

Edelson has, thus, undertaken a major challenge. As a serious proposal, it must be understood as an attempt not only to construct a generative theory of "dream language" but also to answer some of the serious, philosophical questions regarding the nature of the human mind.

Impressed with the generative theory of language and Freud's explicit concern with "meaning," Edelson starts out with a catalogue of similarities between Chomsky and Freud, two pioneering theorists dealing with symbolic systems controlled by humans. His ritual citation of similarities between the methodologies pursued by two of the greatest intellects of our age is, however, nothing more than a result of the temptation to "which we so often succumb in our journals" (Edelson, p. 222).

Vagueness surrounds his ideas concerning the use of the linguistic

---

[7] Cf. Chomsky (1972) on Lévi-Strauss: "No one, to my knowledge, has devoted more thought to this problem than Lévi-Strauss. For example, his recent book on the categories of primitive mentality is a serious and thoughtful attempt to come to grips with this problem. Nevertheless, I do not see what conclusions can be reached from a study of his materials beyond the fact that the savage mind attempts to impose some organization on the physical world—that humans classify, if they perform any mental acts at all. Specifically, *Lévi-Strauss's well-known critique of totemism seems to reduce to little more than this conclusion*" (p. 74; italics ours).

distinction between deep and surface structure, one of the specific properties of grammar singled out by Chomsky for "appreciating the consequences of the operations of the dreamwork" (Edelson, p. 208). "Deep structures [he says] are those abstract, syntactic patterns that underlie the simplest, base, or kernel sentences of the language (exemplified, although this is an oversimplification, by simple—noncompound and noncomplex—sentences, which are active, declarative, and in the present tense)" (p. 216). The concept of "kernel sentence" has been shown to be invalid; and "deep structures" are not simple, active declarative sentences in the present tense. The sentences *John is here* and *Is John here*, for example, are distinguished in the deep structure. The latter contains a marker not present in the former. Though there is some disagreement regarding the precise nature of this marker, its systematic presence is not questioned. Similarly, the sentence *John is here* is different from the sentence *John is not here* because the latter derives from a deep structure that contains the abstract marker *Neg*, which triggers off various transformations that modify the relevant deep structure in appropriate ways. These questions are discussed in Katz and Postal (1964), a source cited in Edelson's bibliography. Edelson uses the term "deep structure" only metaphorically. He seems to believe that *any* gap between the "appearance" and the "reality" of things can justify the postulation of "deep structure." Deep structure in generative grammar, however, is a theoretical construct that has to be semantically justified and syntactically motivated. What specific, empirical evidence is there to justify the postulation of an intermediate, theoretical construct like "deep structure" in a system like "dream language," where, as Edelson himself points out (p. 200), the symbolism seems to be nonarbitrarily motivated. As a matter of fact, the evidence that such a hypothetical construct is needed even in grammar has increasingly vanished (Fillmore, 1968; Lakoff, 1970).

Although Edelson recognizes that any generative theory of dream language would have to be based on the assumption that a dream "yields its meanings only to one who knows its possible 'histories' and 'actual history'" (p. 215), he does nothing to give empirical content to the various processes of combination, rearrangement, and deletion—his putative transformations—which he talks about.

Although he seems to be aware of the fact that a sufficiently powerful theory would be needed to account for his chosen domain, he does not seem to be concerned with the fact that any such theory would need to be constrained in various ways to account for *only* the structures that fall within that domain. Since he gives no instances of the putative transformations within his realm of concern, it is difficult to imagine what some of these constraints might be. In the absence of clearly defined rules and constraints his proposal is bound to appear trivial. It remains only a metaphor.

Metaphor, as a matter of fact, is his chief problem. An example is Edelson's use of the word *generate:* "Thus, Freud claims that, even though no one has ever dreamed or will ever dream a single one of his dreams, he shares with mankind the process by which dreams are generated. Similarly, Chomsky claims that, even though each of the sentences he may devise is novel, he shares with mankind the process by which these sentences are generated" (p. 210f.). In the trivial sense, the observation is, of course, true: both Chomsky and Freud belong to the same species. The point is that Chomsky is talking about the calculus called grammar by generative grammarians that assigns structural descriptions to all and only the sentences of a language, and Freud is not. Chomsky uses the word *generate* to mean *enumerate* (to assign structural descriptions to). The grammar, the calculus proposed by grammarians, assigns structural descriptions to the structures it generates. Clearly, Freud is not implying any such enumeration.

While some of Edelson's suggestions sound initially attractive, they rarely rise above the level of vague analogies. Accepting an out-of-date and demonstrably false definition of deep structure, he suggests, for example, that "wishes" are perhaps analogues to "that part of the syntactic component the rules of which generate such ["kernel"] structures" (p. 216). The part of the syntactic component he is referring to is called "the phrase structure component" in generative theory. The phrase structure rules of a grammar generate the structures to which lexical items are, if they meet certain conditions, attached. There are certain ordering relationships in the prelexical nodes that appear in these rules (Chomsky, 1965) and what they generate is assigned hierarchical structure. Hence it is difficult to see precisely what Edelson is claiming. If he is claiming similarity between phrase structure rules and "wishes," he does not give any examples of possible constituent structure of "wishes" and possible hierarchical relationships among them.

Sometimes, unfortunately, Edelson's analogies are not even attractive. He points out that the dreamwork, which he considers to be the transformational part of the system dreaming, is constrained by considerations of representability, just as transformational rules are constrained by considerations of phonological representability. We fail to understand the statement because there is no convincing evidence that we know of that would show that phonological constraints restrict transformational rules in any way. Since transformations apply—and Edelson seems to be aware of the fact—after lexical insertion, questions of phonological representability could not possibly constrain their application.

Talking about the filtering function of transformations (Chomsky, 1965), Edelson suggests that "defense mechanisms and the proscriptions that motivate their use, operating to control access to conscious representation, [are] the transformational processes of another semiological system" (p. 219). What evidence is there to suggest that defense mechanisms are transformational processes of another semiological system? The notion of "surface structure constraints," for which there is considerable evidence in Perlmutter (1970), seems far more applicable here. This ultimate filtering mechanism disallows certain structures that cannot be filtered out by the transformational rules. "Surface structure constraints" (also called "output conditions") are set up to account systematically for the fact that the blocking or filtering function of obligatory transformations is not enough to rule out certain strings regarded as ungrammatical in natural languages. An example of this is provided by Spanish, where the object pronouns in sentences quite regularly generated by the transformational component must appear in a certain order. If they do not appear in the specified order, the sentence is ungrammatical. This sort of global filtering can be accounted for only in terms of final output conditions. There are, in other words, well-formed deep structures that have no corresponding well-formed surface structures. Perlmutter shows the necessity of such constraints in the grammars of Spanish and French. The difference between transformations and output conditions is that while an obligatory transformation must be applied if its structural description is met, there is no requirement that its structural description be met. Output conditions, however, have to be met (p. 246).

We find the lack of explicit examples and the absence of debatable empirical content particularly disturbing because Edelson is apparently not a stranger to the demands of an empirical theory. His metaphorical extensions of generative theory appear to be empirically untestable. He fails to develop a verifiable generative theory of dream language and in failing to do so he also fails to throw any light on any of the substantive questions mentioned earlier in this section. Since the "propositions" he postulates are devoid of empirical substance, it is impossible to say whether a possible generative theory of "dream language" shares any of the specific properties of generative grammar. Their nonempirical natures makes it difficult to see what contributions he has made toward a general theory of symbolic functioning.

Our evaluation of his proposals is critical because investigations of this sort must be judged on their own and completely within the synchronic context. If we judge these proposals as they stand, regardless of any possibilities that may result, we must, in the interests of the discipline involved, say that out of the three major questions Edelson could have thrown some light on, not even one is seriously approached. He does not seem to succeed in even constructing an empirically verifiable autonomous generative theory of dream language, let alone contributing to a general theory of symbolic functioning. His suggestions amount to neither an explicit description of the relevant domain nor an explanation of it, but merely a skillful notational exercise of a metaphorical nature arising from a conviction that Chomskian linguistics and Freudian theory can be brought together. They may well be, but Edelson does very little to show precisely how.

III

Edelson's audacious undercutting of the status of censorship is based on his rejection of censorship as a motive for using dreamwork; the upshot of such a contention is that, with censorship eliminated, dream distortion and disguise stem solely from the dreamwork (p. 245); in line with this process, of course, indifferent elements may be chosen in a dream because of their visual representability and allusiveness to multiple latent dream thoughts. Ultimately, Edelson's rejection of censorship as a necessary component in dream construction rests on two propositions, one based on textual interpretation and the other related to the law of parsimony. In the first instance, Edelson writes: "My reading of Freud's words is that he tended to give increasing priority as time went on to the intrinsic consequences of choosing a certain way of representing thoughts for determining the form of a dream, and felt less need to postulate the tendentious operation of censorship during a state of sleep as a major contribution to the construction of such a symbolic entity as a dream" (p. 269). But it seems clear to us that the later Freud unequivocably insisted on the centrality of censorship in dreams. Thus in a 1909 addition to his own preferred work Freud declared, "I may say that the kernel of my theory of dreams lies in my derivation of dream-distortion from the censorship" (1900, p. 308, n. 2); further additions in 1911 and 1919 (pp. 234, 142f.) explicitly testify to Freud's strong belief in the importance of dream censorship. Since *The Interpretation of Dreams* underwent considerable emendation as well as elaboration, Freud would certainly (if Edelson were right) have expunged or modified at least some of its many references to dream censorship. Furthermore, in "Revision of Dream-Theory," the last of Freud's major reflections on dreams published during his lifetime, Freud in six instances stresses the value of censorship in dreams (1933, pp. 15, 18–21, 28). In light of this evidence, then, it seems hazardous to maintain that Freud gave increasingly less importance to censorship in dream formation. What change Edelson could have indicated, however, is that by 1938 Freud reassigned the operations of censorship in dream formation from the superego to the ego, although it must be said that Freud himself did not elaborate on this point (1940, chap. 4).

Edelson's second reason for rejecting censorship in dreams is predicated on the law of parsimony: condensation and figurability suffice in themselves to account for dream distortion (p. 268);

collaterally, displacement almost inevitably results from condensation rather than from a motive to disguise (p. 257). Such a position, one may counter, is objectionable for several reasons:

1. Concentrating on dream ideas and thereby attempting to show the superfluity of censorship from a semiological point of view, Edelson neglects the domain of affects and the function of censorship toward them. As Freud (1900) maintained, censorship obviates anxiety and painful affects (p. 267). And again: *"The inhibition of affect, accordingly, must be considered as the second consequence of the censorship of dreams, just as dream-distortion is its first consequence"* (p. 468). One should also bear in mind Freud's explanation of nightmare as a breaking out of affect subsequent to a possible relaxation of censorship.

2. But even remaining in the area of dream ideas, one must state, along with Freud and contrary to Edelson, that at least for three reasons the dynamics of representability do not totally account for the distortion from the latent to the manifest dream:

i. Children's dreams are often undistorted, for they lack censorship (1900, pp. 551, 553f.). If the phenomena of representability necessitated distortion and could entirely account for it, children's dreams should therefore be constantly distorted.

ii. Pictorial representability is by its very nature absent in imageless dreams, which nevertheless are modified by censorship. As Freud (1900) declares quite clearly: "It might have been supposed that condensation and the formation of compromises is only carried out for the sake of facilitating regression, that is, when it is a question of transforming thoughts into images. But the analysis—and still more the synthesis—of dreams which include no such regression to images, e.g. the dream of 'Autodidasker', exhibits the same processes of displacement and condensation as the rest" (p. 597)—such dreams testify to the existence of censorship, however lowered (see p. 542).

iii. The selection of both recent and indifferent material in dreams as substitutes for infantile thoughts can be sufficiently elucidated only in a strictly Freudian sense. Such material has "the least to fear from censorship imposed by resistance . . . the indifferent ones because they have given no occasion for the formation of many ties, and the recent ones because they have not yet had time to form them" (p. 563f.).

3. Edelson overlooks a symbolic factor which Freud adequately answers, namely, that dreams make use of unconscious symbols both because of their use of representability and because they generally escape censorship (p. 349).

4. Freud found that the dreams of healthy people often contain much more characteristic and simpler symbolism than those of neurotics, in whom a more powerful censorship increases dream distortion (p. 374). Strangely enough, Freud's empirical judgments go unmentioned in Edelson's "empirical" hypotheses that would by-pass censorship.

5. In view of the above, Freud's conclusion to chapter 6 of *The Interpretation of Dreams* is all the more forceful: censorship imposes one type of displacement on the dream thoughts, whereas representability necessitates a *fresh* one (p. 507; the distinction also is asserted on p. 339).

Conclusion

Although we have been critical of the psychoanalytic, semiological, and linguistic content of Edelson's proposals, we would like not to leave an entirely negative impression of his work. The task of bringing two theories of distinct domains together is a difficult one. Such a task is directly proportional to the degree of internal difficulties within each theory and to the nature of the issues debated within each domain. Edelson can hardly be blamed for oversimplifying one of the two theories he is concerned with.

In spite of our criticisms and disagreements, Edelson deserves credit for trying to see dream language in the light of Chomskian theory. One hopes he and his students will be able to apply some of his insights to actual instances of dream language. Such real applications might lead to the construction of actual grammars of dream language. The construction of these grammars will allow us to make empirical claims regarding the nature of the human mind. Certainly, speculative explorations of the kind undertaken by Edelson must be encouraged. Their content must, however, be subjected to serious scrutiny because that is the only way empirical hypotheses can be retrieved from such explorations. We, in other words, approve of Edelson's enthusiasm, though we are unconvinced by his proposals. We believe we are right, though our beliefs are irrelevant. The issues, however, are relevant, and therefore our purpose has been to put the issues into the context of an empirical debate.

BIBLIOGRAPHY

BENVENISTE, E. (1969), Sémiologie de la langue (1). *Semiotica*, 1:1-12.
BLANK, R. H. (1958), Dreams of the Blind. *Psychoanal. Quart.*, 27:158-174.
CHOMSKY, N. (1965), *Aspects of the Theory of Syntax*. Cambridge, Mass.: M.I.T. Press.
────── (1972), *Language and Mind*. New York: Harcourt Brace & Jovanovich.
EDELSON, M. (1973), Language and Dreams. *This Annual*, 27:203-282.
FILLMORE, C. (1968), The Case for Case. In: *Universals in Linguistics Theory*, ed. E. Bach & R. Harms. New York: Holt, Rinehart & Winston.
FREUD, S. (1900), The Interpretation of Dreams. *S.E.*, 4 & 5.
────── (1905), Jokes and Their Relation to the Unconscious. *S.E.*, 8.
────── (1913), Totem and Taboo. *S.E.*, 13:1-161.
────── (1916/17), Introductory Lectures on Psycho-Analysis. *S.E.*, 15 & 16.
────── (1923), The Ego and the Id. *S.E.*, 19:3-66.
────── (1933), New Introductory Lectures on Psycho-Analysis. *S.E.*, 22:3-182.
────── (1940), An Outline of Psycho-Analysis. *S.E.*, 23:141-207.
GARDNER, H. (1973), *The Quest for Mind*. New York: Knopf.
JAKOBSON, R. (1971), Two Aspects of Language and Two Types of Aphasic Disturbances. *Selected Writings*, 2:239-259. The Hague: Mouton.
JONES, E. (1916), The Theory of Symbolism. *Papers on Psycho-Analysis*. London: Baillière, 5th ed., 1948, pp. 87-144.
KATZ, J. & POSTAL, P. (1964), *An Integrated Theory of Linguistic Descriptions*. Cambridge, Mass.: M.I.T. Press.
LAKOFF, G. (1970), Linguistics and Natural Logic. *Synthèse*, 22:151-271.
LIBERMAN, D. (1970), *Lingüística, interracción, communicativa y proceso psicoanalítica*. Buenos Aires: Editorial Galerna.
LIENDO, E. (1967), Las relaciones objectales y lo simbolización de la angustia. *Rev. Psicoanál.*, 24:839-897.
MARTIN, M. (1968), *Le Langage cinématographique*. Paris: Seuil.
METZ, C. (1968), *Essais sur la signification du cinéma*. Paris: Klinsksieck.
────── (1971), *Langue et cinéma*. Paris: Larousse.
PASSERON, R. (1962), *L'Oeuvre picturale et les fonctions de l'apparence*. Paris: Vrin.
PERLMUTTER, D. (1970), Surface Structure Constraints in Syntax. *Linguistic Inquiry*, 1:187-256.

PUTNAM, H. (1967), The Innateness Hypothesis and Explanatory Models in Linguistics. *Synthèse*, 17:2–28.
ROONEY, W. (1962), John Donne's 'Second Prebend Sermon': A Stylistic Analysis. *Texas Studies in Language and Literature*, 4:24–34.

Toward a Clarification of the Concept of Narcissism

BURNESS E. MOORE, M.D.

"NARCISSISM," LEWIN (1955) SAID, "IS AN ABSTRACTION, WITH VISIBLE correlates in childhood psychology, in neurosis, in sleep, and in the love life. Narcissism, as a concept, is behind the dream, behind the depression and elation, behind somatic symptoms, etc." (p. 172f.). This succinct statement epitomizes, but does not exhaust, the significance of a concept which remains one of Freud's major theoretical contributions. Presented initially as an extension of his libido theory, the concept had far-reaching ramifications. It contributed to the formulation of a metapsychology, applied first to dreams; led to a deeper understanding of the mechanism of identification in relation to melancholia; pointed the way to the second dual instinct theory; and played a pivotal role in the development of the structural theory. Narcissism was the seed which germinated into ego psychology. The resulting growth in theoretical understanding was prolific, and its applicability to observed clinical phenomena provided the possibility for "the widening scope of psychoanalysis" (Stone, 1954). The latest manifestations of this are in respect to the treatment of borderline conditions (O. Kernberg, 1967, 1969, 1970a) and narcissistic personalities (Kohut, 1968, 1971; P. Kernberg, 1971).

Faculty, New York Psychoanalytic Institute.

Based on a review of the subject given at a symposium on Narcissism at the Boston Psychoanalytic Society and Institute, April 21, 1962, this paper, in condensed form, was presented to the Western Regional Psychoanalytic Meeting, San Diego, Oct. 10, 1972, and to the Psychoanalytic Societies in Topeka, New Jersey, Denver, San Francisco, and Washington.

Nevertheless, the concept remains to this day ill-defined, confusing, and as frustrating to present analysts as it was to Freud himself. Its relevancy and usefulness in alluding to a variety of phenomena and psychopathological conditions, however, have made for an indiscriminate overutilization of the term "narcissistic," compounding a conceptual unclarity which has persisted from the beginning. In psychoanalytic literature "narcissistic" may refer descriptively to a type of libido or its object; to a stage of development; to a type or mode of object choice; to an attitude; to psychic systems and processes; or to a personality type, which may be relatively normal or pathological—neurotic, psychotic, or borderline. As Waelder (1961) has commented, narcissism has a double meaning when used clinically, implying self-satisfaction and inner security or, conversely, the lack of these qualities and a constant need for reassurance. The constructive value of a necessary, even healthful, narcissism may be scotomatized by our view of it as a pathological attribute. Kohut (in Panel, 1961) has emphasized that misplaced value judgments, such as the implication that object love is good and narcissism bad, frequently contaminate consideration of the technical meaning. The stages of narcissism postulated by Freud and necessary for an understanding of his elaboration of the concept constitute another hurdle to understanding. The common words "primary" and "secondary," ambiguous in their double implication of time and importance, confer a confusion in depth when attached to the interrelated concepts of narcissism, masochism, identification, and object love, especially since these concepts have been described at varying times in terms that are inherently inconsistent and sometimes even contradictory.

Because of its seminal importance, narcissism has been a perennial topic for psychoanalytic papers and discussions since Freud's introductory paper on the subject in 1914. In recent years the work of Hartmann, Jacobson, O. Kernberg, Kohut, and Lichtenstein in particular has greatly advanced our understanding of the concept and its implications for psychoanalytic research and therapy. Although, as Kohut (1971) points out, the subject matter of narcissism does not at present justify the comprehensive, textbook type of presentation indicated when a field is more or less settled, it is my belief that the advances made have been significant enough to justify an attempt at "detached assessment and integration in the form of a survey which attempts to round out the newly acquired knowledge and to present it in a balanced form" (p. xiii). In this paper, I shall attempt such a survey with respect to clarification of the concept. In doing so, I shall be repeating the efforts of Bing et al. (1959), Balint (1960), and Pulver (1970). Though some repetition is inevitable, I hope to bring at least a different perspective.

The Historical Context

Although there are allusions to narcissism in Freud's comments at meetings and in earlier papers (1905, 1910a, 1911, 1913), his definitive ideas were first crystallized in his 1914 paper "On Narcissism: An Introduction." This occurred at the beginning of what Waelder (1960) has called the "middle period" of Freud's life, a time of considerable emotional turmoil and of change in his theoretical conceptualizations. He was still holding steadfastly to his earlier ideas while he moved on to new ground. The result is an admixture of the old and the new, with both conceptual and semantic confusion. The transitional quality of Freud's thinking at the time, in addition to certain other complexities to be mentioned, accounts in part for our difficulty in comprehending narcissism. Although Freud himself was dissatisfied with his introductory paper, he never wholly clarified the confusion to be expected when theory is *in statu nascendi*. In several reviews of the development of his libido theory he did mention the significant role which the concept of narcissism played in his gradual formulation of the second dual instinct theory.[1] Except for minor emendations, however, Freud made no subsequent attempt to revise his ideas about narcissism or to integrate them with later concepts, including the structural theory, to which narcissism had also contributed.

The paper "On Narcissism" belongs to the prestructural period when libido was represented as being in conflict with ego instincts.

---

[1] See Freud (1920, pp. 50ff., 61; 1923a, p. 255; 1930, pp. 117–120; 1933, p. 132ff.).

(Nevertheless, Freud described narcissism as "the libidinal complement to the egoism of the instinct of self-preservation," foreshadowing his later recognition of the self-preservative instincts as libidinal.[2] He also referred to narcissism as ego libido.) As Kanzer (in Panel, 1961) has pointed out, discussions of narcissism frequently are still concerned with shifts of libidinal energy only and neglect the fact that libidinal investments and discharges are part of larger complexes involving aggressive energy and structural relationships. In 1914, Freud's terms "ego instincts" and "ego energy" embodied the self-preservative instincts as well as the aggressive drive. Also included were defensive functions which he later ascribed to the system ego. "Ego interest" was sometimes equated with "interest in general" (which had energic implications), with interest in the popular sense, and with what was later designated "attention cathexis"—activities we would now subsume under the functions of the system ego.

It is important to realize, therefore, that the concept of narcissism was introduced in what might be called an undifferentiated stage of Freud's theoretical conceptualization, in which id and ego elements were intermingled in the terms "ego instincts" and "ego interest." There are statements in his paper on Narcissism (pp. 76, 79) and in later papers (1920, p. 57; 1930, p. 119; 1940, p. 149) which presage both Hartmann's concept of the undifferentiated structural stage and Jacobson's concept of undifferentiated psychic energies. Perhaps it was Freud's prescience of the role which psychic energies play in the development and operation of the system ego which led him to use the term "ego" with a number of meanings which now have to be differentiated. Hartmann (1950) took the first step in this direction by pointing out that Freud used the word "ego" at times to refer to the "self" (one's own person) in contradistinction to the object, while on other occasions he referred to the ego as a psychic system in contradistinction to other substructures of the personality. The opposite of "object cathexis" is not "ego cathexis" but "self cathexis," and "self representation" is the opposite of "object representation." Hartmann specified further that he preferred to speak of "narcissistic ego cathexis" for that part of the self cathexis

---

[2] See Loewenstein (1940) for a full discussion of this issue.

localized in the system ego. These distinctions are familiar to most analysts; they have been useful in the understanding of narcissism and are generally accepted, although objections have been offered by Weiss (1957), Kardiner et al. (1959), and Balint (1960).

Freud had at first conceived of the conflict underlying psychoneuroses as being between "the ego" and "sexuality."[3] In the *Three Essays* (1905), libido was established as an expression of the sexual instinct, whereas "the ego" was discussed chiefly in connection with its functions of repression, resistance, and reality testing. He introduced the term "ego instincts" and identified these with the self-preservative instincts and the repressive function in his paper on psychogenic disturbance of vision (1910b). Conflict was then represented as being between two sets of instincts: the libido and the ego instincts, each with energies, cathexes, and interests—a formulation which persisted until after the publication of Lecture XXVI (1916/17). Nevertheless, in the papers "On Narcissism" (1914) and "Instincts and Their Vicissitudes" (1915a) there is evidence of beginning doubts about the validity of this division and indications of his later thinking. For instance, in the latter paper he mentioned that the sexual instincts are at first attached to the instincts of self-preservation and a portion of them remains associated with the ego instincts throughout life and furnishes them with libidinal components. Moved, no doubt, by his examination of love and hate, sadism and masochism, and the vicissitudes of the erotic cathexis in "Mourning and Melancholia" (1917b), he was constrained to review and revise the libido theory in 1920. His old formula about the origin of psychoneuroses out of conflict between the ego instincts and the sexual instincts was not rejected, but the distinction was now regarded as topographical instead of qualitative. He now had to recognize the libidinal character of the self-preservative instincts, but still refused to accept Jung's use of libido as a synonym for "instinctive force" in general, adhering as he had from the first to a dualistic standpoint. He no longer called the contrasting tendencies egoistic and sexual instincts, but life instincts and death instincts. The desexualization of libidinal energies had been advanced as early as the 1914 paper on narcissism, and there are phenomena suggesting the fusion of instincts described in the intervening papers, but the concept of fusion and defusion was fully developed in *The Ego and the Id* (1923b). See Strachey's note, "Instincts and Their Vicissitudes" (1915a), Bibring (1941); Hartmann (1948); Hartmann et al. (1949).

---

[3] The sections printed in smaller type present an elaboration of specific points.

A Summary of Freud's Ideas on Narcissism

In some of his earlier papers Freud used narcissism to explain various phenomena—"the unbounded self-love of children" (1900) and the choice of object in homosexuality (1905, 1910a)—in an analogous way. It is evident from this that he regarded it as a perversion on the one hand and as a passing phase of self-love on the other. He also saw a linkage between narcissism and erogeneity, autoerotism, hypochondriasis, and organ inferiority via the concept of an ego libido arising from the sexual and other bodily organs (1905). His first reference to the subject in a letter to Fliess in 1899, however, implies an inclination to use narcissism as an energic concept to explain the fate of libidinal energies in psychotic disturbances, an idea developed more fully in later writings (1911, 1916/17, 1917). In his 1914 paper he first gave to it "a place in the regular course of human sexual development" (p. 73), conceiving of a primary narcissism, "an original libidinal cathexis of the ego, from which some is later given off to objects, but which fundamentally persists" (p. 75). In various papers, both the ego and the id were considered to be the great reservoir of this narcissistic libido, but at one point in the *Outline* (1940)—his last statement on the subject—(as well as in 1933), he refers to the libido being present in the "as yet undifferentiated ego-id."

The dependency on objects for satisfaction of some of the sexual instincts, Freud (1915a) said, disturbs the state of primal narcissism. The ego takes in objects which are a source of pleasure—by introjection—and expels whatever within itself becomes a cause of unpleasure. Freud's study of mourning (1917b) confirmed his impression that when obstacles interfere, object cathexis can regress to narcissism. In *The Ego and the Id* (1923b) he pursued the subject further. When a sexual object must be given up, the process is made easier by setting up the object inside the ego, bringing about a permanent alteration of the ego. This occurs through introjection, a mechanism typical of regression to the oral phase. "The transformation of object-libido into narcissistic libido which thus takes place [as a result of identification] obviously implies an abandonment of sexual aims, a desexualization—a kind of sublimation" (p. 30). These considerations led Freud to an important amplification of the theory of narcissism:

> At the very beginning, all the libido is accumlated in the id, while the ego [system] is still in the process of formation or is still feeble. The id sends part of this libido out into erotic object-cathexes, whereupon the ego, now grown stronger, tries to get hold of this object-libido and to force itself on the id as a love-object. The narcissism of the ego is thus a secondary one, which has been withdrawn from objects [p. 46].

The system ego was thus seen to be "formed to a great extent out of identifications which take the place of abandoned cathexes by the id" (p. 48). In other words, secondary narcissism—the cathexis attached to the precipitates of lost objects installed within the ego—provide it with the energy for its development and operation, although the phrase "now grown stronger" in the paragraph quoted above implies a prior maturation of autonomous functions of the ego (see Jacobson, p. 259 of this paper).

In 1914 Freud said that "The first auto-erotic sexual satisfactions are experienced in connection with vital functions which serve the purpose of self-preservation" (p. 87). Being concerned with the child's feeding, care, and protection, these pleasurable functions are object-related, a fact which contributes to the development of object libido, but Freud noted that not all of ego libido (i.e., narcissistic libido) passes into object cathexes. Part of it is displaced onto an ideal ego, which, by being possessed of every perfection, recovers some of the lost narcissism via projection. As a standard by which the actual self is measured, the ideal becomes the conditioning factor of repression of libidinal instinctual impulses that come into conflict with cultural and ethical ideas.

Self-regard, Freud (1914) said, has a specially intimate dependence on narcissistic libido: not being loved lowers the self regarding feelings, while being loved raises them. Dependence on a love object that is libidinally cathected lowers self-regard, as does realization of the inability to love. He concluded that "One part of self-regard is primary—the residue of infantile narcissism; another part arises out of the omnipotence which is corroborated by experience (the fulfilment of the ego ideal), whilst a third part proceeds from the satisfaction of object-libido" (p. 100).

In the marked overvaluation of the love object which is characteristic of the anaclitic male, Freud saw a transference of the child's original narcissism to the sexual object. Even for the narcissistic woman, the child, an externalized part of her own body and thus an extension of her narcissism, can be the means for the achievement of object love. In fact, he generalized, parental love—with its characteristics of overvaluation, suspension of the reality principle in the child's favor, and expectation of fulfillment of the parents' wishes—"is nothing but the parents' narcissism born again . . . transformed into object-love" (p. 91).

At the end of the 1914 paper, Freud refers to the connection, through the ego ideal, between narcissism and social phenomena, a link he further elaborated in 1921. Antipathy to strangers, to those who are different, is based on the notion that divergence from self implies criticism and demand for alteration of the self, therefore offending narcissism. This intolerance disappears when a group is formed on the basis of a common quality among its members who then identify with each other. A revered leader, an idea, an abstraction, or particular aspirations may become, as elements of a shared ideal, the binding force for the cohesiveness of the group.

In these descriptions of the vicissitudes of narcissism we can, of course, recognize its contribution to structural differentiation and the operations of the ego. In the main, the transformations of narcissistic energy in respect to sublimation (Freud, 1923b) are applicable to the formation of the ego ideal and the superego as well as the ego.

I have described in some detail those transformations of narcissism that relate to structure formation because they are most relevant to current usage of the concept. Narcissism, however, became an integral part of Freud's libido theory and, as such, was adduced as a partial explanation for many phenomena: the relationship between the behavior of primitive peoples and neurotics (1913); the regressive egoism of the physically ill and hypochondriasis (1914); homosexual object choice and compassion

(1915b, 1918); autoerotism, sleep, and resistance in psychotic disorders (1916/17); exhibitionism, masochism, the evolution of the ego and its relationship to objects and external reality (1915a); the masculinity complex in women (1917c, 1925); the war neuroses (1919); group formation and hypnosis (1921); jealousy and homosexuality (1922); the repetition compulsion, sadism, ambivalence, superego formation, neutral energies, and the problem of anxiety (1923b); the secondary gain in symptoms (1926); humor (1927b); idealization in human life (1927a, 1930); and libidinal types (1931).

These phenomena encompass such diverse elements as clinically observable aspects and attributes of human behavior (biological as well as psychological; individual, social; normal, and pathological), pathological syndromes, and abstractions, i.e., theoretical concepts of genetic, structural, dynamic, and adaptive significance. As Pulver (1970) points out, these complex phenomena each have their own metapsychology, and the ways in which they are related to each other are often vague and obscure. Moreover, the gradual enrichment of psychoanalytic knowledge about development and the elaboration of other concepts (such as the structural theory and the concept of the self) have still further broadened the applicability of the term narcissism to a point which detracts from its explanatory usefulness. Use of the term focuses on an economic factor to the detriment of understanding provided by other concepts. One result—to counter such broad and meaningless use of the term—has been an attempt to narrow its definition, either specifically (Joffe and Sandler, 1967; Pulver, 1970) or indirectly through largely confining its usage to problems relating to the regulation of self-esteem (Kohut, 1968, 1971). I shall have more to say about such attempts at a later point.

In turning to amplifications of Freud's basic ideas by other authors, I shall also deal with certain recurrent and controversial questions.

NARCISSISM AS AN ECONOMIC CONCEPT

Freud made narcissism a part of his libido theory, an economic concept relating to the fate of instinctual energies or drives. Its validity is therefore dependent on that of the economic concept in general, which increasingly has come under attack (Kardiner et al., 1959; Apfelbaum, 1965; and Holt, 1967). Repetition of the arguments would be too long a digression, but I think it is fair to say that even the current literature demonstrates the heuristic usefulness of the concept, a fact generally accepted by the majority of analysts. They apparently agree with Hartmann et al. (1949) that "The psychoanalytic concept of instinctual drive . . . transcends, at present, any definite link to physiological processes, to subjective experience, or to data obtainable from the behavioristic approach. However, the concept of instinctual drive includes all these aspects" (p. 15).

The clinical phenomena Freud considered in support of the general concept of narcissism are all examples of secondary narcissism, which he said arose from the drawing in of object cathexes. Primary narcissism was therefore an assumption, avowedly based not on direct observation but on inference, and its possible nature and the stage of development it represents have been widely discussed. Greenacre (1945) viewed it "as the libidinal component of growth which may . . . become turned one way or another by the vicissitudes of experience at any time in the course of life." During fetal life, the primary narcissism "would appear to be distributed variously throughout the fetal structure, its patterning determined almost entirely by the phylogenetic history of the species, . . ." to be transformed by the enormous sensory stimulation at birth into a "beginning propulsive psychic drive" (p. 45ff.).

Pointing out that primary narcissism and masochism imply that in the primal state the drives are actually turned toward (i.e., aimed at discharge on) the self, Jacobson (1954) considered the avenues by which psychic energy may be discharged during this state prior to the child's discovery of his own self and of the object world. She conceived of "an initial psychoeconomical state characterized by a low level of tension and by a general, diffuse dispersion of as yet undifferentiated physiological energy. . . . After birth, part of this energy would be vested as a basic energetic stock in the nuclei of the future autonomous ego. Under the influence of external stimuli [and periodic hypercathexis of the sensory and motor systems] the undifferentiated forces would then begin to develop into the libidinous and aggressive drives with which the id is endowed . . .

[which turn toward the outside and are] observable as pregenital sexual activity and in biologically prepatterned, primitive affecto-motor and instinctive reflex reactions" (p. 82f.). On this basis Jacobson was inclined in 1954 to dispose of the concepts of primary narcissism and masochism, and Balint and others would also drop primary identification.

Balint (1960) has been meticulous in pointing out the discrepancies and contradictions in Freud's statements which imply primary object love, primary autoerotism, and primary narcissism. While it is true that these contradictions exist, it is apparent that at one time Freud spoke descriptively and at another metapsychologically. Observable autoerotic activity during early infancy would exist only on a reflex basis (van der Waals, in Panel, 1961), but as a psychological phenomenon it would occur as part of the gradual development of self and object representations and their distinction. This is implied by Freud (1914) who pointed out that "a unity comparable to the ego cannot exist in the individual from the start; the ego has to be developed. The auto-erotic instincts, however, are present from the very first; so there must be something added to auto-erotism—a new psychical action—in order to bring about narcissism" (p. 77). Bing et al. (1959) have deduced that Freud was here referring to the ego as an organized structure. In any event, Freud somewhat reconciled the discrepancies in his various statements when he said, "Auto-erotism would thus be sexual activity of the narcissistic stage of allocation of the libido" (1916/17, p. 416). For a similar statement, see Freud (1915a). For a full discussion of Freud's uses of the terms "autoerotism" and narcissism, see Kanzer (1964).

Lichtenstein (1964) believes that "Freud's insistence on distinguishing between a primary and a secondary narcissism is due to his need of a concept that implied the dimension of developmental reversibility" (p. 50).

Van der Waals (1965) agreed with Jacobson's 1954 view; in the earliest stage of infancy, he said, "Psychologically there is not yet a self, nor a nonself" (p. 295), so that primary narcissism does not fit the original psychological concept of self-love. In 1964, however, Jacobson reconsidered the issue, stating "that it is still a very useful term for the earliest infantile period, preceding the development of self and object images" (p. 15). Spitz (1965) regards the nondifferentiated, objectless stage as more or less coinciding with that of primary narcissism, and Mahler (1968) too agrees with Jacobson's later view. She distinguishes two subphases of primary narcissism:

the first absolute, occurring during the first few weeks of extrauterine life, marked by the infant's lack of awareness of a mothering agent and hence equivalent to what she calls the stage of "normal autism"; and a later, less absolute stage, beginning about the third month and coinciding with her "symbiotic stage," when a dim perception of need satisfaction as coming from a part object is still viewed from within the orbit of an omnipotent symbiotic dual unity with a mothering agency. In spite of this agreement, Kohut (1971) has reintroduced the term "primary narcissism" in a different context, using it to designate a stage of libidinal investment of the total, integrated self, as opposed to its parts, following an earlier stage of "autoerotism," when the self is fragmented and narcissistic libido invests "self-nuclei." I think it is unfortunate that Kohut has thus added to our terminological confusion, especially since I find his ideas heuristically useful in understanding the occurrence of somatic and hypochondriacal symptoms in narcissistic patients.

Narcissism and Aggression

The relation between these concepts was never definitively discussed by Freud. Even in the *Outline* (1940) he related narcissism to libido only. Nevertheless, scattered comments throughout his works[4] constitute anlagen of the concept of undifferentiated drive energies developed by Jacobson (1954). She believes that "Freud's significant assumption of desexualized energy . . . [would] be even more convincing if it referred . . . to originally undifferentiated drive energy in the whole self" (p. 82). In that case it would explain the fact that drive fusions appear to result in a prevalence of libidinal drive energy and drive defusions in an absolute predominance of aggressive drive energy. These changes in the proportions between libido and aggression observable in severe pathological states could be better understood in terms of a *structural* regression, which might reestablish the earliest state of diffuse dispersion of energy in the whole self, or *energetic* regression, which might lead to "resexualiza-

[4] Reference to Freud's comments and elaborations of the views of others are presented at the end of this section.

tion and reaggressivization of the neutral energy of the ego or even to partial retransformations of libido and aggression into primary undifferentiated energy" (p. 83).

Hartmann et al. (1949) state that Freud's analogy of self-destruction and destruction of the object to narcissism and object love might have led to an assumption of self-destruction as the form of aggression to be compared to primary narcissism. However, they believe his complex concept of narcissism went beyond this parallel. It included not only "self love" but also other cathexes of the self, one form being the cathexis of the ego with neutralized libido. Similarly, they assumed a "deaggressivized" psychic energy that does not lead to self-destruction but supplies ego and superego with motor power and in particular equips the ego for its function in action. Freud (1914) had partly explained the development from narcissism to libidinal cathexis of the outside world by assuming that the damming up of narcissistic libido in the self, if it exceeds a certain degree, is experienced as unpleasure. Hartmann et al. thought that an analogous hypothesis as to aggression is even more plausible.

By implication Eidelberg (in Panel, 1961) seems to include the aggressive drive, "mortido" or "destrudo" as he calls it along with Federn and Weiss, in his application of the concept of narcissism. In contrast, Waelder (1961) stated that he thought of narcissism in terms of libido only. In his view, if the ego is unprotected by narcissistic libido, it is more vulnerable to aggression. From this survey I would conclude that we should continue to confine the concept of narcissism to considerations of libido but assume a parallel energic flux and transformation in regard to aggression. The outlines of such an analogous hypothesis have been provided by Hartmann et al. (1949), but this subject cannot be pursued further at this time.

In 1914 Freud said, "as regards the differentiation of psychical energies, we are led to the conclusion that to begin with, during the state of narcissism, they exist together and that our analysis is too coarse to distinguish them; not until there is object-cathexis is it possible to discriminate a sexual energy—the libido—from an energy of the ego-instincts" (p. 76).

In discussing the "pleasure-ego" and "reality-ego" stages, Freud (1915a) points out that the external world in the form of parental objects is a source not only of satisfaction, but of frustration (unpleasure) as well. At this point he gives an indication of his awareness of the early operation of the aggressive drive: "When, during the stage of primary narcissism, the object makes its appearance, the second opposite to loving, namely hating, also attains its development" (p. 136).

Later (1923a) he stated that both Eros and the death instincts "have been in operation and working against each other from the first origin of life" (p. 259).

Moreover, it is possibly significant that he added an important amplification to the theory of narcissism (1923b) when he described the disposition of desexualized libido after identification. In taking over libido from the cathexes of the id, the ego "is working in opposition to the purposes of Eros and placing itself at the service of the opposing instinctual impulses. It has to acquiesce in some of the other object-cathexes of the id" (p. 46). In the same connection he refers to another possible consequence of this activity of the ego—instinctual defusion, with the release of aggression consequent to the identification with the father by which the superego arises. In a recapitulation of the libido theory (1930), Freud mentions, in discussing the consequences of his concept of narcissism, that he was led to the death instinct, which, however, was not easy to demonstrate. "A more fruitful idea was that a portion of the instinct is diverted towards the external world and comes to light as an instinct of aggressiveness and destructiveness. In this way the instinct could be pressed into the service of Eros, in that the organism was destroying some other thing, whether animate or inanimate, instead of destroying its own self. Conversely, any restriction of this aggressiveness directed outwards would be bound to increase the self-destruction, which is in any case proceeding" (p. 119). This formulation parallels that which he gave with respect to the relationship between ego libido and object libido in 1914. It suggests that his formulations of narcissism with regard to libido would also apply to the aggressive drive. Perhaps the reason for his difficulty in making this transition is explained by his parenthetical statement that "The desire for destruction when it is directed *inwards* mostly eludes our perception, of course, unless it is tinged with erotism" (p. 120). But "where it emerges without any sexual purpose, in the blindest fury of destructiveness, we cannot fail to recognize that the satisfaction of the instinct is accompanied by an extraordinarily high degree of narcissistic enjoyment, owing to its presenting the ego with a fulfilment of the latter's old wishes for omnipotence" (p. 121). Hence, a component of narcissism long recognized—the wish for omnipotence—here seems to be brought into relation with the death instinct.

Despite the fact that he fits his views into the framework of Federn's (1952) obscure concept of "ego feeling," Eduardo Weiss (1957) has a somewhat similar, though divergent, concept of undifferentiated energies. He postulated a common biological reservoir of energies, not coinciding with the common reservoir of instinctual tendencies, from which a stream of cathexis undergoes bifurcation: one branch feeding the drives in the id, the other in the ego.

Hartmann (1950) assumed that desexualized and deaggressivized (neutralized) energies are closer to one another than the strictly instinctual energies of the two drives, even though retaining some of the latter's properties. He also assumed gradations in the neutralization of these energies, thus approaching closely Jacobson's later concept of undifferentiated psychic energy. In passing, I also note a certain similarity to Federn's (1952) third source of energy, resulting from the living processes of the organism, in regard to which Hendrick (1942) conceived of a "mastery instinct" and Hartmann, neutral energies.

The Nature of Narcissistic Libido

I am sure that it must be clear that Freud, in discussions of narcissism, was often speaking of a form of energy which cathects the self representation, or the person, rather than the ego as a system. But here we are confronted with another question: Does narcissistic libido merely imply the attachment of cathexis to the self rather than to an object, or is there a qualitative difference between narcissistic libido as opposed to object libido? Freud and others have consistently used the phrase "narcissistic libido" in such a way as to suggest that the latter is the case. While it is true that he argued against qualitative differences in instincts, he nevertheless referred to transformations and even spoke of the development of an instinct (1915a). Hartmann's (1950) later conceptualization of the differentiation of the ego and id "out of the matrix of animal instinct" is an extension of this idea, and the changes in energies suggested by clinically observable phenomena may be attributed to the interaction between the developing systems.

Implicit in Jacobson's (1954) description of the effects of the energic flux between self and object representations is the conclusion that the direction of cathexis of such energies—as they become available to the ego from the changing id system—affects their operation qualitatively. Kohut (1971) states categorically—with the emphasis of italics—"Narcissism, within my general outlook, is defined not by the target of the instinctual investment (i.e., whether it is the subject himself or other people) but by the nature or quality of the instinctual charge" (p. 26). In this he appears to differ from Freud, who stated that *"loving oneself, . . . we regard as the characteristic feature of narcissism"* (1915a, p. 133). It seems evident from Kohut's discussion, however, that the quality of the instinctual investment which he calls narcissistic is determined by defects in ego development, so that the cathexis retains an archaic nature related to that which originally invested the self—or selflike objects. Although Pulver (1970) believes that calling such immature object relationships narcissistic obscures the primitive mechanisms used to relate to objects, it can be argued that Kohut is simply emphasizing a genetic viewpoint. In any event, the different quality of the instinctual investment in narcissistic disorders from that present in more mature object relations seems undeniable. Certainly, as Hartmann (1950) points out, maturation intervenes in the development of the sexual drives (for instance, in the sequence of libidinal organizations) and in a somewhat different way also in the development of aggression. It seems warranted to conclude that drive transformations—not the original instinctual energies, which are undifferentiated—do differ substantially in relation to their self or object directedness. Kohut, however, would view the direction of such investment as an effect of the archaic quality of the energies involved rather than the cause. Probably varying proportions of mixtures of sexual and aggressive energies which are neutralized or unneutralized, fused or defused, together with the structural organization achieved, account for the varied nature of normal and pathological phenomena which are usually ascribed indiscriminately to the effect of narcissistic libido.

Narcissism in Relation to Objects and Structural Concepts

Freud's basic ideas about the role of instinctual energies in structural development have been mentioned already. What he described in metapsychological terms has now been substantiated by the increasing body of developmental knowledge derived from direct infant observation (e.g., Mahler and McDevitt, 1968). Nevertheless, as is to be expected, these observations necessitate some revisions of his original formulations. Jacobson (1954, 1964), for example, points out that the terminological confusion of this early period suggests that the system ego is built up and gains strength by being vested with narcissistic libido only. It is apparent, however, that a certain amount of maturation of autonomous ego functions (perception, for example, by means of which a distinction of the self and object world accompanies ever-increasing memory traces of pleasurable and unpleasurable experiences) must have preceded identification and cathectic interchange. "Emerging from sensations hardly distinguishable from perceptions of the gratifying part-object," Jacobson says, the concept of self "is first fused and confused with the object images and is composed of a constantly changing series of self-images which reflect mainly the incessant fluctuations of the primitive mental state" (1954, p. 86). Only when the perceptive functions have sufficiently matured can gratifications or frustrations become associated with the object. When that stage of maturation has been reached, however, frustration, deprivation, and separation from the object serve further to sharpen perception and result in a clearer distinction of self and object; to reestablish the lost unity, the ego must also develop the active capacity for fantasies of total incorporation of the gratifying object. Following actual gratification, self and object images temporarily merge, and perception is weakened in a return to an earlier, less differentiated state of ego formation.[5] Jacobson (1954) postulates highly significant and complicated energetic transformations and cathectic changes between the self and object representations, which greatly stimulate sublimation or, more generally, autonomous ego activity.

---

[5] Spiegel's (1959) observations are particularly relevant to Jacobson's descriptions of the fluctuations in perception coincident with gratification and frustration. Distortions of the feeling of reality, which are related to specific acts of perception of the external or inner world, as well as defensive functions, affect perception itself. Quoting Schilder, "drives are experienced, objects are perceived," Spiegel points out that what is perceived, and especially what is hypercathected, tends to have object quality, whether external or a part of the self. Hence, conflict may develop in distinguishing a part of the self that is intensely cathected from an outside object because of the object quality arising from the intense cathexis itself.

In sublimation, part of the libido vested in the love objects undergoes partial neutralization and is turned to other objects, especially in the area of ego interests. At the same time the shift from infantile dependence to ego independence, in identification with objects, veers libido away from these objects to the self. Thus, part of the object libido becomes transformed into narcissistic libido, which, together with libido withdrawn from erogenous zones, is used for the expanding cathexis of the executive organs of the ego. There is consequently a further building up of the self representation. The development of ego interest also calls away from the love object not only libido, but also aggression, both of which, after fusion, are vested in new objects.

In the mirroring of the self implicit in the Narcissus myth, Lichtenstein (1964) sees a modification of the image due to the surroundings. Such a mirroring, he believes, takes place (through all the sensory modalities) in the mutual responsiveness of mother and child to libidinal cathexes extended by each. The outlines of the child's own image are reflected by the mother's unconscious needs with regard to the child, establishing what Lichtenstein calls a primary narcissistic identity. This is not yet a sense of identity, which requires more structural organization, but a "primary organizational principle without which the process of developmental differentiation could not begin. . . . [It is] comparable to the concept of organizers of the psyche in the terminology of Spitz (1959)" (p. 53). He also associates this primary identity with Spiegel's (1959) concept of the self, which the latter defines as a frame of reference to which specific mental and psychical states are referred, perceived, and judged (p. 96). The primary identity does not, however, "enable the individual truly to cathect an object. Instead, it uses the object as a mirror in which to reflect the outlines of his primary identity . . . during a phase when there was no differentiation between the subject and the object. . . . This type of mirroring is a well-known form of a narcissistic object relation in which the object serves as a mirror for a faltering or undeveloped identity" (Lichtenstein, p. 54). (It is not surprising, if we accept this idea, that narcissistic personalities commonly have parents who were themselves narcissistic.) This type of identity maintenance, he says, must be replaced by one in which there is the capacity to select types of action which will bring a corresponding reaction from the other. Presumably, only when the ego is capable of activity are true object cathexes possible.

Brodey (1965) arrives at much the same conclusion from a different line of reasoning. He points out that Narcissus' intense relationship was not with another, but only with an as-if other, an image of himself reflected from a distance. This externalization "is a defense of the narcissistic, preobject period of ego development" (p. 167). It results in an as-if reality perceived as reality to conform to his own projection. Kohut (1971) views the situation in a similar fashion.

These views delineate some aspects of the process of development of self and object representations, and the beginning of object relations, a capacity integral to ego functioning. Although it is evident that the maturation of autonomous ego functions plays a significant role, my focus has been on the effect of the energies involved, as they affect the cathexis of self and object representations. The earliest stages were characterized by primitive oral-incorporative fantasies, but each successive libidinal stage makes its own narcissistic contribution to ego and superego development.

As one example from the anal stage, Abraham (1920) called attention to the displacement of narcissism evident in an overestimation of the excreta, to which the feeling of omnipotence becomes attached. As the child reaches the phallic stage narcissistic libido is focused and concentrated on the genital. Federn (1952) has even stated that the narcissistic cathexis of the ego is due to an identification of the ego with the male genital. Again, Federn used the term "ego" in an undifferentiated sense, but I think that we may assume that he was referring to the person, the self, in which case his statement would be an expression of the body-phallus equation.

There continues to be agreement with Freud that the castration threat at the oedipal period constitutes the greatest threat to narcissism and gives rise to the most important identification, that with the father. Freud (1923b) made clear that the oedipal identification, the result of an object cathexis, is superimposed on a direct and immediate identification which takes place earlier than any object cathexis, but the object choices belonging to the first sexual period reinforce the primary identification (see Loewald, 1951).

Throughout life, the most intimate relations exist between the genitals and narcissistic libido. The male retains the narcissistic estimation of his penis all of his life, and there is an increase in the cathexis of this organ at puberty. In contrast, Freud (1914) had noted that in girls, puberty is marked by a fresh wave of repression of sexuality associated specifically with the clitoris. Menstruation, which reawakens old castration threats, is the experience which brings this about. Freud stated that the maturation of the female sexual organs is accompanied by an intensification of the girl's original narcissism, which is then invested in her beauty and charm as compensation for social restrictions and the renunciation of her infantile masculinity.

Harnik (1923) observed that this secondary narcissism becomes attached to the body as a whole, contributing to a "genitalization" of the entire body, especially of the face. He concluded that the narcissism of women, in its mature form, reproduces once again the (dispersed) narcissistic distribution of libido which was characteristic of the prenatal period.

In a complete study of the vicissitudes of narcissism in structural and economic terms, I would have to discuss the cathectic changes in respect to self, objects, and ego interests throughout life in both sexes. An example of one phase of such a study is Helene Deutsch's (1925) careful observations of the shifts in cathexis between parts of the body image of the self and objects at various libidinal stages in the development of the little girl. During pregnancy these stages are repeated, and in libidinal relations with the child, this object, an extension of the mother's self, brings back to her some of the narcissism which the woman imparted to her partner in the sexual act. A similar process takes place in respect to organic disease and old age.

Pleasurable sensations connected with autoerotic activities contribute to the cathexis of their perception and to the memory traces of such experiences, from which are built up the images of the body. The ego ideal exerts a dynamic influence in the progression from one libidinal position to another. This change, Kapp (1925) said, occurs through the repression of pleasure in sensation in the affected zone, a process which involves shifts in narcissistic libido. For example, for the giving up of certain anal-erotic sensations there is partial compensation in the gratification from parental approval, but additional gains accrue from the fact that the resulting surplus of libido is directed to another object—an internal one—the ego. Thus, when an autoerotic gratification is given up, the released libido is still employed narcissistically but toward the useful purpose of ego development. Though infantile repression affects perception, distorts self and object representations, and produces amnesia, in Kapp's view it also results in the release of energy by which the ego's defense system fills in the defects with screen elements, distortions, or embellishments.

It is not possible in one paper to describe further the effects of narcissism on ego development or the development of the ego ideal and superego. These have been discussed by Loewald (1951), Jacobson (1954), Annie Reich (1954), Murray (1964), and Blos (1974). In the main, Kohut (1966, 1968, 1971) seems to agree with the formulations of Freud, Reich, and Jacobson with respect to ego ideal and superego formation, but it is my impression that he attaches more importance to the earlier preoedipal stage in respect to the establishment of a stable system of self-esteem regulation. On the other hand, though Reich (1954) regards the ego ideal as earlier and more narcissistic and the superego as a later, more reality-syntonic structure, she emphasizes most the castration threats of the oedipal period as the disturbing force in disorders of self-esteem.

Dynamics of Narcissism

Freud's views about the dynamics of various psychopathological conditions in respect to narcissistic libido can be summarized very briefly. As a result of frustration, object libido is withdrawn to the ego (self) in schizophrenic disorders, whereas in the transference neuroses the libido remains attached to objects in fantasy. In schizophrenia, megalomania corresponds to a mastery of the ego libido, whereas failure to master it gives rise to hypochondria, which is homologous to the anxiety of the transference neuroses. He believed that the restitutive attempts in schizophrenia correspond to the attempts in transference neuroses to deal with anxiety by symptom formation. The significance of the narcissistic object choice was emphasized in Freud's explanations of homosexuality. In melancholia the loss of an object, the choice of which had been effected on a narcissistic basis, is followed by an identification with the object, so that the love relation need not be given up. This represents a regression to a preliminary stage of object choice, the first way in which the ego selects an object. Although part of the erotic cathexis has regressed to identification, another part under the influence of the conflict due to ambivalence has been carried back to the stage of sadism.

These brief statements, derived mostly from the middle period of Freud's work, indicate the trend of his elaboration of theory: from libido only to an ever more complex instinctual concept, which includes the significance of object relations in the development of mental structure. Nevertheless, Freud's tentative and still undifferentiated concepts, as expressed in the 1914 paper on narcissism, seem to have constituted a point of fixation in psychoanalytic thought for a time. Yet, in his description of the vicissitudes of narcissism (1914)—e.g., its transformations into object cathexis and ego ideal—Freud was already moving away from his earlier ideas about quantitative shifts in libido as the cause of pathology. Narcissism began to take its place in the natural course of human development. Implicit is the idea—further developed by Clark (1923), van der Waals (1965), and Kohut (1966, 1971)—that some degree of narcissism (i.e., self-regard or love) is normal and healthy. It also followed, as a result of increasing knowledge of the early role of the mother as a "need-satisfying object" in the structural differentiation of the child, that qualitative changes in narcissistic libido—brought about by ego and superego development in relation to the influence of objects—began in their pathological manifestations to be indistinguishable from ego defects.

The psychic structures are not concrete entities, but are defined in terms of their functions. These functions represent a channeling of psychic energy into an organized mode of discharge determined by the dynamic and adaptive needs of the organism. These structures are characterized, in the words of Rapaport and Gill (1959), by a "slow rate of change." Not only the self (with its constitutional endowment), but objects, primarily, influence the type of energy with which discharge (cathexis) takes place and the direction of its force.

Some Genetic Aspects of Narcissistic Disorders

Currently, the main attribute of patients that is regarded as narcissistic may be described in the words of Otto Kernberg (1967) as "an unusual degree of self-reference in their interactions with other people, a great need to be loved and admired by others, and a curious apparent contradiction between a very inflated concept of themselves, and an inordinate need for tribute from others" (p. 655). While some of these patients may not be psychotic or even borderline, there is a continuum in the severity of their pathology. The main problem, he and others believe, is a disturbance of their self-regard in connection with specific object relationships.

How such narcissistic disturbance is transmitted is convincingly described by Warren Brodey (1965). In the process of differentiation and separation occurring during ego development he assumes that *"what is not directly related to a specific kind of tension building or tension release is not perceived"* (p. 171). The infant's wish carries an unqualified power of expectation, which is unsubstantial in its gratification except as the mother makes it substantial by her comprehension of the need. "The child's cathexis of the mother's functional capacity to relieve his tension at its source ensures her ability to *teach* as she patterns her responses"—but not yet as object. A beginning object relationship takes place when "the 'existent nipple' moves into congruence with the hallucinated nipple . . . [and fulfilling the wish is thereby] perceived and cathected with the energy attached to the wish" (p. 173). But this cathexis of the primordial other is at first without separation. It is an externalization that is a first step in separation. As the mother cathects the infant's beginning capacity for communication, the child's wish ceases to be the only control. Separation is facilitated by learning that the mother can supply his own wishes even before his own attention has been turned to them.

In the preobjectal period an "image mode" of reality testing is developed, based on a pattern of body attitudes, tensions, and affects occurring via physiological reactions and imitation of others, which the child learns to control and then use to predict what his learned behavior will bring as a response. In the "image mode" any loss of information is denied; the world is the product of one's own conduct, held rigid and concrete, as though one's point of view was the only one. It does not grow except as expected. Time is related only to one's own needs and is denied, stretched, and used to manipulate. What is learned is not integrated in an ever-expanding reworking of new sensory and labeled experiences.

If development proceeds normally, an "object mode" of reality testing also develops, by which the child continually redesigns his inner expectations in terms of objects observed to exist substantially. Remnants of unintegrated inner wishes and the satisfactions from them are used as memory, fantasy, and the basis for future expectations. "The omnipotent continuousness with the distanced feeding image begins to be replaced by skills, knowledge, and confidence that life support can be separate yet will not fail" (p. 176).

Both of these modes can coexist and have their functions, and indeed a quantitative matching of each seems important. The image mode carries continuity with the past, organizing the future in terms of the past. The object mode is important to the discovery of what was not expected, especially in a time of rapid change when the capacity to contact change is the only stability.

But in families in which the parents are narcissistic and utilize a defensive externalization in their own relationships, the children are taught by their family experience to use the image mode predominantly. The existent child is not libidinized; he is responded to by his mother as an as-if child—i.e., responded to only when he validates his mother's projection. So the experience of existence itself is altered by the narcissistic relationship. Since the child has no separate existence, his image is wholly governed by expectation and can never be spontaneous. If the child initiates nonmirroring, spontaneous action, the mother experiences separation anxiety, clutches her own image, and withdraws from such object relationship as does exist—thereby becoming even more intensely frightening to the child. By conforming to expectation to prevent severe decompensation in the parents, the child validates his early megalomanic and unbounded expectation that his behavior determines the existence of the world, for by such validation he does hold power. In this situation, no effective communication is established. The existent child feeds off the mother's projected image and is split off from himself. Only those aspects of his inner environment congruent with his mother's cathected image will be organized into his percepts and refined into culturally ordered ways of expression. Those energies of the existent child irrelevant to the experience acknowledged by the mother are random, unorganized, and split off from the pseudopersonality, which is structured to match either negatively or positively the parent's projection. Information that enlarges the Umwelt of the child is supplied only if it makes logical the manipulation. The child's reality and his mode of organizing reality are altered. An identity grows that is unsupported from within. I would add to Brodey's ideas that whether outwardly satisfactory or not, the identity is experienced as empty and false, unvalued by the individual himself, so that he must constantly seek reassurance from others or defensively hypercathect a compensatory grandiosity in fantasy or action.

Rochlin (1953) had previously noted that most serious ego pathology is believed to be related to an empty relationship with the mother during childhood. He emphasizes, however, as does Lippman (1951) and Rubinfine (1962), that the age at which object loss or deprivation occurs has considerable dynamic significance. During the oedipal phase the object most valued is invested with object libido, whereas in the pregenital period, the same object has primarily a narcissistic cathexis. Therefore, while it is true that the shadow of the object falls on the ego when object loss occurs during the oedipal period and thereafter, during the earlier phases it falls heavily on the id as well. Loss of the object before narcissistic libido has been in any great measure transformed into object libido occurs when the primitive identification is still narcissistic, and the ambivalence is preponderantly weighted in favor of sadism as in melancholia. Two courses are open to a child sustaining such early loss: an increase of narcissism and a turning away from reality. But Rochlin (1959) believes that the necessity for object relations, when relinquished, is not met altogether by taking oneself as an object in an exaggerated narcissistic reaction. The ego makes an attempt at restitution. Reality is sacrificed and the object is restored in fantasy and fixed by being made inanimate. Noting that the object, although otherwise frustrating, is often a source of sensual pleasure in the physical care given, Rochlin (1953) states that in providing some autoerotic pleasure, such objects promote a primarily narcissistic relationship.

The reaction to loss is experienced in terms of the developmental phase, especially of the ego, at the time the loss occurs. Regression is a characteristic result, often with arrest of further development of certain ego functions and particularly object relations. There is a tendency to develop animism to a greater than usual degree. The course that identification takes is more apt to have pathological qualities, which will be reflected in the ultimate character formation. Increase in narcissism or its intensification in residual object relations is a common sequel. If the infantile character has a strong fixation in certain pregenital phases, it is likely to be reinforced. If the loss occurs during the oedipal period, this phase will be frozen. Later, the same effect is seen in superego development. It is significant that in the cases described by Rochlin the relationship to objects was characteristically destructive and sadistic, aggressive without any respite, and the same impulses were directed toward the self.

Though Rochlin's studies were primarily concerned with object loss—an actual separation without an emotional substitute—to a lesser degree similar reactions are observed whenever there is a disturbance in the object relationship. Rank and MacNaughton (1950) have noted that early disappointing relationships which produce forbidden, unconscious fantasies regarding the child are reflected in inhibitions of motherliness. These are projected onto the child as the devalued image of the mother in total or in part. The result is that the child invests his libido in the self; his body remains the sole object of love. In a study of moral masochists who showed unusual narcissism, Bernstein (1957) found that during their early years the body attributes and ego functions of these patients were made to serve their parents' narcissistic and partial instinctual needs. These patients had been robbed of the ego gratification that normally is derived from self-accomplishment because their successes were not their own but their parents'. The consequence for many children so conditioned is that failure and defeat become triumph in childhood and a repetitive compulsion in adult life. When a child is made to serve the highly narcissistic needs of parental objects, he regresses to his own narcissistic satisfactions whenever the object becomes disappointing, i.e., cathexis of the object is interfered with. Masochistic relationships in adult life, Bernstein said, are repetitive reenactments of such childhood experiences and fantasies in which the patient has the illusion that he actively controls the situation which he once passively endured.

The genetic observations of Brodey, Rochlin, Bernstein, Rank and others may be interpreted from yet another theoretical viewpoint—that of Margaret Mahler (1968). If the mother has had serious problems in her own separation-individuation, she will not be gratified by her child's individuation. What will be mirrored for her child and become the model for incorporation in his ego structure will be unpleasure and anxiety whenever separation forces his own individuation. He remains bound to her and to the fulfillment of her needs, and his own self remains an alien, unsatisfying as-if object.

Maturational pressures, bodily defects (Niederland, 1965), or the shortcomings of mothering previously mentioned may disturb the normal development of certain narcissistic structures of the personality which, according to Kohut (1966, 1968, 1971), represent transformations of narcissistic libido. Though there may be amalgamations with object love, Kohut regards the appearance of a "grandiose self" and an "idealized parent imago" as "maturational steps *sui generis* in the development of narcissistic libido and differentiated from the development of object love with its own transitional phases" (1966, p. 247). In doing so, he postulates two separate lines of development for narcissistic and object libido, each subject to its own disturbances. Under favorable circumstances both the grandiose self and the idealized parent imago become integrated into the adult personality and contribute important components to the psychic organization. Thwarted in their development by traumata, however, both structures, he says, are retained in unaltered form and strive for the fulfillment of archaic aims. The idealized parent imago remains as an archaic transitional object required for the maintenance of narcissistic homeostasis (1968).

A detailed discussion of Kohut's and Kernberg's work is not required by the purposes of this paper, but a few additional remarks are relevant. Except as a didactic exercise, I do not see the usefulness of Kohut's assumption of independent developmental lines, and I question its validity. In describing the development of the grandiose self and the idealized parent imago, he relates them to disappointment in the self and the object. The introjective-projective mechanisms which accompany such an experience have been amply documented, and Jacobson (1954, 1964) has described the intricate interchange between self and object representations and the effect of each on the libidinal and aggressive investment of the other. Moreover, what appears to be a narcissistic self-orientation is often actually the imprint of the object, who was herself narcissistic. Kohut explains the apparent object hunger of certain narcissistic personalities on the basis that substitutes are needed for the missing segments of the psychic structure; but an alternative view is possible—that the objects which have deprived the child have demonstrated a disregard for his needs and this parental image becomes a part of the structure of the child's mind, a built-in, ungiving, unloving, humiliating part of himself which he would like to replace with other more satisfying imagos. Even so, this self-object does have some libidinal cathexis; it is a masochistic formation which is clung to tenaciously—not an object in an ideal sense, but distorted and cathected with aggressive energy, so that splitting is necessary which, together with denial, interferes with its perception realistically. Meanwhile, the archaic self-objects are clung to tenaciously as the only available substitute providing gratification. This differences of views is significant because Kohut establishes a continuity of pathological and normal narcissism and assumes that the archaic narcissistic structures normally become, or may do so in the course of treatment, higher transformations of narcissism in an essentially normal personality. Like Otto Kernberg (1974), I am more inclined to believe that pathological narcissism is the result of vicissitudes of aggressive as well as libidinal drives and defenses and differs from the "ordinary adult narcissism and from fixation at or regression to normal infantile narcissism" (p. 219).

Narcissism—A Nuclear, Organizing Concept

As psychoanalytic theory developed, narcissism apparently became an anachronism, an obscure and ambiguous semantic and conceptual artifact, confusing despite its seeming usefulness. A revival of interest in the subject as a result of treatment of so-called "narcissistic disorders" necessitated for me an attempt to clarify the concept by a survey of the literature. With this purpose in mind, I have considered the subject first in the context of its place in the historical development of psychoanalytic theory. Freud's ideas about narcissism and its relationship to a variety of phenomena are presented and examined from the viewpoint of later authors, and an effort has been made to integrate the concept with the developmental and metapsychological approaches. Such considerations are essential to a comprehension of the theoretical and technical implications of the subject.

Though the sense in which the term narcissism is used has varied during the course of development of psychoanalytic theory, it is apparent that there has been a continuity. Throughout it has retained the implication of a positive, libidinal feeling toward the self, although it is now recognized that there are parallel, and often intermingled, investments with aggressive cathexes.

In the undifferentiated state of the infant, psychic energy is available for a to and fro cathectic interchange with the mother. This was first conceptualized by Freud as primary and secondary narcissism in apparent recognition of the self reference of the early dyadic unit and the potential of such energic exchange for the development of "normal," adaptive, and satisfying functions of the mind as well as pathological phenomena. As autonomous ego functions—e.g., perception and memory—mature, pleasurable and unpleasurable experiences contribute to a simultaneous differentiation of instinctual drives and structures and cathexis of self and object representations with varying admixtures of drive energies. The cathectic interchanges between objects and child and the resulting communication and learning process instituted may facilitate or inhibit the establishment of a separate sense of identity—a self sufficiently cathected with positive libidinal energy to be stable enough within to withstand the hurts from without. Excessive gratification, and excessive frustration particularly, predispose to a regressive refusion of self and object images, and under the influence of libidinal and aggressive drive energies the fused self-object image may be alternately overvalued or devalued in reaction to the ego ideal and superego, with the reactivation of archaic defenses, such as splitting into good and bad objects, primitive idealization, and projection. Hurts to self-esteem may occur throughout life and lead to a defensive regression to primitive ego states, the severity of the pathology of the clinical states we refer to as narcissistic varying with the earlier preobject pathology.

This brief summary indicates the transformations undergone by the concept of narcissism itself. I have concluded that *it is a nuclear concept which became for Freud an organizing matrix for the construction of psychoanalytic theory, hence an integral part of the whole.* As such, it has a significance which transcends attempts to narrow its definition. Though we may be tempted to abandon the concept as outmoded or to limit its application as Joffe and Sandler (1967) and Pulver (1970) have tried to do, something is lost in such restrictions. Narcissistic, like certain other English words, conveys in brief a meaning which is variable but usually recognizable from its context. It is extraordinarily useful as verbal shorthand if it is not abused. We must, I think, accept it in all of its complexity, attempting to define more clearly each of its aspects as observations expand knowledge.

A review of the concept impresses one with the basic fact that those functions which comprise what we call structures are the result of the constant interchange of psychic energies between mental representations. For psychology, this concept is analogous in importance to the physical concept of the interchangeability of matter and energy. One is also impressed by the genius of Freud's perception and capacity for creative regression, for mirrored in narcissism is the "ego," a remarkable feat of condensation and sublimation.

BIBLIOGRAPHY

ABRAHAM, K. (1920), The Narcissistic Evaluation of Excretory Processes in Dream and Neurosis. *Selected Papers on Psycho-Analysis.* London: Hogarth Press, 1948, pp. 318–322.
APFELBAUM, B. (1965), Ego Psychology, Psychic Energy, and the Hazards of Quantitative Explanation in Psycho-Analytic Theory. *Int. J. Psycho-Anal.,* 46:168–182.
BALINT, M. (1960), Primary Narcissism and Primary Love. *Psychoanal. Quart.,* 29:6–43.
BERNSTEIN, I. (1957), The Role of Narcissism in Moral Masochism. *Psychoanal. Quart.,* 26:358–377.
BIBRING, E. (1936), The Development and Problems of the Theory of Instincts. *Int. J. Psycho-Anal.,* 22:102–131, 1941.
BING, J. F., McLaughlin, F., & MARBURG, R. (1959), The Metapsychology of Narcissism. *This Annual,* 14:9–28.
BLOS, P. (1974), The Geneology of the Ego Ideal. *This Annual,* 29:43–88.
BRODEY, W. M. (1965), On the Dynamics of Narcissism: I. *This Annual,* 20:165–193.
CLARK, L. P. (1923), Unconscious Motives Underlying the Personalities of Great Statesmen and Their Relation to Epoch-Making Events. *Psychoanal. Rev.,* 10:56–69.
DEUTSCH, H. (1925), The Psychology of Women in Relation to the Function of Reproduction. *Int. J. Psycho-Anal.,* 6:405–418.
FEDERN, P. (1952), *Ego Psychology and the Psychoses.* New York: Basic Books.
FREUD, S. (1900), The Interpretation of Dreams. *S.E.,* 4 & 5.
——— (1905), Three Essays on the Theory of Sexuality. *S.E.,* 7:125–243.
——— (1910a), Leonardo da Vinci and a Memory of His Childhood. *S.E.,* 11:59–137.
——— (1910b), The Psycho-Analytic View of Psychogenic Disturbance of Vision. *S.E.,* 11:209–218.
——— (1911), Psycho-Analytic Notes on an Autobiographical Account of a Case of Paranoia (Dementia Paranoides). *S.E.,* 12:3–82.
——— (1913), Totem and Taboo. *S.E.,* 13:1–161.
——— (1914), On Narcissism: An Introduction. *S.E.,* 14:67–102.
——— (1915a), Instincts and Their Vicissitudes. *S.E.,* 14:109–140.
——— (1915b), A Case of Paranoia Running Counter to the Psycho-Analytic Theory of the Disease. *S.E.,* 14:261–272.
——— (1916/17), Introductory Lectures on Psycho-Analysis. *S.E.,* 15 & 16.
——— (1917a), A Metapsychological Supplement to the Theory of Dreams. *S.E.,* 14:217–235.
——— (1917b), Mourning and Melancholia. *S.E.,* 14:237–260.

———— (1917c), On Transformations of Instinct As Exemplified in Anal Erotism. *S.E.*, 17:127–133.
———— (1918), From the History of an Infantile Neurosis. *S.E.*, 17:7–122.
———— (1919), Introduction to *Psycho-Analysis and the War Neuroses*. *S.E.*, 17:207–210.
———— (1920), Beyond the Pleasure Principle. *S.E.*, 18:3–64.
———— (1921), Group Psychology and the Analysis of the Ego. *S.E.*, 18:67–143.
———— (1922), Some Neurotic Mechanisms in Jealousy, Paranoia and Homosexuality. *S.E.*, 18:223–232.
———— (1923a), Two Encyclopaedia Articles. *S.E.*, 18:235–259.
———— (1923b), The Ego and the Id. *S.E.*, 19:3–66.
———— (1925), Some Psychical Consequences of the Anatomical Distinction Between the Sexes. *S.E.*, 19:243–258.
———— (1926), Inhibitions, Symptoms and Anxiety. *S.E.*, 20:3–74.
———— (1927a), The Future of an Illusion. *S.E.*, 21:3–56.
———— (1927b), Humour. *S.E.*, 21:159–166.
———— (1930), Civilization and Its Discontents. *S.E.*, 21:59–145.
———— (1931), Libidinal Types. *S.E.*, 21:215–220.
———— (1933), New Introductory Lectures on Psycho-Analysis. *S.E.*, 22:3–182.
———— (1940), An Outline of Psycho-Analysis. *S.E.*, 23:141–207.
———— (1950), *The Origins of Psychoanalysis*. New York: Basic Books, 1954.
GREENACRE, P. (1945), The Biologic Economy of Birth. *This Annual*, 1:31–51.
HARNIK, J. (1923), The Various Developments Undergone by Narcissism in Men and Women. *Int. J. Psycho-Anal.*, 5:66–83, 1924.
HARTMANN, H. (1948), Comments on the Psychoanalytic Theory of Instinctual Drives. *Psychoanal. Quart.*, 17:368–388.
———— (1950), Comments on the Psychoanalytic Theory of the Ego. *This Annual*, 5:74–96.
———— KRIS, E., & LOEWENSTEIN, R. M. (1949), Notes on the Theory of Aggression. *This Annual*, 3/4:9–36.
HENDRICK, I. (1942), Instinct and Ego During Infancy. *Psychoanal. Quart.*, 11:33–58.
HOLT, R. R. (1967), On the Insufficiency of Drive As a Motivational Concept in the Light of Evidence from Experimental Psychology (abst.). *J. Amer. Psychoanal. Assn.*, 16:627–632.
JACOBSON, E. (1954), The Self and the Object World. *This Annual*, 9:75–127.
———— (1964), *The Self and the Object World*. New York: Int. Univ. Press.
JOFFE, W. G. & SANDLER, J. (1967), Some Conceptual Problems Involved in the Consideration of Disorders of Narcissism. *J. Child Psychother.*, 2:56–66.
KANZER, M. (1954), Observations on Blank Dreams with Orgasms. *Psychoanal. Quart.*, 23:511–520.
———— (1964), Freud's Uses of the Terms "Autoerotism" and "Narcissism." *J. Amer. Psychoanal. Assn.*, 12:529–539.
KAPP, R. O. (1925), Sensation and Narcissism. *Int. J. Psycho-Anal.*, 6:292–299.
KARDINER, A., KARUSH, A., & OVESEY, L. (1959), A Methodological Study of Freudian Theory. *J. Nerv. Ment. Dis.*, 129:133–143.

KERNBERG, O. F. (1967), Borderline Personality Organization. *J. Amer. Psychoanal. Assn.*, 15:641-685.

——— (1969), Factors in the Psychoanalytic Treatment of Narcissistic Personalities. *Bull. Menninger Clin.*, 33:191-196.

——— (1970a), Factors in the Psychoanalytic Treatment of Narcissistic Personalities. *J. Amer. Psychoanal. Assn.*, 18:51-85.

——— (1970b), A Psychoanalytic Classification of Character Pathology. *J. Amer. Psychoanal. Assn.*, 18:800-822.

——— (1971), Prognostic Considerations Regarding Borderline Personality Organization. *J. Amer. Psychoanal. Assn.*, 19:595-635.

——— (1974), Further Contributions to the Treatment of Narcissistic Personalities. *Int. J. Psycho-Anal.*, 55:215-240.

KERNBERG, P. F. (1971), The Course of the Analysis of a Narcissistic Personality with Hysterical and Compulsive Features. *J. Amer. Psychoanal. Assn.*, 19:451-471.

KOHUT, H. (1966), Forms and Transformations of Narcissism. *J. Amer. Psychoanal. Assn.*, 14:243-272.

——— (1968), The Psychoanalytic Treatment of Narcissistic Personality Disorders. *This Annual*, 23:86-113.

——— (1971), *The Analysis of the Self*. New York: Int. Univ. Press.

——— (1972), Thoughts on Narcissism and Narcissistic Rage. *This Annual*, 27:360-400.

LEWIN, B. D. (1955), Dream Psychology and the Analytic Situation. *Psychoanal. Quart.*, 24:169-199.

LICHTENSTEIN, H. (1964), The Role of Narcissism in the Emergence and Maintenance of a Primary Identity. *Int. J. Psycho-Anal.*, 45:49-56.

LIPPMAN, H. S. (1951), Psychopathic Behavior in Infants and Children. *Amer. J. Orthopsychiat.*, 21:227-231.

LOEWALD, H. W. (1951), Ego and Reality. *Int. J. Psycho-Anal.*, 32:10-18.

LOEWENSTEIN, R. M. (1940), The Vital or Somatic Instincts. *Int. J. Psycho-Anal.*, 21:377-400.

MAHLER, M. S. (1968), *On Human Symbiosis and the Vicissitudes of Individuation*. New York: Int. Univ. Press.

——— & MCDEVITT, J. B. (1968), Observations on Adaptation and Defense in Statu Nascendi. *Psychoanal. Quart.*, 37:1-21.

MURRAY, J. M. (1964), Narcissism and the Ego Ideal. *J. Amer. Psychoanal. Assn.*, 12:477-511.

NIEDERLAND, W. G. (1965), Narcissistic Ego Impairment in Patients with Early Physical Malformations. *This Annual*, 20:518-534.

PANEL (1961), Narcissism, rep. J. F. Bing & R. O. Marburg. *J. Amer. Psychoanal. Assn.*, 10:593-605, 1962.

PULVER, E. (1970), Narcissism. *J. Amer. Psychoanal. Assn.*, 18:319-341.

RANK, B. & MACNAUGHTON, D. (1950), A Clinical Contribution to Early Ego Development. *This Annual*, 5:53-65.

RAPAPORT, D. & GILL, M. M. (1959), The Points of View and Assumptions of Metapsychology. *Int. J. Psycho-Anal.*, 40:153-162.

Reich, A. (1954), Early Identifications as Archaic Elements in the Superego. *J. Amer. Psychoanal. Assn.*, 2:218–238.
Rochlin, G. (1953), Loss and Restitution. *This Annual*, 8:288–309.
—— (1959), The Loss Complex. *J. Amer. Psychoanal. Assn.*, 7:299–316.
Rubinfine, D. L. (1962), Maternal Stimulation, Psychic Structure, and Early Object Relations. *This Annual*, 17:265–282.
Spiegel, L. A. (1959), The Self, the Sense of Self, and Perception. *This Annual*, 14:81–109.
Spitz, R. A. (1959), *A Genetic Field Theory of Ego Formation*. New York: Int. Univ. Press.
—— (1965), *The First Year of Life*. New York: Int. Univ. Press.
Stone, L. (1954), The Widening Scope of Indications for Psychoanalysis. *J. Amer. Psychoanal. Assn.*, 2:567–594.
van der Waals, H. G. (1965), Problems of Narcissism. *Bull. Menninger Clin.*, 29:293–311.
Waelder, R. (1960), *Basic Theory of Psychoanalysis*. New York: Int. Univ. Press.
—— (1961), Discussion, Session III, Conference, Institute for Advanced Psychoanalytic Studies, Princeton, N.J.
Weiss, E. (1957), A Comparative Study of Psycho-Analytical Ego Concepts. *Int. J. Psycho-Anal.*, 38:209–222.

CLINICAL CONTRIBUTIONS

Pseudobackwardness in Children

Maternal Attitudes As an Etiological Factor

MARIA BERGER AND
HANSI KENNEDY

In collaboration with Don Campbell,
Sara Lundberg, and Randi Markowitz

FOREWORD BY ANNA FREUD

The successful negotiation of developmental sequences needs in every child's case a happy combination of internal and external circumstances. Where cognitive development and mastery of the

---

The authors are staff members and students at the Hampstead Child-Therapy Course and Clinic, London.

The Hampstead Clinic is at present supported by the Field Foundation, Inc., New York; the Foundation for Research in Psychoanalysis, Beverly Hills, Calif.; the Freud Centenary Fund, London; the Anna Freud Foundation, New York; the Grant Foundation, New York; the New-Land Foundation, Inc., New York; and a number of private supporters.

This paper forms part of a Research Project entitled: "Childhood Psychopathology: Pathogenic Processes and Overt Symptomatology." The project is financed by the National Institute of Mental Health, Washington, D.C. The paper also forms part of the work carried out by the Index Research Group, Chairman, Dr. J. J. Sandler. We are grateful to the therapists, Well-Baby Clinic staff, and the Nursery School staff for making their data available to the Index.

inner and outer world are concerned, the indispensable elements include a large number of factors such as: the intactness of organic and sensory equipment; its environmental stimulation at appropriate periods; on the ego side, the smooth progress from primary to secondary functioning, i.e., from the pleasure principle to the reality principle; on the side of the drives, the transfer of energy from sexual curiosity and scoptophilia to neutralized pursuits; on the superego side, the absence of inhibiting and limiting prohibitions; on the parental side, the presence of positive responses to every forward step. The very multiplicity of factors needed to ensure progress is reflected in the multiplicity of disorders affecting orientation, active mastery, intellectual growth, including the various learning disturbances and school failures. We regard as genuinely backward those cases in which the causes for the defect are located in the basic equipment of the mental apparatus, and we use the diagnostic label of pseudobackwardness when the primary potential for normal development is present, but is interfered with secondarily either by internal conflict or by inadequate and detrimental environmental responses.

The case histories which follow are meant to illustrate the last-mentioned of these possibilities. The life stories and analytic explorations of these children show that at birth and during their first year of life, they did not significantly differ from other infants, i.e., that constitutionally they were well within the norm, with their drive and ego potentialities intact. Moreover, with regard to parental handling, they were neither abandoned, neglected, nor maltreated. There was only one factor missing in their lives and this due to their mothers' own personality difficulties: there was no parental pride and pleasure in the child; accordingly, there was a complete lack of the admiring approval from the parents' side which acts simultaneously as a reward for achievement and as a powerful spur and encouragement toward further efforts in the same progressive direction.

It is a sobering thought that within the complex mesh of influences which shape the life of any individual child, the presence or absence as well as the quality of any single ingredient should have such power to determine the developmental result.

THE PHENOMENON OF "PSEUDOBACKWARDNESS," REFERRED TO IN THE literature as "pseudodebility," "pseudoimbecility," and "pseudostupidity," has attracted the attention of analysts for a great many years. As long ago as 1910, Ernest Jones wrote of "Simulated Foolishness in Hysteria." In the '30s and '40s several analysts, among them Landauer (1929), Bornstein (1930), Oberndorf (1939), and Mahler (1942), described their clinical experiences with such children and their understanding of the relevant pathology. Subsequently Hellman (1954) described her observations of mothers of children with intellectual inhibitions, and Staver (1953), Buxbaum (1964), and Sprince (1967) discussed the part played by parents in certain learning disorders.

These writers are basically in agreement with each other in their main conclusions:

1. These children do not wish to understand, to know, to see; and this defensive "ignorance" pertains especially to sexual matters.

2. These sexual matters formed part of a family secret, mostly a guilty secret, concerning the sexual lives of parents (either as a couple or as individuals), or of close relatives. They involved the child, more or less directly, as an observer or participant (Mahler, Sprince).

3. The parents unconsciously needed the particular child to be "stupid" or "ignorant."

4. The child responded by conforming to his parents' need in order to preserve their love.

Hellman, Buxbaum, and Staver discussed the effects of the mothers' personalities on the functioning of the pseudoimbecile patients. Hellman stressed the effects of the mothers' extensive use of denial and lying on the pathology of these children.

The emphasis in all these papers is on the impairment of the childrens' ego functions and on the inhibition of curiosity and scoptophilia which result from the children's unconscious collusion with their mothers in the need not to know the parental secrets.

In the course of examining cases of learning disturbances recorded in the Hampstead Index we came upon another etiological factor that was striking enough to merit investigation. There were about fifty such cases which varied in their severity and spread. Some were children who had specific difficulties, e.g., with reading or arithmetic; others had a more general learning inhibition. At the extreme end of the scale we found a group of seven children who were considered by their parents, or their teachers, as backward, but who, on testing, proved to have at least average intelligence and who lost their "backward" mode of functioning as a result of analysis. Our attention was caught by the fact that in all these cases one could discern specific maternal attitudes which appeared to have had an adverse influence on the children's development from the start. This study is focused on these children.

For the purpose of this paper, however, we have selected only four cases out of the seven, since these four children were especially well known to us. All four had undergone long analyses. Two of them were observed from their infancy or early childhood onward. In addition, the mothers of two children also underwent analyses with members of the Clinic staff.

CASE PRESENTATIONS

CASE 1

Jane was referred to the well-baby clinic when she was only a few weeks old. From the age of 3 to 5 she attended the Clinic's nursery school. At 5 years of age she was referred for a diagnostic investigation and subsequently went into analysis for four years.

Jane's birth was uncomplicated. Breast feeding was established during the mother's two-weeks' stay in the hospital. However, as soon as Mrs. J. returned home and took over the care of her baby, major problems over feeding began. Jane usually fell asleep after taking a few gulps of milk, only to awake screaming as soon as she was put in her cot. Mrs. J. became depressed, physically exhausted, and quite unable to take care of her child. The doctor arranged for both mother and daughter to be readmitted to the hospital so that care could be taken of both. Jane is said to have thrived on feedings supervised or offered by the nurses, and the mother was advised to supplement breast feeding with the bottle. Mother and baby appeared to settle down and a more satisfactory feeding routine was established. As soon as they returned home, however, and the mother was again unsupported in the care of her daughter, the struggle over feeding was revived; gradual improvement occurred only after weaning and the introduction of solids. Mrs. J. spoke of Jane "refusing" breast and bottle as if she experienced these difficulties as an act of aggression or deliberate withholding. Later she referred back to the early feeding problems by saying, "I tried to do all the right things but could not stand this thing making demands on me."

The mother always complained to the well-baby clinic staff about Jane. For instance, she spoke of Jane's "shyness," calling it a "symptom" she found "difficult to tolerate and hurtful to my pride." There are many references in the baby clinic records to the mother's unfavorable comparisons of Jane with other children, often boys, and to Mrs. J.'s derogatory remarks. She described the baby at 14 months as "unintelligent," and readily expressed a strong wish to get away from Jane. Whenever there was an overt sign of physical hurt, Mrs. J. seemed especially unable to deal with Jane's needs.

From early on the well-baby clinic staff was concerned about Jane's slow development and immaturity, which they linked with inadequate mothering and lack of stimulation. All along, the staff tried to find ways in which to stimulate Jane's physical and psychological development, but somehow the manner in which the mother carried out their suggestions precluded any positive outcome. The mother's inability to answer Jane's emotional needs was striking. While the mother complained of Jane's lack of contact with her, she was not aware of her own lack of contact with her baby.

Jane was late in sitting up as well as in starting to walk and was found to be generally poorly coordinated. She suffered from frequent ear, nose, and throat infections. For the mother, these were signs that there was always something wrong with Jane's body. When Jane was 17 months old, toilet training was initiated. The mother was alternately strict and indulgent, and Jane was late in gaining bowel and bladder control. Her early refusal to feed later changed to excessive greediness and grasping for food, and she developed particularly messy eating habits, all of which irritated the mother.

When Jane was 3 years old, the well-baby clinic recommended

that she attend the Clinic nursery school in the hope that this would counteract some of the adverse environmental influences and offer the child opportunities for new experiences to further her development. Entry into the nursery school coincided roughly with the birth of Dan. The mother, unlike her early reactions to Jane, took great pleasure in her baby son. Dan thrived and was an outgoing, active, and friendly baby. There were no feeding difficulties with him.

Jane reacted to her brother's arrival with a massive regression. Not only did she lose her recently acquired bladder control, but she started to eat and smear feces. The mother reported that while she was feeding Dan, Jane often wandered off, sometimes even outside the house. Mrs. J. did not understand Jane's behavior as a reaction to her breast feeding Dan, but saw Jane's wandering away as clear evidence of her daughter's lack of attachment to her. It seemed that at this time Jane turned to her father and attempted to elicit mothering from him, but he found her too demanding and became irritated by her attempts to cling to him.

Nursery school observations of Jane's play, object relationships, and excessive autoerotic activity confirmed her immaturity and slow development. She was preoccupied with messy sand-and-water play that was not considered age-adequate. She was described as possessive and bossy with her friends; she often withdrew into a corner to suck her thumb or masturbate. Most of the time she appeared clumsy, vacant, drooling, and smelled of urine; occasionally she soiled. She was miserable, unhappy, and unlikable.

There was no significant change in the child's behavior and she did not appear to benefit from the educational opportunities offered by the nursery school during her two years' attendance. The staff became increasingly convinced that Jane was intellectually backward and she was referred for psychological testing. She was found to have a high-average intelligence (on the Merrill-Palmer Test). This unexpected test result led to her referral for analysis.

Although Jane was potentially pretty, at the beginning of treatment her appearance and demeanor clearly reflected her self image of a dirty, messy, stupid, unwanted little girl.

Transference manifestations and fantasies during analysis

strongly suggested that Jane had complied with the mother's image of her and that this devalued self image was later reinforced by conflicts centering on penis envy. It is not surprising that penis envy became the focus of her developmental problems, because her entry into the phallic phase largely coincided with the birth of her brother.

Many of Jane's fantasies expressed her intense wish to be a boy. There was evidence in the analytic material that she had experienced a tonsillectomy, at the age of 4, as castration. For example, Jane would play with a doll which she said was a boy. This boy was then punished for being naughty by the doctor, who did something to his mouth and turned him into a little girl. Jane's wish to be a boy was reinforced when her mother displayed her obvious affection for and pleasure in her newborn son. The fact that the father also was an unsatisfactory oedipal object for Jane further contributed to her inability to make developmental progress. It was not until after one year of analysis, when a great deal of work had been done on tracing the various sources of her intense penis envy, that Jane became established in the positive oedipal phase.

After about two years of treatment the first signs of a more benign image of herself slowly emerged. Jane expressed the fantasy of once having been "a pretty baby in blue socks." She progressively began to refer to herself as a nice and good girl. She expressed genuine surprise when she discovered that she was able to accomplish something without assistance. Until then, in the transference, Jane had often seen the therapist as the mother for whom she had to enact the role of the retarded child. It would seem that only as a result of a great deal of working through in the analysis, Jane could develop a self image that was not a direct replica of her mother's image of her.

The arrival of a second brother during the last year of analysis briefly reactivated some of Jane's earlier conflicts, but did not unduly disturb her. By the end of the treatment this clumsy, late-developer found particular pleasure in such physical activities as skipping, ball games, cycling, skating, swimming. She discovered many other interests: she greatly enjoyed learning to play the recorder; she liked cooking and "making things" and talked about wanting to become a mother. Her achievements in primary and secondary school were average to good. At present Jane is preparing for a career as a social worker.

Jane's case was clearly one of pseudobackwardness in which the interferences with development stemmed initially from the mother's attitude toward her, and only secondarily from the child's own conflicts.

With regard to the question of etiology, it is important to note that when Jane was a baby, the well-baby clinic observers never noticed any sign of protest from her. This degree of resignation could suggest that Jane was a particularly placid baby. It could also point to an early acceptance by the child of the role assigned her by the mother. Such an acceptance may have been the only way open to Jane to retain contact with her mother, who was otherwise "unavailable." Conversely, to protest against this imposed role may have been felt by Jane as a threat to whatever feelings of safety she had, inviting a total rejection, or even abandonment, by the mother. Her security and safety in her environment probably depended on compliance with the mother's unconscious need to perceive her as damaged. But any feelings of safety maintained in this way would be achieved at the cost of developmental progress. We assume that a well-functioning child wishes to please his parents by his success in learning and developing. Jane seemed to have had little experience of being praised and admired, and the effects of her mother's customary disparagement in the face of any achievement could hardly have spurred her development.

The mother's unconscious need to see Jane as inadequate and damaged constantly impinged on her ability to make more realistic appraisals of her baby. Moreover, she saw this firstborn infant as rejecting and attributed hostile intentions to her baby from the very beginning. We suggest that the mother's defensive externalizations made it impossible for her to pick up cues and respond appropriately to her baby. The baby's slow development later confirmed to the mother her view of the child as damaged.

Jane's acceptance of, and identification with, her mother's view of her may have been intensified by the fact that there was no one in Jane's life—prior to her entry into analysis—who had a different image of her. Gradually her own developmental conflicts enhanced this imposed image of herself. Analysis revealed, among other things, how her intense penis envy was bound up with her parents' preference for her brother and constantly reinforced her already vulnerable self-esteem.

CASE 2

Yetta was well known to us from the age of 3 when she was first referred to the Clinic. From then on she and her mother were in contact with the Clinic and were visited at regular intervals by the social worker. From the age of 12 to 18 Yetta was in analysis. Her main referral symptoms were bed wetting, sleep disturbance, excessive clinging to mother, and temper outbursts. Questions about the level of her intelligence, however, had been raised from her first referral at the age of 3.

Yetta was tested on three occasions. (1) At 3½ her IQ on the Binet (Form L) was *88*, and the psychologist commented that she was "a dull little girl, cooperative but never gave the impression of being any brighter." (2) At 8½ her Binet IQ was *92*. On this occasion a different psychologist noted: "Yetta does not seem bright and in some tests she gave somewhat strange stupid answers." (3) At 16½ her IQ score on the WAIS was *98*.

At school Yetta's attainment tended to be below average. At 6, she was not moved up with her classmates. At 8, her teachers thought her dreamy and withdrawn, but doing reasonably well except in arithmetic. At 11, she did not pass the selective examination to grammar school. When she came into analysis she had difficulties in several subjects. In the course of analysis her learning improved so much that she was transferred to a grammar school, where she obtained several "O" levels.

Her analyst, an experienced psychologist, thought that Yetta's real IQ was closer to 115–120. Yetta's intellectual underfunctioning showed itself more during the intelligence testing than at school. In this respect she differed from Jane; but, like Jane, she impressed several trained observers as being dull. To quote from one observation: "Yetta gives the impression of being very dull intellectually and of having just picked up phrases from her mother."

Yetta was the child of an unmarried mother; her father deserted the mother as soon as he knew that she was pregnant. Yetta was brought up by her mother with the help of lodgers, a childless couple who "doted" on the little girl.

Yetta was born prematurely at 6 months, weighing about 4 lbs., and was kept in the hospital for the first 6 weeks. She was breast-fed for 4 months and was weaned gradually to a bottle, which she had till she was 12 months. She did not suck her fingers or a dummy.

In a letter to the Clinic, headed "Complaint," the mother wrote: "Only one thing troubled me—her insatiable thirst. She screamed when we stopped feeding her, so sometimes I had to give her double amount. At that time navel trouble developed so that I was frightened to let her cry too much. In spite of a danger of strangulation the doctor refused to operate on her . . . after a week the navel became alright after all." The "insatiable thirst" may well have denoted the mother's lack of experience, but it also points to her ambivalent feelings toward her baby. The reference to strangulation seems to confirm this.

Toilet training started at 9 months and was carried out "according to the book," i.e., Yetta was held out every two hours. She appeared never to have achieved bladder control at night and enuresis was a major referral sympton. At about 12 months she started to play with her feces, smearing herself, her bed, and the walls. She was not prevented from these activities because her mother did not believe in "interfering with her pleasures." She apparently stopped of her own accord at the age of 2.

Yetta walked at 17 months and started to talk at 2 years. She suffered from sleep disturbance, and at the age of 3 began to refuse to sleep in her own bed. At the same age, she was said to have had "an enormous appetite." She stole food from the larder and from stalls. At that time, her mother began to work, and Yetta was looked after by a neighbor. Subsequently, she was placed in a large nursery. She was reported to be "very attached" and very clinging to her mother, whom Yetta cuddled and stroked when mother was upset.

At 5, Yetta had a long period of separation from mother and home. She contracted pneumonia and spent two months in a hospital and convalescent home. When she returned home, she again went at night to her mother's or the male lodger's bed. This man was highly disturbed. He was said to have been amused by Yetta's overtures to him and permitted her to handle his penis.

Yetta did not know about the circumstances of her birth, which for years remained a "secret." She was merely told that her father was working overseas. Only during Yetta's analysis, at the instigation of her analyst, did the mother tell Yetta the truth.

The mother's attitude toward Yetta's intellectual functioning was highly ambivalent. She reported that she was glad that Yetta was not "an infant prodigy," because her very clever nephew had shot himself at the age of 12 following his parents' divorce and his father's suicide.

Several observers noted that Yetta identified with her mother in her speech mannerisms and use of "wrong words." The mother, too, impressed all the workers who were in touch with her as being dull, yet her dullness also turned out to be a "pseudo" rather than a true dullness. We learned that when she was a child her father had lovingly called her "dumme Liese." As a child the mother had been unable to learn and had been sent to a school for retarded children until it became obvious that she did not belong there. She had almost no education.

There were indications that she needed to have Yetta repeat some of her own experiences. The mother revealed that she herself had been exposed in her childhood to excessive sexual stimulation and had been seduced; and like Yetta, she had been a bed-wetter until she was 10 years old.

The mother claimed that she had very much wanted Yetta. She thought the child was very beautiful and described her as "that wonderful thing that came out of my belly." Later she had fantasies that Yetta would become a "ravishing film star." The child was often photographed, and the mother even managed to attract the attention of journalists to the child. These fantasies appear to reflect the positive side of her ambivalence toward the child. Feelings reflecting the negative side were inherent in many of the mother's worries during Yetta's childhood, for example, that Yetta might suffer from a road accident; in her conflicting wishes about the girl's achievements and future; and others mentioned previously.

It would seem that the underlying motive of the mother's conflicts about Yetta, and especially of the negative side of her ambivalent feelings, was her unconscious need to see her daughter as an extension of the "dumme Liese" image of herself as dull, dirty, and enuretic. Apparently, Yetta unconsciously responded to this image by assuming a psuedobackward style of functioning.

Yetta's analytic material showed that her learning inhibition had several determinants. She had difficulty in history and geography, subjects affected by her preoccupation with the circumstances of her birth and the whereabouts of her father.

The therapist saw Yetta's main problem to be her self-devaluation. She reported: "Yetta feels that nothing can go right for her, and no one was more surprised than she when she won the school prize for improvement. . . . She celebrated the occasion by having an accident in the school playground and hurting her nose. When her improvement in language, history and geography was not matched by her maths results, she felt quite sure that she could never expect that, it would be too much to hope."

Yetta brought her therapist newspaper cuttings of herself. Among them were a number of photographs of herself as a young child in fancy dress in which she had won prizes or competitions. She said that her mother had loved to dress her up. In a whisper she added, "I hated those fancy dress competitions. I wanted to be just me, not all dressed up."

The fact that Yetta had no father was seen as an important reason for her low self-esteem. She hated her name, which was her mother's maiden name. Her mother's ambivalence toward her was seen as another major factor in Yetta's devaluation of herself. The mother's conflicting ideals for her daughter—on the one hand, a fantasy ideal of a film star and, on the other, an unconscious "negative" ideal of a "dumme Liese"—each affected the child. The former presented her with aspirations she felt unwilling or unable to attain (she wanted to be "ordinary"), while the latter contributed to her need to assume the role of a stupid child.

Conflicts clustering around the problem of her self image, the question of paternity, and her ambivalence toward her mother affected Yetta's thinking and learning, and these factors were more significant than the more usual developmental conflicts.

The origins of Yetta's ambivalence toward her mother must have been multiple—the early separations, the lack of a father, and her mother's dullness. The ambivalence showed itself in her conflict over being like her mother or surpassing her. Yetta's identification with her mother's speech, indeed her "backward" mode of functioning, was probably due to her attempts to find a solution for her ambivalent feelings toward her mother. These efforts would have conformed to her mother's unconscious need to have a child as "dull" as she was herself.

CASE 3

Jeremy, who was referred to the Clinic at the age of 6, grew up, like Yetta, in an atmosphere of secrecy. In his case the secret concerned his older brother who was afflicted with mongolism and lived in an institution.

At the beginning of treatment Jeremy presented a picture of real retardation. He lisped, dripped mucus from his nose, could not dress himself or tie his shoelaces. From infancy he drooled continuously and extensively and required medication for lips and chin. His spasticlike hands could barely grasp small objects; his fine motor control was limited. The boy spoke so badly that at one stage his parents had been concerned that he might be "tongue tied" and need corrective surgery. At the start of his analysis his speech was slurred, there was some initial stuttering, and he was difficult to understand. The father was particularly concerned that Jeremy might be limited in intelligence. School reports were not particularly critical, yet Jeremy showed no evidence of readiness to read or write.

At the age of 6, his IQ on the Binet (Form L) was 108, but it was thought to be an underestimate by both the psychologist and the child's analyst. His parents described him as a slow developer. Jeremy started to walk with help as early as 9 months, but could not walk freely for another year. He started to talk late, but when his speech developed at the age of 3, it was fluent and precocious in form and content. Of greater significance, however, was the parents' treatment of Jeremy as a suspected defective. His play was restricted and he was prevented from mixing with other children. He was never expected to meet any age-appropriate demands; for example, at the age of 7 he still stood passively, expecting and demanding of his mother to dress him, comb his hair, wash his hands, wipe his nose, and clean his bottom. The mother felt he was incapable of doing any of these things for himself.

Jeremy disclaimed responsibility for bowel movements, which in fact were most carefully controlled by him; he was late in achieving bladder control; he remained a soiler until the last phase of treatment, when he was 10½. At referral, Jeremy showed massive inhibitions in ego functioning.

The mother had told Jeremy's therapist that she had only wanted one child, preferably a girl, who could be as close to her as she herself had been to her own mother. The first child, a daughter, seemed to have been much loved. However, Mrs. A. did have a second child—the mongoloid boy mentioned above. Jeremy was born shortly after the unexpected death of the maternal grandmother. Mrs. A. was profoundly depressed and suffered from recurring obsessive thoughts that she had killed her mother. She felt impelled to have another child to make retribution for the mongoloid boy, and Jeremy was born two years later.

The pregnancy with Jeremy was normal, though the mother reported that she had been troubled by transient depressive moods. She claimed that she intensely wanted and eagerly awaited the birth and that she did not worry whether the baby might be abnormal. Jeremy was born three weeks prematurely; the delivery was easy. However, from the beginning the baby impressed the mother as somewhat odd or abnormal because of his poorly developed eyelashes and diminutive fingernails.

Mrs. A. had suffered from tuberculosis and was unable to breast-feed any of her children. Jeremy took to the bottle well. Semisolids were introduced at 4 to 6 months and the bottle was given up at age 2, reportedly without difficulty.

Jeremy was always cared for by nannies and au-pair girls, but the mother could not allow any other woman to become close to him. In fact, she selected girls who were soon bound to leave. Jeremy was not supposed to mind the loss of au-pairs or the absence of his parents. The parents themselves denied the importance of separations. For example, when Jeremy was 18 months old, he was sent to the country with a nanny. Mrs. A. instructed this nanny to start Jeremy's toilet training during their absence from home. He began urinating in the pot at age 2 and was dry at night when he was 3, but continued to soil. The mother herself tried to train him, alternating between angry demands and permissiveness. Later she abandoned the attempts to force him because he became furiously upset and she hoped that he would "eventually assume responsibility" when he was ready. Between the age of 5 and 6 he began to be constipated. During treatment the extent of the mother's unconscious collusion with Jeremy's soiling became apparent.

Jeremy's father always thought of his son as a stranger who was better left to his wife's care. He was rather obsessional in personal cleanliness and during Jeremy's treatment it became apparent that he bitterly resented his son's drooling, wetting, and soiling—so much so that he involuntarily shuddered if Jeremy approached him. In fact, the father had very limited emotional contact with his son. He was away from the family frequently.

From Jeremy's birth onward the parents continually looked for evidence of damage. On the father's side of the family, there was a history of mental illness. The birth of the mongoloid son reinforced fears of hereditary defect for which the father felt responsible. He looked at Jeremy's odd development with anxious trepidation, and found his worst fears confirmed by Jeremy's behavior. The mother, intensely guilty about her "abandoned" mongoloid son, had a distorted view of Jeremy, and thereby encouraged his passivity. Her fear of being "unkind" to Jeremy was so great that she failed to appreciate his pleasure in mastering tasks, achieving control, and becoming independent. She could hardly believe, for example, that he might want to walk to school on his own, or wash and dress himself. At the time of referral Jeremy seemed to have developed in ways that realized his parents' worst fears; he seemed hopelessly effeminate, infantile, and intellectually defective.

Jeremy's therapist had the impression that the mother could not tolerate a masculine child and that her permissiveness with regard to the boy's anality masked her aversion to phallic sexuality. In his infancy she dressed Jeremy as a girl; she still bought him petticoats at the age of 3; she provided him with a dollhouse he did not want. She was terrified by Jeremy's temper tantrums and tried to avoid them by giving in to his wishes at almost any cost. Signs of aggression in Jeremy aroused her fears that he might become a criminal. Yet, at the age of 7, Jeremy's aggression was anything but age-adequate in expression, quality, or quantity. He had outbreaks of rage when frustrated at home, but otherwise he was pathetically passive and restricted.

Jeremy was not supposed to know about his mongoloid brother, who was never mentioned by the parents. However, during treatment there was ample evidence of fantasies about this brother and of Jeremy's identification with him. He frequently presented himself as a stupid, defective, clumsy, neglected child who, in fantasy, was ultimately sent away and killed.

Secrets and mysteries were recurrent themes in his treatment. The connection between his soiling and the secret surrounding his brother became clear. More and more often, a reference by the therapist to Jeremy's soiling or to his fear of rejection, would be followed first by resistance, then by material about mysteries and secrets. Sexual curiosity was perceived as dangerous by Jeremy, who clearly showed his fear of looking at, or knowing about, forbidden things.

At the start of treatment, Jeremy's self-esteem was depressingly low. He considered his body as bad (smelly) and not functioning properly (it could not retain feces). He felt he could neither do nor learn anything. This view of himself accurately reflected his parents' view—that he was a child who needed to be constantly looked after and handled physically, yet who remained distressingly distasteful.

During treatment Jeremy's fear of failure and its consequences began to emerge in his accounts of John, his other self, a boy who was afraid to try, because if he failed, he would be punished by being sent away and destroyed. This explained why Jeremy did not allow himself to try anything until he was certain of a high degree of competence.

In addition to seeing himself as a passive, dependent, soiling child, Jeremy perceived himself as tyrannical, violently aggressive, and omnipotent. He felt isolated and ignored by his parents and peers. He retreated into self-isolated fantasies or regressive anal gratifications via toilet and body care. During analysis he revealed that he both feared and wished to be his parents' defective child.

His work improved considerably in the course of analysis. At the end of treatment Jeremy showed an ability to undertake hobbies, to master games requiring concentration and competition, and to learn new skills. All this confirmed that his tested IQ had, indeed, been an underestimate.

The parents' intense guilt over the conception and subsequent abandonment of the mongoloid son heavily impinged on Jeremy's development from the start. The ongoing fears that he, too, would become abnormal had a later counterpart in Jeremy's fear of failing and being sent away or destroyed. However, there were other factors which also affected the mother's feelings about this son. Originally, she had not wanted another child, and particularly not a boy. Jeremy was conceived to help her cope with her guilt feelings about the death of her own mother and about the birth and abandonment of the mongoloid child.

The mother's negative attitude to Jeremy's masculinity, coupled with her preoccupation with the question of his normality, entered into her tolerance for his soiling and his general incompetence. Jeremy complied with her unconscious demand that he remain a passive baby. Her handling of him conveyed to him her image of an inadequate child. The father's ambivalent attitude to Jeremy reinforced rather than counteracted this image. Apart from these impingements, the mother's physical illness and depressed states during Jeremy's infancy interfered with the early mother-child relationship. To a large extent she was an emotionally unavailable object. In addition, the departure of his first nanny (who left suddenly two months after returning with him from the country) interrupted an intense relationship with a mother substitute. The subsequent coming and going of au-pair girls repeatedly undermined any stability of relationships he may have experienced.

CASE 4

Clement's referral to the Hampstead Clinic, when he was 10 years old, was instigated by his headmaster. Clement worried excessively about his work; although he seemed to be trying his best, his scholastic achievements were rather poor. His parents alternated between the view that Clement was mentally retarded and the view that he was "morally retarded" and did not apply himself sufficiently to his work.

The father had had a previous marriage which was dissolved after only a few months. The parents wanted to avoid repeating such a mistake and waited several years before they married. Clement was a planned and much wanted baby, but there were problems from the beginning.

Both parents were emotionally unprepared for the care of their first baby. They were totally unsupported by relatives, since Clement was born abroad in an American hospital. Already at birth he did not fit in with his parents' prearranged plans. Mrs. C. showed signs of preeclamptic toxemia toward the end of pregnancy and birth was induced. Breast feeding, too, presented difficulties and had to be supplemented. Clement had colic during the first three months, cried a lot, and both parents resented the disturbed nights. The mother felt tired and depressed and found it difficult to cope with the baby, especially when the family had to move six weeks after Clement's birth. Although a proper sleeping pattern was soon established, Clement continued to be a poor feeder. The mother expressed guilt about having forced him to eat; she had always worried he was not getting enough. Now she regretted that she "had not done what one does with animals; let them eat and leave what they want."

While the mother-child interaction during the first year established a significant pattern for later development and was characterized by the mother's disappointment in her "inadequate" baby and the baby's apparent noncompliance with his mother's expectations, the major pathogenic influences in Clement's life occurred in his second and early in his third year.

Except for a brief separation from mother at 6 months, when the parents went on a holiday, and at 16 months when the mother went to the hospital for her second confinement, the mother always looked after Clement herself.

Clement's toilet training was described as "a great struggle." Although it was started in Clement's first year, he did not become toilet trained until he was $3\frac{1}{2}$ years old. In fact, he gained bladder control at more or less the same time as his younger brother, but continued to wet his bed intermittently until 9. Irrespective of the accuracy of the developmental history, there is ample evidence in the analytic material relating to the effects of the tremendous battle with mother over toilet training.

The problem of gaining bladder control was undoubtedly increased by the fact that Clement developed phimosis. The mother had constant difficulty in retracting the foreskin, a circumstance which must have caused considerable discomfort to Clement and involved extensive examinations and manipulations of his penis. Eventually he was circumcised at the insistence of the family doctor, but afterward the mother wondered whether the operation had been necessary. Although she stayed with him in the hospital, Clement is said to have reacted with great distress to the treatment.

These experiences, colored by unresolved anal conflicts, may even have led to a premature entry into the phallic phase, and certainly contributed to the intensity of his castration anxiety. The combination of sexual stimulation, pain, and attack on the penis shaped the form of the subsequent phallic and oedipal conflicts.

Following the operation Clement experienced his mother as even more omnipotent, rejecting, and now also as castrating; and the mother, too, probably now saw her "inadequate" son as even "more damaged." There is ample confirmation from the analytic material that the experiences surrounding the circumcision constituted a major sexual trauma for Clement. The excessive handling of his penis, both exciting and painful, mobilized a massive aggressive response at a time when he already felt rejected by his mother because of the arrival of the new baby. The operation, and especially the anesthetic, was experienced as an assault by his mother on him and his body.

At first, Clement's revengeful hostility found expression in messy and destructive bevahior, but this was met by his parents with severe reprimands and physical punishment, which carried the threat of total abandonment and loss of love for Clement. The rigid standards held up by his parents eventually became internalized and acquired enormous reinforcements from aggressive and sadistic instinctual sources. This punitive, harsh, and sadistic superego largely contributed to Clement's unhappiness and his inhibited and restricted functioning.

When Clement was 16 months his brother was born. He was in

the care of his grandparents for 12 days and, although on this occasion he showed signs of distress over the separation, according to the parents there were no signs of jealousy afterward. Much stress was laid on the good relationship between the brothers and by parents and teachers, but the analytic material certainly did not bear this out. Clement's deep-seated hate and envy of his brother was an ever-recurring theme in the analysis and was only thinly disguised at the beginning. In part this was a displacement of his hostility and anger toward his mother for having produced this child and for ostensibly favoring the baby.

The parents described the younger brother as an altogether more satisfactory, bigger, and easier baby; and comparisons must have been made from the earliest time. Physically, the boys were soon of the same size and, as the baby was always developmentally advanced while Clement's development began to lag during his second year, the parents commented that they often thought of their two sons as twins. Clement walked only when he was about 2 years old, while his brother did so when he was just over 1; and in this way the developmental gap gradually narrowed. Clement's speech development was so retarded that his younger brother was said to have talked first. This delayed speech development may well have been linked with the enormous aggression he was trying to contain. Speech certainly became in due course an "aggressivized" activity. In analysis some of his most guilt-ridden material was "unspeakable" and had to be brought in writing. His speech was always difficult to understand, it was slurred, and it was often inaudible.

The younger brother quickly became more successful in almost every area, and especially in his scholastic achievements. While Clement attacked other children as rivals, or provoked their attacks on himself, his brother made friends wherever he went—thus confirming Clement's idea that his brother was better loved by everyone. The unfavorable comparisons with the brother became an integral part of Clement's life. They not only increased, and kept alive, his hostility and murderous wishes; they had a devastating effect on his self-esteem. He felt that his brother was not only better loved but also superior in every respect.

Clement started school when he was 5 and had four changes of school in the next four years. From the beginning he was unhappy and unsettled and his progress was slow. This was usually attributed to his difficulty in adjusting to the many changes. However, his scholastic achievements remained poor. At the time of referral he was in a form *below* that of his younger brother. Yet, tested on the WISC, he had a verbal IQ of 131 and a performance IQ of 91.

Both parents were irritated by Clement's lack of interests and disparagingly referred to him as "bored and boring." Although the mother was well aware of her disappointment in him, she felt guilty about her irritation, boredom, and impatience with him. There is some evidence to suggest that these attitudes in the mother stemmed from her own unconscious conflicts around penis envy.

Clement clearly experienced his mother as a seducer and attacker, both aspects being reflected in many of their interactions. His highly ambivalent relationship to her not only was based on his need to repeat the early sexual trauma, but also was a way of contacting her, getting close to her, and trying to get her undivided attention. Symbolically, he appeared to relinquish possession of his penis to her; unconsciously, the mother appeared to demand and respond to this. Throughout Clement's development, even during the analysis, the mother appeared to seize every opportunity "to handle" his body. As she was a trained nurse before her marriage, she could readily rationalize these interactions.

In spite of an open preference for the brother, the father, at times, showed sympathy with Clement on the basis of an identification with him as a solitary, withdrawn, and depressed person. As the more compliant partner in the marriage, he at first left the care and upbringing of the children to his wife. He was unable to give her adequate support and help. In later years he began to play the role of martinet; in accordance with his wife's wishes, he became the strict and punitive father who put all the emphasis on discipline. Thus, for Clement, father reinforced mother's rejecting and denigrating attitudes, and failed to provide a satisfactory object for masculine identification.

At the beginning of treatment Clement was a severely inhibited and very depressed boy. His frail appearance, his awkward movements, his inability to communicate, and his initial anxious overcompliance all added to the picture of severe impairment of functioning. The diagnostic assessment raised the question whether he was organically damaged. In spite of his good intellectual potential, indicated by the result of the intelligence test, Clement presented a picture of slow and delayed development from earliest childhood.

It is likely that the mother's disappointment in her baby, based in part on unrealistic expectations about birth and the mothering role, affected her handling of her firstborn. These early experiences probably interfered with the baby's feeling of omnipotence. Furthermore, the experiences surrounding the birth of his brother and the traumatic circumcision caused such severe narcissistic depletion that development henceforth was interfered with by his lowered self-esteem and highly ambivalent object relationships. Clement's aggression, which may at first have been largely reactive, became intolerable and conflictual in the face of his later experiences of retaliation and threatened abandonment by his mother. This forced him into a role of passive submission toward the mother on the basis of a sadomasochistic interaction with her and was at the root of his deep-seated conviction of being unloved, inferior, stupid, damaged, evil, and unlovable. The complete lack of understanding of his difficulties and dilemmas of that time led his parents to react to manifestations of disturbance and stress, which emanated from feelings of rejection and low valuation, in a manner which reinforced them. In the end he completely identified with his parents' disparaging picture of him.

Clement's learning problem was intimately linked with this devalued self image and his inability to compete with his brother; but he also had a problem with concentration. The latter was linked more directly with his sexual problems, his fight against masturbation, and the intrusiveness of his sadomasochistic fantasies. These conflicts were in turn condemned by the superego and thus secondarily contributed further to his devalued and denigrated self image.

Discussion

It is apparent that none of these four children grew up in an environment conducive to healthy development. Their social backgrounds differed, but there were some common and striking features in their emotional backgrounds, most notably their mothers' attitude toward them. This attitude, whether overtly or covertly conveyed, was highly ambivalent on the part of all four (indeed, all seven) mothers and it contained a striking need to denigrate the child. Moreover, this attitude appeared to be prevalent from birth onward and, as far as could be ascertained, in some cases was already present during the pregnancy. It may also be significant that three of the children were firstborn babies (six out of seven in the original sample); one, Jeremy, followed the birth of a mongoloid brother.

One can infer that these mothers' fantasies about and expectations of their babies affected their mothering role from the very beginning. Several of the mothers had a fantasy that they would produce a damaged child. Yetta's parents were not married, and the father deserted the mother during the pregnancy. Jeremy was born three weeks prematurely, and his mother thought that his faint eyelashes and thin fingernails were evidence of mental abnormality. Clement's mother had definite, inflexible expectations of her baby and found him wanting right from the start when he arrived a few days too early and there were slight complications at delivery.

These mothers perceived their children from earliest infancy as damaged or inadequate. With the exception of Jeremy (who was not breast-fed), there were difficulties in feeding. None of the three mothers enjoyed breast feeding and none felt that her baby enjoyed it. All three mothers felt that their crying and dissatisfied babies rejected them and made too many demands on them.

Almost from the beginning the mothers' concern about the physical growth of their babies was matched by their fears about their children's limited intelligence. Although there was no real cause for such anxieties insofar as the early development of the children did not appear significantly deviant, these mothers seized on any unusual aspect in their children in a derogatory and damaging manner. The degree to which maternal attitudes influence the actual developmental processes is, of course, open to speculation. In all our cases the early development was somewhat slow. One may question how far this reinforced the mother's idea that her child was backward, and how far these developmental lags were responses to maternal attitudes and expectations. It is likely that there was a mutual interplay between the two factors in that lack of pleasure and pride in their babies and inadequate maternal stimulation and encouragement may have exacerbated whatever initial difficulties the babies may have had.

It is important to note that the denigrating maternal attitudes centered on only one child and did not extend to the other siblings. In every case in which there were siblings the mothers compared the "denigrated" child unfavorably with them and often showed overt preference for the siblings. This was more prominent in the original sample of seven cases, where Yetta was the only child without siblings. Although we have relatively little information about the fathers' attitudes to these children, the fathers tended to share and reinforce the mothers' negative attitudes rather than to counteract them. Yetta, of course, never met her father; Jeremy's and Jane's fathers were frequently away from home because of their professions. In fact, none of the fathers seemed to have actively participated in the care and early upbringing of their children.

Some insight into the origin of such ambivalent and denigrating maternal attitudes could be gained from the analyses of two of these mothers. Their pathology centered around a severely devalued self image and the conviction that they were incapable of achieving or producing anything good. It is likely that the attainment of motherhood mobilized conflicts and intensified their anxieties.

In our small sample of cases we can discern a pattern: the mother assigns a specific role to her child, who is perceived as a not-quite-good-enough baby, an inadequate and damaged product. While three of the mothers almost constantly looked for evidence to confirm signs of damage in the children, Yetta's mother strenuously tried to defend against this by denial and reaction formation. There was little evidence of overt guilt in these mothers about having damaged their children. Rather, they used the children as a vehicle to rid themselves of unwanted aspects of their self images. The role assigned to the child might be viewed as an externalization of those aspects of the mother's denigrated self that she wanted, defensively, to disown. Another important factor may have been the mother's need to perpetuate, in the relationship to that one child, the denigration she herself had experienced from her own mother.

The children we studied appeared to have been unusually compliant in accepting the role allotted to them by their mothers. We assume that this compliance was motivated by a wish to preserve a sense of safety and retain the mother's involvement on whatever basis of mutual interaction existed. In the absence of positive emotional involvement by the fathers, this probably was the only way out for these children.

The analyses of these four children revealed that their main pathology centered around a severely devalued self image and depleted self-esteem. The other presenting symptoms can be viewed as attempts to adapt to this basic problem. Jeremy was encopretic; Yetta and Jane were enuretic; and Clement remained enuretic well into latency. All four children were described as solitary, sad, and unhappy. Their tendency to cling to early body pleasures (soiling, wetting, masturbating) can in part be understood as an attempt to find some pleasure and satisfaction, but this inevitably perpetuated their low self-esteem.

While the functioning of all the children substantially improved with treatment, considerable vulnerability in the area of self-confidence and self-esteem remained. This was least in evidence in Jane, the youngest child in our sample. This suggests that the analysis of the sources and influences of a devalued self image may have greater success in changing the self representation if the denigrated role has not yet been fully taken over by the superego. One could also assume that all four children benefited from some by-product of analysis, such as experiencing the therapist as a new object valuing the child and offering alternative and more beneficial identificatory ideals. Moreover, in their contacts with the Clinic, the mothers' attitudes were sufficiently modified so that they could allow their children to progress. They did not appear, however, to have been profoundly changed, and this seemed to have been true even of the two mothers who were analyzed.

In her study of mothers of children with intellectual inhibitions, Hellman (1954) stated that "the mothers' capacity to understand their children was confined to certain areas only, areas in which the child played the role unconsciously assigned to him. . . . To keep the child passive and stupid was a necessity for these mothers" (p. 266). It was linked up, as Hellman illustrates, with the mothers' need to deny the impact of their secrets on their children.

Two of our children grew up with the burden of family secrets. Yetta had to cope with the secret of her paternity as well as with her own secret, sexual experiences with the lodger. But even her secrets were not the only, or even main, cause of her distorted personality development. Nor was the secret in Jeremy's family (the existence of a mongoloid brother) the only reason for his "backwardness." The secrets played, of course, a part in Yetta's and Jeremy's inhibitions of curiosity and therefore in their inability to learn, but they formed only one aspect of the generally pathological attitudes shown toward these children. And there were, to our knowledge, no special secrets in any of the other cases.

Our findings are in agreement with those of Hellman insofar as the mothers in our study also needed to keep their children passive and stupid. However, we found that this need arose from deeper-seated motives than a need to preserve a secret. The fact that they saw in their children undesirable aspects of their own selves seemed to us to be crucial. For some of the mothers, their "damaged" children represented their "castratedness" or stupidity; for others, their entire despised self images.

That such impositions of parts of their own self representations upon their children can be carried out by fathers as well as mothers is illustrated by Sprince's case, a boy whose pseudostupidity "was based on a conviction that his father viewed him as part of himself" (1967, p. 106). Underlying this conviction there was a history of sexual play between the father and the child.

In her study of 17 cases of intellectual retardation, Nancy Staver (1953) hypothesizes that in each case the mother had some unconscious need for the child not to learn. She found that some of the mothers themselves had intellectual inhibitions and appeared to encourage their children, whom they identified as parts of themselves, to develop such inhibitions. In at least one of our cases (Yetta), intellectual inhibition was both the mother's and the child's way of adapting to reality.

In researches based on simultaneous psychotherapies of mothers and their children, Johnson and Szurek (1952) described the impact of unconscious parental expectations on the pathology of their children. They observed a specific superego defect in the child which was "a duplication of a similar distortion in the organization of a parent's own personality" (p. 342).

Berta Bornstein (1930) and Ilse Hellman (1954) discuss the link between difficulties experienced in the oral phase and intellectual inhibitions. The equation of oral intake and the intake of knowledge was recognized as far back as the writings of Abraham (1927), Fenichel (1937), Glover (1925), and Strachey (1930). Subsequently many analysts stressed the role of oral fixation in reading difficulties and the link between conflicts over oral aggression and such difficulties (M. Klein, 1931; Blanchard, 1946; E. Klein, 1949; Pearson, 1952). The tendency of these and other contemporary authors is to stress multiple causation of learning difficulties rather than to connect them only with oral conflicts.

Among the children of our study, three (Jane, Yetta, Clement) had early feeding problems of one kind or another. Of the three, only Yetta had difficulty in learning to read (Jane's analysis may have forestalled the emergence of such a difficulty). Even in Yetta's case, however, it was the *generally* disturbed mother-child relationship which had repercussions on the child's development and learning rather than just the feeding aspect of the relationship.

Summary

In the four cases we have described, as well as in the remaining three that were studied, the inhibitions of ego functions were far-reaching. We have defined their pseudobackwardness descriptively, taking as a point of departure the parents' or educators' view of the child. We found, however, that the child's presenting himself in this way was due to his unconscious compliance with the image imposed on him by his mother. To be sure, all the children had neurotic conflicts, but it was not the magnitude of their conflicts which accounted for their generally "backward" way of functioning. We assume that quite early in their development these children adapted to their mothers' perception of them, in order to ensure their mothers' cathexis and to preserve feelings of safety. In that sense these children may be said to have developed as distorted personalities rather than as neurotically disturbed children.

BIBLIOGRAPHY

ABRAHAM, K. (1927), The Influence of Oral Erotism on Character-Formation. *Selected Papers.* London: Hogarth Press, pp. 393–406.
BLANCHARD, P. (1946), Psychoanalytic Contributions to the Problems of Reading Disabilities. *This Annual,* 2:163–187.
BORNSTEIN, B. (1930), Zur Psychogenese der Pseudodebilität. *Int. Z. Psychoanal.,* 16:378–399.
BUXBAUM, E. (1964), The Parents' Role in the Etiology of Learning Disabilities. *This Annual,* 19:421–447.
FENICHEL, O. (1937), The Scopophilic Instinct and Identification. *Int. J. Psycho-Anal.,* 18:6–34.
GLOVER, E. (1925), Notes on Oral Character Formation. *Int. J. Psycho-Anal.,* 12:131–154.
HELLMAN, I. (1954), Some Observations on Mothers of Children with Intellectual Inhibitions. *This Annual,* 9:259–273.
JOHNSON, A. M. & SZUREK, S. A. (1952), The Genesis of Antisocial Acting Out in Children and Adults. *Psychoanal. Quart.,* 21:323–343.
JONES, E. (1910), Simulated Foolishness in Hysteria. *Papers on Psycho-Analysis.* London: Ballière, Tindall & Cox, 1st ed., 1913, pp. 141–153.
KLEIN, E. (1949), Psychoanalytic Aspects of School Problems. *This Annual,* 3/4:369–390.
KLEIN, M. (1931), A Contribution to the Theory of Intellectual Inhibition. *Int. J. Psycho-Anal.,* 12:206–218.
LANDAUER, K. (1929), Zur psychosexuellen Genese der Dummheit. *Z. Sexualwiss.,* 16:12–22, 87–96.
MAHLER, M. S. (1942), Pseudo-Imbecility. *Psychoanal. Quart.,* 11:149–164.
OBERNDORF, C. P. (1939), The Feeling of Stupidity. *Int. J. Psycho-Anal.,* 20:443–451.
PEARSON, G. H. J. (1952), A Survey of Learning Difficulties in Children. *This Annual,* 7:322–386.
SPRINCE, M. P. (1967), The Psychoanalytic Handling of Pseudo Stupidity and Grossly Abnormal Behavior in a Highly Intelligent Boy. In: *The Child Analyst at Work,* ed. E. R. Geleerd. New York: Int. Univ. Press, pp. 85–114.
STAVER, N. (1953), The Child's Learning Difficulty As Related to the Emotional Problems of the Mother. *Amer. J. Orthopsychiat.,* 23:131–141.
STRACHEY, J. (1930), Some Unconscious Factors in Reading. *Int. J. Psycho-Anal.,* 11:322–331.

"Hysterical Materialization" in the Analysis of a Latency Girl

ROBERT EVANS, M.D.

FERENCZI (1919) PROPOSED THE TERM "MATERIALIZATION" FOR CERtain hysterical phenomena which intrigued him because they implied a capacity for "a decided increase of innervation, which the normal neuro-psychic apparatus is incapable of manifesting," in contrast to the paralyses, anaesthesias, and paraesthesias, which are characterized by "interrupting or disturbing the normal afference of sensory and efference of motor innervation as regards consciousness" (p. 91).

Directing his attention to the alimentary tract, Ferenczi chose for special study such phenomena as globus hystericus and certain forms of constipation. He noted a case of globus described by Bernheim, in which palpation disclosed an actul tumor projecting in the area of the oesophagus, but, when oesophagotomy was

---

A revised version of a paper presented at the Wednesday Meeting of the Hampstead Child-Therapy Clinic, London, July 24, 1974. This work was supported, in part, by a grant from the Foundation for Research in Psychoanalysis.

Dr. Evans, who was at the Hampstead Child-Therapy Course and Clinic, London, is now at the Yale Child Study Center, New Haven; the Child Guidance Clinic of Southeastern Connecticut, New London; the Juvenile Court for the State of Connecticut, New Haven; and High Meadows, Hamden, Connecticut.

Owing to special circumstances, I wish to acknowledge my great indebtedness to two supervisors, Dr. Max Goldblatt and Mrs. Hanna Kennedy, who supervised different phases of this analysis.

performed, "no malformation existed at this level" (Ferenczi, 1923, p. 105). In one of his own cases, Ferenczi (1919) analyzed a peculiar constipation from which a male patient suffered from time to time. The analysis indicated that this patient was compelled to "materialize" an unconscious homosexual fantasy by molding a "faecal penis" in his rectum on occasions when he particularly wanted to make a determined stand against some consciously hated male opponent (p. 94f.).

> When in a case of globus hystericus the unconscious wish for fellatio causes a lump in the throat, when in real or imaginary pregnancy the hysteric makes a 'stomach-child' out of the contents and wall of the stomach, when the unconscious homosexual moulds the rectum and its contents to a body of definite size and shape, we are dealing with processes that do not correspond in nature with any of the 'faulty perceptions' known to us. We cannot call them hallucinations. . . . Neither can we speak here of an illusion in the sense hitherto customary. . . . The subject of an illusion is passive, while on the other hand the hysteric himself creates the stimulus, to which he can then give an illusory misinterpretation. . . . It might be called a *materialization phenomenon,* since its essence consists in the realization of a wish, as though by magic, out of the material in the body at its disposal and—even if in primitive fashion—by a plastic representation, just as an artist moulds the material of his conception or as the occultists imagine the 'apport' or the 'materialization' of objects at the mere wish of a medium [p. 95f.].

Ferenczi (1919) believed that the ideas implicit in his term shed light also on the organic basis of artistic endowment. "Hysteria is, as Freud says, a caricature of art. Hysterical 'materializations,' however, show us the organism in its entire plasticity, indeed in its preparedness for art." He wondered whether one might not consider the symptomatic "autoplastic tricks" of the hysteric to be prototypes not only for the performances of actors still making use of the body, but also "for the work of those creative artists who no longer manipulate their own bodies but material from the external world" (p. 104).

I was struck by the peculiar appositeness of Ferenczi's term, and of the ideas implied in it, to the material brought by a little girl who was in analysis with me from age 8 to 10. In presenting her case, I shall focus on the "materialization" phenomena, and, by including the exchanges between us in considerable detail, I hope to convey not only a description of the phenomena themselves but also some idea of the way we used them in the analysis.

Case Presentation

THE DIAGNOSTIC PICTURE

Claire came to the Clinic with multiple complaints centering on dramatic tantrums that I understood to be essentially "hysterical." Yet I hesitated to stress the hysterical elements, because of Anna Freud's (1965) warning that, in diagnosing childhood pathology, we should not overemphasize the links between infantile and adult neurosis or assume that a particular type of infantile neurosis will prove to be a forerunner of the same type in adulthood. Nevertheless, the material seemed to fall together convincingly under that broad heading. Furthermore, now that the analysis is over, I venture to assert that Zetzel (1968) would have considered Claire to be a "good" hysteric, as a little girl anyway, whatever the future may hold for her. Certainly she met the criteria of the verse that introduces Zetzel's paper: when Claire was good, she was very, very good; and when she was bad, one was well advised to step very softly indeed.

Claire grew up in a close and stable family with enduring values and a gift for enjoying mutually shared pleasures and support. Her parents were well-to-do, cultivated, and intelligent, with wide-ranging interests that embraced politics, art, music, literature, and travel.

Her father, a quiet, gentle man of 40, was in the diplomatic service. Sometimes he seemed to be a bit overwhelmed by his five children, and occasionally he gave the impression of being retiring and diffident. But this was deceptive: in reality, his highly structured personality had a core of resolute determination in all matters save one, and his easygoing, warm ways with his children did not interfere with his coming across to them as a solid, dependable, and enduring support.

Claire's mother was a lively, ebullient, and intelligent woman of

35, who had given up a promising career of her own when she got married, and had since, except for the demanding round of entertaining required by her husband's career, devoted all of her time to her children, managing skillfully their complicated school programs and their formidable series of private lessons in music, dancing, swimming, sailing, and riding. She was high-strung, and her voice tended to become penetrating and strident when she was coping alone; but when she was with her husband, tension and anxiety subsided, and the note of managerial agitation was relinquished in favor of a warm and reciprocal partnership. Their marriage appeared to be very stable.

Claire had three beautiful, talented, and socially gifted sisters. At the time of assessment Alison was 14, Jennifer was 12, and Susan was 10. Claire, at 8, was fast losing her ability to adapt to their custom of bossing her about, as well as her tolerance toward her paragon of a brother, Richard, who, at 6, was already a football hero, an intellectual giant, and a social lion.

Although she was undoubtedly the cleverest of the lot, Claire did not believe it for a moment, and she exhausted herself and her family with her intense competitiveness and her inexorable perfectionism, which, predictably, never allowed her to achieve results that pleased her. At the piano, for example, her considerable talent was spoiled because, in her frenzy to play as well as Alison, she would slam down the lid in a fury at the slightest mistake. For a few years, she had managed her problems with Richard by "appersonating" him as a kind of twin, teaching him, bossing him about, and sharing his baths and his room. But this arrangement was fast coming to an end as Richard struck out for himself into a new school world and declared himself to be no longer available for Claire's ideas of an ideal relationship.

These upheavals took place in a big, rambling house with a large garden. It was a child-oriented house, pleasantly chaotic and noisy, swarming with the children, their friends, and a large staff of cooks, housekeepers, nannies, maids, and gardeners. The parents were at the disposal of the children, and were generally overpermissive in matters of sexual and aggressive expression. They could not bring themselves, for example, to moderate the open masturbation of the girls or their "game" of delivering passionate "movie kisses" to anybody within reach, especially their father. The mother was incredibly patient with aggressive and demanding outbursts, especially from Claire, with whom she was strongly identified. Nevertheless, there were expectations, and the children were imbued with such standards as honesty, fairness, and consideration toward others.

Although there were warning signals, Claire's earliest experiences did not prepare her parents for the dramatic upheavals of her eighth year. She began as a happy chubby baby, with no complications except for constipation, which commenced at 3 months when she was changed from breast to bottle. This problem, which was expected to be a transient one, proved to be stubbornly persistent so that laxatives twice a week became routine.

Otherwise life was good to her, her sisters mothered her delightedly, and she was generally a contented toddler, the center of everybody's attention, until Richard was born when she was 17 months old. The sisters dropped her instantly in favor of the baby, and she was provided with a new nanny, who also quickly showed an obvious preference for Richard. Claire's screams shook the rafters when the nanny tried to feed her, and her mother had to take charge. She devoted a great deal of attention to Claire from then on, making a point, she hoped, of not allowing her to feel displaced by Richard.

But Claire was not to be altogether appeased by these gestures, and, by the time she was 3, she was making no secret of her wish to take Richard's penis away and put it on herself. Shortly after her fourth birthday, following a case of measles, it was discovered that she was near-sighted, and eyeglasses were prescribed. As with the constipation, there was something peculiar about this symptom which went beyond its organic basis. Claire frequently discarded her glasses and was thought of as being only moderately near-sighted. Yet her mother had to be careful not to embarrass her by calling attention to a friend approaching across the road, since, even with the glasses on, Claire could not distinguish objects at such a distance.

During this period, Claire apparently was working out her "twinship" arrangements for coping with her feelings about Richard. She called him "my Dickie," ordered him about, and was generally content when he was with her. Her nursery school teacher described her as "popular, well-balanced, cheerful, active, intelligent, dependable, and of a sweet disposition." There were a few rumblings of somatic outlets in the form of bouts of tonsillitis and skin allergy, but the complaints that brought her to the Clinic really did not concern her parents greatly until they began to burgeon over the course of the year following her seventh birthday.

That autumn Claire was sent to the junior school. Richard remained in the infants school, and she was not allowed to visit him. She began to lose weight and became quite thin. She could not go to sleep at night and constantly kept leaving her room to come down to her parents. She developed a large repertoire of physical ailments, such as stomachaches, headaches, joint pains, upper respiratory problems and the like, which led to extensive medical examinations of all kinds, including head X rays. By the time she came to the Clinic, Claire's family thought of her as a hypochondriac who loved to take medicines and retire to her bed with her drawings and books, holding court there whenever she could attract an audience. They referred to her as Elizabeth Barrett Browning.

Claire had managed to miss about a third of her last term in school by these maneuvers, but when she got to school she worked very hard, achieved good results, and so impressed her teachers that they found it difficult to believe that she had a serious problem. Claire had two ways of coping at school. One was evidently to exert rigid controls. The other was her ability to elicit special support from her fat, gentle teacher who was putty in her hands. Claire had to give her effusive kisses on coming and going, to the considerable annoyance of her mother, who had also to listen to endless paeans of praise to this lady at home. The mother was sorely tried by another school ritual: the instant she reached the gate, Claire greeted her with a formidable tantrum. Her mother was especially sensitive to being observed in such circumstances, and she was so embarrassed that she devised a temporary remedy: she contrived to have a sweet ready in her hand, and, the moment Claire opened her mouth to howl, she would pop it in.

At home Claire became increasingly tense and irritable, and, by the time of the assessment, she virtually ruled the household with dramatic tantrums and retreats to her bed. Whenever she became aware of the slightest flicker of inattention during one of her lengthy narrations, for example, screaming ensued and objects began to fly. Endless complaints that her siblings, especially her brother, were picking on her made every mealtime a nightmare, and it was to be expected that at some point she would leave the table and withdraw to her room to nurse her wounded dignity. In the intervals between tantrums, she was cloying in her fulsome praise of her mother. "You are the very best, the kindest mother in the whole world," she would say. A moment later some slight from Richard or some deficiency in herself would be blamed on this kindest of mothers and Claire would fly into a raging tantrum.

Claire was enchanting to look at, with dark hair, great blue eyes gazing out with a sweet and open expression behind the spectacles, and a winning smile. Having heard the history, I was prepared for a rather seductive approach, but she was more subtle than that. Her gestures and her general manner were pleasingly feminine, and she was gentle and considerate in her attitude, but her mind was on the pressing concerns of her daily life and she clearly wanted help. She spoke eagerly, if a bit shyly, throughout both hours of the assessment, talked frankly about her worries, and brought an abundance of material about her relationship to her family, her nanny, and her teacher; about her fears and weaknesses; and about her ambitions and her hopes for the future.

Claire made two significant complaints that had not been mentioned by her parents: boredom and sensitivity to perceptual impingement. Both concerned school. As an example of the boredom, she cited a recent discussion of the Rosetta stone. She was terribly interested when the teacher told the class about it, but then came the children's part of the job, to write down the complete story. As soon as she sat down to write, she said, she became preoccupied with the thought that she would never finish and that was when the boredom began: she would find it very difficult to set down the story because she always began to think of other things that she would rather be doing. The other problem concerned her reaction to the loud voice of her male French teacher. He had a marked accent and she did not always understand him very well when he talked English anyway. But he was also given to shouting and that was the worry: she considered him to be a nice man and knew that he would never hurt her, but when he shouted, his loud voice startled her terribly.

My enthusiasm for working with this charming and articulate little patient was enhanced when she came in the next week to hear the result of the diagnostic conference and to make final arrangements for the analysis which was to begin in the autumn, following the imminent summer holiday. After we had discussed everything, Claire drew a pool of water with five elegant penguins standing about. One was poised at the edge of the pool, and she explained that he just wanted to look all around before he plunged right in.

THE COURSE OF THE ANALYSIS

A few months later this lovely little girl was snarling her way through every hour, arrogantly domineering, swearing like a fishwife, issuing bossy orders, and cutting off every sentence I tried to utter with a peremptory "Shut up!" "Oh God," she would say, "I can tell you're about to start one of your boring lectures again. Do come off it." Her characteristic response to an interpretation was to take it as the starting point for an argument or for a tirade of denigrating scorn. Her attitude toward time was typical. One day, when she had arrived in the consulting room early, she said crisply, "Don't look at your watch—I don't care what time it is. When I get here first and you come in second, you're late!"

It hardly sounds like an ideal atmosphere for doing analytic work, and yet Claire did eminently good work and slowly developed a first-rate treatment alliance. Her inquiring mind was at work from the beginning, assessing what she could expect of me and what uses she could put me to. Even in her stormiest periods she rarely lost sight of her goals for very long. Reflecting on a holiday she said, "One of the things I hate about your being American is that you might go back before I have finished with you—you are very useful to have around except when you talk garbage." As time went on, she even allowed me to know about an improvement: the partial analysis of her inhibition at the piano had enabled her to give an excellent performance at her lesson, and she said of the change, "What do you think I come here for? To get my problems solved, of course."

The material unfolded in an orderly manner, the conflicts with their typical defensive stances being experienced with varying intensity at various stages. Low self-esteem, longing and envy, including penis envy, appeared first and continued. Anal material was more heavily defended and did not achieve full expression until well into the second year, at which time superego pressures and her masturbation conflict became especially severe.

Both positive and negative oedipal modes entered the transference from time to time, but they were muted, and were quickly submerged in phallic and prephallic concerns. Although this oedipal avoidance was rooted in very early experiences, there were convincing indications of a powerful contributory stream deriving from later traumatic visual experiences, attributable to primal scene encounters or other encounters with an erect penis. It seemed clear that the higher level manifestations would not be analyzable until there had been a full opportunity for the assimilation of insights into self-esteem regulation on phallic and prephallic levels. This indeed proved to be true: oedipal strivings with a new mood of reciprocity and "give-and-take" attitudes did not fully emerge until the last three months of the analysis.

THE "MATERIALIZATION" PHENOMENA

Claire was an articulate child, with a highly developed capacity for putting thoughts, wishes, fantasies, and conflicts into words. She brought many direct verbal statements of problems, with pleas for help, as well as abundant material in the form of dreams, stories, opinions, and observations. But her verbalizations were characteristically supplemented by graphic modes, which took the form of drawings and, for long periods of time, of enactments and other phenomena which I have called, following Ferenczi, "materializations."

These modes were typically dramatic, were often artistic, and were always imbued with emotion and absorbed concentration. Claire seemed to breathe life into an enactment or a creation so that the thought, the fantasy, the wish, or the conflict did indeed appear to "materialize" before one's eyes. Although she often accompanied these expressions with verbal associations, it was as if she could not achieve a full assertion with words alone, and one often felt, as Ferenczi noted, that one was in touch with the organic basis of art in the making, as she manipulated her body and its contents or material representing them in her creations. In addition, the dramatic modes were frequently used as the first approach to material of which she was not fully conscious, and, characteristically, they became the first steps in working through material, whether or not it had been previously approached.

I shall give a few examples that appeared in the context of longing, of envy, and of traumatic visual experience, and then go on to the long phase, spanning more than six months, during which, as the resistance to the emergence of anal material subsided, Claire regained access to the derivatives of this plastic medium and exploited them to the full.

Early in the analysis, when Claire was struggling with envy of my other patients, and especially of a little boy whom she had inadvertently seen with me, she brought in her costume for a school play which she had written and in which she was to play the part of a little French lad. She began to remove her clothes in order to give me a demonstration. As she pulled off her blouse, she said severely, "This is not a sexy show, you know." I replied that it looked rather like one and wondered whether she might want to pull a big chair away from the wall and use it for her dressing room. She did so and, after careful preparations, came out in vivid red trousers and a bright green shirt. Totally without self-consciousness, she removed her eyeglasses and stood before me with graceful impudence, one hand on her hip—the very incarnation of her current fantasy. I wondered about the magic wish involved and she grew impatient. She said that the transformation took place because she had taken off her eyeglasses—glasses made you look more like a girl. Obviously I was not playing the part assigned to me and, unwisely persevering, I had every sentence chopped to bits. "I really am quite fed up with you, you know," she said. "You bore me and besides I have an awful cold."

A few months later Claire had been able to tolerate a few interpretations of penis envy, but she was still smarting under their impact, and she came in to tell me that she was going to be in another play, only she did not intend to talk about it because I would only say that it was connected with robber dreams and willy problems. But she talked about it anyway: she was going to take the part of a 19-year-old boy who, in collaboration with a man and a woman of 30, has planned to kidnap a little boy and his sister. First they rob all the jewels from the children's mother and then the plan goes wrong—they are obliged to kill the children.

The following day Claire collapsed on the couch with her thumb in her mouth, saying that she was very tired. But she had brought in a large bag containing her costume, and she soon jumped up and prepared her dressing room behind the chair. When she came out she looked uncannily like a little boy. Dissatisfied with my response, she brought out an Indian breechcloth that she had been working on. She stripped off her pullover and vest as well as the shorts she was wearing, and soon was standing naked except for her pants. I said that she seemed to want me to see her without any clothes. She replied that I was talking nonsense again.

As she tried to fit the breechcloth, Claire became more and more awkward and seemed to have lost all ability to visualize the problem in design involved. I thought that often happened when she was having willy problems—when she thought of having no willy, she became "stupid," believing that willies were what caused people to be bright. Totally absorbed and not deigning to reply, Claire carefully glued a large cardboard knife to the front of her breechcloth.

Many months later, already deeply involved in the work with the plastic "anal medium" to be described, Claire added another dimension to her preoccupation with willies, an aspect that partook of Greenacre's (1953) concept of "penis awe" and moved through various facets of her conflict, including a strong implication of traumatic visual experience.

One day I was sitting in my chair, with my feet up, reading, when Claire arrived. She stood in the doorway taking in the spectacle, and her mouth fell open in what looked like astonishment. As she gazed at me, the astonishment subtly changed to awe, and the awe to fear—a wide-eyed, staring, fearful look came over her face. After what seemed to be an interminable time, she closed her mouth, folded her arms, and, leaning against the doorpost, continued to gaze at me. I said, "Do come in," and she ignored me.

Claire opened her little purse and took out a handkerchief which she threw over her eyes for a moment. Then I noticed that, along with the handkerchief, had come a tiny Japanese parasol. She examined it for a full five minutes, holding it a couple of inches in front of her eyes, turning it this way and that. Finally she opened it, twirled it a bit, closed it, and put it back in her purse. She took out next a "chap lipstick," applied it to her lips, afterward returning it.

Suddenly she began to move the zipper of her purse back and forth, running it more and more rapidly. Claire got out the little umbrella once again and repeated the whole process. Then she began to do games with her fingers, twining them in and out, reversing them, and folding one arm around the other. She conveyed an impression of profound self-involvement, and then managed a contortion in which just one finger stuck out which she wiggled.

The last part of the hour was devoted to drumming various tattoos on the doorpost, after which she looked at the clock on the mantel, squinting mightily. Finally she came all the way in, going up to peer at the clock from a distance of a few inches. She gave me an intent look and walked out. Not a word was spoken.

Claire's second year in analysis followed a massive disintegration of behavior during the summer holiday, in the course of which she had reverted to her old methods of coping at home, to the distress of her family who had begun to enjoy her considerable improvement. She came in with formidable tics, the most impressive one consisting in a peculiar, sudden throwing back of her head, her eyes rolled up into her skull so that only the whites showed. It gave an odd impression: it was quite involuntary, and at times almost continuous, but it also conveyed a message, seeming somehow to say, "Oh God, I'm with that stupid ass again—it's more than can be borne." (The words I have used to try to capture the flavor of this distressing symptom are quoted from some of her actual comments made in various contexts.) The other tics were ghastly nasal, grunting, snuffling sounds which went on constantly when she was doing close work, interrupted at intervals by the eye gesture. She left her eyeglasses off for some weeks, and, when she addressed herself to a list or a drawing, her nose almost touched the page—it seemed impossible that she could see what she was doing.

Her anxiety mounted and Claire began to stuff into her mouth and noisily to chew enormous quantities of liquorice in a manner that could only be described as disgusting. "Me first," she said, snatching a cup of water from my hand and gulping it down greedily as I was about to pour it onto her neglected plant. "Stubborn, isn't it?" she added, when she noticed that the plant did not absorb the water very readily.

As the days passed, Claire literally "became" the desperate little girl, frantically begging to be loved and cared for in spite of a firm conviction of being unlovable, a state of mind which she actualized by making herself truly as disgusting as she imagined herself to be. After an interpretation of her guilt feelings, the tics grew less obvious and finally disappeared altogether, to be replaced by provocative nastiness and sharp kicks to the shins, administered under the table where we sat across from one another.

One day Claire came in rather cheerfully, but thunder was just around the corner. She began to spatter a piece of drawing paper with drops of ink from a new pen, a gift from her mother. Glancing through a case full of pencils and pens that she had brought with her, she said darkly, "*She's* pretty well equipped." It turned out that she was taking care of the case for her sister, Susan, who had gone shopping with mummy. When I said that she felt left out, she screamed that she hated shopping anyway, and began to kick me. But for the first time she allowed my meaning to sink in when I said that she was treating me just like mummy. It was a turning point in the analysis, and the anal material broke through.

Claire began to do dashing pictures of fireworks. She would viciously scribble on a piece of paper with crayons, producing a large Guy Fawkes fire with rockets and Catherine wheels and sparklers bursting all around. Then she would dip a large brush in black paint and furiously paint over the entire surface. As she did so, the fireworks emerged with stunning effect because the wax crayon marks did not hold the paint. They were to be "invisible" until the black paint was applied and she made them "go off" with enormous explosions, gazing in the air to admire their effect. It was impossible not to "believe" in them.

Claire developed a new technique; she held a brush over her shoulder and then brought it down with a smart flick of her wrist, causing the paint to splatter on the paper. It was fascinating to observe the mixture of impulse with the control that literally forced her to turn the splattering paint into an interesting design, and I compared it with the paintings of Jackson Pollock. Claire said that he must be a very *young* painter if he did work like that. When I said that she certainly was fascinated with all kinds of explosions, including the explosive words that she used all the time, she said, her voice trembling with disgust, "Wees and poos and shut up!"

In the following week Claire experimented with "turning things into other things." She asked for a candle and began melting crayons into a paper cup. She was totally preoccupied with this "filling of the pot" and seemed to be almost oblivious of my presence. Yet I was supposed to be there—very much so—and, from time to time, she emerged to engage me. Occasionally she turned out all the lights to test out whether she could find me in the dark—it was very scary, she said, rather like those awful ghost feelings that came to her at night. Within a few days her cup was full, and she was immensely proud of the huge new "supercrayon" that she had made out of the little ones. She had to bring her mother into the room to admire it and was terribly disappointed when she got only a perfunctory and indifferent comment.

Claire plunged back into her experiments and the theme moved to the next logical connection—stinks. She talked about how intrigued she was with investigations, especially investigations into how things turned into other things. As she burned plasticine in the candle flame, a ghastly odor permeated every corner of the room. Who would ever dream, she said, that the smelly bit had once been a piece of plasticine? Immediately she popped a biscuit into her mouth and I wondered whether she had never asked that question about food—what happened to food after she ate it? Practicing her brand of pseudostupidity she said that food, of course, turned to crumbs. I said that it did not, and she knew it; food turned to B.M. "Why can't you say the word right out?" said Claire.

The next week Claire allowed me to make some links. When she resumed her preoccupied melting of crayons, I spoke of how a very little child sometimes became so interested in his poos that he did not even need to talk to people—he could just talk to his poos. When she turned the lights out, I spoke of the fears of the little child that important objects might go down the toilet—like being lost in the dark. She even allowed me to link her arrogant orders with the "poo power" that the little one gets as he sits on the pot. She said that I was exactly like Hitler—mad—and she glared at me furiously when I said, "Do you mean potty?"

A week later Claire found her true medium—melted candle wax—and the most intense period of the materializations began. She started on the object which was to become an anal baby, then to metamorphose into a breast and a phallus, until it finally represented the entire analytic process. She dripped candle wax onto a piece of drawing paper until the entire surface was covered. As the wax cooled, she added more and an object began to take shape. It was a real mess, but it was a "something."

She had been in bed for three days with a cold, Claire said. Her nose was terribly stuffed, but she could not be bothered to blow it. She added to the theme of constipation by managing to clog up the sink with a piece of burning paper that she had anxiously quenched there, but when I called her attention to the connection, she said loftily that she could not imagine how I could suppose that poo matters could possibly apply to a 9-year-old.

As Claire melted her wax, however, she admitted a thought or two: "There *was* a time when I had trouble in the loo. My nanny took me in and we had to give up because it didn't want to come out. So I went to bed and we had to wait till the next day or the day after that until it was ready." She continued her work and, as she spilled a bit of wax from time to time, she would say, "Oh God—it went just where I didn't want it to."

As Christmas was approaching, Claire sang as she worked, "Go tell it on the mountain, that Jesus Christ is born today." Other December birthdays intruded into her thoughts—Alison's, her father's, that of her beloved hero, Jimmy Osmond. She cut herself off. "Why am I talking about birthdays?" she said impatiently. "What does it all mean?" She gazed at the wax object and said dotingly, "I wonder what I should call it. I just can't think of a name." She talked of a book she was writing about a fabulous boy called Jimmy. He began as Richard, she said, but she changed the name. She told of Jimmy's incredible character, of his possessions and skills. He was also very much in love with a girl whom he met at school through a game called the "kiss chase" in which the girl chased him, caught him, grabbed him around the neck and kissed him.

A week later Claire flew into the room brash and loud, calling me a silly old cow. I said that I had been thinking about her wax object and about her experiments and I thought that I might have a clue. She was suspicious, but she ordered me to go on. I said that little girls were terribly curious about what made mummy's tummy swell up and they wondered constantly about how babies were made. If they were in the poo period, they often thought that a baby came out like poo. I really thought that wax thing might be a sort of poo baby. Claire shrieked her disbelief and called me a silly old cow again. I thought that the silly old cow must be mummy. Long ago, when Richard was born, Claire must have been very impressed by the way everybody was going "ooh" and "ah" over the new baby. Probably she felt neglected and thought that the new baby was taking her place. She denounced everything I said, arguing about each point, but insisting impatiently that I go on.

The following day, as Claire was taking the poo baby out of her locker, she handled it carelessly and it dropped to the floor. She moaned and said that she would have to repair all that damage now. She was very impatient; intending to bang her hand down on the table with a great crash, she managed to hit the poo baby right in the middle. She decided to repair the damage by cutting off a piece of the edge. (It made no sense from the technical angle; it would have been much simpler to repair the injury with melted wax.) I said that she was really *after* that thing: she dropped it, she hit it, and now she was cutting off a piece. She screamed at me. I said that she was really not that angry with me—I wasn't the silly old cow. The anger was coming from that far-off time when mummy brought the baby back—she wanted to hurt it and take something from it as well. Claire snarled at me to shut up. I said that I really did not think she fully understood how angry she had been. Nowadays she talked about her lovely, darling mummy and talked baby talk to her. But I thought she must have been terribly angry when she saw mummy getting fat and bringing that baby in—she wanted to crawl into mummy's lap and be a baby herself. Claire howled.

By the next day Claire's mood had changed. She stood on a chair to get out the poo baby and handed it to me gently, asking me to take it to the table. A day later she was waiting at the top of the stairs for me and she said in a gentle and wistful tone, "Did you expect me to be standing there?" She was receptive to my comments as she industriously continued her melting. I thought that a little girl of 17 months must have had quite a hard time trying to get used to a new baby. We knew some of her thoughts, but we had not really looked sufficiently into how she must have longed to make a baby herself. She was kissing, licking, and nibbling a large biscuit as she worked, and I wondered if the little girl had not decided that it was something mummy ate. Possibly she ate and ate herself and then was disappointed that all she got was poos. Claire said, "Well, I can have a baby at about 18." I replied that of course this was true, but a tiny girl did not believe that for a moment—she just felt small and worthless. She looked very thoughtful and said, "You know, this is the very first time that I have *really* listened to you."

The following week was the last before Christmas. On the Thursday Claire came in with a large bag of sweets; staring into the flame as she melted her wax and reaching out from time to time, without ever turning her head, she stuffed a soft cream cake into her mouth. It was the most intensely concentrated mood of the poo series, and the wax object grew steadily as she added layer after layer to create a mound in the center. I turned my head to look at it and she said, "Don't tell me it looks like a bloody baby!" It actually looked quite like a puppy at the moment and I said so. Claire grew interested and said brightly, "It really does look good, doesn't it? It's a good thing we kept it up after that time it dropped to the floor." She took my hand in both of hers when she told me good-bye, saying warmly, "You know, I really *am* sorry we are stopping today."

Claire came back saying that the fortnight's holiday had seemed to her like "a million weeks away from Hampstead." She got out the wax object, lighted up her candle, and started to work. There were days of intense, ambitious application, alternating with others on which she made helpless and irritable appeals for me to make things "right."

One day Claire came in complaining about some stupid men teachers and I noticed a sign on her forehead that displayed the letters SFBSKG. It meant School for Beautiful, Smart, Kind Girls and was prophetic of storms to come.

Claire grew excited about a new baby boy born to her old nanny, Martha, whose breasts had become so big that mummy had to take her on a "bra hunt" to search for a garment that would accommodate them. She added to the bulk of the wax object, noting with satisfaction that it was getting heavier and heavier. When it was finally finished, she said, and weighed about a ton, she would take it down to show it to her mother. But afterward she intended to bring it back to the consulting room because only there could she be sure that it would not be broken.

Claire became concerned about her nasty, bossy attitude and said that she did wish she could control it—those horrid things just seemed to pop out against her will. To my vast relief she did bring some control and the kicks under the table ceased altogether. She dashed off an impressive autograph and tried to outline the letters "Claire" by dripping wax on them, managing to produce a mess. As she discarded it she spoke sadly of Inky, her old lost puppy, who had been sent away because he barked too much—it wasn't fair because he really couldn't help it. When she ruined another autograph, I said that she thought of herself as a messy, smelly poo baby. She began to feel sorry for me because she was convinced that I was bored with her and had to sit there anyway. The wax object began to look like a breast.

The next day I made one of those interventions whose implications had not been thought through with any conscious plan in mind, but which turned out to have far-reaching effects. There were a number of such happenings during my work with Claire—she seemed to evoke them—and she characteristically experienced the incident, whatever it was, as an interpretation and incorporated it into her work. On this occasion, her candle gave out; when I looked into the storage locker, I discovered that I had no splendid phallic replacement such as she was accustomed to use. I hesitated to offer her the only one left: it was a hideous candle in the shape of a hamburger which had been sent to me as a joke from America. It was repulsively realistic, with layers of meat, cheese and roll molded in vividly colored wax. I thought that it would be intrusive, but it seemed preferable to interrupting the work and I handed it over.

Claire was enchanted. She gave the hamburger a great kiss and lighted it up, whimpering apprehensively when she spilled a bit of wax in the process of adding to the big wax object. The following day she accidentally dropped a bit of debris into the hollow formed by the melting wax and tears came to her eyes. I said that she was very fond of that hamburger and was sorry to hurt it. She called me a cow, but she listened carefully as I talked about how dirty and smelly she felt when she thought that everybody had dropped her when Richard was born. It had not been so bad when she had had control of Richard, but now he was nasty and teased her and refused to do what she said. Suddenly she looked up at the clock on the mantel, a good ten feet away, and said, "Does that say 5 minutes past 5?" I wondered if her problems with her eyes could, in part, have something to do with her feelings, and she thought that I was taunting her.

The next week Claire flew in, again brash, loud, and bossy, reversing roles and trying to trick me into revealing "secrets." The layers of the hamburger came apart and she irritably commanded me to fix them together again, saying in a superior way, "Please don't look so high and mighty." But she was still working and once she flung out, "How could I possibly want a poo baby—wouldn't it be rather dirty?" The big wax object was subtly changing shape again—it began to look like a phallus.

A week later Claire arrived in a formidably nasty mood—the "shut ups" and the epithets were continuous. I irritated her enormously, she said, with that horrid grin on my face. She melted some wax onto her construction and then moved on to charcoal, discarding piece after piece as no good. I said that I had noticed that about her: she was always pleased with a new piece of equipment and then it became useless. She set a piece of paper alight and became frightened, screaming as she threw it into the sink. How she envied two girls she had met, she said, because of their analysts. Both analysts were very young and they were not stupid, but best of all they were female. On the next day there occurred the silent hour that I have described, when she came into the room to discover me with my feet up.

A day later Claire grew impatient because the candle that she was using (not the hamburger) had burned down in such a way that the wick could not get sufficient oxygen. I suggested that it might be smothering and would probably burn better if she took off a bit of the wax. She grabbed a knife and began to hack away at it viciously, looking at me balefully and saying, "It's mine; I can destroy it if I want to."

The following week Claire continued to add to the big wax object, now unequivocally phallic, but most of her attention went to the hamburger candle. It had such a large surface area that the burning wick had made a deep hole right down through the middle and this distressed Claire terribly. She had been so careful with it, she said, she simply could not understand how it had happened. I said she was afraid she had injured it. That was ridiculous, she said, why had it happened? I told her I believed that it was due to the shape of the hamburger and not to something she had done to it. Why didn't I get a proper candle in the first place, she asked. I said, in that case, it wouldn't have been a hamburger at all. Claire laughed, saying that the United States certainly produced the stupidest people in the world, except the Osmonds. For the rest of the week she worked away assiduously at the hamburger candle. She bored holes into the various layers and inserted new wicks. She took the layers apart and tried to make new candles out of them, constantly seeking my help.

She had decided to tell me something, Claire said: she kept a problem book at home in which she had written down her chief worries and she wanted me to see it. The first problem was the disagreeable habits that she got because of me; she did not know exactly how it happened, but she was sure it was because of me, like the eye thing (the tic)—she did not have that before she knew me. The second problem was how tired she felt in the morning, and the third was how she kept putting off her homework. She wrote the problems down and then got to thinking about how she could work with me better; so she decided to show them to me.

Claire started the next week with more work on the hamburger candle and then returned to the big wax object, melting wax on it as she talked. Before the end of the week it had begun to represent the entire analytic process. She was wearing a large medallion bearing the legend "Truro Agent," a secret organization of girls that she could not discuss with me, she said. The knob came off her locker and, as she tried to refit it, she became furious with me because the threads would not catch. She hurled the screwdriver across the room and took out the big wax object. Turning suddenly, she let it slip through her fingers and it dropped to the floor, a big piece of the edge breaking off. She was distraught, shrieking for me to help her and refusing to allow me to do so. It was very important, she screamed, and it was my fault—I should have caught it.

Claire spent three days making repairs and, by Friday, she was talking about how pleased she was with the result; she was really rather glad that she had broken it because she was so proud of the repairs. I said I knew she was proud of the repairs, but I thought she was still disappointed that it needed repairs at all, however good they were; after all, the wax thing was very important to her. She said that it certainly was; all of her thoughts went right into that thing.

I said that I had been thinking a lot about her problem book, and it did seem to fit together with the broken wax thing and her feeling that she had damaged something that was precious to her. Could that not be because of the "habits" that she was so worried about? After a bit of repudiation Claire admitted that she worried a lot about having injured herself by masturbation and that she did indeed believe that it made her crazy. With great relief she talked about it in detail, all the while boring more holes and inserting new wicks in the remnants of her hamburger candle. When she finished, she asked me to shut the curtains because she hoped that lighting up the wicks would create a bit of cheer in this room and make everything light and lovely. I thought she was saying that what we had been trying to understand made her feel embarrassed, and perhaps sad and depressed, and that she wanted some bright lights and longed for the day when those problems would be understood and over with. Claire heaved a great sigh and said that I was quite right. When the many wicks were lighted, she looked up wistfully and asked me if I liked the effect. I thought perhaps she felt so guilty and ashamed because of the habits and other things that she really thought she was not lovable anymore and was asking me if it was so. She nodded shyly.

The next week Claire moved further into this conflict and added some others. First she produced some "fingers" by dripping candle wax onto her forefinger, letting it dry and then slipping it off; it was supposed, while the wax was on, to feel like an injured finger in plaster. Gradually she extended the process to her whole hand, and when she removed the coating, there materialized a "hand" that was both eerie and ghastly. It was remarkably lifelike (or perhaps one should say deathlike), conveying the impression of some horrible plague, bulging and pitted as it was from the solidification of the drops of greenish-blue, red, and white wax. As if to make sure that the conflict "got into" her analysis, she also, from time to time, held her hand over the big wax object so that the excess dripping from her fingers would fall onto it and become a part of it. She slipped into and out of a sort of "narcissistic trance" as she worked, occasionally flinching in pain as the hot wax dripped onto her skin.

The hands encompassed many meanings. There were two versions: the unmitigated "successes," which pleased her enormously, had the thumbs rigidly extended; the "failures" had the thumbs closed modestly alongside the fingers. She left a "success" prominently displayed in her mother's kitchen after showing it to her father and evoking dismay and revulsion. She then organized a sort of Lilliputian "women's lib" movement, trying to enlist three girls whom she had met in the waiting room. They were indeed entranced with the hands; and when they tried out the technique and found the wax too hot for their own skins, Claire undertook to create hands for them in her sessions, presenting to each one a splendid specimen. The SFBSKG organization—the relatively gentle School for Beautiful, Smart, Kind Girls—passing through the intermediate stage of the more militant Truro Society, had become a fiercely warlike band of Amazonian man-haters, at least in *her* fantasy. As she saw it, when she needed a man, the tribe was to descend upon the unfortunate victim and hold him down, struggling but helpless, while she delivered her kisses.

But Claire left a pathway open. One day she inadvertently created a "failure" and asked me if I did not agree that it was unattractive. I said it looked like the others to me except for the position of the thumb. "Well," said Claire, "I don't like it. Do you want it? If you don't, I'm going to throw it away." When I reminded her that she had been breaking wind and complaining of the stink and probably wanted to know whether I was willing to see *her* thrown away, she marched back to her locker and tossed the "failure" carelessly in. A day later she allowed me to talk about her terrible guilt feelings about the masturbation and responded by relating some sadomasochistic fantasies. She said that I was embarrassing her terribly. I thought that was a pity because she would then be tempted to use the embarrassment to convince herself that I was punishing her for what she felt so guilty about. Suddenly she took off her glasses and noted the time on the clock.

Claire began the next week in a nasty, man-hating mood, but she allowed me to interpret the acting out as her wish to be the better mother, equipping her friends with willies. By Thursday she had stopped making hands and was eagerly seeking links as she returned to her big wax object. When I called her attention to how she had thrown the "failure" indifferently into her locker after offering it to me, and was now endangering it by carelessly piling a lot of things on it, she said that it was a failure after all, and she didn't care. I thought she *did* care—that was the one she secretly wanted to be admired. She sniffed disdainfully as I rescued the hand and put it in the storage locker for safekeeping. Still struggling a day or so later, she said, "How tall are you, for God's sake? Six feet? You are a boring old man." But she acknowledged her desperate wish for help in controlling her masturbation and, when I said that she wanted her mummy to stop her, she replied, "Well, the right person *could* stop me!" She became more and more depressed and spent the entire next week in bed. Her parents noticed her low spirits and thought that she was feeling guilty because she had appropriated her sister's friend.

When Claire returned, her mood was very different. She wanted me to forget all of her nastiness and she participated fully in the work, bringing explanatory fantasies that she had worked out for herself at home. She had been thinking about willies, she said, and had decided that, in the olden times, both boys and girls had them. But the boys were nasty and took away the girls' willies. No, they didn't like the girls better without willies—they just took them away to be nasty. As she talked, she added more wax to the big construction, which by that time had taken on a monstrous phallic shape. She wanted it to be as big as the room, she said. The following week was the last before the Easter holiday and, looking at her materialization carefully, she agreed with me that it was indeed beginning to look more and more like a giant willy.

TERMINATION: THE LAST THREE MONTHS

Claire returned from the Easter holiday in a mood of warm reciprocity, and I heard not one single "shut up" from that day onward. The big wax construction came to the table every day, and she always added a few drops of wax to it at some point during the hour, but she was no longer obsessed with it. Her mind was on other things.

Claire brought with her an enormous stuffed panda called Dumpy, a gift from her sister Alison. I had seen him once, briefly, right after the Christmas holiday when he was without a name, and Claire had said then that if I was very good, she might name him Robert. However, Dumpy was short for Dumpling, and she had decided that it better expressed her tenderness for the endearing creature.

Dumpy was dressed in Claire's clothes and he came to her sessions almost every day, the exceptions being occasions when he was sick. At the end of every hour she always turned to him to ask if he was ready to go and, from time to time, she caught him up in her arms to give him a big kiss. It was important that I appreciated the beguiling ways and the accomplishments of this child of ours. Claire constantly invited me to share in her doting affection for him as she felt under his pinafore to determine whether she ought to change his nappies; or as she held him by both arms with his feet on the floor and showed me, bursting with pride, that he had learned to walk. Claire had become a mother.

I had been looking for an opportunity to introduce the notion of my leaving at the end of the term, but I was unable to do more than plant a seed on the first attempt. Claire had been surprised that I sent her a postcard from London instead of from America during the holiday, and I wondered whether she had not thought that I might go back some day. Immediately she began to paint a Union Jack and I said that she was telling me that I ought to be an

Englishman. Of course I wouldn't go back, she said; I would have to stay in England to help sick children because that was my job. She grew silent, looked at the clock, and recited a bit of doggerel: "All was silent, and nothing could be heard except the ticking of the clock. Until Claire interrupted the silence by saying, 'All was silent, and nothing could be heard except the ticking of the clock.' Until Claire interrupted the silence by saying 'All was silent. . . .' " She smiled and I said that she seemed to be arranging matters so that everything would be the same forever and ever.

The next week, stimulated by a casual remark of her mother's, Claire gave me an opening to discuss the termination directly and, during the rest of the term, she participated fully in discussions of the best course for her to follow—whether she ought to continue with another analyst or to try out handling things on her own. She decided on the second alternative and she convinced me that she was right. I had helped her, she said, she was much happier, and she wanted to find out whether she could manage without me. Besides, she was very busy and, really, two years of missing one's favorite television programs was a long time. "Then," she added, "if I have more trouble, I can always ask to come back to another analyst, God help me."

I heard nothing to indicate that her plan was unsound. I became convinced that she was quite ready for a year or so of analysis-free latency. Furthermore, I really felt confident that she would ask for help in the future if she needed it. Her parents were in agreement. They were delighted with the changes in her attitudes, and they subtly altered their own approach: Claire no longer demanded the center of the stage at home, and they were no longer obliged to think up excuses to the other children for special concessions to her. She was quite able to hold her own with both her sisters and her brother without reverting to tantrums or somatic retreats.

Claire plunged back into her analysis with a will, well aware that she had unfinished work to do. She drew some steep mountains. "But they really aren't as steep as they look," she said. "If you just glanced at that picture, you would think that those mountains were impossibly steep. But when you get up close, they really aren't all that tall." I said I thought she was talking about willies. The first time she saw one she exaggerated its importance enormously, just like the mountain. Now that she could look at it better, it didn't seem all that marvelous after all—it's just the way a boy is made.

Later in the week, when the material clearly indicated a continuation of the same theme, Claire tried to brush aside an interpretation and than caught herself. "Oh, I guess we can talk about it," she said, "I've done all that work on it, I might as well finish the job." She had come across an old pad of graph paper, the cover of which displayed the Leonardo drawing of a naked male figure with arms and legs extended to show the proportions of the human body. When I gave it to her during the first months of analysis, she had been profoundly shocked and had quickly popped gummed labels over the "rude willy and bosoms." When she found it again, she said, "Oh, there's that picture! Leonardo da Vinci did that. We learned about it in school." I said that it no longer seemed to look so rude, and Claire pulled the labels off at once.

On another occasion Claire fell to thinking about death. She could not imagine anybody really being dead, because life goes on, after all. She liked the notion that people are born again as another person or as an animal or something like that. In considering her own rebirth she still wanted to be born a boy because she wanted to know how it would feel to smoke—women could not smoke because it was bad for the baby inside. I thought it was pretty well established that smoking was bad for anybody, but there surely was no more reason for a woman not to smoke than a man—after all, a woman was not pregnant all the time. I thought it was another example of her listing things that women could not do and men could. It might have been true in the olden times, but no more. Claire said thoughtfully that perhaps it was true—in the olden times there really would have been a reason for wanting to be a boy.

But Claire was a true daughter of her generation and compensatory ideas found their way into her approach to the avoided aspects of her oedipal conflict. She advanced toward it in a manner that was quite typical of her, and that fully confirmed the assumption that it was inaccessible to real mastery before the analysis of her self-esteem problems on phallic and prephallic levels had carried her a considerable distance.

On the day Dumpy learned to walk, I reminded Claire that long ago she had cooked me a fine roast beef dinner and afterward had taken very tender care of the baby doll. Perhaps, I said, she had in mind being my wife. "Oh, but you weren't married then," she replied. "You only got married early in 1973." Dumpy sat on the table between us and, from time to time, she kissed him and offered him chocolate.

Two weeks later a chance happening gave Claire an opportunity for further explorations in displacement. She was terribly upset because the mother of her best friend, Samantha Hargraves, had died the night before. Claire did not know Mr. Hargraves, who had been divorced for some years, and she thought that Samantha ought to go and live with her father. Claire had been thinking a lot about it and worrying about it and a thought had come to her mind: *I* was really Samantha's father and was just not admitting it—I hadn't liked the name Hargraves and so I took the name of my new wife which was Claire Evans.

I thought that her concern about Samantha was very special: Samantha was going to do something that she would really like to do, and it was a bit less scary to think about Samantha. I reminded Claire of the death thoughts about my wife some time ago and she grew quite sad and pensive. She thought I ought not to expect her to discuss it anymore; after all, if a grownup's best friend died, he wouldn't be expected to talk about it right away. I thought everybody needed a chance to talk about things like that. Claire said, "That's what grownups always tell children, but they really wouldn't do it themselves." She looked out of the window and suddenly drew back in terror as a large pigeon landed on the ledge. She said that it was his great eye staring at her that made her uneasy.

That pigeon was one of a host of birds that came to the ledge every day to receive Clair's bounty. Early in the term she constructed a bird feeder out of balsa wood. She actually had had the idea before the Easter holiday, she said, but then it did not seem to be the right time and she gave it up, but now she had come back to it and she felt that it was just the thing to do. When it was finished, she brought a bag of bread every day, broke it up lovingly, and put it on the ledge.

Claire waited patiently and meanwhile fell into the custom of reserving a piece which she toasted in her candle flame for herself, for me, and for our children—we lived in very olden times and she baked the bread at the log fire while I went into the forest to kill a deer for supper.

Finally the birds discovered this bountiful mother and they eventually grew sufficiently courageous to come to the ledge to eat while she stood delightedly watching them. It was indeed quite an experience to observe this greedy little "me first" girl taking such unselfconscious pleasure in her own nurturing impulse. She even came without Dumpy one day, saying that her sister Susan was in low spirits and that she had left him to cheer her up. Most pleasing of all was the fact that there was not a hint of a false note, not a trace of sentimentality.

One day Claire put a bit of extra bread on the ledge as she was leaving, saying that the birds might be coming back, after she had gone, to eat the rest of the feast—they wanted to celebrate the recovery of one of them who had been sick. I knew that the analysis was over.

Discussion

Ferenczi believed that his concept of materialization and the theory of development to which it led him shed light on the "mysterious leap" from mind to body in hysteria. Rangell (1959) thought it was an "intriguing phrase," but that it brought one no closer to solving the mystery. Besides, he rather felt that the mystery had been overemphasized with regard to conversion: "this leap, while mysterious, is no more mysterious than many another psychophysiologic or somatopsychic or even intrapsychic event" (p. 656).

Rangell argued against the exclusive association of conversion with hysteria. He proposed a conceptualization in which conversion would be regarded as a process that could occur "along the entire gamut of psychopathology, at any stage of libidinal or ego development. Though covering a wider range of phenomena than hitherto generally employed, the focus is still on the distorted use of physical or somatic innervation for the symbolic expression . . . of repressed psychic products" (p. 660).

Claire's material lends some support to this argument. It seems likely that she made use of a multi-determined anal symptom for symbolic expression of conflict long before one could appropriately speak of phallic dominance or of "hysterical organization." The tendency to constipation began during her first year, and her rigid adherence to rules and her perfectionistic strivings at the time of assessment suggested the existence of considerable anal fixation. In retrospect, it is plausible to assume that Claire used the conversion process in connection with varying drive organizations over a considerable period. By the time she came for assessment, however, there is no doubt that she had achieved phallic dominance and that the rigidity and perfectionism had been incorporated into phallic-narcissistic strivings. The eye symptoms, which intensified and declined during the course of the analysis, revealed clear evidence of roots in very early experiences, the residuals of which carried over with increasing intensity and changing meaning as phallic dominance proceeded.

As for the term materialization itself, it has seemed peculiarly felicitous to me in conveying a basic sense of an active process at work. In this case it was especially instructive to observe the slow transition, within the anal medium, from mess to "something" to unequivocal fecal baby, breast, and phallus, each phase, I thought, being convincingly representative of conflict which had been dealt with, at one time or another, by plastic molding of body products. In this sense it conveyed more than the term conversion, because it gave one an "organic feel" of the transitions from psychic to somatic and back again, and exposed the developmental aspects quite clearly. Perhaps materialization too should be separated out from its association with hysteria.

In any case, after working with Claire over a long period, I should not want to discard the term, even if the clarity of the material she brought, as I suspect, should prove to be quite rare. Materialization is probably an "old-fashioned" notion and its plastic connotations might be criticized as suggestive of a "product" rather than a process, not to mention the invitation inherent in a concrete and beguiling term to be less than thorough in seeking a full metapsychological understanding of symptomatology. Perhaps, with its implication of "a decided increase of innervation," it might be understood as a special instance of conversion.

Ferenczi broadened the meaning of his concept to embrace a wide range of phenomena, many of which were no longer immediately involved with bodily alterations. A number of the examples cited from Claire's analysis were materializations only in this extended sense. In both kinds of material—that which involved the body and that which did not—the essence of her experience was almost perfectly captured by the concept. It is difficult to convey the utterly convincing effect of Claire's contributions in this mode—the "suspension of disbelief" that she evoked as her inner reality found its way into whatever creative opportunity was at hand.

As a mode of communication, materializations like Claire's are not, of course, unique, nor do they differ fundamentally from the ways in which all children bring analytic material. As Ferenczi (1919) pointed out, many of the "expressional movements that accompany the emotions of the human mind—blushing, pallor, fainting, anxiety, laughter, crying, etc.—evidently 'represent' important happenings in the career of the individual and of humanity, and are therefore 'materializations' of a similar kind" (p. 96). What made Claire's materializations so enlightening to me was their quality of exposing process and means as well as content, together with the accompanying attitude of total involvement and commitment. She was indeed like an artist at work as well as being a serious analytic patient.

With regard to content, I would especially emphasize the clarity with which the components of Claire's low self-esteem emerged. Her transference manifestations were dominated throughout the analysis, up to its terminal phase, by experiences of shattered self-esteem, expressed first in terms of longing and then of envy, precursors of envy, and extensions of envy, to encompass an enormous range of attributes, qualities, advantages, and prerogatives.

Faced daily with the explosive manifestations of these aspects of envy, I often turned to Joffe's study (1969) for both enlightenment and reassurance. Joffe singled out envy as a clinically significant reaction to painful discrepancies between self and ideal self, differing, for example, from the depressive response. Joffe characterized the depressive response as being dominated by helplessness, hopelessness, and resignation, whereas, in the response of envy, hope is not lost and the "envious person's narcissism receives an increment from the *fantasy of one day possessing that which he does not have.*"

> If the envy response fails, we may get the development of one or other pathological reactions, of which one of the most important, from a clinical point of view, is depression. Other responses include psychosomatic disorders and paranoid states, but there is a whole spectrum of possibilities. On the other hand, envy may itself act as a spur to development, particularly when it is not associated with the need to destroy (in fact or in fantasy) the admired and idealized object. Here the balance between envy and the admiration to which it is so closely related is of crucial importance [p. 544].

It seemed to me that Claire might have sat for this portrait, with its manifold possibilities for hope and despair. Happily, she was one of those fortunate ones whose destructive impulses are counterbalanced by genuine warmth and tenderness. It was also no small matter that her natural gifts included beauty, intelligence, and artistic vision, and that she was blessed with a loving and supportive family, ready and eager to foster her growth. The alternative was therefore open to her to master her envy and to profit from it as a spur to development. Some of the ways in which she went about this task will have been apparent in the clinical material.

One could raise the question why Claire was so much more vulnerable than her siblings to the development of pathology requiring intervention. In fact, her female siblings did develop some rather stubborn problems, but apparently handled them adequately, at least from the practical point of view, by the available opportunities for mastery at school and in the family. One can only speculate about why Claire could not use the same opportunities.

In the first place, her first serious rival was a boy, who was especially precious to the family after the arrival of three girls. Secondly, she was so tiny at the time of this momentous event that developmental considerations alone would lead one to assume greater vulnerability. Her sisters had already had the opportunity to work through some of their feelings during Claire's own infancy, and they probably also enjoyed such compensatory privileges as being allowed to hold the newly arrived Richard, experiences in which Claire was too small to participate. Her sisters, at the time, were already well advanced into phallic-oedipal concerns, while Claire, immersed in anal matters, was especially vulnerable to the implication that she was rejected as dirty and smelly. The last assumption was amply confirmed in the analysis, most graphically, perhaps, by her messy wax autograph.

Besides all of these more or less convincing bits of evidence, there is an impressionistic one that seems crucial. I had the strong feeling that Claire's mother coped with powerful conflicts in the area of self-esteem regulation which paralleled those of her daughter. I have assumed that these were activated by the birth of her first son and by her resonant response to Claire's distress. She was, in any case, intensely sensitive to Claire's conflicts—sometimes to the point of being paralyzingly sympathetic—and one often sensed that she relived her own strivings through her daughter's experience and thus unconsciously supported the pathology. I formed the impression that she herself used Claire's analysis to come to terms with these issues, at least sufficiently so as to impose no barrier to Claire's recovery from her current distress.

Predictions should perhaps be mentioned in spite of their notorious inaccuracy in childhood pathology. I have presented Claire's material as illustrative of the analysis of internalized conflict in a child whose family had, relatively speaking, a remarkable stability. Anna Freud pointed out that, even after taking account of the favorable immediate outcome of this work, one still had to regard Claire as a highly disturbed child who suffered intensely from the two major traumas of her life: the birth of her brother and her primal scene experience. What the future holds for her is certainly not foreseeable. Nevertheless, for the time being, it seems appropriate to conclude that her analysis fulfilled its purpose in enabling her to return to the main stream of healthy development.

BIBLIOGRAPHY

FERENCZI, S. (1919), The Phenomena of Hysterical Materialization. *Further Contributions to the Theory and Technique of Psycho-Analysis*, London: Hogarth Press, 1950, pp. 89–104.
——— (1923), 'Materialization' in Globus Hystericus. *Ibid.*, pp. 104–105.

Freud, A. (1965), Assessment of Pathology. In: *Normality and Pathology in Childhood.* New York: Int. Univ. Press, pp. 148–212.

Greenacre, P. (1953), Penis Awe and Its Relation to Penis Envy. In: *Drives, Affects, Behavior,* ed. R. M. Loewenstein. New York: Int. Univ. Press, pp. 176–190.

Joffe, W. G. (1969), A Critical Review of the Status of the Envy Concept. *Int. J. Psycho-Anal.,* 50:533–545.

Rangell, L. (1959), The Nature of Conversion. *J. Amer. Psychoanal. Assn.,* 7:632–662.

Zetzel, E. R. (1968), The So Called Good Hysteric. *Int. J. Psycho-Anal.,* 49:256–260.

The Mirror Dream

CHARLES FEIGELSON, M.D.

>The crystal spies on us. If within the
>four walls of a bedroom a mirror stares,
>I'm no longer alone. There is someone there.
>In the dawn, reflections mutely stage a show.
>JORGE LUIS BORGES

IN HIS PAPER ON THE "UNCANNY" (1917), FREUD REFERS TO RANK'S (1914) concept of the double as originally representing an insurance against the destruction of the ego, "an energetic denial of the power of death." Freud elaborates, "This invention of doubling as a preservation against extinction has its counterpart in the language of dreams, which is fond of representing castration by a doubling or multiplication of a genital symbol" (p. 235). That doubling can be used as a defense against loss is inherent in the concepts of both Freud and Rank. In 1920, Freud referred to a child who made an effort to deal with a brief separation from his mother by making his own image alternately appear and disappear in a mirror.

The process of mental duplication or doubling is intimately bound up with the mirror mechanism of mirror dreams. The literature on mirror dreams is sparse. Elkisch (1957) described the behavior of three psychotic patients who used the mirror as a defense against the fear of loss of self. Miller (1948) wrote that mirror dreams occur in "narcissistic types of patients" when the integrative function of the ego is increased, and that these dreams represent a struggle of the ego to master reality. Kaywin (1957) understood one of his patient's mirror dreams as revealing a negative self image. Eisnitz (1961) summarized his study of three

---

The author is a member of The New York Psychoanalytic Society and Institute.

cases by stating, "The mirror dream represents an attempt at defense against narcissistic mortification from the superego, from the analyst, or from reality. In the case of the superego threat, the threatening part of the superego is split off and projected to the mirror." Omnipotent voyeurism masters the projected image which is then safely reintrojected as a protector of narcissism (p. 477). In a paper on the metaphor of the mirror, Shengold (1974) wrote, "The mirror's magic . . . stems from its linkage with the narcissistic period when identity and mind are formed through contact with the mother; the *power* of mirror magic is a continuation of parental and narcissistic omnipotence" (p. 114). Myers (1973) described a recurrent element in the manifest content of certain dreams in which a patient sees himself in the dual representations of both observer and observed, and related this to the primal scene as well as to the presence of a mirror in the parental bedroom.

Using clinical material from five patients, I shall attempt to explain the mirror mechanism in mirror dreams as a narcissistic defense against object-related conflicts.

Clinical Illustrations

PATIENT A

A 30-year-old woman lawyer entered analysis with symptoms of work inhibition and depression associated with intense preoccupation with her physical attractiveness. During a period in her analysis when material dealing with her childhood relationship to a 3-year-older cousin, a surrogate sister who lived next door, began to emerge, Ms. A. told of the following experience: she had gone shopping for a coffee pot and as she started to make her purchase, she began to feel a sense of discomfort that she identified as guilt. She fell into a momentary reflective state, thinking "would she [the cousin] approve" of her buying this. While still in this state, she began to feel that her cousin would have criticized her choice of restaurant or makeup. These choices had given her pleasure.

That night, she dreamed that she was in the waiting room to the analyst's office and looking in a mirror. There she saw reflected from inside the office the image of the analyst sitting on the couch necking with the female patient who comes before her; she felt shocked, but was aware of feeling jealous. Still looking into the mirror, she was now looking at an image of herself putting on a dowdy black hat and fixing herself before coming into the office so that her feelings of shock and jealousy would not be seen.

Associations led to her previous session when she had seen a new woman patient just before her appointment and had felt jealous. It led her to the jealous rivalry with her cousin who she felt was more beautiful than she; the patient recalled spending hours watching this cousin as she dressed and made herself up in front of the mirror. Ms. A. had actually tried on a colorful and sexy dress the evening before and felt that her cousin would have been jealous and critical. Associating to looking in the mirror, she immediately felt a sense of embarrassment. It was vain, she said, going on to latency memories of how she would dress up in a G-string, stand before a mirror dancing, and become sexually excited looking at her image in the mirror.

After Ms. A. had seen the new patient, she experienced guilt feelings while shopping. The jealousy and rivalry were projected onto the image of the cousin, whom she clearly replaced in standing before the mirror. In the manifest dream, Ms. A. was dowdy, but the latent wish was to be in the cousin's place, beautiful and sexy; it was this thought which evoked the recall of the latency masturbatory equivalent in which she used the mirror.

In this mirror dream Ms. A. duplicated: she became like the childhood rival and displaced her. The analysis of this material led to the emergence of rage and death wishes toward cousin and mother, feelings which alternated with immense fears of loss and being alone. As the fear of being alone reappeared in her current life, she recalled early childhood fears of sleeping alone and the many nights her fears were assuaged by sleeping with this cousin. Less frequently, she would go to her parents' bedroom.

Ms. A. began to have morbid thoughts about what life would be like after her parents' death, and then reported a second mirror dream:

> I am in a building looking out a window onto a beautiful scene of trees, grass, and parklike setting. I see my reflection in the window

glass and I look youthful and virginal; then I again look on the scene and it is no longer sunny, but dark and stormy, everything drenched in rain.

Associations led to a reverie state she had had last summer. Waiting for her boyfriend in Copenhagen, she was seized by sudden curiosity and a desire to go and see the apartment where her parents had lived before she was born. Again she became embarrassed when she associated to the reflected image of herself in the dream, and again brought up the latency masturbatory dance. The embarrassment was about the sexual excitement, but she also recalled that in dancing before the mirror she was able to overcome feelings of loneliness, much as she had in sleeping with her cousin. The parklike setting had reminded her of Copenhagen; and the dark scene of the hallway in her childhood home. Then she remembered that her parents' bedroom had double French doors with French glass in them; when she went to their room, she saw a reflected image of herself in the glass (seeing herself on the surface of the mirror thus warded off the dark and stormy scene beyond).

Through this dream, the mirror mechanism became clear. It not only revived the memory of the stage for the primal scene experience, but, metaphorically, it showed the model of this patient's defense. The reflected image of herself represented her preoccupation with her body, here viewed as a defense against seeing beyond it into the dark and stormy room. The memory of looking at the image of herself in the glass of the doors protected her against the memory of the loneliness, of being the excluded one.

Both mirror dreams were preceded by preoccupation with loss. In the first, it was loss of the analyst to the new patient and loss of the cousin/mother by virtue of her own death wishes toward them. Before the second dream, Ms. A. was preoccupied with losing her parents. Day residue experiences of some change in her state of consciousness acted as stimuli to the mirror dream. In the first, it was the reflective state in the store; in the second, the reverie experience. The mirror mechanism served as a defense against the experience of loss; it protected the object of her aggression by a heightened preoccupation with herself (withdrawal).

The mirror dream also led to specific masturbatory experiences in which mirrors had been used in the past. This was the source of the embarrassment which she felt in associating to the dream mirror experience.

PATIENT B

A 20-year-old woman college student came for analysis because of problems in her relations with men. Like patient A., Miss B. was given to long, ruminative preoccupation with her body and suffered from intense penis envy. During a menstrual period when she felt particularly depressed and unattractive, she reported the following dream:

> I first felt that my teeth were broken and looked in a mirror and felt reassured when I saw that they were alright. Then I felt that my hair was messed up and again looked in the mirror and felt reassured.

During her period, her bodily preoccupation and fear of loss of attractiveness were always present. She could not associate to the feeling that her teeth were broken, but the hair reminded her that until age 5 or 6 she had had long blond hair which her mother had forced her to cut, and since that time she felt she had not looked as nice. Feeling reassured in the dream gave her a sense of physical well-being—that she had what she feared she had lost. Miss B., too, became embarrassed when asked to associate to the mirror and recalled adolescent masturbatory experiences in which a mirror had been used.

A state of consciousness involving diminished attention to the outside and heightened awareness of her body preceded the mirror dream, which reassured her against the experience of loss. She denied her castration and restored her long blond penis. In the dream experience of feeling reassured, she was able to ward off the aggression against her mother, whom she held responsible for her castration and menstruation.

PATIENT C

A 43-year-old married woman had been in twice-a-week psychotherapy for two years for a depression which followed the tragic death from meningitis of her 4-year-old adopted daughter.[1] At that time, she had a 2-year-old adopted son who was now 4, and subsequently adopted another girl, now 2. It was very difficult for her to accept her daughter's death and Mrs. C. often hoped for a miracle that would bring her back. She dreamed that she was lying on a sofa. A young woman was sitting or standing next to her, stroking her arm, and the patient felt something homosexual was involved. Then she was in her bathroom in her chemise, but when she looked in the mirror, she was naked, younger, and her breasts were distorted as though twisted over to one side. When she looked down at herself, she was wearing her chemise. When she looked in the mirror, she was naked. She thought it was a miracle.

The young woman stroking her arms reminded her of the way her little boy, age 4, stroked her. The person in the mirror seemed like a little girl. The breast distortion reminded her of her dead daughter who was born with unilateral gynecomastia and thus had one-sided breast development as an infant.

The therapist told the patient that the miracle in the dream was seeing her daughter alive again. Mrs. C. said that on the day of the dream, she had had a dental appointment which she had to postpone. Two years earlier, on the day her daughter died, she also had had an appointment with this same dentist, which she had had to break when her daughter was rushed to the hospital. The patient then began to experience the grief and sadness.

The mirror dream again defends against the experience of loss. While I do not have all the associative material, I include this dream because, like the others, it suggests bodily preoccupation and some alteration in consciousness (lying and being stroked) as a stimulus to the dream.

PATIENT D

A 28-year-old physician was in analysis for potency disturbances. He felt depressed by the thought of his younger brother's forthcoming wedding to his father's secretary. In talking about the anticipated wedding party, he was able to make himself feel better when

---

[1] My thanks to Dr. Martin Willick for this example.

he daydreamed that he as the physician, the son with the engaging personality, would be the center of interest. It was extremely painful for Dr. D. to give his brother his due because his brother's being in the limelight meant that he himself was excluded. His concern about the loss of his parents' and family's interest during this time was extreme and on a childish level. It evoked many childhood memories of intense envy of the 4-year-younger brother and of feeling displaced by his baby brother. The day after the wedding, Dr. D. dreamed:

> I was in a box at the opera or theater, seated to the left of Rose [a female colleague of his]; then, as if standing for royalty to come in, I was standing in the box with my penis pressing against the bar; suddenly I am looking at myself in a mirror and cannot see the stage. I am simultaneously looking at my face in the mirror and having an emission; my face looks unresponsive, showing no signs of having the emission and I am feeling concerned that it should not be seen.

This dream was incompletely analyzed. I use it in this paper only as another example to illustrate that concern about loss acts as a stimulus to a mirror dream in which the use of the mirror and the attendant self-absorption again ward off the primal scene experience. This was inferred from his associations to the stage at the opera or theater in the dream and the wedding scene, which led him to fantasies of watching his brother sadistically make love to his new bride. In the dream the mirror blocked his view of the stage.

Unlike the other patients whose immediate associations to their mirror dreams led to their masturbation, Dr. D. let a few days pass before he introduced his adolescent masturbation into the analysis. Wearing mother's stockings, he would look at himself in the bathroom mirror, fantasying that he was a woman ballet dancer with foot on the bar (towel rack). This obviously complex activity is mentioned here only as a further illustration of the relationship between mirror dreams and earlier masturbation practices in which mirrors played an important part.

PATIENT E

A 26-year-old artist had been in analysis for one year when he went home to another city to visit his parents over the Christmas holidays. Roughly one year before he began analysis, he had suffered a transient psychotic episode under the influence of drugs. At that time, he experienced an extreme remorse and conscious feelings of guilt over having made a girlfriend pregnant and having refused to marry her. She had returned to her home in another country at the time of his psychotic experience, which lasted two to three weeks and for which he was hospitalized.

The night he returned from his holidays and before he resumed his analytic sessions, he felt a painful sense of loneliness and smoked pot, putting himself into a sleepy reverie, the content of which he could not remember. He then fell asleep and had the following dream:

> I was in a room without windows, it had rounded, low ceilings that were breastlike in shape; my grandmother was there with two hats; she gave me one and I tried it on and looked at myself in the mirror; I liked it a lot, the way I looked; I looked handsome and masculine (I could only see my torso and face); the mirror seemed like a floating space in front of me. A few seconds later, I looked again and I didn't like the way I looked, I had an awkward unmanly expression on my face.

In connection with the experience of looking at himself, he felt some sense of embarrassment, but it reminded him of his recent visit to his parents where he spent hours looking at photographs of himself and his family. He had especially enjoyed looking at a photo of himself taken when he was 3 or 4; he was wearing a trenchcoat and looked manly, just as in the first image of himself in the mirror. The night of the dream, he had felt weak and unmanly and tempted to masturbate, but did not for fear that it would increase his sense of weakness. He felt his mother regarded him as weak and was critical of him—the way he dressed and lived—and her criticisms of him always frightened him. He remembered that especially during the years from 6 to about 11 it was very important for him that his mother or sister admire him, particularly how he looked.

In this dream, he attempted to re-create the experience of feeling admired as a way of warding off his mother's critical attitude. He as the looker was identified with the admiring mother who was not separated from him and the mirror image was himself.

Before going further with the analytic material, I want to emphasize the changed state of consciousness and the separation experience that preceded the dream, as well as his embarrassment in associating to the mirror.

In the next few days following the dream, the patient brought much material including a mirror dream he had had just before his psychotic experience:

> I am in a house that I helped an architect build; I had a tremendous feeling that he condemned me for the pregnancy. I was on a balcony overlooking a two-story living room; there were some other people there and then they were gone. As I looked out into the room, I felt completely physically, perceptually dizzy, like zooming in and out: I was saying, "Help me." Then I was looking in a mirror, as if through prism eyeglasses; the effect was that I saw many images of myself as if the mirror was shattered. Then I turned and tried to look in the mirror again. I could not see the mirror; as I moved, it moved, like it was at a right angle to me; it felt like the mirror was made by my mind, a hallucination, like a mirage. I yearned to look into it.

Shortly after this dream, the patient became psychotic. Prior to the break, he had felt weak, impotent, and masturbated a lot with extreme feelings of guilt. The night of the break, he was working on a collage of a house with a small person inside. While working, he began to notice his hand and to see it as beautiful as he worked; he then saw his hand as a work of art in itself (what had been involved in the guilt-ridden masturbation was transformed into a maker of beauty and then became beautiful itself; a regressive defense against the guilt), and this feeling spread to encompass his entire body. He was a work of art to be looked at and admired—there were no more feelings of guilt, inferiority, or impotence.

In analyzing this fascinating material, he spoke of how throughout latency he had sought his mother's admiration by joking and performing for her, and how in his adolescent masturbation, he would sit or stand while holding a mirror and look at the mirror image of his penis as he masturbated. With the mirror, he felt masculine and that he had a beautiful penis; without the mirror, he felt guilty and weak and his penis looked smaller. The admiration and recognition served the functions of relieving guilt and reassuring him that everything was intact. The mirror served the same functions; he became the admiring mother and the mirror image became himself.

Without citing all the analytic material on which my conclusions are based, I would say that his becoming psychotic was a regressive attempt to deal with oedipal guilt in connection with the pregnancy and reflected his inability to deal internally with the loss of his girlfriend. In the dream preceding the psychosis, the mirror mechanism failed. Looking at the multiple images of himself was an exaggerated, desperate effort to duplicate the mother-child union as well as a representation of his fragmenting ego. Even this failed and he felt "completely physically, spatially, perceptually dislocated." He was unable to hold onto the internalized good mother—the mirror disappeared.

I might add that the major thrust of the transference in his analysis had to do with repetitive efforts to win my admiration. When this wish was frustrated, the patient developed guilt feelings usually in response to conflicts over aggression and masturbation. I was impressed by his intense need for my admiration to protect himself against a severely punitive and archaic superego.

The patient equated the mirror with his canvas on which he could create his own reality. What he painted there in his dream was a self-portrait, a duplicate of himself as he wanted to be. This may be one of the motives of artists who repeatedly paint self-portraits.

The patient solved his conflict in the reality of his life by creating artistic happenings or "environments," as they were called in the '60s. These were artistic representations where the artist created an environment in which he would be part of the scene (one was a gigantic outdoor bathtub with himself lying in it) and the viewer would admire him as part of "the picture."

Discussion

In his work on narcissism Heinz Kohut (1971) introduced the concept of the "mirror transference," which is pertinent to mirror dreams. In the transference patients A, D, and E insisted on having the analyst's admiration, on being the "gleam in his eye." Patient A regressed to this need in response to a conflict over aggression which was mobilized by oedipal transference fantasies. Patient D wanted admiration from the analyst as a way of protecting himself against the experience of envy and aggression toward a sibling. Patient E resembled most closely the type of patient described by Kohut. This patient manifested a persistent, intense need for the analyst's total admiration. Invariably, the frustration of his wishes resulted in intense feelings of guilt. He seemed to need the analyst's admiration to protect him against his punitive, archaic superego. While narcissistic phenomena were evident in these patients to a considerable degree, I could not separate the narcissistic needs from the object conflicts. They seemed to work together like the heart and its blood. Each could be understood individually, but functionally they were inseparable.

Kohut mentions that while mirror dreams may occasionally occur in the analysis of transference neuroses and may then symbolize self-scrutiny, they usually are found in the narcissistic patients when a major part of the grandiose self is in the process of being mobilized in relation to the analyst. My own formulation differs with his and is described below.

In presenting the clinical material, I emphasized that each patient was consciously preoccupied with loss or separation at the time of the mirror dream. In the associative material, there was reference to some alteration in consciousness toward inner processes—a shift that one might conceptualize as a reflection upon the self, either the body, some bodily sensations, or the mental self. These self-preoccupation phenomena are directly expressed in the mirror dream as a concrete looking at the self (or some part of it) as in the notion of the mirror's surface expressing a state of reflection.

The mirror dreams in each analytic case (case C was a psychotherapy patient with another analyst) led to childhood or adolescent experiences in which mirrors were used in masturbatory acts. From the standpoint of the clinical usefulness of mirror dreams, this is important. None of the masturbating practices involving mirrors had come into the analysis prior to the mirror dreams.

The mirror dream as well as the mirrors used in masturbation served a guilt-relieving function. There was in each analytic case a current conflict which mobilized rage or hostility to some object, either through sibling rivalry, penis envy, primal scene, or oedipal rivalry. The guilt resulting from the object-directed aggression might be dealt with in other ways. In these patients, the aggression (death wishes) mobilized fears of object loss. It is this fear that stimulates use of the mirror mechanism. Eisnitz described the mirror mechanism as a protector of narcissism in which the punitive superego is projected onto the mirror, turned into a protective superego, and this protective image is then reintrojected, thereby relieving guilt and protecting the patient's narcissism. I believe this is a correct formulation, but not complete.

I venture the following explanation: a conflict, usually oedipal in nature, is triggered by some event in reality or mobilized by the transference. This conflict becomes even more charged in these patients who in addition to the usual oedipal anxieties suffer from a more than usual fear of object loss. A regression ensues. On a psychosexual level, it reaches the oral level; on the ego level, it extends to a period when separation-individuation has started, but has not yet been completed.

The mirror in the mirror dream seems to me to represent a highly polished surface of the dream screen (Lewin, 1946). One might visualize a movie screen where events and characters are portrayed as the more usual kind of dream representation. If one visualizes a movie screen where these characters are portrayed and in one's mind's eye places a mirror on it, then he comes to the surface of the screen itself. In this, I see the mirror as an extension of the screen itself.[2]

The work of Margaret Mahler (1968) helps us to understand the mirror experience in the dream. The experience is one in which the looker is also looked at. Yet, the looker experiences the image in the mirror as "me" and yet not "me." It represents, I believe, a revival of experiences that the person must have had in the separation-individuation phase of development. At some point before separation-individuation is complete, the experience of an object (mother) as "me" and yet not "me" seems inevitable. Before an object experienced as part of the self can be experienced as separate, the

---

[2] Eisnitz (1961) also mentions this in his paper on mirror dreams.

notion of it being "me"—yet not "me" probably occurs in alternating phases, much as the dream mirror experience of it being "me"—yet not "me" (but a mirror image of "me") does.[3]

I assume that the ego regresses to a state in which the internalized image of the self is split from the internalized protective mother image. In the mirror dream, the looker represents one image, the mirror image the other. What the mirror dreamer has resurrected in his dream is an ego state in which good, protective mothering reassures the self in a state of incomplete separation. The regression in this way acts as a protector against guilt or against the internal image of a critical mother or father. The incomplete separation experienced through the mirror imagery serves as a protection against the fear of loss (or destruction of the object). In this respect, I refer particularly to the dream of patient E in which he could not effect this union and became "completely physically, spatially, perceptually disoriented."

In the mirror dream, a manifestly narcissistic type of defense, through regression, is invoked to ward off a conflict with an object. To be sure, when the dream is successful, it also protects the person's narcissism. One might say that in the concrete representation of the mirror dream, the narcissistic defense is represented by the surface of the mirror. Herein is expressed the surface preoccupation; derivative in consciousness is the absorption with the self that is experienced as a changed state of consciousness in which attention is shifted from the outside (reality) to the inside (one's body, inner sensations) for purposes of avoiding an object conflict that is represented by the mirror's depth. In Carroll's *Alice Through the Looking Glass*, the oedipal theme is reached when Alice goes through the mirror's surface, enters and explores the room beyond, and dethrones the Red Queen.

The surface versus the room beyond model was brought to my attention by the clinical material of patient A who, standing in front of the glass doors to her parents' bedroom, saw her reflected

---

[3] A patient not described in this paper said in associating to the mirror experience: "It is me and yet not me." He was in analysis for homosexuality which could be acted out only when he was in a state of consciousness in which he felt himself to be "me—yet not me."

image—an experience that in her memory clearly warded off the primal scene.

In patients A, B, and E, the mirror dream's wish-fulfilling function is clear. The projected image of the self represents the self as one would like to be. This aspect of the clinical material has not been stressed since it is not specific to mirror dreams.

While the defense mechanisms of regression, projection, introjection, and denial are involved in the mirror mechanism, I have wondered if an unnamed mechanism—duplication—may be involved as well. We usually think of a psychological phenomenon in which something is added or created to protect against loss or castration as denial. It is a form of denial when the child creates an imaginary companion, attributes a phallus to his mother, or is reassured by seeing his teeth intact in a mirror dream. The double or the fantasy of having a twin is a duplication. In each instance, the person duplicates himself or part of himself and thereby protects himself. The artist patient sees his mirror as a canvas on which he duplicates an image of himself as a protection against anxiety. Children normally see the outside world in terms of themselves—a kind of duplication. Anthropomorphizing is a duplication. Duplicating, a normal childhood experience, may, I suggest, be retained as a mechanism of defense, and make up part of the inner network of the mirror mechanism in mirror dreams.

Duplication should be distinguished from denial and projection. Denial represents a disavowal, not a re-creation in terms of the self. To deny the woman's genital would involve eliminating it from perception. To me, it seems that seeing her as possessing a penis is a re-creation in terms of the self. In projecting, we attribute something of the self to someone or something outside the self in order not to know about it in the self. In duplication, we continue to know about it in the self while also attributing it to the outside.

Summary

1. Clinical material of several patients who had mirror dreams is presented. Their preoccupation with loss and changed state of consciousness were experiential derivatives that stimulated the mirror imagery.

2. Mirror dreams are a clue to masturbatory practices in which mirrors are used.

3. The mirror dream represents a regressive partial reunion with the protective mother to allay guilt and reassure against object loss in response to aggression mobilized by an object conflict.

4. The mirror surface represents the narcissistic defense, whereas the object conflict is found beyond the surface in the mirror's depth.

5. A new mechanism of defense—duplication—is proposed.

BIBLIOGRAPHY

BORGES, J. L. (1970), *Dream Tigers.* New York: Dutton, p. 60.
EISNITZ, A. (1961), Mirror Dreams. *J. Amer. Psychoanal. Assn.*, 9:461–479.
ELKISCH, P. (1957), The Psychological Significance of the Mirror. *J. Amer. Psychoanal. Assn.*, 5:235–245.
FREUD, S. (1919), The Uncanny. *S.E.*, 17:217–256.
——— (1920), Beyond the Pleasure Principle. *S.E.*, 18:3–64.
KAYWIN, L. (1957), Notes on the Concept of Self Representation. *J. Amer. Psychoanal. Assn.*, 5:293–301.
KOHUT, H. (1971), *The Analysis of the Self.* New York: Int. Univ. Press.
LEWIN, B. D. (1946), Sleep, the Mouth, and the Dream Screen. *Psychoanal. Quart.*, 15:419–434.
MAHLER, M. S. (1968), *On Human Symbiosis and the Vicissitudes of Individuation.* New York: Int. Univ. Press.
MILLER, M. L. (1948), Ego Functioning in Two Types of Dreams. *Psychoanal. Quart.*, 17:346–355.
MYERS, W. A. (1973), Split Self-Representation and the Primal Scene. *Psychoanal. Quart.*, 42:525–538.
RANK, O. (1914), *Der Doppelgänger.* Leipzig: Internationaler Psychoanalytischer Verlag, 1925.
SHENGOLD, L. (1974), The Metaphor of the Mirror. *J. Amer. Psychoanal. Assn.*, 22:97–115.

Childhood Memories As Contents of Schizophrenic Hallucinations and Delusions

MAURITS KATAN, M.D.

THE TITLE OF THIS PAPER REFERS TO THE INFLUENCE OF CHILDHOOD experiences upon schizophrenic symptom formation, a phenomenon for which the psychoanalytic theory has so far found no solution. This phenomenon has puzzled me for more than twenty years. My puzzlement increased when Niederland (1959) compared the methods of child rearing used by Schreber's father with the contents of some of Schreber's psychotic symptoms and found a clear relation between them. Niederland convincingly demonstrated that Schreber's early childhood experiences resulting from his father's upbringing made their appearance almost half a century later as contents of his schizophrenic symptoms.

In my discussion of Niederland's paper (1960a), I stressed that his findings contained a specific problem: why did these memories become conscious as the contents of schizophrenic symptoms instead of simply being recalled as childhood experiences? Particularly conspicuous was Schreber's complete unawareness of the fact that he was dealing with memories of his own childhood. He conceived of these memories as newly created events caused by a persecutor such as Flechsig or God. Niederland's remarkable discovery thus gave rise to a problem which successfully resisted all attempts at explanation.

Dr. Katan is Professor Emeritus, Case Western Reserve University, Cleveland.

In a recently published book (1972), Schatzman attempts to view Schreber's *Denkwürdigkeiten* in a totally new light. By imitating Niederland's method, Schatzman arrives at new conclusions about Schreber. If these conclusions can be proved to be correct, Schatzman will have found a solution to the problem that I was unable to solve. In the Preface, Schatzman acquaints the reader with his viewpoint: "If an odd experience of the son seems recognizably related to a procedure of his father, I call the experience an *image* or transform (i.e., the product of transformation) of that procedure." From this statement I draw the conclusion that Schatzman conceives of the *Denkwürdigkeiten* as a "transform" of the childhood experiences to which Daniel Paul Schreber was exposed by his father. It is clear that the title of Schatzman's book expresses his conviction that Schreber believed his father, through his peculiar methods, had been persecuting him for the purpose of murdering his soul.

This conviction leads Schatzman to the peculiar idea that Schreber was not psychotic, that his supernatural revelations were not the result of a mental illness. His father's persistent influence upon Schreber's thought processes kept Schreber from finding a more normal way of expressing himself. What his father had taught him as a child prevented him later on from recognizing that his strange relationship to God was a reexperience of his childhood relationship to his father. This last idea Schatzman calls his thesis. Clearly, Schatzman's thesis covers precisely that subject which I regard as posing a problem. Schatzman's reasoning does not convince me that he has found the solution to it.

Schatzman (p. 10) criticizes Freud for not having made use of the writings of Schreber's father. Similarly, a very erudite colleague asked me whether I could explain Freud's lack of interest in the father's writings; Freud would have been so much better informed (according to my colleague) about Schreber if he had taken note of these writings. To this colleague it sounded almost unbelievable when Anna Freud informed him that her father's library did not contain a single copy of the older Schreber's publications. One has to keep in mind that Freud had already formed his theory about the paranoid form of schizophrenia before he read the *Denkwürdigkeiten*.

There are of course compelling reasons why Freud presumably

had never thought of consulting the father's books. On this point I do not want to be misunderstood. It is certainly true that the father's methods of child rearing must have exerted a tremendous influence upon the mental development of his son. How can one find out in what ways and to what extent the father's influence left its marks on Schreber's mind? How did the son conceive of his father's treatment? *All this we can learn only from the son and not from the father.*

There may be an even more important reason why Freud would not have wished to read a book by Schreber's father, assuming he had known of its existence. In my opinion, Freud had no incentive to read statements made by the father, for he did not want to be influenced by any material that did not come from Daniel Paul Schreber himself. To Freud it was essential that his mind be in tune with Schreber's state of mind at the time when Schreber wrote down his thoughts. It is fully permissible to compare this situation with that of psychoanalytic treatment. The analyst's mind is in a state of "evenly suspended attention" (Freud, 1912). This state enables him to use his mind as an extremely sensitive receptive organ that reacts to the patient's associations. One can imagine how Freud's sensitivity would have been harmed if he had prepared himself by first reading the older Schreber's publications. Inadvertently he would have been influenced by this information, which would then have rendered his mind less receptive to the overall picture offered by the patient (Katan, 1966).

Freud, without any knowledge of the father's writings, did exceptionally well. He was the first to construe that the complicated delusional features of God were the offspring of certain characteristics of Schreber's father. Freud connected Schreber's ambivalent attitude toward God with Schreber's childhood ambivalence toward his father. He quoted Schreber's belief that God did not understand living human beings and was used to having contact only with cadavers. This makes it very easy for the reader to conclude that the father required a *Cadavergehorsam* (the type of obedience demanded in the German army) from his children.

Next, Freud conceived of Flechsig as representing a brother, with the assumption that this brother was older than Schreber. Indeed, Schreber did have a brother who was 3 years his senior.

The women were not forgotten either. The front realms of God pictured the feminine part, obviously representing Schreber's mother; the back realms were his father. Again Freud leads the reader in the direction of making his own interpretations. The picture of God floating on top of the forecourts of heaven is a primal scene observation, the intercourse most likely being a coitus à tergo. The speaking birds that were too stupid to know the difference between "Chinesentum and Jesum Christum," or between "Santiago and Karthago," were obviously "revenants" of his sisters, who were kept stupid by the father.

There is more to admire. Freud interpreted "murder of the soul" as an act of masturbation. This interpretation renders another remark of Freud's very valuable. He related Schreber's obsessional thinking, by which he wanted to convince God that he had not lost his intellect, to Schreber's anxiety about losing his intellect through masturbation. Schreber as a child must have had a masturbatory problem.

After this review, I ask: Did Freud really need any information provided by an outside source? Was he not building a construction of Schreber's childhood which in no way is contradictory to but is even more informative than what the father's books might have brought to light? My answer is: Freud demonstrated that a construction can provide more complete insight into Schreber's childhood development than all the books written by the older Schreber could do!

Following closely Freud's method of interpretation (1911, chap. 2), I have previously (1959) published some constructions which I now want to make use of. (I am very glad I wrote them at a time when I was still completely uninformed about Niederland's research.)

Schreber was one of "those wrecked by success." Even before he assumed the presidency of a higher judicial court, a number of his dreams revealed how this honorable appointment had started to unsettle his mind. One of his dreams showed that he desired to be a woman submitting to intercourse. After assuming this office, he competed with the other judges, who with a single exception were all older than he was. At the moment when he had sufficiently demonstrated his superiority, he was completely exhausted and had to be hospitalized in Flechsig's clinic. After some months of hospitalization, during a four-day absence of his wife, who had until then visited him daily, a night of six nocturnal emissions marked the beginning of his psychosis. He then discovered that Flechsig was starting to persecute him. Freud made the interpretation that Schreber's homosexual wish was satisfied when he had these emissions. The absence of his wife robbed Schreber of her protection against the influence of the men in his surroundings.

According to my experience, in every case of schizophrenia the outbreak of the psychosis proper occurs after the patient has an orgasm comparable to Schreber's.

Once Schreber's psychosis had begun, he tried desperately not to become sexually stimulated again. My 1959 article deals with the first two chapters of the *Denkwürdigkeiten*. In chapter 1, Schreber describes the structure of the hereafter, a structure that would enable him to postpone any sexual activity until after his death. In chapter 2, Schreber narrates how Flechsig, through the abuse of God's rays to his own advantage, prevented this plan from materializing. Conspicuously, these persecutions started at a time before either Schreber or Flechsig had been born. They occurred between the ancestors of the two families. I drew the conclusion that the descriptions of the hereafter on the one hand, and of the period before Schreber and Flechsig were born on the other, portrayed two different aspects of Schreber's childhood experiences.

This conclusion was based upon some constructions I succeeded in making. The first were based on chapter 1 of the *Denkwürdigkeiten*, which focuses on Schreber's relationship to God. Generally, God established contact with the nerves of men only after death. After a period of hibernation, the nerves of the dead men were awakened by God to a heavenly life. They then had to undergo a process of purification and simultaneously to learn the "ground-language," which was the language spoken by God. During this process of purification, the nerves, also called souls, were transformed into feminine creatures. Yet the purification not only involved the loss of masculinity but clearly betrayed an anal cleansing as well. From an anal point of view, the masculine genital could be used for dirty acts such as masturbation, and enemas were administered not only to clean the bowels but especially to prevent soiling.

Certain traits of the "ground-language" show characteristics similar to those of the purification process. This language, the one spoken by God, was a somewhat old-fashioned but nevertheless powerful German, which was characterized by its great wealth of euphemisms. Any word containing a trace of foreign extraction was dropped and exchanged for a purer German expression. I concluded that the ground-language had been submitted to the process of purification, this process being similar to the treatment to which the souls were subjected. The words of the ground-language were revealed to Schreber by the voices.[1] Schreber denied having any previous knowledge of this language or of its origin. The words were not his own invention, were not used by other people, and were partly of a scientific, especially of a medical nature. Additional examples that could be cited make it clear that it was the language spoken by Schreber's father. The euphemisms contained in the language are extremely instructive regarding the father's attitude. For instance, souls who were undergoing the process of purification, which was called a test, were called tested souls, although in reality they were untested; punishment was called a reward.

The souls still in the process of being tested were devils. These devils were different from what devils are commonly assumed to be, for they were very God-fearing. Instead of repeating the description of the various features of these devils, I cite part of my conclusions (1959):

> We have a mental picture of a father who does not punish his son for the sake of punishment, but for the child's own good—a father who wants to drive the "devil" out of his son, who wants to make his son pure so that he will not masturbate again and will not spread "repugnant odors" or, even worse, soil himself. . . . Such a father deserves the name of hypocrite. Under cover of having his son's interests at heart, he submits him to a treatment of relentless testing and tongue-lashing, which Schreber so appropriately called the "ground-language." I think we are not far wrong in calling this upbringing sadistic [p. 337]. No doubt the little Schreber learned at that time to speak the "ground-language": he learned to obey the

---

[1] The "voices" were hallucinations of a very special type. Séglas (1927) named them *hallucinations verbales psychomotrices*.

"somewhat old-fashioned" but "powerful" German which was characterized by its great wealth of euphemisms [p. 336].

The devils form an important part of this picture. They are projections of Schreber's own forbidden instincts. "Once they are projected, Schreber tries to deny their vicious character by saying they are already very 'God-fearing'" (p. 339). When the father caught his son in one of his sinful acts, he would have called his son a devil and have wanted to drive the devil out of him. I concluded that under the influence of the father's continual testing, which clearly started in the anal phase and extended through the phallic phase, the son must have felt that his father was continually keeping an eye on him.

I have yet to speak of the world order. Under the aegis of this order, God could "take a nerve attachment to a living man and inspire him with fertile thoughts about the hereafter." This could become very dangerous if the nerves of this man became inordinately excited. These nerves would then exert such an attraction upon the nerves of God that God would not be able to free Himself and accordingly God's existence would be threatened. Does not this delusional description portray a perfect picture of young Schreber reacting with sexual excitement to his father's behavior and in that way threatening his father's authority?

I think my reader will join me in my conclusion that Schreber's father was far from successful in the upbringing of his son. The father, through his relentless testing, tried to regulate his son's anal activity, and, more important, he tried to instill so much anxiety in the child that he would not masturbate at all. The result, however, was just the opposite: the father's methods excited the child sexually, and this excitement in turn created continual problems. It would lead too far to explain my assumption that Daniel Paul Schreber became a severe obsessional neurotic, although one who could at least take advantage of his neurosis to the extent of carving out for himself a prominent judicial career.

Next I turn to my construction about Schreber's relationship to his brother who was 3 years older, a construction based on chapter 2 of the *Denkwürdigkeiten*. Schreber's hope that he would be able to abolish his masturbation until the hereafter was wrecked by

Flechsig's attempt to murder Schreber's soul. Long before both Schreber and Flechsig were born, an ancestor of Flechsig's had attempted to murder a Schreber soul. In this I see Schreber's effort to date back to a prenatal time an occurrence between himself and his brother, who was represented by Flechsig. Freud interpreted soul murder as meaning masturbation. A construction which I derived from the following statement by Schreber (1903) will inform us better regarding this point: "Both the Flechsigs and the Schrebers were members of 'the highest heavenly nobility,' as the phrase went: the Schrebers in particular bore the title of 'Margraves of Tuscany and Tasmania,' for souls, urged on by some sort of personal vanity, have a custom of adorning themselves with somewhat high-sounding earthly titles" (p. 24). I conceived of the adornment with titles as being of the order of children's play in which two boys engage in boasting, each of them trying to outdo the other by assuming still higher titles. Previously I explained that the "earthly" advantages which the devil promised in exchange for a man's soul were of the nature of genital masturbation. Thus I decided that the jealousy also revolved around the genitals—which boy could boast of having the biggest penis and therefore masturbate better. These occurrences never became known to any outsider.

Another part of chapter 2 deals with the formation of a plot against the patient. God had granted Flechsig certain privileges as a reward for his high moral standards, and Flechsig abused these privileges by taking advantage of Schreber. I deduced that Schreber had shown signs of extreme nervousness because of his sexual excitement. Schreber's father had "granted" his oldest son the privilege of acting as guardian, which means that he had assigned him the task of watching his younger brother in order to keep him from masturbating. Schreber's brother misused the privileges which his father had granted him by performing a homosexual attack on his younger brother. From the delusional material (Katan, 1959, p. 370) I was able to enlarge my construction. The sister who was next in age to the older brother discovered what had gone on between the two boys and told their mother. In the discussions that followed, the older brother showed himself very resistant and refused to give up his privileges unless his mother and his sister would assure him that they would not divulge anything to the father. The mother was so afraid of the father's wrath if he heard about what had happened that she readily convinced the older daughter that she must not tell the father. Once these conditions had been accepted, the brother promised not to repeat his homosexual attack on Daniel Paul. The younger Schreber felt indignant about what he regarded as a plot against him. Especially because of the mother's attitude, the older brother now escaped a well-deserved punishment. On the occasion of Daniel Paul's complaints, his mother explained to him that she could not continually be with him to protect him against his brother, that the other children also needed her attention.

These constructions not only reveal how young Schreber reacted to his father's treatment but also bear witness to the fear which the father's attitude instilled in the mother and children. I have already mentioned that the father's methods, contrary to their intended goal, precociously stimulated young Schreber's sexuality and resulted in his masturbatory activity.

I regard the "ground-language" as one of the most revealing subjects in the *Denkwürdigkeiten*. This language not only portrays accurately the hardships to which the father insensitively subjected his son. It demonstrates as well the scorn which Daniel Paul felt for these methods of upbringing and his ridicule of the father's pomposity and use of a purified language. "Soul murder" was not a word chosen by the son to designate the harm done to him by his father. *The word was used first by the father* when he tried to impress upon his son the damage done to his mind by masturbation. According to the father, *the child through his sinful habit was murdering his own soul!*

I believe that *my* constructions do not contradict the facts which, thanks to Niederland, have become known about Schreber's father. Therefore I conceive of this information regarding the father as corroborating the correctness of my constructions.

How can we use the newly acquired knowledge of Daniel Paul Schreber's reactions to his father's methods of child rearing? A new conclusion has to be drawn. The night of numerous nocturnal emissions marked the beginning of Schreber's psychosis proper. The patient tried desperately to prevent a repetition of this excitement which would result in an orgasm. Nevertheless, the *Denkwürdigkeiten* contains evidence of the daily recurrence of sexually stimulating situations. Here my constructions are of help. *They reveal that these exciting situations were based upon Schreber's childhood experiences when he was stimulated by his father as well as by his brother.* His relationship to his brother dominates the period of his beginning psychosis. Schreber felt persecuted by Flechsig. At this point many problems arise. I shall concentrate upon what I consider the two most prominent ones. Which psychotic reactions were used by Schreber to ward off the danger involved in an orgasm? And why was his brother replaced by Flechsig, and his father by God?

I start with the danger situation. After the night when Schreber's desire to be a woman submitting to intercourse was satisfied in his dreams, he no longer was able to maintain reality testing. The fulfillment of this desire meant acceptance of castration. As a result of this castration danger, Schreber surrendered his reality testing. However, his becoming psychotic did not in itself guarantee that the same desire would not return (Katan, 1954, 1974). If in his psychotic state the same desire should be satisfied again, he would no longer be able to escape castration.

What changes does the surrender of reality testing create in the mind of the patient? His reality as far as it is connected with the danger situation will disappear. This implies that the reality ego, which maintains the function of reality testing, no longer exists; neither will the objects which contribute to stimulating the patient's feminine desires exist anymore. It is not only the representations of the male objects that will drop out of the picture. Schreber's wife, for instance, by leaving him for four days, no longer afforded him protection against the homosexual attraction of Flechsig and his male retinue. Mrs. Schreber became the target of her husband's aggression; she was the first to become a person who was only "fleetingly" alive, "made there" by a wonder.

Accordingly, surrender of reality testing leads to a regression to the undifferentiated state (Hartmann, 1939; Freud, 1940; Katan, 1940) of that part of the total personality which is involved in the danger situation. Such a conclusion would mean, for instance, that neither ego nor objects would exist. There is no separation between self and outside world, between consciousness and unconsciousness; secondary process thinking is not possible.

Yet the occurrence of psychotic symptoms seems immediately to contradict the existence of the undifferentiated state. Indeed, the undifferentiated state can be maintained only as long as stimuli are absent. For instance, how will a beginning homosexual danger be warded off? For this stimulus does not disappear when the reality ego dissolves itself. What reaction does this stimulus evoke in the state of undifferentiation?

In order to find a solution to this problem, I turn to the beginning of normal development. At this early stage, various stimuli force the undifferentiated state to undergo a change. These stimuli are a threat to the state of primary narcissism which is inherent in the undifferentiated state. A primordial ego develops, which acts according to the pleasure-pain principle. It considers everything pleasurable as belonging to the self, and everything disagreeable as belonging outside of the self. By reacting in this way, the primordial ego strives to maintain a state of primary narcissism.

This description is useful in understanding what happens in a psychosis. A part of the total personality has regressed to the undifferentiated state. However, this form of flight away from a danger is unable to cause a dangerous stimulus to disappear. The patient has been tempted to yield to a homosexual stimulus, and this stimulus has already begun to create a genital excitement. That part of the ego which has surrendered reality testing has been transformed through regression into a primordial ego as it exists at the beginning of mental development.

At this point it is necessary to make a distinction between the vicissitude of the excitement already formed and the vicissitude of the homosexual stimulus. The excitement has to be discharged; the homosexual stimulus must be prevented from again creating such a sexual excitement.

Let me focus, first, on the process of discharge. In the undifferentiated state, only primary process thinking is possible. I wish to emphasize that the functioning of this process becomes observable to any clinician who is willing to keep his eyes open. The absence of an orgasm as a sign that the genital excitement has reached a climax proves that the ego has been able to prevent such a result. This result came about because the ego surrendered its reality testing on the basis of the expectation of the havoc which would be created by such an orgasm. However, the excitement has not disappeared and exerts its influence on the undifferentiated state. Through the process of displacement, it makes itself felt in another organ, one which is remote from the genital area. *The result is that the displaced stimulus, which is the derivative of the sexual excitement, is perceived as a hallucination in one of the sensory organs and is no longer felt as originating in the genital area. The hallucination is a discharge phenomenon.* Generally, certain features are connected with the hallucination, pointing to the genital origin of the hallucinatory perception. Sometimes hallucinations are perceived in the motoric sphere instead of in a sensory organ, and there are other occasions when an orgasm cannot be prevented. Without discussing these "exceptions," I can assert that they do not constitute any obstacle to this theory. They can all be brought within its frame.

The hallucination impresses the observer as being a psychotic defense mechanism. But is this correct? Does the reality ego, when it dissolves itself, know that the hallucination will follow? The hallucinatory reaction appears because secondary process thinking in that part of the personality is no longer possible. The state of undifferentiation enables the energy contained in the excitement to find its way, by means of displacement, to other sensory organs. These organs will be chosen according to previous fixations. Thus it appears that the ego does not participate in this hallucinatory process of discharge, and, according to my view, this process should be called a reaction—not a defense.

The discharge of the excitement does not mean that the homosexual stimulus has also disappeared. In 1974 I tried to make clear that the defensive quality of the hallucination is limited. The hallucination prevents a dangerous orgasm from occurring, but it is unable to prevent the genital stimulation from being renewed. In order to support the discharge function of the hallucination, a delusion frequently follows, which tries to take care of that part of the danger situation which is not covered by the hallucination. This delusion tries to prevent a genital stimulation from occurring at all.

The explanation, based on my new insight, is that after the sexual excitement has been discharged through a hallucination, the homosexual stimulus is still present. The primordial ego wards off the stimulus by accusing its originator of being the persecutor.

Let me give a brief example. Chapter 6 of the *Denkwürdigkeiten* contains a description of a series of hallucinations, each of which deals with the destruction of a part of the universe. This series of hallucinations is followed by the delusion that the world has come to an end. The men whom Schreber saw around him were only "fleetingly made there" and existed only as long as they were within the range of his observation. He thought they were revived from death for this brief period of time. I explained (1949) that this delusion served the purpose of preventing these men from stimulating Schreber genitally. I deduced that after a period of approximately two years Schreber was able to suppress his erections. As a result he discovered that the men around him were not dead at all. The genital urge had been forced to regress to an anal level. Although Schreber still felt persecuted, the persecutions assumed an anal character.

I shall now discuss the remaining problem: why, in Schreber's psychosis, was his brother replaced by Flechsig, and his father by God? My constructions clearly reveal that Schreber as a child was sexually stimulated by his father and his brother, resulting in solitary masturbatory activity as far as his father was concerned, and in mutual masturbation with his brother. When Schreber became psychotic—he was then over 50 years old—these childhood events were revived. His father and his brother had both been dead for many years. The question arises: were God and Flechsig transference figures standing for Schreber's father and brother? Such a statement seems to be immediately contradicted by the well-known fact that the schizophrenic patient, at least in that part of the personality which is psychotic, does not form transference relationships.

I have stated (1974) that cases of schizophrenia offer an unparalleled opportunity to study the psychotic mind at the moment of transition from a situation in which the ego is still governed, although tenuously, by a more realistic attitude toward a state in which the ego has surrendered reality testing. I repeat, in this latter state the reality ego has ceased to exist.

I shall therefore consider the situation in which Schreber was not yet psychotic and the presence of Flechsig recalled to Schreber the childhood event when he was seduced by his brother. In this early, still reality-oriented situation Flechsig was indeed a transference figure representing the brother. In this transference situation, a displacement took place in the id from the brother to Flechsig. However, in a transference, both id and ego are involved. The ego participates in the feelings for the therapist, which feelings originate in the id. In the regular analytic treatment of a neurotic, the analyst can interpret this transference, and through this interpretation the neurotic patient's ego will gain in strength.

Schreber's ego, however, as soon as the psychosis started, had to face the insurmountable castration danger resulting from his feminine homosexual transference feelings for Flechsig. As soon as this transference relationship led to a genital stimulation, the ego dissolved itself. With this dissolution of the reality ego, a regression to the undifferentiated state took place. Through this regression, the transference situation ceased to exist. Yet the genital excitement which had already started to develop could not be undone by the process of regression. The existing genital excitement was discharged through a hallucination, in the content of which "Flechsig formerly was named as the primal instigator of soul murder." The content of the hallucination pointed to Flechsig as being the persecutor. In connection with the hallucination, perhaps even independent of its content, Schreber accused Flechsig of having destroyed the wonderful plan for the hereafter. The chain of events as I have just described it, beginning with transference feelings for Flechsig, ended with the formation of a persecutory delusion, Flechsig being the persecutor. Through this delusion, Schreber tried to prevent an eventual transference situation involving Flechsig from leading to a genital stimulation.

Nevertheless, one has to conclude that the combination of hallucination and delusion does not form a psychotic reaction which for long will destroy the formation of transference phenomena. Schreber's permanent hallucinations became daily occurrences which continued almost uninterruptedly. This fact proves that genital stimulations are continually renewed so that the psychotic reactions have to be repeated accordingly.

I conclude that the nonpsychotic part of the personality still maintains a contact, although a limited one, with the outside world. In this part, transference relationships are repeatedly renewed, and as soon as they assume a stimulating influence, a hallucination will result. Every separate one of these transference relationships will be destroyed by the psychotic reaction formation.

I now feel sufficiently prepared to come to grips with the problem I formulated at the beginning of this paper. One might ask whether a contradiction exists between the psychotic reaction formations which prevent the development of genital excitement on the one hand, and their contents referring to memories of sexual events in childhood on the other. Freud (1915a) emphasized that the hallucinatory sound of knocking or throbbing was derived from his patient's clitoral sensation of throbbing as a sign of her sexual excitement. Similarly, in Schreber's case, the references to childhood sexual events in the contents of his hallucinations and delusions served as a warning that a repetition of the orgastic experience which had ushered in the psychosis proper should be avoided at all costs.

A final problem remains: why does the patient not recognize the various features contained in his hallucinations and delusions as constituting a return of his own childhood memories? Earlier I stated that in order for the psychotic defense mechanisms to develop, the preceding transference relationship must be thoroughly destroyed. The existence of this transference relationship is an essential prerequisite for the recognition that these contents of the psychotic symptoms are memories of childhood events. This prerequisite was absent in Schreber's case. The primary process had taken over, bringing with it the absence of a time regulation in the unconscious. The patient then experienced these events as occurring in the present and caused by Flechsig.

I now expect to be reminded that the patient's mind is not totally psychotic. A greater or lesser part remains in which an ego is still present, and this remaining part maintains some contact with reality. Why does this part of the ego not recognize its own memories? The answer is very simple. This part was not involved in the danger situation and therefore is unable to understand what went on in the psychotic part. Just as we do not understand our dreams, so the more normal ego parts of the psychotic personality are unable to gain insight into these intricate processes.

In my deliberations I have touched upon two new subjects. Can the schizophrenic patient be analyzed? Are dream and psychosis similar processes, or are they different?

I hope I have made it clear that, as I see it, the psychotic part of the patient cannot be reached by our efforts. Our therapeutic endeavors should be directed toward the nonpsychotic part of the personality. We should try to increase the strength of the ego, remembering that this ego is present only in the part which is not psychotic. We hope that an increase in ego strength would enable the ego to master conflicts which it previously was unable to do. This would mean that the ego would become less susceptible to situations in which it originally was forced to surrender reality testing.

To me, it still remains a problem whether one should try to strengthen the nonpsychotic ego through psychoanalysis or whether one should instead attempt to obtain some results through management of the patient. Shortly before the death of Frieda Fromm-Reichmann, I attended a psychiatric meeting at which she described her method of treating schizophrenic patients. I believe that her method was a form of management, in the application of which she excelled. It would seem, from the method she applied, that she was trying to establish a mother-child relationship with the patient in which she presented herself as the mother who was willing to accept the child under any and all circumstances. Of course, such a method also would have its drawbacks, but in view of the severity of the illness, this type of treatment is certainly preferable either to an analysis with very slim chances of succeeding or to drug treatment which would render the patient unfit for any metapsychological understanding by the observer.

The comparison between dream and psychosis leads to a deepening of our insight into both phenomena. They have the primary process in common. Yet this primary process is used quite differently in the dream than in the psychosis. The dream takes place during sleep, the psychosis in waking life. "A dream can be described as a piece of fantasy in the service of the maintenance of the sleep" (Freud, 1925, p. 127). I have changed "working on behalf of" in the English translation to "in the service of." I do this not only because Freud uses the words "in the service of" but also because "in the service of the ego" has become the commonly used connotation for a defense mechanism. Thus the ego, in order to defend the sleep, applies primary process thinking. In order to use secondary process thinking, the ego must wake up. The dream may have the same content as a delusion, but, in contrast to the dreamer, the psychotic is unable to deal in waking life with his conflicts by secondary process thinking. Accordingly, the psychotic is forced to regress toward primary process thinking.

Therefore, what the ego of the dreamer, by relying upon the primary process, does out of relative ego strength, the psychotic in waking life does out of ego weakness!

I hope my discussion has made it clear how far apart Schatzman's view is from my own. The word "soul murder" belongs to the ground-language, and this word denotes the opinion of Schreber's father about the disastrous effects that masturbation will have on the child. Accordingly, I think the title of Schatzman's book results from a misconception.

I shall not discuss differences of opinion with other authors. Let me point in this respect to Freeman's article (1970) on Arlow and Brenner's theory about psychotic development.

In this paper I have strongly emphasized the value of constructions. We cannot do without them in the analysis of the neurotic patient. They form the foundation for his improvement (Katan, 1939, 1969). To point out the value of constructions is perhaps the most important task in our supervisory analyses. In our evaluation of the psychological insight of the creative writer, it is necessary to form a solid construction of some of his works. And in the schizophrenic patient, although in my opinion a construction will not have a therapeutic effect, it will open up surprising insights into the abnormal functioning of the human mind. Thus the construction, instead of being a cerebral endeavor—an opinion held frequently by those who try to cook their meal on the analytic stove[2]—is essential for the entire field of analysis. Through his constructions, the analyst reveals himself to be in the service of helping the patient as well as in the service of furthering science.

[2] I believe this description is an approximation of a remark of Freud's. I am unable to locate the exact place.

BIBLIOGRAPHY

FREEMAN, T. (1970), The Psychopathology of the Psychoses. *Int. J. Psycho-Anal.*, 51:407–415.
―― (1974), The Prepsychotic Phase and the State of Partial Regression. Read at the Hampstead Clinic, London.
FREUD, S. (1911), Psycho-Analytic Notes on an Autobiographical Account of a Case of Paranoia (Dementia Paranoides). *S.E.*, 12:3–82.
―― (1912), Recommendations to Physicians Practising Psycho-Analysis. *S.E.*, 12:109–120.
―― (1915a), A Case of Paranoia Running Counter to the Psycho-Analytic Theory of the Disease. *S.E.*, 14:261–272.
―― (1915b), Instincts and Their Vicissitudes. *S.E.*, 14:109–140.
―― (1925), Some Additional Notes on Dream-Interpretation As a Whole. *S.E.*, 19:125–138.
―― (1937), Constructions in Analysis. *S.E.*, 23:255–269.
―― (1940), An Outline of Psycho-Analysis. *S.E.*, 23:141–207.
HARTMANN, H. (1939), *Ego Psychology and the Problem of Adaptation*. New York: Int. Univ. Press, 1958.
KATAN, M. (1939), Der psychotherapeutische Wert der Konstruktionen in der Analyse. *Int. Z. Psychoanal.*, 24:172–176.
―― (1940), Die Rolle des Wortes in der Schizophrenie und Manie. *Int. Z. Psychoanal.*, 25:138–173.
―― (1949), Schreber's Delusion of the End of the World. *Psychoanal. Quart.*, 18:60–66.
―― (1954), The Importance of the Non-Psychotic Part of the Personality in Schizophrenia. *Int. J. Psycho-Anal.*, 35:119–128.
―― (1959), Schreber's Hereafter. *This Annual*, 14:314–382.
―― (1960a), Discussion of Niederland (1959). Abst. in *Psychoanal. Quart.*, 29:302.
―― (1960b), Dream and Psychosis. *Int. J. Psycho-Anal.*, 41:341–351.
―― (1966), The Origin of *The Turn of the Screw*. *This Annual*, 21:583–635.
―― (1969), The Link between Freud's Works on Aphasia, Fetishism and Constructions in Analysis. *Int. J. Psycho-Anal.*, 50:547–553.
―― (1974), The Development of the Influencing Apparatus. *This Annual*, 29:473–510.
NIEDERLAND, W. G. (1959), The "Miracled-Up" World of Schreber's Childhood. *This Annual*, 14:383–413.
SCHATZMAN, M. (1972), *Soulmurder: Persecution in the Family*. New York: Random House.
SCHREBER, D. P. (1903), *Denkwürdigkeiten eines Geisteskranken*. Leipzig: Mutze.
SÉGLAS (1927), In: G. Jelgersma, *Leerboek der Psychiatrie*, 1:87. Amsterdam: Scheltema & Holkema.

An Unexpected Result of the Analysis of a Talented Musician

JEROME D. OREMLAND, M.D.

FROM ITS VERY BEGINNINGS, PSYCHOANALYSIS HAS BEEN INTERESTED IN talent and creativity. The understanding of exceptional abilities has closely paralleled the understanding of symptoms and pathological character traits. Because of this relationship, there has long been a concern as to the fate of exceptional abilities during therapeutic psychoanalysis. Initially, psychoanalysis tended to see insight as a threat to talent and creativity.

With more biographical and direct clinical study, there has been a trend toward understanding exceptional abilities as having origins separate from, though at times intrinsically involved with, pathological structures. Kris (1952) led the way by emphasizing the relationship of exceptional ability to flexibility in psychic organization. Weissman (1971) noted that psychoanalytic terminology tends to "accentuate the unintended conception that creativity and infantile neurosis, rather than creativity and infantile development, are inseparably interwoven" (p. 402). Greenacre (1957) cautioned against emphasizing the narcissistic aspects of creativity. She described the artist's greater varieties and flexibilities in object

---

Chief of Psychiatry, San Francisco Children's Hospital and Adult Medical Center; Faculty, San Francisco Psychoanalytic Institute.

I wish to thank Dr. Phyllis Greenacre, Dr. Calvin F. Settlage, and Dr. Albert J. Solnit for many specific formulations which elucidated a number of perplexing clinical issues and substantially increased the theoretical scope for understanding them.

relationships, "collective alternates," and related this to innate extraordinary sensorimotor-conceptual endowment. Jacobson (1964) proposed that the intermittent unity characterizing the creative person's involvement in his creative work reflected a drive "elasticity and fluidity" which enables him to "hypocathect temporarily all other objects" and related this capacity to "a particularly favorable vicissitude of their orality" (p. 81). Erikson (1954) vividly described the creative capacity "at the height of consummation [as the ability] to identify with father, mother, and newborn child all in one" (p. 49).

The relationship of talent to creativity is complex and unclear. The *Webster's New World Dictionary* (1960) defines talent as "a special, superior ability," and creativity as causing "to come into existence; originate." Etymologically, talent comes from the Greek *talanion*, a balance, a thing weighed. *Talentum* was a Roman unit of weight or money, suggesting the relationship of talent to the ability to discriminate, but also giving it a commercial connotation; whereas creativity probably comes from an Indo-European base, *kere*, meaning to cause to grow.

General usage reflects these meanings and tends to differentiate between talent and creativity around the crucial dimension of originality. Although there is obvious overlap, talent tends to emphasize a highly developed skill, while creativity squarely emphasizes originality.

This paper reports on an unexpected result of the psychoanalysis of a young musician whose talent hid creative ability. As his oedipal conflict unfolded in the analysis, it could be seen with unusual clarity that his playing the music of others, talented as it was, was in large measure involved in neurotic conflict in that it expressed and at the same time inhibited exhibitionistic desires. As the conflicts moved toward resolution, his ability to use his talent was severely interfered with. During the working through process, he discovered within himself a creative ability—he began to compose.

Case Presentation

Tom had just turned 20 when his father called, asking if I would see his son. The father was very worried about Tom's excessive use of marijuana.

Some eight years earlier when Tom was 12, the father had been in psychotherapy with me for severe alcoholism. He was a hearty, good-natured, very overweight man whose profession required much travel with long periods away from home. He had fully experienced the Depression, was constantly fearful of unemployment, and all but worshipped the idea of the "Good Job." He had a strong tendency toward an obsequiousness with professionals and educated people. His therapy with me was permeated with respect for my authority and wishes that I guide him. Hostility was always indirect, passive-aggressive, or displaced. He had strong beliefs, was politically conservative, and was always quick to stereotype. Although he was involved in an obvious father-son relationship with his employer, he felt intense contempt for people who were "weak" and "parasitic." This largely expressed itself as contempt for "colored people," welfare recipients, and to a lesser extent, "youths who don't take advantage of what is given to them."

I saw the father for three and a half years in twice-a-week psychotherapy. During that time, he lost his job, separated from the family, and had several turns in jail for drunken driving and other misdemeanors associated with drunkenness. Despite the tumultuous times, he regularly continued his therapy, and we were gradually able to put his life back together. He regained employment, maintained sobriety, and rejoined his family when Tom was 15. Since the completion of his treatment more than five years prior to my first seeing Tom, the father has remained sober, advanced steadily at work, and on rare occasions called me to have a "chat."

The mother, a pediatric nurse, was industrious, efficient, managing, and conservative. She shared her husband's beliefs, but without the rancor or vehemence. She had a strong sense of "place" and a feeling of "God's will" in the order that she desired. Tom was their only child.

INITIAL EVALUATION

Tom explained that although seeing me had been his father's idea, he was himself very eager to seek help, sensing that his drug use was "way out of control." He was an unusually handsome, well-built, young man, who had a good deal of his father's likableness and engaging qualities. As in his father, underlying his eagerness to please were depression and contempt.

He explained that he was a "rock 'n' roll musician," a trombonist, playing with a very well-known rock group. He was a part-time student of music at a nearby university. It was clear that he was a serious musician who studied hard, practiced hard, and played with care. I was struck by his wide knowledge of the history of music, composition theory, and musical form. He had an exceptional ability to conceptualize his interests, his feelings, his musical aspirations, as well as a discerning criticism of fellow musicians.

He told me that his major interest was jazz, which he characterized as endless variation; and his chief dislike was rock, which he saw as endless repetition. He lamented having to work in rock, but asserted that "the fact of the matter is, there are no jobs in jazz." At that time, the mid-60s, there was a tremendous, ever-increasing, apparently never-ending demand for rock. His group was one of the best, widely acclaimed locally, and gaining national recognition.

He deeply regretted the situation in music at that time. With bitterness, he gave an all too vivid, yet poignant picture of the world of the rock musician—set upon set, flashing lights, screaming girls, "everyone high on something; no one real; never sure when you're real." The total emphasis was on volume and the bizarre. "I couldn't do it without grass" was presented, not as an excuse, but as a simple fact. He emphasized the need to blunt his mind in order to stand there hour after hour, immersed in the din.

He rather ashamedly indicated that he was still living at home, even though there was constant fighting, mostly centered around his attacking his parents' "bigotry" and their nagging concerns about his "style of life"; however, he frequently stayed at the apartments of fellow musicians, especially after a "gig." He indicated that he had the best of both worlds, "the straight and the hip," in that "she [mother] keeps my clothes clean, feeds me when I want her to, I can use her car when mine breaks down, I often borrow money from her, and never repay her." In general, "I do what I want to when I want to." This was presented in a self-critical way, emphasizing his distaste for the unbridled quality to his "selfishness." "I give to no one. I don't know if I can."

After some exploratory sessions, I suggested analysis, to which he eagerly agreed. We met four times a week, with occasional interruptions necessitated by tours, until the completion of the analysis nearly five years later.

THE BEGINNING OF ANALYSIS

In the first sessions, Tom commented on his feeling that "You know more about me than I do."[1] This continued to come up in many forms throughout our work together. Most often he described it as "sort of like talking to an uncle or an old family friend." Several times early in our work, he remembered his mother during the height of the difficulties in the family, praying to God with him to "help and strengthen" the father. Later they prayed together to God that Dr. Oremland could help the father. He remembered at those times being intensely curious about me, wondering what I "did to" the father. He recalled vague fantasies of my being some sort of hypnotist, forcing his father to do certain things and punishing him for not doing others.

Gradually Tom clarified his main concern: feeling cut off from people and life itself. Friends, girls, his studies, music, all had lost meaning to him.

He described intense resentment toward his parents, mostly his father, and had some awareness of difficulties with anyone in authority over him. His feelings toward peers were a mixture of contempt and longing. He knew he used arrogance and indifference

---

[1] Only some of the many ways, *expected* and *unexpected*, in which my having seen his father in therapy affected the transference, the countertransference, and, indeed, the whole course of the analysis will be detailed. I shall emphasize only those aspects which are most centrally related to the understanding of the development of Tom's talent and the eventual uncovering of his creativity. Other significant areas (e.g., the quick transference tie of Tom's marijuana addiction to his father's treated alcoholism; the fact that my knowing the father seemed to give Tom increased license to be angry with his father who was then less easily damaged), although of technical and theoretical interest, will not be discussed here.

as powerful tools, at times consciously. Other times, however, it was as though these attitudes seized him. He then felt a "glass wall" descending between him and others.

Marijuana both put him in contact with and separated him from people. Its use went far beyond the need to get through concerts as first described. He feared he was "addicted to it" as he sensed his fear of being without it. In a striking way he noted the parallel to his music.

His seeking therapy had been precipitated by a specific incident with a girl. He recounted how following the nightly concerts, routinely the girls would line up before the musicians pleading to be taken home by them. He would select one (sometimes several), take her to a fellow musician's place, go through the motions of sexual play and intercourse, to awaken the next morning scarcely aware of who she was or what had happened.

One night when he was having intercourse, the girl pleaded, "Tell me you love me." He looked down and for the first time saw her face. He said, "I love you . . . ," realizing that he did not even know her first name. He immediately stopped, got dressed, and silently walked into the night. All he could think was, "What has become of me? What am I? I feel nothing."

Early the next morning, he went to his favorite place, a very beautiful grove of redwood trees near his home, to watch the sunrise. He took a large dose of LSD, something he rarely did, hoping "I could reach out, break out of it, feel something." He found himself zipping up his jacket, putting his hands into his pockets, and curling up into a ball. He began to sob uncontrollably, but there were no tears. That evening he talked with his father, unable to tell him what he felt, but saying he needed help in controlling his use of marijuana.

Gradually the sessions became repetitious with severe denouncements of his parents and society at large. He blamed his parents for having given him various fears, and strongly intimated that they had in many ways crippled him. He complained bitterly of being kept dependent by his family, especially his mother, and about "the hypocrisy and ignorance" of his father. Throughout this was the implication that I agreed with him and an expectation that I, through my influence, would change them.

THE SUPERPARENT FANTASY

This hope was elaborated into the theme of my being "the superparent" who would change the parents so that "she won't need me" and who would change the father so that "I won't feel such contempt for him." As this was identified, he sensed his enormous fear of leaving home and his dealing with this by tempting his parents to throw him out. His provocative behavior, the marijuana, the social views, and his sexual life reassured him that he was highly different and independent from his family.

As we clarified the extent of his fears, the superparent fantasy took on new meaning. He remembered that early, perhaps even at age 3 or 4, he had had a recurrent feeling that he was his own father; he also described a somewhat formalized "daydream" in which he saw himself as the parent to his parents. In early childhood, he had had a recurring fantasy of talking "man-to-man" with his father's employer to get him to improve his father's position and effectiveness. This fantasy of getting the employer to help the father mounted as the father's drinking became more noticeable and interfered with the family's functioning.

At this time in our work, Tom began to understand that the fantasy of my being some kind of hypnotist to his father was a reedition of his old fantasies. In short, he always saw the father as needing "strengthening" from another man, at first himself, then himself through the employer, later God, and still later "the magical Dr. Oremland," with the implied hope that Tom himself would thereby be "strengthened." Now again, Tom would through me "strengthen" the father, thus solving his conflicts over his father's passivity and his mother's possessiveness. It stunned him when he saw the parallel between his imploring me to solve the problem and his mother's praying to God.

As the material about his contempt for the father's "ignorance" and "weakness" developed, the central part that music and his instrument played in his life presented itself.

THE INSTRUMENT

Tom began playing the trombone when he was 7. The particular instrument was selected largely on the basis of availability. There was a trombone in the family which had been left there by a former neighbor. When Tom expressed interest in music, his mother suggested he use that instrument because they had it. He quickly showed unusual talent for music and the instrument. His mother was very encouraging and protective of his interest. His father was afraid it would "sissify" him.

By the time Tom was 10, the family situation was openly unstable. The father drank very frequently. Often there were violent outbursts, usually directed toward Tom and his music, after which the father would leave home, not to return for several days. This behavior justified and cemented the closeness between Tom and his mother, and the trombone became the major symbol of this bond. Tom consciously sensed its power to anger the father and please the mother. It gave him a feeling of control over them, even to knowing that he could drive the father from the family. When Tom was 12, the father was asked to leave, apparently for good.

ADOLESCENCE

As Tom approached age 13, he gained an enormous amount of weight. Although he constantly dieted, his belly became pendulous, nearly covering his penis, and his hips became large and rounded with folds of fat. Most distressing were the enlarging nipples and the developing breasts. He became the typical prepubertal fat boy (Stolz and Stolz, 1951). His misery was furthered by a markedly delayed puberty.

At school Tom was the object of intense teasing. Even clothed, he was teased about his "teats." Gym came to epitomize his horror. His intense shame of his body and his poor coordination made him the scapegoat of the class. He was nicknamed "Tillie" and was always the last to be chosen for any team. Even the gym teachers joined in the taunting. He remembered one saying, "Well, the class is co-ed." His father added to the torment by calling him "sissy," "fatty," and "Mommie's boy."

One time, during the height of this fat period, when he was about 14, a group of boys invited him to play with them. Tom was fearful to accept for he knew they had been leaders in the torment. However, he agreed, half hoping that this heralded a change in attitude. They all met after school at a nearby playground. Suddenly they pounced on him, stripped him naked, and ran off with his clothes, yelling, "Look, no balls at all." He was paralyzed with fear, humiliation, and anger. His only thought was a wish that he could disappear. He longed to be dead. He never, even during the analysis, was able to recover the memory of how he got home. It was as though his "mind stopped working."

BLUES AND JAZZ

During this time, Tom's father was fired from his job, was recognized as an alcoholic, frequently spent time in jail, and was in regular treatment with me. Jeers of "Your father is an alky" added further humiliation. Tom began to have fantasies and dreams of his father being killed in horrible ways and suffering agonizing deaths. At the height of this, one time he awoke in the middle of the night, terrified and unable to breathe. He was sure he had killed his father. This changed to the idea that the father had crashed his car in a drunken stupor. Tom was sure he had had a nightmare, but could not remember it. He tried to sleep, but could not. He lay in bed sobbing. Suddenly be became horror-struck by the thought that he would have to live with his mother for the rest of his life. He was gripped by fear of her, wondering if he could ever free himself from her. He felt he had no one, anywhere.

His main solace was his trombone, and his playing took on a new quality. As he said, "I spoke to it and it spoke to me. When I couldn't stand it anymore, I would play. When I played, I cried into it." Gradually he found the blues and mournful jazz and knew it was "my music."

AN IMPORTANT CHANGE

When Tom was 15, his father returned home in control of his alcoholism and again became successful in his profession. Tom greeted his return and recovery with mixed feelings. He resented his intrusion into their lives and keenly felt betrayed by his mother's "taking him back." However, there was also a feeling of relief.

When Tom was 17 he rejoiced over some beginning signs of puberty. Gradually he noticed that his body was thinning and shaping. He felt "reborn." He also noted that he was gaining a coterie of friends, primarily because of his trombone playing. He was playing in dance bands at school, and in some small jazz combos professionally.

By the end of his senior year Tom was markedly successful socially, highly sought after by boys and girls, though never really trusting any relationship. Always there was the lingering fear that at any moment they might turn on him. By 18 he was fully pubertal, had a remarkably excellent physique, and was regarded as unusually handsome and talented. Although he knew his shyness reflected tremendous social inhibitions, he sensed its appeal. He knew that providing music for others to dance kept him from becoming involved.

THE FIRST GIRLFRIEND

As the initial hope that his coming to see me would change his parents faded, Tom fully sensed that he needed them to change so that he would not have to leave them. As he experienced the extent of his fear of leaving home and the role his provocative behavior with his parents played in helping him deny his anxiety, the fighting at home lessened.

He became friendly with his group's singer, Katie, a girl some 6 years older than he. He laughed as he recognized that she, like his mother, was a nurse. He felt it was an accomplishment when he decided to live with her. He moved in, at first hiding it from his family, and later excessively exhibiting it before them. He saw it as evidence of improvement, really a cure, and felt sure that he had completed the analysis.

Clearly, the overriding quality to the relationship with Katie was overt nurturing. She repaired his clothes, bathed and fed him. She stroked him and openly admired him, his body, his penis, and his music. They talked a great deal about feelings and emotions, and he felt a great complementarity between his analysis and what he was learning and experiencing with her.

As I pointed out some of the mothering aspects and indicated that he was making us into ideal parents, Tom became increasingly critical of me, gradually turning more vituperative. He indicated that I was jealous of his youth, his talent, and his future. As he acknowledged his making me first into an ideal and later into a jealous father, he began to fear that I might want him all to myself. I interpreted how I, the jealous father, was becoming an engulfing mother. As I pointed out the passive implications of these thoughts, he discussed fears of femininity.

Tom repeatedly and painfully remembered the events of his "fat period" and his hatred of the "big-breasted, fat-hipped monster." Over and over he bitterly recounted the experience of being stripped naked. All that he wanted to hide had been exposed. He sensed how accurately their jeering reflected his own inner feelings about himself, especially the "no balls at all."

Concurrently, a variety of problems with Katie developed. At times he felt that she was keeping him from gaining experience with other girls, and other times that he could not survive without her. During the sessions he would have elaborate fantasies of being the great "stud." He talked of the various musicians who "screwed every girl they could," and dreamed of tours which would end in huge orgies in which he had many girls. The provocative exhibitionistic quality was very clear, as was a developing fear that I was about to "kick him out of analysis." The relationship of this to his feeling that *he* had kicked out his father, with its multiple reversals, was readily apparent.

AN UNSUSPECTED ASPECT OF THE EARLY RELATIONSHIP WITH THE MOTHER

As Tom talked increasingly about his earliest years, the main emphasis was on his father's absences and possible infidelities. As he elaborated these ideas, he interwove stories of the sexual feats of musicians on tours, emphasizing the ubiquitous infidelity of musicians to their wives and his own struggle in being faithful to Katie.

I introduced the idea that the fantasies about his father's infidelities were related to Tom's having been left alone with his mother, and the feeling of freedom and excitement when his father was away.

When Tom talked with his mother about this early period of his life, he was surprised to learn that she had returned to pediatric nursing shortly after he was born. She attributed this to economic reasons, which Tom, at first, readily accepted, because it supported his ideas of his father's incompetence. As this was discussed in our sessions, he began to question its necessity. He had no memory of housekeepers or baby-sitters. Hesitantly he pressed his mother for information and discovered that even as a very small infant, when he was no more than 2 months, until he was about 3 years, he had been left with a neighbor, the neighbor who eventually left the trombone for him. At age 3 he was placed in nursery school.

Now his father's coming and going took on a new dimension, for Tom began to think about his being left, rather than being left with his mother. He realized he had emphasized his father's leaving in order to hide intense feelings about having been left by his mother. There were thoughts that the trombone, in a curious way, symbolized a reunion with the woman whom he had been left with, a "true" mother.

Although these ideas undermined his conviction of his singular importance to his mother, Tom could not shake a sense that he had a peculiar specialness to her and a confused feeling that she was like a man giving her son to a woman to care for while he (she) worked. This led Tom to question for the first time why he was an only child. Originally he was sure that his mother's having him "was all she needed." For a long time he had had the idea that once having him, she no longer needed his father. Now he wondered why once she had him, she rejected him and became "like a man going off to work."

As Tom pursued these thoughts, he remembered, when he was older, waiting alone for his mother to come home from work. Now he recognized that he felt like a woman waiting for the man to return. During this time, the feeling as to who was father and who was mother, who was husband and who was wife, who was child and who was spouse became more and more confused.

As these themes interwove and reached clarity, Tom realized that the fantasy of his father's infidelities and his intense interest in his fellow musicians' infidelities were related to "her infidelity." He desperately wanted "her infidelity" to be vis-à-vis his father (her love for him). Sadly he acknowledged that "her infidelity" was vis-à-vis him (going to other children). Implied was his own "infidelity"—a longing for the caretaking mother. These ideas were greeted with rage, interest, and a feeling of increasing control over his own promiscuous desires and fantasies.

As Tom discussed these various "infidelities" he sensed a relationship to his early "good boy" behavior. The "good boy who practiced" brought oedipal closeness to the mother, with anticipated oedipal fury from the father. He realized that there had been self-emasculation (abetted by his mother) in order to remain close to her, and saw his late teens as a struggle to gain independence and regain his masculinity. Clearly, his fat period and delayed puberty had been unbearable, but somehow deserved punishments. He felt it an actual castration as he watched other boys develop while he became grotesquely feminine.

Tom sensed that his overeating, like the trombone playing, provided a feeling of controlling (producing) his father's anger. The father's anger over the fatness, like the anger over the practicing, cemented the closeness to the mother and justified Tom's looking to her for solace. There was some glimmer of awareness that the obesity allowed him a relatively nonsexual, essentially infantile, safe closeness to her; more so, he saw it as having made him into a caricature of his "passive, feminine father." Sadly, he acknowledged that he had gotten rid of his father, but in the process became "like him—a worse punishment I can't imagine."

THE TROMBONE AS A PENIS

As these ideas about the "good boy who practiced" were approached, new meanings of the significance of the trombone emerged. He saw the trombone as a detachable penis, discarded and left (hence permissible) for him to use, allowing him to deny and thereby protect his own penis. This was augmented by the fact that it had been urged on him by his mother, who actively endorsed his playing with it before her. At the same time his being the "good boy" (castrated) assured that neither of them needed acknowledge this interplay or that the trombone tormented the father. To Tom it seemed something which she prized more than the father. It was not until the analysis that he questioned whether it might have been more prized by her than he was. His father helped deny its phallic meaning by labeling it "sissy."

These memories were clearly related to one facet of his current performing. At that time the emphasis in rock was on "far-out" dress and hair styles, with each group competing to be more of a "freak-out" than the next. While Tom's group followed this fashion, Tom's dress and appearance were distinctly "clean-cut" and conservative. He was clean-shaven, his hair trimmed, and he wore Edwardian velvet suits. Both he and the members of the group recognized that this gave their group specific appeal. In our sessions, we could sense that he was again the "good boy"—the highly sexually provocative, yet asexual, almost feminine innocent —involved in a "dangerous game."

As this was clarified, we noted a change in his playing. In his extensive solos, Tom increasingly experienced a thrill and a contempt when he would hear the orgastic cries of the girls. At times, he would add a little hip wiggle at the proper moment and would all but "bring down the house" with cheers and screams. He was amused when he recognized the implications of the musicians' jargon for a successful solo, "Getting it up." A failure was labeled "I just couldn't get it up."

A DIFFICULT PHASE

We had nearly completed the second year of analysis when these ideas became central themes. Tom felt he had to leave Katie, because he believed that their relationship helped him avoid experiences with other girls. Sadly they decided to separate.

By this time Tom was an acknowledged "rock star." His playing was highly "charged," extremely versatile, and reaching new heights, which brought him critics' acclaim and great prestige within the group. His "stud" fantasies enormously increased and he began again taking girls "home" from the concerts. Although he feared a return of the feeling of unrelatedness, he sensed that it was hostility rather than unrelatedness that he was experiencing with them. He openly described his delight in having them do various demeaning things with him and having them at his "beck and call." With this, his concern that I was critical of him increased.

The tone of the sessions changed markedly. At first subtly, then openly, Tom was contemptuous of me, especially of my work, which he saw as slow, picky, and uninteresting. I pointed out his "cocky" attitude and his competitive demeaning of me. He frequently was late for appointments, often arriving very sleepy and disheveled. He asked for different appointment hours, and tours required blocks of cancellations. The general feeling was that I must accommodate him.

The tours began as exciting adventures, but quickly became dreary, timeless ordeals. The group traveled together, and was plagued by poor management and the shoddy dealings characteristic of this type of show business. There were constant delays, hideous hotels, all-night parties, and ever-present drugs. Many of the tours were to small towns, where the local police reacted harshly to the musicians. Their rooms were constantly searched; they were often frisked, and sometimes arrested on any pretence. The group's use of drugs was always very high, and Tom's use of marijuana again increased. Amphetamines and cocaine were widely used by the group, and it became difficult for me to ascertain the extent of Tom's drug use.

As sessions became irregular, it was difficult to identify themes. Tom was continuously angry that I let "the straights" treat him the way they did, and he saw me as one of "them." Coupled with this was intense fear that I would abandon him because of his hostile provocative behavior.

As his general physical and mental deterioration became more apparent, I interpreted it as a request that I intervene in his life and take over. Strongly implied was that I should insist that he leave the group and music in general. Tom wanted me to stop his playing, as he wished his father had been strong enough to do. He wanted me to take care of him without his instrument, a wish that his mother might have cared for him for himself rather than as a phallic replacement. At times, he realized that he was testing me to see whether I was the mother who left him or the "mother" who cared for him.

THE LIMP TROMBONE DREAM

One day during this tumultuous period (after about 2¾ years of analysis), Tom reported a dream, which was rare in his analysis.

This dream was remarkably short, frightening, and vividly remembered. In the dream he opened his trombone case and looked at the instrument. As he picked it up, he noticed that the bell was badly dented. He was so upset by the dream that when he awakened, he had to check the instrument to make sure it was undamaged. Throughout the day he felt that something awful was about to happen.

During the following sessions, he was morose and depressed, strongly maintaining that there was little to discuss. The next week, he reported a second dream: "I was playing my trombone to a full house. I was playing very well and had really 'gotten it up' [the solo was being expertly projected]. I noticed that my trombone was beginning to droop. I couldn't believe it; first the bell and then the whole thing. It looked like a Dali painting. I blew harder and harder, trying to inflate it, but it became hopelessly limp in my hands."

The next months were extremely trying. Without question he was "losing my lip," and he and the group were very upset. He had no control over his instrument and dreaded every performance. He incessantly blamed me for interfering with his playing. I pointed out that he was retreating from being "the star," provocative, powerful, and desired, to becoming needy and helpless. I related this to his mounting sense of taunting me and his fear of my reprisal. I indicated his wish to return to being the dependent, castrated "good boy."

Although his distress was severe and his anger with me intense, at no time did he threaten to stop the analysis. In fact, all the factors which had previously made for irregularities now disappeared, and he tenaciously and consistently held on to the sessions.

MASTURBATORY THEMES

Tom began to describe "a masturbatory quality" to his practicing when he was younger and even more so in adolescence. He reflected back on his loneliness as a child and the long hours of practicing while he waited for his mother to return from the hospital or shopping. Practicing truly was a tie with her, a having her there with him when he was alone. Masturbation, which began in his late teens, was compulsively tied to "girlie" magazine pictures. The *unacknowledged* fantasy was that the girl in the magazine pictures was watching him, admiring what he could do as he slid his hand up and down his erect penis. In fact, the picture often was propped right next to his penis and he would watch the girl watching him. Later he reenacted this directly with Katie and in the analysis became aware of the relationship of the practicing to the masturbation. Both expressed his wish to be watched and caressed by his mother. Now he asked which mother, his mother or the mysterious never-to-be-known mother?

Tom began to experience exhibitionistic desires on the couch with fears of erection, and ideas that I was looking at him, admiring his body. He felt young and small as he experienced what he called "inrections" in which his penis "shriveled up" before my gaze. One time he had a quick fantasy on the couch in which I said, "O.K. Show me how small it is." In this fantasy, he opened his pants and there was a large erection, which immediately became small and then large again. I walked over to him, suddenly grabbed his penis, and tried to rip it off.

Tom knew that the large-small oscillation referred to the trombone and was amused as he remembered that when he was a small boy erections had been called "boners," further confirming his conviction that the trombone represented a penis. In addition, he strongly experienced the vacillation between his wanting me to admire him and his fear of my jealousy and retaliation. He knew the "rip it off" was also a holding on to it. He openly desired me to masturbate him as an acceptance of his masculinity and at the same time a taking it away. His masturbation, like the early practicing and later performing, was a holding on to a totally admiring, ever-giving, completely available mother. There was a strong implication that the analysis itself reflected a similar "innocent exhibitionism and hanging on."

As the many facets of this material presented themselves in different contexts over the next several months, Tom played very little and practiced even less. Essentially he was being carried by his group, doing the setups, minimal managerial functions, and minor playing. His criticism of me was intense, and for the first time there were long silences. Inquiries into his thoughts produced little, and interpretations of his disillusionment with me and angry withholding were agreed to.

ORIGINAL TUNES

His disillusionment slowly changed into stark depression with strong feelings of having lost all and feeling nothing but despair. Repeatedly Tom described a "black void" within him. Once during a particularly bleak moment, he said, "It is so real, I can almost reach out and touch it." The hour was tense as he openly berated me for "ruining" his playing. With stifled sobs he expressed his longing to play, to turn to the instrument, but knew he couldn't. At one point he said, "I need someone so badly, I don't know what to do."

Throughout the course of the analysis, indeed as far back as he could remember, Tom frequently had tunes running through his head. As he grew older, at times, he would share these with a fellow musician, who might in turn share his with him. Often this would become a back-and-forth interchange, each elaborating on the tune of the other, interweaving them to develop a melody or a theme. Music was a kind of language reserved for certain friends.

In the analysis, characteristically, the tunes could not be described or communicated to me, although occasionally Tom was tempted to whistle one. It was clear that he often used the tunes running through his head to tease me, at times to separate himself from me, sometimes to tantalize me, and occasionally to lose himself in.

During this bleak period the tunes assumed an enormous importance. Frequently an entire hour was spent in silence, his mind filled with tunes. One time he said, "They're almost a private language with myself." He advanced the idea that long before he began playing his instrument, really since very early childhood, "tunes had filled a void." As he considered this, he realized that a change was taking place. Previously the tunes had been those of others; now he noted that they were original. "They [original tunes] come into my head when I am alone at home; they're there sometimes during the sessions; they occur to me at the oddest times; they just appear in my head." He began writing them down and orchestrating them as numbers for the group.

Tom experimented with using jazz in classical forms and undertook some major compositions. He "found" a trio repeatedly going through his head, thinking that it must represent a bringing together of his family. He laughed when he thought it should be a quartet to include me. The trio was eventually performed at a university recital, with moderate acclaim. At the same time, he worked very hard on numbers for his group, which they used enthusiastically in concerts. They cut several records containing many of Tom's compositions, which received excellent reviews.

During this difficult period Tom realized that his talented playing, although at times containing highly artistic improvisations, had largely been an embellishment of the music of others. In essence, he elaborated on the tunes of others, using another's instrument to delight his mother and destroy his father. The talented playing was an expression of sexual and aggressive exhibitionistic desires, hidden and made safe in that they were not his, but another's. As this was worked through, his talent gradually returned.

A LOSS

By this time Tom was living alone, dating, playing, recording, touring, and composing. One day he came in agitated. His trombone had been "ripped off." Immediately, the words "ripped off" reminded him of the fantasy that I had "ripped it [the penis] off." As he continued, he alternated between nearly uncontrollable hostile outbursts and silent sobbing. He began searching the various pawnshops in the hope that it would turn up, but to no avail. He reluctantly began to accept that he would have to buy a new instrument and begin building "my lip" all over again, a complicated process involving many hours of practice to develop the mouth musculature to the specific characteristics of the new mouthpiece. Vehemently he berated me, insisting that I could not possibly understand such a loss. We discussed his fear of having to select the instrument alone; after all, his old one had always been there, left for him. In this context, we considered his fear of developing on his own.

TERMINATION PHASE

As his loss was discussed, Tom talked about ending the analysis and what it would feel like not having me. One day, after a few weeks, he proudly declared that he had found the right horn. He brought it with him, not to show me, but because he would not let it out of his sight. He was even sleeping with it. He set the case on-end on the floor at the foot of the couch. When he lay down, he was surprised to see it standing there between his feet. He began to laugh, saying that it must look like an erect penis to me. Quickly, he became serious, then sad as he described how different the instrument felt to him. Whereas the old trombone was a part of his body, the new one had to be mastered and controlled.

In the fourth year of the analysis, Tom showed steady improvement in all areas. He was playing with several groups, was highly sought after for his technical skill and his original songs, and was recording and composing. He found himself moving away from the "good boy" image in the group, and was letting his hair and beard grow. He sensed that he was "getting older" and could no longer rely on being the entertaining, highly sexual, innocent-looking boy.

AN IRREPLACEABLE LOSS

One day Tom soberly explained that his father had suddenly become seriously ill and was being operated on that morning. That evening he visited his father. When he saw the various tubes coming out of his father's body, he had an intense urge to pull them out. His first thought was that it was a desire to kill him; but he also sensed it was a desire to make him all well. He felt an intense urge to kiss his father, and did, and they both cried. His father, who knew he was dying, said, "I was such a fool to waste these precious years fighting with you." Tom replied, "Don't blame yourself; all three of us were blind." He visited daily, needing to be with his father as he progressively worsened. During the painful vigil, there was the occasional fleeting thought, "Die already, can't you do anything right?" followed by the most severe self-reproaches. The father died one week later.

During the next weeks, Tom repeatedly had to remind himself

that his father was dead and that he would never see him again. Somehow it did not seem so different. His main memories were of his father's being away. When he thought of his father as dead, which was mainly during our sessions, Tom cried softly. One time he said, "I'm glad you knew him and that you liked each other. It helps me to think that the ideas you have about him are not just the hateful ones I told you." I indicated that this thought was in part an expression of his own positive feelings which he feared to acknowledge.

The next two months were marked by increasing despondency and low productivity. For the first time Tom began drinking. I interpreted that by becoming like his father, Tom could preserve him and at the same time not acknowledge the intensity of his hostility toward the father. He agreed, saying that it was also a pitiful bid to his mother to take him back and care for him as she had for his father. Most clearly he saw it as a wish to begin analysis again, out of his fear that we were coming to an end. He then acknowledged having felt a momentary exhilaration when his father died and he thought, "Now Dr. Oremland can be my father." Of special importance was the intense feeling that drinking made him his father who eventually would be saved by Dr. Oremland. By taking all four of us back to those terrible times when his father had been in treatment with me, he expressed the wish that we could all begin again.

TERMINATION

Tom had now completed nearly five years of analysis, and was playing well, dating, composing, and teaching. His marijuana use was extremely moderate, as was his drinking. He was asked to join a major group on an extensive international tour, playing and composing for them. After weeks of discussion, we decided that this was a good time to end our work together.

In our last session, Tom thought back on how long he had been seeing me and sensed a confusion. He knew it was nearly five years, but at the same time said, "You seem like a family friend, sort of always there." He continued, "I think of our work together in four parts. First I came to complain about my parents and get you to change them. I remember how furious I was at your implying that maybe I needed to change in order to leave them. The second part was the time with Katie. I was sure you were jealous of me and wanted to split us up. I felt totally confused. The third part was the most difficult and unclear. I felt unbearably alone. The fourth part was when my father died. I so much wanted you to replace him as a father. I really was afraid to be a man." He laughed and said, "It's like the classical form of the symphony—four movements."

Discussion

Two particularly interesting aspects of this case are the changing significance of the instrument and music in Tom's life as it was reconstructed in the analysis, and the emergence during the analysis of the ability to create music.

Tom's Talent

The treasured instrument was presented to him in latency, age 7.[2] It quickly and intensely became invested with conflictual aspects of his relationship with his father and mother. In the analysis, Tom placed the trombone in the center of this interaction, seeing it as the symbol of his "bond" with his mother and the "bone of contention" with his father.

It seems that Tom's mother's relationship with his father changed once she had used him to have a child, a son. Shortly thereafter, she returned to work, leaving Tom with a substitute mother. In latency, Tom's trombone became a source of pride for the mother. In this way, on one level, Tom's talented playing was "the result of demands of . . . the parents [mainly the mother] using him as an

---

[2] Phyllis Greenacre, commenting on the timing of the emergence of Tom's talent, noted that "quite a number of children show promise of artistic ability of one kind or another in latency. . . . [Such talent] often goes into eclipse with puberty, and may or may not emerge toward the end of adolescence or later." Strikingly, with Tom each developmental event always changed, usually enhanced, but never "eclipsed" his ability. However, it must be remembered that Tom had a prolonged and distorted latency due to a markedly delayed puberty—a fact that complicates the understanding of his adolescence.

extension of themselves in an attempt to realize some expansive ambitions [largely phallic-exhibitionistic strivings] in which they have felt themselves frustrated" (Greenacre, 1957, p. 56).

It was interesting to study the choice of the instrument. The instrument is itself suggestive: a trombone has expanding characteristics and it had been given to him by his mother. Later, we realized the importance of its having been left for him by the neighbor. Tom had always had the definite feeling that the trombone joined him to and delighted his mother. It was a surprise to learn that it was, perhaps, another "mother" whom he was joining. The importance of the instrument was soon enhanced by the power it gave him over his father.

It was clear that Tom's contempt for his father, directed at his "bigotry and ignorance," was contempt for the father's (and his own) passivity. Throughout Tom's life, in fantasy he often "replaced" his father. In latency and preadolescence Tom's trombone playing was directly linked to the father's demise. When the father was forced to leave the home disgraced, Tom had his ultimate success; his talent was developing.

Nature dealt Tom a cruel blow. Instead of adolescence bringing manhood, a delayed puberty and Tom's defensive hyperbulimia produced a grotesquely feminized body, a caricature of the despised (castrated) father. A punishment was being actualized. All men (peers, teachers, his father) turned on him for what he had done. The *turning on him*, the exposing of what he was, was epitomized by the never forgotten and yet never fully remembered episode of exposure and humiliation on the playground. There was no possible mitigation or resolution of what had happened. Being exposed was the ironic punishment for the exhibitionistic delight in playing his trombone for his mother. This was clearly represented in his adolescent masturbation, at first without fantasies, later with images obsessively tied to "girlie" pictures. In the analysis of the masturbation, he could see the wish for his mother's slavish admiration of his functioning penis, and understand the central place this wish occupied in his playing.

At one point during this painful adolescence, the wished-for death of his father was experienced in repetitious fearful fantasies, culminating in the nightmarish idea of his having killed the father.

Oedipal panic ensued, and with it sudden fear of the mother. He truly had made himself alone. With this, his playing changed from a constant attempt to please others to an inner sobbing. Blues and mournful jazz became his music as he cried out to the world his utter despair and loneliness.

At the height of this, his father returned home, changed by the magical Dr. Oremland. Tom felt betrayed by his mother, but relieved, sensing that the return and presence of the father helped him feel safer with his impulses. Though openly resentful of his father, he felt freer of his mother and markedly decreased his overeating. With physiological adolescence, his body changed rapidly; he felt "reborn," but the scars remained.

Playing allowed him to engage in, and yet be protected from, relationships. He played the music of others so that others could dance, while he felt alone and separate. This became a profession and a way of life. As the public's interest in jazz and blues waned, Tom was forced to play rock. The old exhibitionism and competitive hostility thinly disguised by "innocence" supervened. At this point, his music expressed sexualized contempt, rather than mournfulness. Again, he found himself the "innocent" young man titillating and controlling females. Girls fought for him and needed to possess him; yet all he could find in them was an empty servicing of himself. In despair, he turned to his father for help.

In the analysis, as incestuous exhibitionistic desires began to emerge as a central theme, his playing became "charged." This closely parallels Greenacre's (1957) description of the masturbatory component in talent. In some "the remarkable performance is the result of neurotic conflict with the development of special achievement usually on a somewhat compulsive basis as part of an effort to overcome or counteract a masturbation addiction" (p. 56). The punishment for the incestuous exhibitionistic desires became epitomized in the "limp trombone" dream, after which his playing deteriorated and he was left feeling he had nothing and was alone.

TOM'S CREATIVITY

The discussion thus far has detailed the specific facets of Tom's conflicts which gave exceptional qualities to Tom's skills; his playing was talented. The understanding of his creativity is more elusive.

Where did the original music come from? Tom said, "The tunes are in my head and they keep coming." He was able to systematize them, write them down, elaborate upon them, improve them, and present them. Their being recognized, accepted, enjoyed, and encouraged provided important secondary gratifications. He became a successful composer.

The Meaning of the Trombone

In general the material was strongly oedipal with limited preoedipal elaboration. The transference was largely understood and accepted within the vicissitudes of the relationship with the father, even though there were frequently very clear maternal aspects to the transference. There was a relative paucity of oral factors, even though so much depended on his mouth and his very breathing. Yet there were suggestions of important links between the mystery of the trombone and the mystery of the original music.

Tom discovered that his most cherished memory, that he had had his mother alone, never happened in reality. In its place, he found a mother who was functionally more a father, and a shadowy, unknown "stranger" mother. With this revelation, the oedipal interaction took on an additional complexity. Tom was providing his masculine-striving mother with a sham penis (the trombone) as a protection of his own. This sham penis played a central role in his oedipal struggle.

The limp trombone dream epitomized the incestuous, exhibitionistic motivations and the punishment for them. As the trombone playing lost its defensive function, it was severely interfered with. It was then that he sensed the "black void" inside. At one point during the depth of his despair, "the void" was nearly personified. "I can almost reach out and touch it," he said. It was during this tension-filled hour that he began to realize that his pervasive despair was closely related to an intense longing. He wished to turn to his instrument, but could not. Gradually he conceded that he longed for "a someone."

One can only speculate about the early "stranger" mother, and wonder about the significance of her having left the trombone for him. In this, perhaps, is some glimmer of Jacobson's (1964) "particularly favorable vicissitude of his orality." I suggest that the trombone functioned *primarily* as a transitional object representing the reunion—an oral reunion—with the giving "stranger" mother, and *secondarily* as the phallus for the masculine-striving mother.

Viewed in this dual way, the practicing during his latency and the playing during his adolescence and young adulthood take on an additional meaning. The phallic mother, while enjoying his sham penis, unknowingly encouraged and promoted reunions with the "stranger" mother. Perhaps this is an important factor in understanding why the neurotic structure enhanced rather than interfered with his playing. Her need allowed him primary gratifications. When this synergism was disturbed in the analysis, his playing deteriorated.

Superimposed on this repeated reunion with the "stranger" mother, distorted in the analysis by the fact that I had "saved" the father, is a theme of "strengthening" and implied rebirth. Throughout Tom's life there was a recurring theme of his hope to be reborn out of a "strengthened" parental figure.

There was the very early wish to be the father to himself, which evolved into the fantasy of being the parent to the parents. This developed into the early latency fantasy of seeking out the father's employer to help the father. The mother participated in these "strengthening" fantasies by praying with Tom for God to "strengthen" the father and later for God to "strengthen" me so I could "strengthen" the father. I eventually became the man who "strengthened" the father. In the *hypnotist fantasy* we can see the wish for the powerful father encouraging and scolding the child. Tom came to be changed by the very man who, by "strengthening" the father, had given him a new father.

These fantasies present an unusual variation of the family romance experience. Greenacre (1958) has noted that the response to the family romance is "especially strong in gifted" people. In Tom's version of the family romance, he became the father to himself, to the father, and to the family. In this context, it was striking to learn from Tom that I, as the father's therapist, "participated" in this family romance experience, and subsequently to observe it as a major transference theme in his analysis.

The specific quality of *precocity* in these early fantasies is of special interest in the study of Tom's talent.[3] If seen as an attempt to ward off loss (being the parent to the parent reduces the danger of again losing a parent), such precocity could be an early indication of a developing defensive mode, namely, using a special skill (a talent) to an exaggerated extent in coping with the anxiety associated with a host of developmental issues while other aspects of development are neglected and distorted.

The analysis of the "strengthening" fantasies revealed many complex derivatives of primitive introjection. Although it varied in accord with the developmental level and the *stage* of the analysis, "strengthening" was a condensation of oral incorporation and oral, anal, and umbilical (direct intra-abdominal) insemination. I propose that these "strengthening" fantasies screened and expressed a hidden, repeated, wished-for insemination of, and desire to be reborn from his union with, the inner "void"—the lost, introjected (though not integrated) "stranger" mother. Tom strove to be reborn from the union of himself as his own father with the introjected lost mother.

However, more central in the analysis was Tom's increasing realization of the twofold meaning of the trombone. As a sham penis, the trombone warded off intense castration fears. This was vividly actualized when his trombone was stolen, and he was forced to find and master a new one. In its transitional object functions, the trombone linked Tom to the "stranger" mother. In this regard, perhaps, his general feeling that I knew more about him than he knew about himself and his statement in the last hour, "You seem like a family friend, sort of always there," was a transference reexperiencing of the unknown "stranger" mother, *screened* by the event of my having treated the father. I, like the trombone, came to represent that primary union.

As the analysis brought Tom close to experiencing the sense of castration and the loss of the "stranger" mother, depression ensued. The "black void" that appeared at the time was the symbolic representation of something once there now missing, a loss never

---

[3] I am indebted to Dr. Calvin Settlage for stimulating this line of thinking.

mourned, and closely related to the sense of pervasive loss and feelings of emptiness which had typified his presenting symptoms. I suggest that the "black void" symbolized at one level castration, and at another, the lost "stranger" mother whom he longed to reach out to and, as he said, "touch."

The Tunes As Transitional Phenomena

The loss symbolized by the "black void" had been hidden by the trombone and at the same time mitigated by the trombone itself. As this was clarified, Tom sensed that throughout his life, long before he had begun to play his instrument, *tunes* in his head "filled the void." This suggests that the tunes in his head also served the function of transitional phenomena, "rich in . . . protean possibilities . . . promoting a kind of psychophysical homeostasis as individuation progresses" (Greenacre, 1969, p. 158).

There has been considerable research on very early infant and even prenatal reactions to various sounds and rhythms. Salk (1973) has reported a series of investigations demonstrating the newborn infant's marked responsiveness in a variety of ways to maternal heart beat rhythms. His work on the very early acquired preference of mothers, right- and left-handed, for holding their newborn infants in their left arms is of particular interest with regard to transitional phenomena. As mothers, without conscious awareness, attempt to provide a continuity of experience from inside to outside their bodies, they tend to give their babies not only a continuation of uterine warmth and support, but also of the *rhythmic pulsations of their hearts*, coupled at times with rhythmic patting, jiggling, rocking, and a large variety of rhythmic sounds and utterances. The infant's responsiveness to such rhythmic movements and sounds, can be regarded as primitive forerunners of a whole host of transitional phenomena.

An appreciation of the role of rhythmic sounds and movements in leading to or becoming transitional phenomena may increase our analytic understanding of the response to and the creation of rhythms (Kohut, 1957; McDonald, 1970; Noy, 1968). Viewed in this way, music with its central organizing principle, the tempo—the beat—probably is among the most complex of all the artistic endeavors in that it calls upon developmental elements ranging from the most primitive to the most subtle and sophisticated.

I hypothesize that the tunes in Tom's head were the residues of longings for the "stranger" mother. As transitional phenomena, they provided him with a sense of her appearing when she was needed, mitigating loss. In this regard, it is especially interesting to study the important functions the tunes served during the analysis in the various manifestations of the transference. At times he teased me with them (not sharing them [her] with me); often they competed with me (he was more interested in them [her] than in me); and at times they separated him from me (he would become lost in them [her]).

Even though Tom's overriding feeling was that I was the ineffectual father who had to compete with the perfectly attuned, ever-present mother in order to become a part of his life, we could see in these interplays a condensation of several other significant developmental levels. "Being lost" in the tunes was clearly a reexperience of the regressive union with the "stranger" mother. The teasing with them was more complicated. At times, it was a playing off the "stranger" mother against his mother. The passive experience of being handed from one to the other became the active process of choosing one over the other. However, at times, the teasing seemed designed to establish a differentiation between the "stranger" mother and the tunes themselves. My (her) "competing" for his attention vis-à-vis the tunes helped establish and, in effect, master a sense of their being related, *but* separate.

I propose that it was in relation to the composite internalized, though partially integrated, representation of the early "stranger" mother that Tom's creations arose. The analysis, by reactivating and helping him work through the early loss and allowing him to mourn, changed the nature of his tie to the lost "stranger" mother. This changed his relationship to these transitional phenomena, accounting for the emergence of the creative capacity. Prior to the analysis, the tunes needed the quality of belonging to another in order to protect him from loss. As a result of analysis, they could be his own tunes. Essentially the analysis shifted the transitional object (the tunes) from being more of her and less of him to being more of him and less of her. The quality of originality came as the construct became more "the me" and less "the not me." I see his expressions, "The tunes are in my head and they keep coming, they occur to me, they appear in my head," as metaphoric descriptions of his sense of integration of the self representation, yet with the quality of separateness—a space between inner and outer. This would be in keeping with Winnicott's (1967) proposal that much of the creative process takes place in a special psychic "location" derived from the developmental evolution of transitional phenomena.

This suggests that a critical component of the anxiety associated with Tom's being creative (another way to state this would be the anxiety necessary to overcome in order to be original) stemmed at a deep level from separation anxiety, his fear of being alone. This was intertwined with and masked by higher level anxieties related to castration, fear of loss of love, and various social concerns.

This view of Tom's creativity adds a further dimension to understanding his *talent*. Prior to the analysis his talented renditions were, by and large, skillful elaborations of the tunes of others. In structure, they were compromise formations which hid and at the same time revealed, among other things, Tom's innovative contributions, which were *encumbered* by his need to use something from another. The creativity, though hidden in the talent, was at times given relatively undisguised expression in his jazz improvisations, which very early were recognized as being exceptional. He could allow himself these brief creative moments because improvisation by its very nature is spontaneous, not reproducible, and quickly becomes hidden in and a part of the product of others, hence relatively safe.

In summary, as the analysis progressed and his castration and abandonment anxieties lessened, aided by various identificatory components, the nature of his relationship to his instrument and his playing changed. Tom was able to shift in many areas of functioning from various kinds of holding on to another to a freer use of aspects of himself. This increased individuation was epitomized in his music when he discovered his own tunes developing[4] within himself.

---

[4] "Developing" accurately reflects the essential passive quality Tom always emphasized when he attempted to describe the emergence of the tunes. Another

Tom's enhanced ability to tolerate loss was vividly put to test during the analysis when his instrument was stolen and he had to find and master a new one, and most critically when his father died. At that time, he insightfully extricated himself from his (and his mother's) regressive desire to replace loss by holding on to her and from his regressive desire to replace loss by holding on to me. This was reworked finally in an attenuated form in the termination process.

Yet even in this carefully studied case, critical questions remain unanswered. Was there a particular element in the nature of the relationship to the "true" mother and the biological mother which resulted in Tom's having unusual access to transitional phenomena, an ability which ultimately became involved in neurotic conflict and was subsequently "freed" by the analysis? Or is there in Tom an innate constitutional capacity with increased sensitivity (Greenacre, 1957; Noy, 1968) which resulted in Tom's experiencing, in a way different, the vicissitude of his unique development?

Postscript

Tom's analysis terminated over four years ago. I have several times read about Tom in the newspapers and seen him on television. About one year ago, I heard directly from him. He was engaged to a girl, two years younger than himself, a singer with a group. He was working with several groups, playing, recording, and composing. He told me that rock jobs were on the wane and more and more he was playing blues and jazz in small clubs and on concert tours. His "classical compositions" were never completed, though he continued to study composition and himself teaches both

---

important part of this creative process was the way Tom "played with" the tunes. He would take his tune, change it, turn it around, and try it in endless variations before he discarded it or developed it into a theme. Only later came the active part—the "working them over" or the "working them up." The process by which the tunes were transformed into compositions of varying complexity required a remarkable balance of discipline, intensity, and scholarship as the tunes were elaborated into themes and orchestrated for performance.

composition and trombone. In short, he was a reasonably successful, moderately creative, talented musician.

Summary

The analysis of a young, talented, professional musician is presented. Factors which influenced his choice of instrument and the function it and music served in his development are discussed in detail.

As the many defensive purposes the instrument and music served were uncovered in the analysis, at a point heralded by a striking castration dream, his talented playing was severely affected. In the ensuing months, the analysis reached a greater clarity, and for the first time he discovered an ability to compose.

The various psychological meanings of his instrument are discussed. The change from playing the music of others to creating original music is viewed in terms of dynamic shifts related to transitional phenomena. Several hypotheses are offered with regard to the genetic origins of the patient's unusual abilities, and certain distinctions are made between his talent and his creativity.

BIBLIOGRAPHY

Erikson, E. H. (1954), The Dream Specimen of Psychoanalysis. *J. Amer. Psychoanal. Assn.*, 2:5–56.
Greenacre, P. (1957), The Childhood of the Artist. *This Annual*, 12:47–72.
—— (1958), The Family Romance of the Artist. *This Annual*, 13:13–31.
—— (1969), The Fetish and the Transitional Object. *This Annual*, 24:144–164.
Jacobson, E. (1964), *The Self and the Object World*. New York: Int. Univ. Press.
Kohut, H. (1957), Observations on the Psychological Functions of Music. *J. Amer. Psychoanal. Assn.*, 5:389–407.
Kris, E. (1952), *Psychoanalytic Explorations in Art*. New York: Int. Univ. Press.
McDonald, M. (1970), Transitional Tunes and Musical Development. *This Annual*, 25:503–520.
Noy, P. (1968), The Development of Musical Ability. *This Annual*, 23:332–347.
Salk, L. (1973), The Role of the Heart Beat in the Relations Between Mother and Infant. *Sci. American*, 228(5):24–29.
Settlage, C. F. (1972), Cultural Values and the Superego in Late Adolescence. *This Annual*, 27:74–92.

STOLZ, H. R. & STOLZ, L. M. (1951), *Somatic Development of Adolescent Boys*. New York: Macmillan, pp. 367–394.

WEISSMAN, P. (1971), The Artist and His Objects. *Int. J. Psycho-Anal.*, 52:401–406.

WINNICOTT, D. W. (1953), Transitional Objects and Transitional Phenomena. *Int. J. Psycho-Anal.*, 34:89–97.

——— (1967), The Location of Cultural Experience. *Int. J. Psycho-Anal.*, 48:368–372.

Discussions on Transference

The Treatment Situation and Technique in Child Psychoanalysis

JOSEPH SANDLER, M.D., PH.D., D.SC.,
HANSI KENNEDY,
AND ROBERT L. TYSON, M.D.

THIS PAPER IS A VERSION OF A CHAPTER OF A BOOK, NOW IN THE COURSE of preparation, on *Treatment Situation and Technique in Child Psychoanal-*

Dr. Sandler is a research psychoanalyst at the Hampstead Clinic, and Director of the Index Project. Mrs. Kennedy is a research psychotherapist and Dr. Tyson is a research psychoanalyst at the Clinic. The material for this paper was gathered at the Hampstead Child-Therapy Clinic, an organization which is at present maintained by the Field Foundation Inc., New York; the Foundation for Research in Psychoanalysis, Beverly Hills, California; the Freud Centenary Fund, London; the Anna Freud Foundation, New York; the Grant Foundation, Inc., New York; the Andrew Mellon Foundation; the National Institute for Mental Health, Bethesda; the New-Land Foundation, New York; and a number of private supporters.

The project which is partly reported in this paper was supported by a grant from the Foundation for Research in Psychoanalysis, Beverly Hills, California. The authors wish to express their profound indebtedness to Anna Freud and to all the child analysts and therapists who contributed to this project.

Copyright © 1975 Joseph Sandler, Hansi Kennedy, Robert L. Tyson.

ysis. This work is the outcome of our realization that developments in the technique of child analysis at the Hampstead Child-Therapy Clinic have not been adequately documented. In 1968 the Hampstead Index Group initiated a project aimed at crystallizing and recording some of the specific views and experiences of senior child analysts and therapists at the Clinic. The project began with weekly meetings chaired by one of us (J.S.), in which Anna Freud participated actively, and which extended over a period of two and a half years. Most senior staff members attended and participated in all or some of the meetings, which were tape-recorded. These recordings were later transcribed and edited.

In order to provide a suitable format for the discussion, a section of the Hampstead Index (Treatment Situation and Technique) was used as a basis, and material indexed under the relevant index headings was extracted and made available to the research group. The Index allows access to various aspects of the psychoanalytic treatment of a large number of individual cases seen and treated at the Clinic over a period of some twenty years. Anna Freud (1965) has described the Index as a "collective analytic memory" which can be viewed as a "storehouse of analytic material which places at the disposal of the single thinker and author an abundance of facts gathered by many, thereby transcending the narrow confines of individual experience and extending the possibilities for insightful study, for constructive comparisons between cases, for deductions and generalizations, and finally for extrapolations of theory from clinical therapeutic work."

The Index is divided into ten major sections, and each section has an appropriate Manual aimed at providing therapists with possible headings and definitions to assist them in indexing a case. Cases are usually indexed after the first year of treatment and reindexed annually for the duration of the analysis. The current version of the Manual on Treatment Situation and Technique contains the following sections:

I. *Attendance and Interruptions*
   A. Attendance
   B. Interruptions, Reaction to
   C. Change of Therapist

Discussions on Transference

    D. Other Changes in Treatment Situation
    E. Changing Frequency of Sessions

II. *Attitudes and Relationship to Therapist and Treatment*
    A. Treatment Alliance
    B. Resistance to Analysis
    C. Fantasies and Expectations about Treatment
    D. Use Made of Insight and Self-Observation
    E. Reaction to Interpretations
    F. Transference
       1. Predominantly of Habitual Modes of Relating
       2. Predominantly of Current Relationships
       3. Predominantly of Past Experiences
       4. Transference Neurosis
       5. Summary of Transference
    G. Other Uses Made of Therapist and Treatment Situation

III. *Child's Modes of Expression*
    A. Ways of Bringing Material in the Session
       1. Mainly through Verbalization
       2. Mainly Nonverbally
       3. Through a Mixture of Verbalization and Other Ways
       4. Changes During Analysis
    B. Acting Out
    C. Behavior on Coming and Going

IV. *Interpretations and Interventions*
    A. Introducing the Child to the Idea of Treatment
    B. Clarifications, Confrontations, Explanations, and Reassurance
    C. Aids to Interpretation
    D. Significant Interpretations
    E. Selection and Timing
    F. Working Through
    G. Restrictions
    H. Physical Contact and Gratification
    I. Specific Modifications of Technique
    J. Extra-Analytic Contacts and Procedures
       1. Contact with Child Before and After Sessions

        2. Contact with Child Outside Sessions
        3. Contact with Parents
        4. Contact with Others
        5. Modification of Environment
        6. Use Made of Extra-Analytic Material
    K. Termination of Treatment
V. *Aims and Results of Treatment*
    A. Aims of Treatment
    B. Changes in the Child during Treatment
    C. Gains and Achievements during Treatment
    D. Assessment of the Child
    E. Follow-up After Termination

Meetings were held on all these topics, and a book containing the gist of the discussion is close to completion. The present paper reflects the pertinent points which emerged in relation to II.F. *Attitudes and Relationship to Therapist and Treatment:* Transference.

The digestion, integration, and editing of the transcripts of the recordings have been extremely difficult and complex tasks, but we believe that we have succeeded in doing justice to the discussions. Many of Anna Freud's comments have been reproduced verbatim, while the contributions of the other participants have been incorporated into the text.

Transference

The term "transference" has been derived from adult analysis and refers to the way in which the patient's view of and relations with his childhood objects are expressed in his *current* perceptions, thoughts, fantasies, feelings, attitudes, and behavior in regard to the analyst. It should be noted that especially in the analysis of children, transferences may reflect aspects of present-day relationships with important objects, in particular the parents. For the purposes of the Hampstead Index the term is used in a relatively wide sense to include, for example, various forms of "externalization" in which the therapist may represent different aspects of the child's personality, e.g., aspects of superego, introjects, of instinctual strivings, of the child's self representation.[1] However, when the processes of externalization play an important part in determining the relationship of the child to the therapist, instances of this are usually indexed elsewhere (for instance, in the *Ego: Defense* and *Superego* sections) and only cross-referenced to the transference section.

It has been found convenient to divide the Transference section into the five subsections given above. These are not hard and fast categories. Difficulties arise here, as elsewhere in the Index, if theoretical concepts are approached as "absolutes" into which one attempts to fit the observed clinical material. In a sense it is the clinical observations which are the "absolutes" in this context, and the indexer does the best he can to make use of a set of theoretical categories which may be relatively imprecise, but adequate for the clinical purposes of the moment. Clearly, the five categories overlap, and this becomes evident in the course of the discussion which follows. Although the material of the discussions is organized around these categories, the reader will find that the issue repeatedly arises of how one can make a finer distinction between the various subsections. Because the term transference is often used extremely loosely, it is often treated as a single phenomenon, but our own experience has convinced us of the clinical value of establishing a number of subcategories in the effort to maintain a degree of precision in a very complex area. The discussion reported below is also incidentally concerned with a number of larger questions, such as the specific features of transference phenomena in children as compared with adults.

1. Transference Predominantly of Habitual Modes of Relating

Material entered under this heading refers to modes of relating to, and attitudes toward, the therapist which can be considered to be

---

[1] In *externalization* any aspect of the person is attributed to the external world. It should be noted that in the Index the term *projection* is used in a restricted sense. It refers to the attribution to another person of a wish or impulse of one's own toward that person, and felt by the subject to be directed back against himself (e.g., "*I* do not hate *him,* he hates *me*"). Projection has, therefore, been regarded as a specific instance of the wider class of externalizations.

habitual and characteristic for the child. What is sought for here are those aspects of the child's relationships to people (or to special groups of people) which are not in any way specific to the therapist, but insofar as one can speak of the child's personality having been formed are aspects of *character*. These modes of relating are often seen in the very earliest sessions of treatment, and may later become transference (in a stricter sense). Examples of such habitual attitudes are the tendency to make sadomasochistic relationships, the tendency to placate, and the like.

The sort of material included in this section can be exemplified by the case of a child who is frightened of policemen or doctors, or anyone in uniform or in authority, and who begins treatment by being frightened of the analyst. This might occur, for example, when a patient who habitually externalizes onto adults critical aspects of his superego relates to the analyst in the same way as to any other adult. This would be a "character transference," so to speak.

The distinctive features of this form of relating can be brought out further by considering the example of an adult patient who appears late for an analytic session. This may be the consequence of a specific transference situation arising in treatment, in which, for example, an anxiety about a homosexual attachment to the analyst has been activated. On the other hand the lateness might reflect a characteristic tendency in the patient to be late, which shows itself in the analytic setting as a symptom. Psychodynamically, such fixed patterns are, of course, based on earlier relationships (or defenses against earlier object-directed impulses) and can be understood, in the course of the analytic work, in this way. Nevertheless, what is important here is that these residues of earlier relationships have now spread to the world as a whole and may be regarded as having attained a degree of autonomy. The analyst is confronted with the technical problem of how to facilitate the revival of the earlier relationships and to catch them in their "live" as opposed to their "fixed" form.[2] Anna Freud gave an example:

---

[2] In "energic" terms it could be said that the character transference involves a cathexis of a whole category of persons to whom the patient relates in a habitual fashion. During the course of treatment we hope to be able to find a change in the

This point can be seen in treating a child who forgets and loses everything. He forgets everything in the consulting room, which might have a very definite transference meaning. Most analysts would say, "Of course, you wanted to stay with me and so you left your cap or your penknife or pencil." Then the analyst may hear that the child leaves his cap and penknife and pencil everywhere: in school, on the bus, and at home. Then it can be seen that it simply isn't true that he wants to stay with all these people.[3] The whole thing has a completely different meaning and only comes into the analysis as a fixed symptom. The point is that when one first sees that piece of behavior there is no way of knowing at the time whether it is the one or the other.

Children have an ongoing dependent relationship with the parents in the present. Naturally this complicates the task of distinguishing between a fixed pattern of behavior used with parents and adults in general and the specific revival of a past experience within the context of the treatment situation.

An illustration from the treatment of Kenneth B. is an example of the transferring of "habitual modes of relating." Kenneth was 5;10 years at the beginning of treatment and the case was indexed when he was 7;8 years old.

Kenneth's great problem when he commenced treatment was his fear of involving himself in relationships in case he should be

---

quality of the relationship so that it is the specific person of the therapist who becomes cathected *in a more focused way* in the transference. We are referring here to technical problems relating to the transformation of character transferences into more emotionally loaded transference relationships. An example of this might be found in the treatment of the child who habitually mistrusts everyone and commences analysis by mistrusting the analyst. The analyst might then point out the child's mistrust and suggest that he may have good reason for being like this because he may have been let down by grownups in the past. However, in our view, it is an error to treat these *habitual* modes of relating as if they were full-fledged transference manifestations or even aspects of a transference neurosis, even though they are categorized as forms of transference in the broadest sense of the word.

[3] Later Anna Freud commented: "This patient was one of the children to whom I referred in my paper 'About Losing and Being Lost' [1967]. He demonstrated by losing inanimate possessions how 'lost' he felt in regard to his parents. He lived with his father who paid insufficient attention to him and had actually 'lost' the mother to whom he was deeply attached (except for rare visits)."

abandoned. He defended against his anxiety by being as unpleasant as he could, thus inviting the object to reject him. The therapist felt that although the necessity to invite rejection had been diminished by treatment, Kenneth may still have a tendency to retain this defense against close relationships.

An interesting point in the example of Kenneth is that habitual modes of relating can serve as defenses against anxiety. When one or another of these modes appears in relation to the analyst, an opportunity arises to show the patient the nature of his defense. For instance, one may show the patient the contradiction within himself between the *wish* to be emotionally involved with the analyst and the *fear* of being involved, and what he does to protect himself against involvement.

A further clinical illustration is from the Index card of Esther L., who was 8;10 years at the beginning of treatment and whose case was indexed at 9;11 years.

> One of the main features of Esther's object relationships was her need to defend herself against anticipated disappointments and rejections which she had previously experienced on both preoedipal and oedipal levels. Her parents had given a history of her past tendency to form friendships with children who would reject her. In treatment she showed a marked degree of self-sufficiency, and it became apparent that this as well as her need to keep herself busy with a variety of activities were her ways of avoiding the rejection and the disappointment she expected if she would ask for help or attention. As the analysis of this defensive attitude proceeded, Esther gradually became able to make demands on her therapist, and she re-created a situation in which she would provoke rejection or experience disappointment by making requests that could not be granted.

Esther's initial defensive posture is a good example of a habitual mode of defense used in relation to the analyst as well as to all her current objects. The defense was against disappointment and rejection, and with analysis of the defensive attitude, the underlying wishes were regressively revived in relation to the analyst, on whom they became focused. The difficulty in distinguishing between "habitual modes" and other revivals of the past is compounded when *everything* that happens between patient and analyst is called "transference."

The inclusion of "habitual modes of relating" in the Transference section of the Index is somewhat ambiguous. Historically, Freud used transference to refer to the spontaneous development within the analysis of a libidinal relationship revived from the past. Later authors have broadened the concept of transference by including various modes of relating, among them relatively autonomous habitual defensive attitudes as they appear in the analytic setting. Therefore the manifestations indexed in this subsection are not transferences in the earlier or stricter sense. They can be brought under the rubric of "transference" only if the term is used in the widest possible way. However, the provision of a section for this type of material points to an important clinical distinction between habitual "character" attitudes and the transference which evolves in the course of the analysis. It should be emphasized that although "habitual modes" are not specific to the transference relationship, they may involve a great deal of intense affect and action directed toward the therapist.

2. Transference Predominantly of Current Relationships

This heading refers to the displacement of current wishes, conflicts, or reactions into the analytic situation, or onto an involvement with the person of the therapist. These current preoccupations may be largely reality-related (one example would be the child's regressive reaction to the birth of a sibling), or may be a product or manifestation of the child's current age-appropriate level of functioning (e.g., the appearance of oedipal strivings as a consequence of the child's progressive development). The essential criterion for entries under this particular heading is that the preoccupations of the child relate to a real object (or objects) *in the present* and their manifestations in the analysis represent an extension or displacement from that present relationship. The relation to the therapist has the predominant quality of a displacement or "extension" in the present rather than of a "revival" from the past.

This latter distinction cannot always be clearly maintained or easily made. The therapist attempts to gauge the distinction in terms of the *predominant* quality, by the feel, flow, and development of the material. It cannot be assessed only by the feeling of something being very real in the "here and now," because this is in any event typical of all transference reactions. The child who enters a new phase of psychosexual development will obviously differ from the child who has regressed *within* the analytic relationship. Thus a child in the oedipal phase may bring oedipal feelings and conflicts into the analysis, where they should be seen as extensions of current involvements rather than as a revival of the past. In this case, the current oedipal relationship with the parents is displaced or extended into the analysis rather than being reactivated.

The point at issue is the distinction between the revival of something from the past within the analytic situation and *as a consequence of the analytic process* on the one hand, and the extension *into* the analysis of something currently active in the patient's life, on the other. Current relationships extended into the analysis include regressive as well as phase-appropriate manifestations, a form of "spillover" into the analysis.

One of the forms of "transference of current relationships" is of particular interest and should be distinguished from the phenomena indexed under the subheading "transference of past experiences." This form is consequent on the "permission to express" offered by the analytic situation. For example, a child of 5, after some hesitation, allowed himself to shout at the analyst, obviously enjoying the experience, though somewhat frightened by it. After a while he remarked that "Mummy would never let me shout like that at home." This need be neither regression in the analysis nor transference. However, it can be considered to be a spillover of an impulse which he feels is prohibited at home, but as the prohibition has not yet been fully internalized, he can allow himself to express his wish to shout in the treatment room. It would seem that he could respond to a different, externally provided ideal for himself (the therapist indicated that she could accept in an uncritical way the child's wish to shout), one which allowed him to feel safe and free from the threat of punishment in his relationship to the therapist. It may be a relief to the child to bring such material in relation to the analyst, someone who is not such an important and highly invested object as is, for example, the mother. The permissiveness of the analytic situation allows more open expression, not because the analyst has really become the most important person in the child's life, but because he is a less important person.

The difficulties involved in classifying material under the heading "transference of current relationships" are well illustrated by the example of Andy V., a boy who was 2½ years old at the beginning of treatment and 3;2 years at the time of indexing.

> When his father started a new job which entailed his absence from home one night each week, Andy was markedly negative toward the therapist, particularly on Fridays, and often told the therapist to shut up, that he did not like him. This was seen as anger at the father's absence transferred to the therapist.

In this example, the child felt angry with the father for going away. The therapist felt that Andy was angry with him before the weekend break because he transferred some of his feelings from a current situation with the father onto the analyst. Here a current situation impinges on the child, anger is aroused, and a similar situation in the analysis stimulates anger toward the analyst.

It was questioned whether this example was transference of a current problem at all, or whether it was a defense, by means of a displacement, against his angry feelings toward his father. It would be a displacement only if Andy managed to lessen his anger with his father by doing what he did in treatment. Also, what may appear at an early stage of the analysis as a manifestation of current problems may come to be understood differently later, for example, that the anger with the deserting father covers an earlier anger with the abandoning mother.

A further blurring of the distinction being discussed may occur when the child acts something out with the parents as a result of the analytic work. It may be difficult to know whether this is acting out as a consequence of the analysis, or whether the child is bringing some aspect of his current interaction with the parents *into* the analysis. Obviously the spillover phenomenon operates both ways.

The case was discussed of a little girl who was referred for analysis because of a profound reaction to the birth of a second child. During treatment, when a third baby was on the way, she became extremely angry about the new child "inside mummy's tummy." This is certainly a current situation, but it also involves the whole of her disturbance in which the revival of the past is contained. One could say that the predominant situation here is a current problem which was carried over into the analysis. The patient hammered the (male) analyst's abdomen because she was clearly so angry about the pending arrival of the new child. However, her disturbance had begun with the arrival of the first sibling, and it would normally be expected that the past experience would be relived in some way in the analysis. It would appear that both a current and a past (revived) reaction to the mother's pregnancy entered into the analytic material. Anna Freud commented:

> But what brings into the analysis material about the wish to destroy the baby? If the mother had not now been pregnant, would the material in the analysis at this time have turned to the anger about the previous pregnancy of the mother? Or is it the current event at home, the mother's present pregnancy, which brings the whole thing into the analysis? I think that with children the material is quite often activated by a current event, so that it really comes into treatment like an intrusion. That is one of the reasons why the whole procedure of child analysis often appears to be less orderly than that of adult analysis. It is not only determined from inside, but is also determined by outside events very much more than with adults.

It was felt that the example from this case illustrates the problems raised by the fact that regressive manifestations shown at home may themselves involve a revival of the past, and are then displaced onto the person of the analyst or onto the analytic situation. This would be different from something which might emerge spontaneously in analysis as a result of the analytic work.

As an example of this the case of Kenneth B. (referred to in section 1) was cited.

> When Kenneth felt anxious about his parents' love, he would ask for oral satisfaction, e.g., one month before his second sibling was due, he began to insist on having orange juice in the waiting room every day before his session.
>
> [Anna Freud said:] This is a spilling over of the behavior, because surely at that time he had regressed and was more orally demanding at home and elsewhere, and this spilled over into the

treatment. This spilling over is, of course, what is meant by the extension into the treatment situation. It is not a defense in the sense that by demanding the orange juice at the Clinic he succeeds in being less demanding at home.

This is a good example to illustrate the need to indicate whether the behavior in question occurs only under specific circumstances, e.g., at home or in the analytic situation, or whether it occurs everywhere and with everyone. In the latter case, it would be understood either as a habitual mode of relating or as a manifestation of regression.

The next case was discussed because it illustrates the complexity of childhood transference manifestations. Ilse was 4;11 at the start of treatment, and her case was indexed when she was 6½ years old.

> On occasions Ilse's fear of her father was transferred onto the therapist, with the roles reversed. She would scold the therapist for her naughtiness, shout at her, or take the part of a most exacting teacher (her father taught her Hebrew and English at home), and demand obedience. Ilse transferred to the therapist various aspects of her current oedipal relationship with her father, including her wish to be admired by him and her sexual wishes for him (e.g., she wanted to exchange kisses with the therapist and sought excitement in physical approaches; she also wanted to make a baby with the therapist and was disappointed at not having her passionate desires reciprocated).

It was thought that this illustration contained two separate examples of the transferring of current relationships to the analysis. In the first example the child scolds the therapist and takes the part of a most exacting teacher, and in this way transfers into the analysis her fear of the father, while reversing the roles. What is extended into the analysis is something which has arisen at home. The way she deals with it in the analysis, by reversing roles, raises several questions. Is the reversal of roles a defense against her feelings about the father analyst? We may also understand this slightly differently. The child did not have the opportunity to reverse the roles at home as she did in the analysis, and she may have been trying something out in the analysis that she would have liked to have done at home. Such a piece of behavior may also be understood as the child's chosen mode of expression, i.e., as her only way of creating a situation in the analytic hour which could reflect the conflict inside her.

The second instance of the transferring of a current relationship in this child seems to be a more straightforward displacing of developmentally appropriate oedipal wishes into the treatment situation.

The discussion went on to the observation that, from the point of view of the treatment situation and technique, there seemed to be a parallel which could be drawn between the prelatency child and the adolescent, because they share an intensity of developmentally appropriate reactions and conflicts (in comparison with the normal latency child). Current developmental turmoils may spill over into the analysis or be defensively deflected there. There is a special technical problem with adolescents in that the therapist has to "fight for the past" because of the adolescent's enormous fear of regression. The problem is whether or not the therapist can get a revival of the past in the transference so that it can be analyzed fully, because negative feelings arise in the patient as soon as regression threatens, and enormous resistances may appear.

To sum up, the patient may express feelings in the analytic situation in regard to the analyst which can be designated as the transference of current relationships and problems. These may appear in treatment as a kind of spillover into the analytic situation, but such spillovers might also occur elsewhere. Alternatively, we might witness something more than a simple spillover in that the patient might deflect attitudes, relationships, and problems into the analysis as a defense against experiencing them outside. This may come about because the analyst is "safer" at the moment, since direct expression (for example, to the parent) is too threatening in some way. In the course of treatment, the emergence of intense feelings about the analyst and of conflicts within the analytic situation is then accompanied by a diminution of their expression outside the treatment. What looks like a manifestation of transference neurosis in this respect is not so at all; nor is it transference in the more narrow sense, that is, a specific revival of the past. In none of these examples does it appear that the analytic process in itself plays a crucial role in the timing of the emergence of such material. In all of this, due regard must always be given to the child's age and developmental level, as these factors will always influence the nature of the transference relationship.

3. Transference Predominantly of Past Experiences

Material indexed under this heading refers to the way in which past experiences, wishes, fantasies, conflicts, and defenses are *revived* during the course of the analysis, as a consequence of the analytic work, and which now relate to the person of the therapist in their manifest or latent (preconscious) content. In this section the transference manifestation can be considered to be a derivative of the repressed, one which, due to the analytic work, emerges in regard to the person of the therapist. It will combine present reality (including the person of the therapist) with the expression of a revived wish, memory, or fantasy, e.g., a preoedipal wish for the exclusive possession of the therapist.

A clinical example entered under this heading in the Index was taken as a starting point for discussion. It refers to the analysis of Karen C., 12½ years at the beginning of treatment, indexed at 15 years of age.

> Karen turned the sessions into a repetition of her anal-sadistic relationship with her mother through which it was possible to recognize her longing to reestablish this kind of intimacy. She bribed the therapist with gifts of food as mother bribed her. She enacted being sick in the session, with the therapist tending to her, and imagined the therapist ill and nursing her. Karen tried to seduce the therapist to anal games, even to the extent of lying on the floor "as I did when mummy gave me suppositories." Anal material was brought together with stories of illness and praise of mother who never failed her when she was ill: "She would do anything for me, wipe my bottom or stay in the lavatory with me all night."

This first example was regarded as ambiguous because the behavior, as described, might equally well have been regarded as a general mode of relating to people at that particular time. The crucial point would be whether what was described arose as a consequence of the analytic work or not, and this is not made clear in the example. It would have fitted the Index heading (Transference Predominantly of Past Experiences) more clearly if it had indicated, for example, that Karen now experienced the revival of earlier anal wishes in the course of the analysis, that Karen, although having a fixation point[4] at an anal level, was no longer interacting *with her mother* in the manner described previously. If this were true, Karen's behavior with the therapist would not reflect her current relationship to the mother but could be regarded as a consequence of the analytic work and the analytic process. On this basis it would have been justifiable to distinguish this example as a transference of a past experience rather than as a displacement from something in the present. Anna Freud commented:

> One should keep in mind the development of the transference in this case. It cannot be said that this girl regressed to anal-sadistic behavior. She lived on that level with the mother for a very long time and still did at the time of the analysis. She disturbed the mother at night; she woke her up either to demand food or to accompany her to the toilet, or to wipe her bottom, and so on. She disturbed any event in the family by vomiting, or by getting a sudden stomach upset. These were her symptoms. It was not merely a question of something which had become repressed and unconscious and which had then been revived in the transference. It was really that, with the development of the analytic work, the symptoms were drawn more into the transference. That of course was greatly helped by the mother being enabled, through her own treatment, to stop this interaction, because the mother had kept this situation alive by playing her part in it. Karen's analyst did not play that part, and so the whole thing became amenable to treatment.

One of the elements which complicates the distinction between

---

[4] Anna Freud distinguishes between *fixation* at a particular level (the child then functions currently, in regard to some aspect of his personality, at that level) and a *fixation point* at one or other level of development. While *fixations* may change, a fixation point, once established, never disappears, although the child may develop past it. The fixation point represents a point in development to which the child will tend to *regress* if conflict or pain become too great, and is also thought to exert a "backward pull" on the child.

the transference of past experiences and transference of present problems is the fact that the child develops a growing libidinal attachment to the therapist. Facilitated by this attachment, a current conflict at home might then more readily spill over or extend to the therapist. This is because current conflicts usually involve past patterns of behavior which have been taken up or absorbed into subsequent developmental phases. For example, this may be shown by the way in which a sadomasochistic relationship in the anal phase becomes structured and then persists. Subsequently it is absorbed into the structure of the oedipal phase and "colors" it. This is not an arrest in development, because the child goes on to achieve phase dominance in the next phase. It is not, strictly speaking, a fixation, nor is it a fixation point, because fixation points are "silent" and the concept of fixation points is intimately linked with that of regression. We are speaking of none of these, but rather of a sort of persisting influence, as described above, of an earlier phase on a later one. In the course of the analytic work such earlier patterns find a more direct expression in terms of their repetition in the transference. It is not, however, absolutely clear whether we can regard such expressions as being a "revival of the past" in the transference in the sense in which we see it in the treatment of adults. The point here is that a pregenital pattern may remain in the oedipal or postoedipal phases, finding more *intense* expression during the course of treatment, rather than being "released" or "regressed to" in the course of the analytic treatment.

The next clinical example to be discussed, which illustrates more clearly the revival of the past in the transference, was from the case of Esther L. (referred to in section 1).

> During her resistant silences, Esther communicated her feelings of sadness, loneliness, and neglect by means of sniffing, finger sucking, her facial expression, and general appearance. This became particularly noticeable at a time when, following a holiday and a change of treatment room, she felt that she had been rejected by the analyst and replaced by another child. Her defensive self-sufficiency increased, she kept herself very busy with drawing, and could scarcely speak at all. However, she revealed the feeling she was trying to deny in these nonverbal ways. When these feelings

were linked to those she had following the birth of her younger sister, she responded very slowly and gradually by seeking the therapist's attention in various nonverbal ways. She dropped things or could not find them unless the therapist helped her. She waited in the dark in the treatment room until the therapist turned on the light.

The example of Esther was felt to be a good one because the interruption of a holiday and the disturbance caused by a change of room led to a clear revival of feelings in the transference. These feelings were an aspect of the repetition of her past experiences around the birth of her younger sister. There were no discernible current extra-analytic factors which could have been responsible for the observed changes in the analytic material, but the changes in the analytic setting, as described, had a clear relation to the change in the child's material.

In regard to the example of Esther Anna Freud said:

> I think it might be a better example if it were explained what the child is actually doing. She not only seeks the therapist's help and attention, but her defense of self-sufficiency changed to an earlier state of helplessness. What the child repeats here in the transference is a bit of her history. Prior to this we had no clear understanding of what the self-sufficiency and overactivity meant. How did she acquire them? One had no way of finding out until she repeated in the transference the experience of being neglected and deserted, defending against it by her overactivity and self-sufficiency.

This example appears to show that when a defense comes to be transferred to the analytic situation and is meaningfully interpreted within the transference, an earlier mode of reaction may become accessible to analysis. If one looks at it from the viewpoint of transference of a defense, then the example, as given, may illustrate a defense against the revival of feelings from the past, with a repetition, in this case, of the same defenses against the same feelings related to the *same* conflicts. One could, of course, also view this material as representing the use of a current defense against past feelings arising in the transference, so that it could be called a "defense against the transference," rather than a "transference of defense."

The question then was raised of the *choice* of defense used to deal with the repetition of past feeling states and experiences, as they are reexperienced in the course of analysis. The child may also use a relatively *new* defense, one which was not available to him in the original situation, but which can now be employed to defend against the revival of the past experience. For example, adolescents will frequently employ intellectualization as an age-appropriate defense against revived earlier conflicts such as concerns over violence and aggression, although at an earlier developmental level intellectualization is not an age-appropriate defense.

Such considerations have important technical implications because it might not be appropriate to link a defense with an early conflictual childhood experience, if the defense was a later acquisition. It seems that analysts often fall into a routine of interpreting a defense as being part of the reconstructed original experience.

Anna Freud concluded the discussion with the following comment:

> The chronology of the defense organization is a very interesting subject to study. One way to approach it would be to look at the analyses of adolescents who dealt with their problems mainly by intellectualization. I mean by this, the changing of personal problems into a discussion of world problems. One might then see what methods were used previously when the child had to deal with the same problem. One might then make a comparative study.

4. Transference Neurosis

By transference neurosis we mean the concentration of the child's conflicts, repressed infantile wishes, fantasies, etc., on the person of the therapist, *with the relative diminution of their manifestations elsewhere.* This concept stems from adult analysis. The occurrence of full transference neurosis in child analysis is a controversial subject and is of special research interest.

In adult analysis a distinction is generally made between transference neurosis and other transference manifestations. In child analysis, there is usually significant transference involvement, but the evidence for transference neurosis, at least from the material recorded in the Hampstead Index, appears to be relatively sparse. It is possible that what is included in the Index under the heading of "Transference of Past Experiences" may be considered by others to be transference neurosis. On this point, Anna Freud said:

> To me the difference between transference in children and in adults is the following: what the adult transfers and revives in the transference neurosis are object relationships of the past and relationships to a fantasy object, whereas the child, even in matters of the past, has this past relationship or fantasy firmly fixed to the persons of the parents. Therefore he has present-day objects (as opposed to past and fantasy objects) involved in his neurosis.[5] The question then is—how far does the child transfer past relationships and fantasies *from the present-day objects to the analyst?* That is how I always saw the distinction. I think the child very rarely transfers everything in the analysis because the objects at home are still the more convenient ones, since they are still important to the child. I therefore think it is largely a matter of quantity, i.e., of *how much* is transferred. If one had an adult patient in a similar situation, almost all his problems would very soon be grouped around the analyst, around such issues as the holidays of the analyst, the analyst's other patients. It would be comparatively unimportant for the adult patient's transference what he had been enacting at home. We call it a transference neurosis when, shall we say, three quarters of the patient's transference repetitions are now focused within the analysis. I do not think that the appearance of transference material in a young child's analysis diminishes in any way the interplay with his current objects at home, or rather the living out of the neurosis at home. Here I am speaking quantitatively, but I think that if we speak of qualitative differences we have to look at the differences between real objects and fantasy objects in the child and the adult.

It was agreed that the transference neurosis, to the extent that it can exist in child analysis, may be blurred by the degree to which the parents are still available to the child patient and needed by him as real objects. Instead of borrowing the concept of transference

---

[5] This has a number of technical implications. For example, the therapist would tend to interpret the transference to the analyst from the mother of the present, *before* referring to the past.

neurosis from adult analysis (and imposing the concept on child analysis, searching for the child analytic analogues to the adult transference neurosis) it may be more worthwhile to separate out whatever significant elements apply and are appropriate. Also, the process involved in what we understand to be transference neurosis in adults may occur for only very brief periods in child analysis. For example, a process may last one or two days in child analysis which, were it to last for one or two months, might more readily be equated with an adult transference neurosis. It is very likely that we may spend time looking for distinctions significant for adult analysis when they have no exact counterpart in the child analytic situation, and vice versa.

There are similar questions about the occurrence of transference neurosis in adolescents. One possibility is that a full transference neurosis (in the adult sense) is not really possible for an adolescent because he is currently striving to break the ties with the parents and is acting out these relationships with others, externalizing his conflicts in this process. Perhaps the crucial point is the adolescent's need to distance himself from the parental objects. However, toward the end of adolescence, the patient might go through transference developments which are more like the transference neurosis as seen in the adult.

There are analysts who firmly believe that in children a transference neurosis can exist from the very beginning of treatment, that only transference and transference actions should be interpreted, and that this is the only "true" approach to the technique of child analysis. This view was seen by us as an oversimplification. Anna Freud commented:

> In past teaching, it was understood that the appearance of a transference neurosis was a very gradual process which built itself up as a reaction to interpretations, to the analyst's "speaking to the patient's Unconscious," and to the patient's growing positive attachment to the analyst. Thus the whole range of the patient's feelings are gradually brought into the new relationship, in all possible forms. Nowadays some people seem to think that the moment the patient enters the room he has a transference neurosis, and this assumption does away with a great mass of detailed information about the patient.

The first clinical example considered by the group under the heading of Transference Neurosis was from the treatment of Katrina L., aged 6;1 years at the beginning of her analysis, and indexed a year later.

> As treatment progressed Katrina became more able to express her feelings and conflicts in the treatment situation. She showed herself as a provocative, controlling child with many regressed behavior patterns and fantasies characteristic of much younger children. It was interesting to see that as this evolved her parents reported that she was more "perfect" both at home and at school. After some six months of treatment the parents said that her previous hysterical attacks had practically stopped; that she was at ease and seemed to enjoy life, had stopped being aggressive and provocative at home, stayed for all her meals at school, and was able to enjoy going to other children's parties.

The behavioral improvement occasionally seen early in analysis has often been called "transference improvement." We may also see a defensive "flight into health," but in Katrina's case the therapist noticed her improvement only after about six months of treatment, following progress in the analytic work.

In this case the regressed behavior previously seen outside treatment was limited to the analytic sessions, whereas now the behavior outside improved markedly. The regressed behavior in the session can be understood either as the transference revival of something from the past, or alternatively as the consequence of a "permitted regression" in the treatment situation. In the first case, the relationship to the therapist undergoes a development, the material produced shows an evolution, there is a concentration of unconscious wishes and object investments on the person of the analyst, and something is revived from the past. This becomes all-absorbing and all-important for the patient. As a consequence, the importance of enacting or living out conflicts involving people outside is no longer so great since the therapist is, for the time being, the prime recipient of the early object relationship. In the second case, i.e., that of "permitted regression," one might conceive that a gradual development of a more tolerant situation in the analytic setting allows the child to feel less under pressure and less constrained, and to feel instead, "here I can regress." [6] This may then allow the child to live out the regressive wishes in the session and be able to keep them in check outside. It was felt that this is an important point not sufficiently developed in the psychoanalytic literature.

Katrina's therapist saw the developments in her transference material as indicative of transference neurosis, taking into account not only the intensity of the child's transferred feelings but also the changes which occurred outside the analysis. However, the question still remains whether Katrina's transference to her therapist had the same quality of total involvement which one may see in the case of an adult patient who, for example, falls head over heels in love with his analyst. It is conceivable that the "license" given in the analysis could account for all the phenomena and changes described.

A permissive attitude in the child analytic situation is an important factor in allowing internal controls to relax. This may lead to behavior and material which is, descriptively speaking, "regressive," but does not constitute a regression in the usual sense of the word. The child may be in a situation at home and at school in which he is frightened to give in to infantile impulses or reactions, which are then consciously or unconsciously held back. He "works" to maintain himself on a more mature level of functioning. Given permission and a feeling of security within the analysis, he may "let his hair down." This is not, intrapsychically, a *return* to or a *revival* of infantile wishes, modes of functioning and expression, but rather a *release* of something currently present and "imprisoned" as a consequence of the child's fear of the reactions of external authority. There is a significant qualitative clinical difference between this and regression "proper." Of course, some children (and many adolescents) will defend against the emergence of infantile tendencies, whatever the reason for these. Very often, such patients, by using projection and externalization, will perceive

---

[6] I.e. "Here I can allow myself to behave in a less controlled and more childish fashion" (see the reference to "permission to express" on page 418). Anna Freud remarked: "One of my early child patients, an obsessional, called her analytic hour her 'rest time.' All day long she had to make a great effort to keep her inner 'devil' in check, but in the hour she could let him out."

the analyst as a representation of an internal superego figure, and will resist any tendency to "regress" in either of the forms described above.[7]

Another example of what was indexed as transference neurosis comes from the case of Arthur H., aged 12;4 years at the beginning of treatment. His age at the time of the second indexing was 15½ years.

> Arthur's analysis pointed to a most intense relationship to the therapist with many transference features, even in the face of very real external conflicts in the home. For a long time he maintained an image of the therapist as an idealized parental figure. By the middle of the third year of his analysis there were many pointers to the development of what could be understood as a "transference neurosis."
>
> Arthur came to admit that if he allowed himself to experience pleasure he might "lose" or "spoil" it. He initially rejected the transference interpretation that he felt the therapist could not tolerate his rivalry of Arthur's success or pleasure. However, Arthur subsequently revealed the following: often when he was enjoying something such as football, he would have a sudden image of the therapist, would feel awkwardly self-conscious, and his pleasure would stop.
>
> Arthur was told that the therapist would be leaving the country in six months' time. Working toward termination, Arthur verbal-

---

[7] Some analysts conceive of patients wanting to regress, or actually regressing to a supposed ideal state in which there is an all-embracing idyllic relationship between mother and child. This would represent a Nirvana for the child or a sort of ideal "symbiotic" state in which there are no unsatisfied demands, no painful feelings, and no frustrations. In our view, the idea of such an ideal state is a fiction, even though we may expect that, in normal circumstances, the very young infant will experience states of well-being following on the gratification of his needs; but this state would be one which is constantly disrupted by stimuli from within and without. However, some analysts have built theories of treatment on the idea that nearly all pathology results from disruptions of the earliest state of well-being, and believe that the analyst can subsequently provide the gratifications that the patient is presumed to have missed early in life, and that subsequently the patient's demands will diminish, and the patient will retrace his development along healthier lines. This idea is reminiscent of Franz Alexander's theory of the "corrective emotional experience." It is a view with which we thoroughly disagree, as far as analysis proper is concerned.

ized his fear of hurting the therapist's feelings, which made clearer his equation of "giving up old objects" and "killing them off." Arthur then presented himself as "troubled" only in the treatment, whereas outside he had achieved a great measure of self-confidence and assurance in his relationships. This was understood by the therapist to be part of a transference neurosis because it was a revival in the analysis of old, previously analyzed, feelings of being abandoned.

The striking fact that it was Arthur's image of the therapist and not the image of the mother which spoiled all his pleasure speaks for the presence of a transference neurosis in this case. It was thought to be a possible characteristic of the transference neurosis that the patient reports thinking and daydreaming about the analyst outside the analytic hour and the analytic setting.

Arthur missed a session in his analysis for the first time when he stayed at school to play football. Throughout the following weekend, Arthur felt miserable and anticipated the therapist's criticism for his absence. That Arthur was able to play football was, in the first place, due to the process of the analysis; and his feelings of guilt and fears of retaliation were also related to the treatment situation. It was suggested that Arthur's expectation of punishment because of guilt feelings was related to a conflict which was currently emerging in the transference—the anticipation of criticism appeared in the context of the analysis and he expected censure because he felt guilty about the pleasure he had experienced when he had been away from the therapist. This differentiates it from the so-called "negative therapeutic reaction" in which the patient punishes himself or fails because of an internal unconscious sense of guilt. Although it is important to attempt to make this distinction, it is not always easy to do. Clinically, both elements are frequently present to some extent. In Arthur's case, the preceding analytic work enabled him to make an attempt to break the tie to his mother. Therefore both the repetition of the conflict in the transference and the guilty reaction to an actually attempted break (with some degree of success in the attempt) are found in his reactions.

Because of Arthur's age (he was almost 16), it is doubtful if his material throws much light on transference neurosis in younger children. The capacity to develop a transference neurosis requires the ability to contain an internal conflict, and this ability is a developmental task which is only gradually achieved. In younger children, the facility with which conflict is externalized interfered with the development of a transference neurosis because the analyst is also used for other purposes. In adolescents, a further problem arises which is connected with the need to sever the ties with the parents. Thus regressive dependency in an intensive relationship with the analyst is feared.

The child analyst is commonly confronted with a situation in which a patient's problem emerges in relation to the analysis, but it is unclear to the analyst whether the problem should be understood as a development in the transference based on the ongoing analytic work, or whether it is related to a change in the availability of the primary objects. Child analysts frequently see an intensification of the child's feelings toward them when the mother is absent for a holiday. For example, consider the first eight weeks of treatment with a 9-year-old girl. She began analysis with the anxiety that her mother would lose her and forget to collect her at the Clinic—but the mother always did appear. These anxieties were interpreted as indicating that she felt her mother did not particularly care for her. After a few weeks the child said happily that she had found a way around her worry by coming to the Clinic herself. In this way she saved herself from the fear of waiting and the anxiety that her mother would forget her. Shortly after this session she arrived at the Clinic too early. She then became extremely worried that her analyst had forgotten her completely and was pale with fear. On the one hand she had dealt with her problem in relation to her mother, but on the other the anxiety appeared in the transference a few days later, centered on the analyst. Of course, it often happens that the child masters anxiety in one place and it appears, immediately thereafter, in another place. In the present case the "other place" was the relationship to the analyst, but the anxiety does not always shift to the analyst.

During analysis the parents may be involved with early conflicts in many ways. Such early conflicts may continue to be very live issues between the mother and the child. The conflict may have continued in its original form throughout, or it may have been modified in one way or another in the course of the child's development. Thus, for example, a conflict over soiling may persist as such, or it may reappear in a new edition such as a struggle over cleaning teeth or washing. Or a new level of expression may be found, for example, when a conflict appears to be around phallic exhibitionism, but an associated sadomasochistic struggle with the parent is the real continuing issue. The availability of the primary objects to the child also complicates the recognition of what is transference in yet another way. The child in analysis has the problem of dealing with his thoughts and feelings about his parents as they emerge in the analysis. The child only gradually develops the capacity to contain conflicts, fantasies, and impulses within the analytic setting. The younger he is, the more he has a natural tendency to action, and to carry the products of the analytic work straight home. This affects the interaction of the child with his parents and makes it difficult for the analyst to sort out reality, transferences, defense, and enactment.

For this reason it is important for the therapist to be guided in his interpretations by the *current* feelings of the child. Material should be considered, and if necessary interpreted, not only in relation to himself, but, where appropriate, also in relation to the parents of the present as well as the parents of the past. In a sense one could say that the child analyst in his interpretations has to take up a variable position between himself, the present parents, and the internalized parents of the past.

Throughout the discussion of transference neurosis in child analysis it was evident that the isolation of a conceptual entity of "transference neurosis" was a more difficult task than would be encountered in psychoanalytic work with adults. When a piece of analytic material from the past (as well as from the present) becomes alive in relation to the person of the therapist, we are faced with the fact that people other than the therapist may become involved, and this is much more frequent in the analysis of children than in adult analysis. Moreover, the frequency of the child's apparently regressive response to the implicit "license to express" offered by the analytic situation may also complicate the problem of delineating a transference neurosis in child analytic work.

5. Summary of Transference

In this subsection of the Index therapists are asked to give a summary of the stages through which the various aspects of the transference have moved and developed during the analysis, e.g., changes in the type of transference conflict and in the object which the therapist has come to represent for the patient. The description of these changes is of value in obtaining an overall picture of important elements in the patient's developmental history through their link with the analytic work as it unfolded in the transference and in the therapist's interpretations.

The example of Kevin C., aged 13 at the beginning of treatment, indexed for the third time at 18;1 years, may be used to illustrate the sort of entry placed in this subsection.

> In the course of the third and fourth years of treatment, the main emotional involvement in the boy's life was with his girlfriend with whom he clearly repeated his early mother relationship. The analytic material was mainly concerned with the girlfriend, even when she lived in another town. The transference material seemed to be an extension of this.
>
> The picture changed only at the end of the fourth year when the material centered directly on the relationship with the therapist and now became the place where the resistance was strongest. The oedipal conflict, both negative and positive, was transferred onto the therapist and worked through with her. The material now brought about home and school could be taken as a displacement away from the transference.

On occasion, the development of the transference is reflected in the patient's involvement with a person in his contemporary life. Kevin brought such material in the third year of his analysis, in regard to the absence of his girlfriend. This material, quite clearly a repetition of an aspect of the early mother relationship, could be seen as transference to the girlfriend, but could also be regarded as a manifestation of the patient's resistance to the development of similar feelings toward the therapist. In the latter case, his feelings toward the girl would be seen as a displacement or extension of his unconscious feelings toward the therapist. The technical problem arises of how much to interpret the repetition of the past in terms of the relationship to the girlfriend (using the feelings and fantasies about the absent object as a path toward the reconstruction of the patient's unconscious processes and fantasies) and how much to take the material up directly as a resistance toward the realization that such feelings are really felt toward the therapist. It is certain that therapists differ in their technical approaches in this respect. Adolescent patients bring a great deal of relevant material in the displaced form described above, and they can often stay in treatment only when this is tolerated by the analyst, and not interpreted as a resistance to experiencing the transference in the present. The latter point is illustrated in Kevin's case. It should be emphasized, however, that we may be discussing a special technical procedure used in the treatment of adolescents, appropriate because of the adolescent's fear of regression and his need to loosen his tie to the primary parental objects.

A further example has been taken from the indexed material on Tina K., aged 16;5 at the beginning of treatment, indexed at 18;9 years.

> Transferred feelings and attitudes played the most important part in the analysis. The therapist's appearance reminded Tina of her mother's appearance, her continental origin and age. This stimulated seemingly passionate, mainly positive desires from the very beginning of the analysis. Tina expressed her homosexual wishes toward the therapist in letters, dreams, and fantasies. Her attachment to the therapist was first understood and interpreted as a defense against her hostile wishes toward the therapist, and also as the result of a fear of rejection, reminiscent of her mother's rejection which Tina experienced in early childhood. An attempt by the patient to express more hostility gave way to intense feelings of depression. Her fear of losing the love object was excessive, but the libidinal aspect of Tina's feelings toward the therapist, her wish for physical contact, her curiosity about sexual activities, and her intense jealousy of the therapist emerged in the treatment and played a central part in it. Her need to see the therapist as a "perfect" person was interpreted in its defensive aspects and linked with her feeling that as a small child she had to see her mother as perfect in order to defend against disappointment. The homosexual transference was seen as a defensive one. However, during the

second year of treatment, the transference became a predominantly clinging and dependent one. This was reminiscent of the relationship of a very young child to her mother. Tina's need to interrupt treatment at this point was partly the expression of her fear of reexperiencing loving, tender, and dependent feelings, originally disrupted by an abrupt separation from her mother. All of this was reenacted and reexperienced in the transference.

It was suggested that this example gave a good picture of the roles assigned to the therapist in Tina's analysis. One could point to elements of the real relationship, of the extension of current relationships, and of the repetition of the past. However, Anna Freud pointed out that a different view could be taken. She commented:

> This is a good example, but it also highlights the difficulties of apparent transference in the analysis of an adolescent. What Tina showed might well be an adolescent "crush" on the analyst, a passionate sudden involvement with a person who becomes idealized. For Tina, this was a real relationship. I wonder if there really was any possibility of showing her the repetition of the past in her current feelings, and if so, if such an interpretation would diminish the intensity of her passionate feelings.

It would be worthwhile to attempt to make a distinction between the "crush" phenomenon and the transference. While the adolescent "crush" serves developmental needs, the transference in child analysis is usually (but not always) a revival of the past. In Tina's case, it is possible to see the "crush" side by side with transference manifestations. At times she also appears to be using the adolescent "crush" as a resistance.

The example of Edward G. was then considered. He was 3;1 years at the beginning of treatment, and was indexed at 4;11 years.

> Throughout treatment Edward in the main transferred onto the therapist aspects of his relationship to his mother. There was no clear progression of the transference through definite phases, but rather a tendency for certain transference features to occur in certain situations. When intercourse fantasies were predominant, the therapist was seen either as the castrating, phallic mother, or as a positive oedipal mother, depending on how intense Edward's

castration anxiety was. When Edward feared his mother's absence, the therapist was seen as the faithless, rejecting mother. She was also seen as the denigrating, rejecting mother when Edward's fears of his impulses to mess were uppermost, or when he felt unable to become the big, phallic man who could please and win the mother. Occasionally when Edward identified with the sadistic aspects of his father, the therapist was seen as the denigrated mother who was a "silly nitwit."

The description is typical of a 3-year-old in that the material described depends on spillover from the relationship to the parents. Strictly speaking, it is the mother of the present who is the transference object for the mother of the past, while the therapist may become a transference object *by displacement from the mother.*

The Index entry for Susan M., 3;9 years at the beginning of treatment and indexed at 4;9 years, is a further example of transference material from a child of the same age level as Edward, i.e., between 3 and 4 years.

Generally speaking, Susan has transferred the oedipal features of her mother relationship (envy, jealousy, rivalry, and feminine identification) onto the therapist, while the preoedipal features of the anal phase (such as whining, clinging, and domineering) have been much less marked. Sometimes characteristics of oral dependence have been transferred, as in games of being the therapist's baby. Since the negative feelings belonging to the ambivalence of the anal phase have continued to be enacted directly with the mother, the transference has tended to be positive up to date. Susan's initial fear of the therapist and of being alone with her was seen to be a transference of her fear of being seduced by the father, determined by her sadistic conception of intercourse. This fear disappeared after interpretation. She then for the most part transferred from her oedipal father her wish to be loved and admired, to please by being clever and competent, and her desire to be given a penis and babies.

The first part of this example can be seen as a splitting of the ambivalent feeling toward the mother, leaving the negative feelings directed toward the mother and the positive toward the therapist.

The two examples of Edward and Susan show that it is not difficult to give a descriptive account of what happens in the transference. However, it is more difficult to identify and distinguish "splits" in ambivalence, elements of real relationship, repetitions of the past, and so on. With adolescents, in contrast to younger children, we face the additional problem of how to characterize those differences which are *specific* to adolescence, which change the nature of the way in which the transference is developed and handled by the adolescent. There are special features of transference applying to children under the age of 5, discussed in more detail in section 2. On the other hand we should be careful not to ascribe too much to the child's age or stage of development in our considerations. This may lead us to neglect other important factors.

The question of the resolution of transference (or, as a member of the group put it, the "myth of the resolution of the transference") should also be considered in writing a summary of transference development.

By the "resolution of the transference" we imply that an active conflict involving the person of the analyst—one which represents the externalization of an internal conflict of some sort—should have receded as a consequence of the analytic work. There should, we hope, also be a more realistic assessment by the patient of the therapist as a person, and the ties that *remain* to the therapist should ideally be less emotionally laden and conflictual.

As an example we may consider a boy who had lost his father and was treated by a male analyst. Two years after termination his mother reported that the analyst had played a very large part in the boy's thoughts shortly after termination, and he had wanted to contact his analyst whenever he felt unhappy or upset. Now, however, he has made many relationships and is getting on well with his peers at school. Only when things go very badly or very well does he currently say that he would like to talk to his therapist, but only to tell him about it. Between such moments the analyst seems to be a benign figure for him, not a person who is very heavily cathected, as his emotional investments have moved to others in his daily life.

Anna Freud remarked:

> I think what we are talking about here is really a resolving of the real relationship, and not the resolving of the transference. In a

case such as this one, of a fatherless boy where somebody else takes over the father's role as well as being the analyst, the relationship is very mixed.

Reference was made to various views which contrast the transference and the "real" relationships. It has been pointed out that there are difficulties in keeping these two kinds of relationship separate and apart, that it is dangerous to neglect either of the two, and that they really make sense only in relation to each other. In our discussions it was emphasized that the issue is not one concerning the social relationships between patient and analyst, nor is it one concerning the management of these relationships as such. The problem refers to the two sides of the relationship formed by the patient with the analyst, one the "real" relationship, being, so to speak, between one person and another. The other aspect is the distortion of the relationship through the transference. Of course, such mixtures exist in relationships outside analysis. However, in the psychoanalytic situation the focus is much more on the transference aspects of the analytic relationship, and the analysis of these aspects is a major tool in the analytic work.

BIBLIOGRAPHY

FREUD, A. (1965), Preface to J. Bolland, J. Sandler, et al., *The Hampstead Psychoanalytic Index.* New York; Int. Univ. Press.
────── (1967), About Losing and Being Lost. *This Annual,* 22:9–19.

On Termination in Child Analysis

HEIMAN VAN DAM, M.D., CHRISTOPH M. HEINICKE, PH.D., AND MORTON SHANE, M.D.

TERMINATION IN CHILD ANALYSIS RAISES MANY CRUCIAL ISSUES BOTH for clinical work and the conceptualization of child development. Anna Freud (1970a) clearly states the problem: children "should be considered cured as soon as the developmental forces have been set free again and are ready to take over. But as appealing as this solution is in theory, in practice it is not at all easy to determine when precisely this welcome change in the child's personality is taking place and where exactly in his structure it is operating" (p. 14). In this paper we attempt to develop some guidelines that may help child analysts to determine where and when this "welcome change" has occurred. In addition, we shall consider some technical problems during the termination phase.

A child analysis can be terminated under varying circumstances. While Anna Freud (1970a) focused on causes for premature terminations, we shall concentrate on more ideal circumstances—namely, when parents, child, and child analyst are in agreement

---

The authors are associated with the Los Angeles Psychoanalytic Institute and the Department of Psychiatry at UCLA School of Medicine.

Presented at the Annual Meeting of the Association for Child Psychoanalysis, Palm Springs, California, March 1972, and to the Child Study Group, San Francisco Psychoanalytic Institute, June 1972.

about the termination. In other words, we shall discuss when the analyst can be satisfied that a reasonable result has been accomplished.

The literature on the termination of treatment contains only few contributions dealing specifically with child analysis (Kohrman, 1969). The majority of papers is concerned with developing criteria for the termination of adult analysis (Hurn, 1971; Pfeffer, 1963a, 1963b). Yet, most of these criteria are not directly applicable to children, as an examination of those most frequently discussed demonstrates.

"Removal of symptoms" (Freud, 1937) is a less reliable criterion in work with children than it is with adults. Symptoms often disappear in children since the child is a developing individual in whom changes are going on at all times (Anna Freud, 1970b). Furthermore, the real relationship with the child analyst, a reliable adult who listens noncritically and empathetically, is more likely to bring about symptomatic improvement in a child than in an adult long before an understanding of the underlying causation can be achieved.

The criterion of the removal of defenses and resistances by interpretation (Hoffer, 1950) also is more complicated in child analysis. For instance, a reaction formation in a latency boy may serve as a defense against unresolved anal conflicts. Yet, the same boy may need to use reaction formation as a phase-appropriate defense against his phallic impulses toward girls. In such instances, we try to undo only excessive and crippling defense activities. Moreover, as we shall demonstrate, special age-appropriate defenses also may come into play in the termination phase itself.

Other frequently mentioned criteria—genital primacy (Freud, 1937; Balint, 1950), the capacity for work, and the capacity for mourning—also have to be modified considerably if they are to be utilized as criteria for termination in child analysis. Moreover, the evaluation of whether the general aims of an analysis—the gaining of insight, working through, resolution of the transference, and the finding of new adaptations—have been accomplished presents special problems in the analysis of children.

Although many valuable criteria for termination have been developed, one cannot escape the impression that for both adults and children a systematic approach to the question of how to arrive at the decision to terminate is still lacking (Rangell, 1966; Firestein, 1969). Moreover, we doubt that the search for specific criteria is really a useful endeavor. Rather, we believe that a child's readiness to terminate must be evaluated from a multiple aspect view. The tools for such a procedure are readily available in the Developmental Profile developed by Anna Freud (1962).

A Multiple Aspect View of the Child in the Decision to Terminate

The application of the various viewpoints contained in the Profile forces the analyst to pay equal attention to all of the child's areas of functioning. In addition, by virtue of this broader and comprehensive viewpoint, much of what otherwise would remain preconscious in the analyst, his so-called clinical intuition, enters into his judgment about termination. Finally, he may discover and become aware of some of his own blind spots.[1]

When a child's functioning at the beginning of his analysis and during the pretermination period is compared by means of the Profile, the analyst becomes aware of the many qualitative and quantitative changes, whether they occurred in the areas of the drives, the ego, the ego ideal, the superego, the various lines of development, or in the areas of genetic, structural, or dynamic interactions. While it is assumed that an analysis leads to a greater availability of more advanced forms of functioning, we often see that early structures and modes of functioning are still present at the end of an analysis. The unevenness of the results of our analytic efforts becomes quite apparent. In addition, the Profile allows for an assessment of the many developmental changes that are brought about not solely by analytic efforts, but also by the impact of such factors as the real relationship to the child analyst (A. Freud, 1974).

For the child analyst in particular, the dilemma of too little or too much analysis is a real one. Is it best to free the child from the

---

[1] In his discussion of this paper, Dr. James Anthony correctly supplemented these remarks by stressing the continuing importance of the analyst's feelings toward the patient and the analysis in setting the termination date.

regressive pull of the analysis so that the analytic progress made can be integrated with the age-appropriate developmental forces? Or is more analytic work necessary before the progressive developmental forces are sufficiently freed to insure continued progress following the termination of analysis?

In setting the termination date for an adult patient, the analyst is less concerned with developmental forces and relies primarily on the patient's general functioning (including the overcoming of the initial symptoms). In child analysis, on the other hand, the rapidity of ego and drive development may necessitate periods of integration, sometimes without analysis. Moreover, developmental forces and reintegration after termination may move the child to adaptive levels at which the persistence of some symptoms may no longer be viewed as a serious matter. The assessment of a child's status along the lines of Profiles at the beginning of analysis, at termination of analysis, one and two years after analysis has been terminated, demonstrates this quite well (Heinicke, 1965, 1969). We do not imply that in clinical practice it is necessary to write out a Profile; rather a knowledge of the various viewpoints of the Profile will lead to an organized, broader picture of a child's functioning. This, we suggest, should be obtained before the analyst decides to terminate.

CASE ILLUSTRATION

Certain aspects of the case of Peter, age 9, will be used to illustrate how we use the various Profile considerations and concepts to arrive at the decision to terminate a child's treatment.

One of Peter's symptoms was inadequate progress in schoolwork, especially arithmetic. A general stubbornness pervaded much of his learning. Serious fights had ensued around the father's attempt to drill him on his times tables and other homework. Peter also had a flinching tic, as if someone was about to hit him. He cleverly provoked fights with his brother and his peers, so that his parents would get into arguments not only with each other but also with the neighbors. He was unexpectedly violent when he could not have his own way, and a sudden attack on a girl in his classroom precipitated the teacher's making the referral.

After a period of once-a-week treatment, an analysis was

initiated and continued for three years. The parents were seen by another therapist.[2] As is true in many cases, when termination was considered, one could still detect components of previously seen fixations and conflicts. In this pretermination phase Peter's wish to terminate was evaluated in terms of the various Profile considerations. At the end of the analysis, a more systematic Profile was written out by both the child's analyst, one of the authors, and by one of the coauthors who had seen and evaluated the child and parents at the beginning and end of treatment. In addition to his own contacts, this outside analyst had available to him the psychological test findings at the beginning and end of treatment and the description of the first three and last ten therapeutic sessions with the child. The findings reported here integrate the Profiles of both the child's analyst and the independent analyst evaluator.[3] While all sections of the Profile were written up, we present the material in the order that best captures the essential qualities of this boy.

One of the most important considerations in making the judgment about Peter's adaptation, and the related judgment about termination, was the concept of the *balanced availability of defenses and affects.* Initially, Peter showed a defensive imbalance, excessively relying on a frightened, anticipatory cautiousness whenever he met anxiety-provoking situations and on a defensive identification as if he were a waif or a scavenger. He avoided all schoolwork that looked difficult, and showed excessive externalization of controls in the sense of depending on others to make him do his schoolwork and stop him from demolishing his younger brother.

Confronted with his male therapist, Peter seemed frozen and wondered: Is it all right to paint here? Is it all right to throw the ball here? Later he reluctantly admitted that he had received his report card, but added, "I didn't look at it." His predominant interest was in making up for what he felt his parents had not given him. He acted like an abandoned child. He looked for coins in all

---

[2] We wish to thank Mortimer M. Meyer, Ph.D. and Lillian Weitzner, M.S.W. for their assistance in the evaluation and treatment of this family.

[3] It was possible to make this extensive evaluation because Peter's treatment was part of a research project.

the fish ponds and wishing wells of local restaurants and was ready to salvage out of the waste paper basket things which the therapist had thrown away. Peter's doleful questions about the size of the analyst's house were intended to make the analyst feel that he should share his riches. Actually, Peter could not really ask for things directly. Most important, there was initially no sense of fun or laughter in this generally depressed and repressed child.

Toward the end of treatment, this imbalance had changed. The anticipatory cautiousness, the denial of his academic difficulties, the defensive identification with the scavenger or waif were all absent or at least greatly diminished. More importantly, the repressive nature of his defense organization had changed to allow him a spontaneity of feelings and a greater sense of pleasure and a real sense of humor. For instance, after having successfully defeated his father in a bowling game, he repeatedly took on the analyst in a similar game during the sessions. His ability to laugh as the analyst completely missed all the pins was viewed as an important sign of progress.

We had reservations in regard to this flexibility in Peter's functioning because he continued to use externalization of control as a defense. At the end of the analysis, he still looked to his parents or his analyst to make him do certain things, especially his homework. Yet, by comparison with the beginning of the analysis, this defense had lessened sufficiently so that one could anticipate that it would continue to decrease as part of the reintegration after the analysis and thereby come within the bounds of a balanced defense organization.

Another important aspect to assess is the *quality of ego integration*. Is the child's ego functioning still characterized by great rigidity or is it very labile? (Frankl, 1961.) We ask ourselves whether in the context of increasing adaptation, certain areas of malfunctioning have remained and are not likely to be subject to much change, even in the period of reintegration that typically occurs after analysis. Analytic work often reveals that certain areas of functioning may serve as useful indicators of the extent and quality of ego integration, for instance, Peter's tic and his reading difficulties. As long as Peter's tic remained, one would question the quality of his ego integration. After much analytic work and working through a great variety of material, and after extensive therapy with Peter's parents, it finally was possible to reconstruct the following incident. When the child was 4 years old, the father, in a fit of rage, pulled the string on Peter's jacket so tight that Peter was choked to the point of changing his facial coloring. After the meaning of this episode was reconstructed and linked to other determinants, the tic was no longer seen.

Similarly, as long as Peter's reading remained far below his potential, setting the termination had to be questioned. It was not until the type of material illustrated around competitive bowling had been repeatedly worked through that his reading and general academic work improved considerably. Again it is important to stress the extensive analytic work that had preceded this phase of treatment. Even so, through the construction of block towers which would only go just so high, one could understand that he had not adequately resolved all his competitive feelings toward his father. Nevertheless, termination now seemed feasible since we hoped that these slight inhibitions of his success would be resolved in the period of postanalytic integration.

The balance between the progressive and regressive drive and ego forces in the child is another important guideline used in setting the termination. Making *genetic assessments* for this particular purpose requires that one recall the pattern of working through that has occurred during the analysis. One needs to focus on an intrapsychic conflict dominant in a given period of treatment, including how it showed up in the transference. Then one examines the sequence of conflict themes. In Peter's analysis these themes were related to important childhood experiences and fixation points. As in other analyses, we noted that there was initially a regressive movement from one critical experience involving a fixation to another, until eventually a turning point in this pattern of regressive recapitulation was reached and developmentally more forward-looking phallic material increasingly appeared.

To give an example, in Peter's case, the reconstruction of his early acts of actively exploring his environment and the reconstruction of his achieving toilet training represented these important turning points in his analysis. The mother, in order to deal with her own depression, precipitated by her husband's losing his job, left the boy in the care of the father while she herself sold domestic goods. Struggling with his own rage at her departure, Peter found that his provocative messing, urinating, and hyperactivity turned a somewhat withdrawn but caring father into a raging figure. After these experiences with the father in the anal period (in the setting of separation-individuation) were reconstructed, both the fear and the counterphobic pleasure of wrestling with the oedipal father emerged in the treatment for the first time. This was dynamically linked to regressive conflicts involving Peter's anger at a mother who did not pick him up on time. Peter felt that if he expressed his anger, she, just like the father, would slap him in the face and not feed him the next day. Further working through of this oral material allowed him to challenge his father again on the phallic level, this time in card games such as Black Jack. He was so successful at this that the father actually abandoned the game. As Peter told of this, trucks again suddenly bashed into each other. As the fear of the consequences of his beating his father on the oedipal level could be related to his fear of being beaten as a soiling child, Peter drummed on his belt buckle and then near his genitals. And just as this competition in card games represented more forward-looking phallic material, so associated phallic material like the bowling followed. Other regressive links were of course also represented. Thus, the identification with the ragelike father could be linked to a much more archaic rage that Peter felt when his mother became pregnant when he was 3.

To summarize, a turning point in the balance between regressive and progressive forces could be detected in the pattern of the analytic material. As Peter continued to elaborate the more advanced components of his conflicts and functioning, one could expect that a definite move to phase dominance in the next developmental period would be consolidated.

Viewing this same material from the point of view of *drive development*, questions of phase dominance, libido distribution, object relations, and aggression had to be related to considerations of the emerging adolescent development. How would the progressive forces freed by the analysis interact with the challenges of a new developmental phase? We considered whether it would be best for Peter to struggle unaided with this as part of the normal move toward independence or whether further analytic work was needed to allow this adaptation.

Assessment of *phase dominance* revealed that Peter had clearly entered the adolescent libidinal development. In view of the fact that he was in treatment during latency and the beginning of adolescence, it was not easy to distinguish whether the indications of the oedipal conflict and the related phallic derivatives were the expected revivals associated with the onset of adolescence or represented residuals not likely to lessen and be resolved as part of adolescence. Examples of turning to the strong phallic mother and passively seeking direction would not favor such resolution. In contrast, his forward-looking phallic response to the interpretations of the oral-regressive material during the termination phase suggested that the move toward independence from the mother would predominate. He moved from childish games to mature chess competition with his father and his analyst. In the evaluation by the outside analyst, Peter showed himself as independent, self-assured, and able both to separate from the mother and yet be reasonable in relation to her demands. He obtained several jobs and showed an increasing adolescentlike determination to do things by himself.

In regard to *libido distribution,* his self-esteem had improved considerably; in general, he made one feel that he liked himself. His narcissism seemed healthiest in the phallic body area. The tics had disappeared, and he was competent in a variety of age-appropriate sports. This was perhaps best reflected in the bowling contest with the analyst, including his ability to laugh at the analyst's failure in this game.

Peter now derived considerable narcissistic gratification from his ego achievements and object relationships. His academic work had improved, and he felt confident that he "would make it." His chess play was excellent, and he read easily. He had formed some friendships and, most important, was less dependent on external sources to replenish his narcissism; a quality of desperation and depression was no longer present.

A timidity in reaching out to peers could, however, be noted, and could be related to instances of feeling like "a dumb shit." This is what he had more or less written on his school desk at the beginning of treatment. One could perhaps also relate his sloppy dress and casual behavior to this self concept of being "a shit," but it seemed to us to be part of the adolescent developments.

The assessment of the narcissistic supplies in relation to the superego structure showed both the greatest gain and an area of concern. The inner representation of a ragelike jealous father had lessened sufficiently to allow Peter the inner strength "to take him on." But there was also evidence that his own jealousy of the father was projected, perceived in retaliatory form, so that at times he might again feel harassed rather than self-confident.

The evaluation of Peter's *object relations* revealed inner object expectations focused on a feeling of being loved by the mothering figure and more generally by people. There was a quiet assurance about this expectation, but also some evidence of a feeling: "It wasn't enough." Despite a strong transference and a successful termination phase, including extensive work on his longings, a sense of wanting to maintain continuity was clearly expressed. Peter was therefore encouraged to contact the analyst who specifically mentioned follow-up interviews. Peter made it clear that he wanted to be contacted. This indeed revealed a residual expectation that people show their care by keeping after him.

The closer and more affectionate relation to his mother and other women was now associated with the arousal of erotic feelings, which at times he still perceived as threatening. The father could not be completely trusted as a protecting person, even though open rivalry as well as intimate conversations now occurred. Peter sensed that the father's jealousy could still lead to a sudden loss of control. To defend against this potential lack of protection Peter needed to protect himself; he still had to put a certain brake on the level of his success. In chess he would suddenly "give up" the queen. Yet, to put this into context—and this is of course exactly the kind of weighing of factors that experience with the Profile encourages—Peter's inner relationship to his parents had changed greatly in the course of treatment. We therefore expected that these oedipal residuals would largely be resolved in an adaptive direction in the posttreatment phase.

With regard to *aggression,* Peter now showed a fairly age-expectable level of aggression. The continued need to quarrel with and downgrade his brother revealed his remaining feeling that others received more or intruded upon what he had. But the level of aggression was within the normal range of brotherly encounters, and we anticipated that the intensity of its manifestations would subside in the posttreatment phase.

We were more concerned about the fact that Peter's tendency to rush through work or not to work at all had persisted, and that residuals of infantile longing were connected to fantasies of wishing to be gratified without having to work so hard. But at termination manifestations of this passivity were rare. Moreover, the temper tantrums and the previous inclination to provoke fights and attack girls, which had also been dynamically associated with these longings, were no longer in evidence.

The *turn to new partnerships,* especially with peers, is of particular importance at the psychological entrance into adolescence. Has the child at the end of the analysis formed new object ties or changed his old ones so that they now reflect a true partnership? At the time of termination, the sadomasochistic components in the peer relationships ought to be of less importance than a genuine give-and-take and a consideration for the partner. This is especially significant because of the loss of the real relationship with the analyst at termination. Peter's sadomasochistic peer relations were now minimal, he had several friends, but an intense partnership was more a potential than an actuality.

Viewing Peter's development in terms of *dynamic and structural assessments (conflicts),* we concluded that much of Peter's functioning was now relatively conflict-free. This was most readily deduced from his low level of anxiety and the lightness and spontaneity of a whole new set of feeling experiences. For example, he showed delight in the success and defeat of others; or he could with real humor blame the other person for not getting his own tower up higher. This attitude, though, also indicated the persistent residual of "Why should I work so hard to get it up there when I have gotten so little." In Peter's fantasies, his brother and the analyst were rich; he still turned to eating to curb the emergence of such primitive fantasies as that he had destroyed his mother's breast and the family's favorite house. Humorously he referred to himself as a dirty greedy pig. We must reemphasize that the Profile considerations are likely to reveal such qualitative residuals of early conflicts and fantasies. But the weight assigned to the persistence of these residuals is determined by their role in the total personality functioning. The overall assessment indicated that Peter had resolved many of his conflicts and was moving to increased ego autonomy.

At termination the most visible set of conflicts concerned his taking a masculine, competitive stance in relation to his father. Confronted with the full intensity of this competition—and that he could permit himself to experience this was of course a tremendous gain—he could still, through an identification with his father, experience the dread of going out of control. Like his father, he might choke someone or provoke external control. More specifically a conflict between the internalized jealous father and the successful son rival still inhibited his building the tower all the way up. It was safer "to go just so far" to avoid castration. The imagined lack of control on the part of the father was clearly accentuated by being regressively linked to the image of the wild, messy kid who, at the age of 3 while riding his tricycle, had destroyed a fence. Links between castration anxiety and being dumb (as a sign of castration) could also be inferred. But, most important to note, these residuals were inferred only in the projective psychological testing, were not obvious in the evaluative sessions with the outside analyst, and had all been actively interpreted and subject to therapeutic progress during the analysis. This emphasizes once more the importance of the total context in which certain qualitative material emerges. Taking this into account, the above-stated conclusions about Peter's conflict picture could indeed be maintained.

Whether these conflicts would be further resolved or accentuated in a maladaptive direction depended also on the *parental environment.* Both parents had had the tendency to abandon Peter and his brother, the mother by escaping into work and the father by escaping into unemployment. These were no longer present; and the mother's tendency to attack her husband as a generally inadequate male who could not limit his son was now very greatly reduced. The father's inability to support Peter's developing masculinity, however, was of greatest concern to us. The father still had an intense need to be superior to his own twin brother—a need that Peter activated and kept alive. The father was still struggling with his guilt about his physical attacks on Peter in the past. Moreover, he was still incapable of taking those steps toward success that the family expected—becoming a partner in his business and buying a house. These traits of the father might activate internal dangers in Peter and make it difficult for him to succeed. Since the father wished to continue his therapy and since it was possible that the factors impinging on Peter could be changed significantly, the final evaluation of Peter again had to await follow-up.

The first follow-up interviews and testing were done a year after termination, and Peter was again evaluated from the multiple aspect view of the Profile. In almost every respect the developmental questions raised at termination were resolved in a progressive rather than a regressive direction. Clear phase dominance in adolescence was revealed by his heterosexual interests, friendships with girls, and his distancing himself from his parents' control. His achievement in school (as well as his IQ test performance) led to a new experience: inner pride supported by open praise from his parents. While he was not as ambitious as his parents wanted him to be, he was at ease and no longer saw himself as "a dumb shit." There was no evidence of the inhibition of academic achievement and competitiveness, and the implied further resolution of the oedipal conflict was supported by other observations. Most impressive was the balance in his defense organization and especially the greatly reduced reliance on others to assume responsibility for him. This was consistent with other indications of effective ego integration. Tics, twitches, and restlessness had permanently disappeared. His attention span was impressive, as was his capacity for self-observation.

But we had to raise the question whether his relationships to his parents represented a normal developmental distancing consistent with his general tendency to "cool" things or whether this distancing was defensive in relation to a deep sense of disappointment, an avoidance of getting into their quarrels, and would ultimately leave him with a sense of loneliness. His capacity for relationships to girls, a partnership with one boy, and a moving expression of warmth and gratitude toward the therapist all revealed his capacity and need for object relations. He also made it clear that he wanted to be able to maintain contact with the therapist and, by implication, that he was disappointed in what his parents had offered him. The mother did indeed seem too restrictive in regard to allowing girlfriends in the house. Yet, her warm, caring feelings for her son continued. The follow-up brought to light a recurrence of marital conflict that would not be supportive. The revival of an earlier family situation was noted. The mother was out working, was late, and the father found himself having to do the pots. On this occasion she again pointed out that she had to work because he was not an adequate provider. He, on the other hand, showed her how she constantly demanded more and more and humiliated him. Nevertheless, they had been united in buying a house. It was also significant that because of their own previous therapy, these encounters were now more easily resolved.

It was in similar conflict situations when the father had taken care of Peter, between the ages of 2 and 4, that he had actually attacked his son. In view of the father's failure to resolve this conflict, Peter may have been forced to seek a more protective figure outside of the family. This was no doubt one reason for his open wish to maintain contact with his male analyst. Further contacts would have to determine to what extent Peter could distance himself from his parents and make new relationships.

Technical Problems During the Termination Phase

In the termination phase of both adult and child analysis, one analyzes ongoing conflicts, the specific meaning of the termination in terms of the patient's past conflicts and experiences (Arlow, 1971), and the giving up of the analyst as a real object. In this section we shall illustrate some additional features which are specific to termination in child analysis and which we believe have not been sufficiently stressed.

Prelatency, latency, and even early adolescent children may react to the stress of termination, the impending loss of the analyst as a real object, with age-appropriate defense mechanisms, which, by adult standards, are nevertheless immature mechanisms. As will be demonstrated by case material, these defense mechanisms may interfere with working through, the final resolution of the transference, and insight (Kohrman, 1969). The extent to which this holds true varies of course from child to child, and depends on his previous experiences with actively decathecting object representations, for instance, on the vicissitudes of the separation-individuation process (Mahler, 1965). The latency child is already actively involved in making considerable cathectic shifts in his relationships to objects outside the family. Each of these situations represents an active developmental shift forward, as a result of which it is not experienced primarily as a loss. The unique object loss associated with termination calls for particular defenses which deal with giving up the analyst and permit closure of the analytic process. Anna Freud (1971) also refers to the real relationship and wonders who will inherit it after the analysis is terminated. As the case material will demonstrate, at times there may be some unexpected heirs because the child decides that issue and not his analyst. Termination also has other positive values for the child. It frees him to engage in many activities which he had to forgo due to his analysis. It also frees him from the regressive pull of the analytic work, and gives him the opportunity to develop further without the aid of the analyst, for example, by establishing new object ties (Solnit, 1960) and the formation of new sublimations.

However, in this section we wish to stress the pain and pressure created by the impending termination, which may give rise to individual as well as age-appropriate ego reactions. Each child's individual reactions have to be analyzed. In addition, the analyst needs to deal with the age-appropriate reactions, which range from the most primitive reactions, such as somatization and denial, to the most advanced ways available to a child's ego of coping with the impending change in his outer reality. The analyst verbalizes what the child himself is not yet capable of doing. Of course, this verbalizing is most helpful in strengthening the ego in its tasks. However, the analyst's effort may meet, in a certain sense, with limited success. As a result, the question of whether the child has adequately worked through the stress of termination may remain open (Wallach, 1961). One is reminded of the theoretical and technical problems surrounding mourning in childhood (Shambaugh, 1961; Furman, 1964; Wolfenstein, 1966; Nagera, 1970; Miller, 1971). The answer varies from child to child, depending on his past experiences, his current level of development, and what, as a result of this development, is available to his ego. Accordingly, the length of the termination phase has to be related to all of these factors. For instance, Anthony (1970) permitted a patient a full year for termination because of the possibility of a residual suicidal tendency.

CASE ILLUSTRATION

In describing how one child dealt with termination, we shall demonstrate what could be analyzed in terms of past conflicts and the transference situation; and what had to be understood in contrast to the usual adult model of termination.

Amy A. was 10½ years old when she began analysis. Her mother, who was herself in analysis, could no longer ignore the increasing distress of her youngest child. At the age of 7 Amy developed facial and bodily tics which became increasingly severe. She was excessively worried about her grades, complained of stomachaches, was a finicky eater, was intermittently constipated, had to sleep with a menagerie of stuffed animals, was too polite, and was extremely self-conscious about her skin, teeth, hair, and small stature. The initial interviews with the parents revealed that Mrs. A. had suffered a miscarriage of a 5-month male fetus at some time during the six-year period between the birth of her eldest daughter and the birth of the patient. This contributed to the mother's need for closeness to Amy. She found it difficult to let Amy grow up in certain ways. For example, she wiped Amy after bowel movements until she was 5, cuddled her frequently, and allowed her in the parents' bed with little restriction throughout the latency years. Amy's father, too, was doting and seductive. The parents quarreled often, each accusing the other of being too indulgent. They also argued about other matters, so that occasionally the child overheard talk of divorce.

In spite of the ample evidence of unresolved oedipal and preoedipal conflicts, Amy had attained several latency accomplishments. She did very well in school, albeit abetted by her obsessive-compulsive neurotic conflicts and character structure. She knew how to please demanding teachers and could be engaging with girlfriends and even with boyfriends, although she was only 10 years old. Amy was an accomplished dancer and musician, and was talented, though restricted, in art and acting. She hid her regressive behavior from her peers, allowing the open expression of fears and tears only at home. With considerable effort she also controlled her tics in public.

Amy's psychological development was seriously interfered with by a trip that her parents took when she was 8 years old. She was cared for by a couple, Carmen and Carroll. Carmen was overly strict and insensitive to the child's regressive demands. She threw out Amy's favorite teddy bear after the family dog chewed off a part of the face—an event that proved traumatic. The child blamed Carroll for not coming to her rescue on this as well as on several other occasions. She timidly kept her anger to herself and entertained daydreams of appropriating his power by trading places with him. Amy's parents were disturbed by her regressive clinging and easy tearfulness after their return and correctly attributed it to her experiences while they had been away.

During her first hour with the analyst, Amy sat immobile, revealing shortly that she was trying to follow the advice of a psychologist who once tested her; he had told her that by sitting quietly, she could control her twitches. The analyst told her she was free to move about in the hour as she wished. After this her bodily and facial tics became obvious, entering into the analytic dialogue from then on. She was able to express herself in words and was open and trusting, although she was clearly inhibited in expressing affect and in her voluntary movements. Amy's precocious capacity to verbalize was evident from the beginning of her analysis.

Throughout the three years of analysis, Amy's physical movements remained inhibited. This characteristic, augmented by a trustful magical transference, imparted to the analytic material an adultlike quality. She saw the analyst as a wizard, whose strength she would acquire by trading places with him as she had daydreamed of doing with Carroll. An unconscious belief in her parents' omnipotence was worked through. As a result, superego anxiety diminished so that the aggression and forbidden preoedipal and phallic-oedipal identifications that underlay most of the tic formations were revealed. By the end of the first year the tics had essentially disappeared. Amy's continued, although diminished, access to the parents' bed kept in the open much primal scene material and related oedipal fantasies which were experienced regressively in oral and anal terms. In addition to being the magical, omnipotent, abandoning, preoedipal mother, the analyst was also seen as a knife-wielding, attacking father. However, this knife came more and more to resemble a loving penis as Amy attempted to resolve her castration wishes and penis envy.

Amy's progress in giving up her neurotic fixations and conflicts could be seen not only in the process of working them through in the transference, which led to a diminution of her symptoms, but also by significant indications of resumption of progressive development. As time went on she demonstrated, with less regressive interference, that she had more fully moved into the phase of preadolescence. She was able to become increasingly objective, both about her mother's clingingness and her father's seductiveness. Her relationships with peers increased in strength so that the process of object removal reached age-appropriate levels. She related to her teachers less as parents whom she had to please and fear and more as ideal figures whom she wished to emulate.

Termination Material As Defense and Content Rather Than As an Indication for Termination Per Se

Amy's interest in termination was expressed early and continued intermittently throughout the analysis. It was consistently dealt with as analytic material until the middle of the third year of treatment when an ongoing evaluation of her total functioning led to its realistic consideration at that time.

Right from the start Amy had wondered how long analysis would take. Her sister had been in therapy three times a week for several years and was still seeing the doctor once a week. Her mother had been in such a prolonged analysis that Amy both wished for and feared an analysis without end. In the seventh month of analysis she verbalized her fear of losing the analyst if her tics stopped. This statement served to illustrate her mode of clinging to her mother through illness. Termination material came up again in the second year when she expressed fears that her friends might discover she was going to a psychiatrist. This was connected with shame about conflictual childish things, like sleeping with her mother or her teddy bear. She wanted to stop by tapering off, not suddenly going from four times a week to nothing. The analyst reminded her of how upset she had been when Carmen had suddenly thrown away her teddy bear. This memory had served as a screen for earlier experiences and fantasies of people suddenly disappearing, e.g., fears of her mother stealing away in the night. Pointing out the link between her wish for gradual termination to avoid sudden object loss seemingly diminished Amy's fear of a traumatic separation. She was then able to express her anger at being forced to come so often. Two months later she tearfully pleaded with her mother to help her cut down to twice a week. However, it became clear, to both patient and analyst, that this was a defensive turning to her mother in order to avoid discussing the "hot feelings" she experienced after being French-kissed by a boy at a party. Heterosexual and homosexual genital excitement emerged after the patient's attempted avoidance was interpreted.

In the summer of the second year of analysis, termination came up again; this time as an attempt to turn passive into active. Amy was facing feelings of being deserted both by her sister, who was leaving for college, and by her analyst who was leaving for summer vacation. But as she left for camp that summer, Amy said something that made the analyst think for the first time that termination might be a possibility at some vague point in the future. She said, "I'm beginning to analyze myself. I ask myself questions about what I am thinking, like I think you would do." After returning from vacation, she continued from time to time to be able to ask herself what she was thinking. She even had a dream that she was a psychiatrist helping her girlfriend. Her defense against separation by identification with the analyst thus had its adaptive and progressive aspects. She was then $12\frac{1}{2}$ years old. As will be demonstrated, however, when the actual termination occurred many forms of regressive ego functioning came into play instead of clearly progressive moves. Thus, although the patient could respond to a vacation with relative ease, she perceived and responded to termination quite differently.

The Pretermination Period

Throughout this period the analyst is engaged in assessing the patient's analytic progress. The overriding consideration is the patient's potential for continued progressive development, in the absence of help from the analyst.

As has been indicated, Amy was in the third year of her analysis when pretermination assessments became prevalent. For instance, for the next six months she continued working with increased self-awareness and diminished defenses of isolation of affect, motoric inhibition, and repression. She was able to enlarge the distance from her parents, asking her mother not to hold her hand and her father not to keep her up at night with long conversations. Her father indirectly brought up the subject of termination by praising Amy for her improvement. This was motivated in part by his neurotic jealousy of her having another man to confide in. Amy responded to her father's attitude with feelings of disloyalty, which had to be worked through repeatedly. A few months before the termination phase actually began, Amy said that she thought of her boyfriend a lot more than she thought of her analyst. She worried that the analyst, too, might respond with jealousy, become angry as a result, and then get rid of her.

Amy's ability to deal openly with conflictual material was further demonstrated when her father became seriously ill. She was able to see her wish to take her father's place with her mother, and confront her death wishes toward her father at a time when he was in fact threatened by death. She described her ambivalence as being split down the middle, adding that this was better than being split across the waist, because then she would worry only with her body and not be able to think of the worry at all. She knew she was referring to her tics. In addition, Amy kept most of her concerns to herself, resisting her mother's seductive invitations "to talk it all out."

In spite of some definite, though mild, bodily defects, her pride in her own body had been growing steadily. This was augmented by minimal pubertal changes. She had not yet begun to menstruate. Essentially, her pride grew out of increased self-esteem. Her standards for herself became less stringent. In Amy's case, it was actually a sign of improvement when her grades fell from her usual all A's to an occasional B or even C. Amy's acceptance of herself seemed to make her more attractive to peers of both sexes.

Termination

Following an hour in which Amy reported a dream of jumping over a wall and not being able to get back, she asked how she could stop treatment. She said everything was going well. A week later she again asked to cut down her hours because they interfered with dances and parties. She became tearful at the thought of having to keep coming when she felt all better. But in the same hour, she said she would not want to stop right away. A year seemed too long and she settled on nine months. This was easily interpreted because her neighbor was pregnant at that time. A few weeks later she marveled that there was still so much she had to relate that she could just go on forever. A short time later, she injured herself in school; this accident was clearly related to conflicts over feeling better and more independent, on the one hand, and unconsciously longing for her mother's care, on the other. The analyst could link this incident with her thoughts about wanting to stop the analysis. She said, "I'm not thinking about stopping. I'm thinking about *thinking* about stopping." In other words, her beginning anxiety about leaving the analysis led the patient to an intellectualized distancing of the problem. A few hours later Amy had to deny her dependency needs and use reversal of affect and projection. She was scornful of a small boy who held his mother's hand as he left the analyst's office; she called him a "faggot mama's boy." A little later, she could acknowledge her pain about termination only via displacement, a screen experience in *statu nascendi* (Kennedy, 1950). She said she hated finishing a book that she was reading. She began to cry at the endings of books because she wanted them to go on. Yet, alongside this displacement, there was a momentary acknowledgment of the pain connected with termination; for in the next hour, she said, though aided by the analyst, that she hated the idea of stopping and of not being able to come back at all. Simultaneously, Amy's capacity for sublimation increased; she was able to produce art objects that were creative and original enough to be bought by an art gallery.

When she brought up termination again she was told that it was possible that she might look forward to a time when she actually could stop. She objected again to the passive experience of being told about termination by stating, "It's okay when I say it, but when you say it, it really scares me." This way of dealing with her anxiety did not last but a moment. In reaction to the ever-increasing threat of termination she became interested in having a pet and spoke of buying a talking myna bird. Though interpreted, this defense of displacement and regression continued well into the posttermination phase. Yet, side by side with it, Amy was able to speculate on how it would feel not to have regular appointments. She decided she could never really know until it actually happened, and she imagined that talking about it would give her at least some idea. During a rare silent hour she became very aware of the clock ticking. Her eyes began stinging, but she attempted in her old way to deny the impending tears. But then she acknowledged feeling sad, lonely, and angry, and even felt pride at allowing herself to have these feelings so freely.

Amy did not want to stop at the summer vacation, which was less than a month away. Therefore, we mutually agreed on a date one month after the vacation if all went well. She responded by saying that she felt good about stopping and good about herself because she was able to stop. Yet, a few hours later she used magical thinking to deny that she had ever been told she was ready to stop. She invented a game in which, by moving her hat forward, she could go back in time to four weeks earlier. This followed an unhappy mood in which she felt once again ugly and deformed and unable to terminate. This feeling was not only due to her belief that she was being rejected by the analyst; it was also a guilty reaction to feeling free of the stigma of needing treatment, as compared to her mother who was still in analysis.

A few hours before the vacation Amy saw the analyst driving with a lady and this produced new material. She wondered if the person could be the analyst's "other girlfriend." She then explained that her father would joke about having been with his "other family" when he returned home from a business trip. She was reminded of her previous thoughts of being the analyst's girlfriend. The analyst suggested that, in view of her father's jokes, the possibility of being a married man's girlfriend might seem feasible. In other words, the pleasure derived from this denial in fantasy triumphs over the pain of attempted mourning.

In the last hour before the summer vacation, Amy struggled with her feelings of being abandoned, comforting herself with the rationalization that some day she would have a husband of her own age or a few years older. It seemed that facing this vacation, as prior vacations, was much easier than facing the termination that would soon follow it. During the vacation she developed a tic of moving her thumb, which disappeared again when she resumed treatment. This tic was interpreted as a way of magically returning to the beginning of the analysis.

The remaining nineteen hours of treatment were concerned mainly with the theme of stopping and Amy's defenses against and reactions to this event. She began cracking her toes more frequently and related this to burping—making unpleasant noises that would irritate adults. In this way, she compared termination with rejection out of anger. At that time a teacher gave her the assignment to write about a humorous episode from her childhood. She said, "I cannot remember much—and what I can remember is not funny," thus heralding a trend to the increasing use of repression as the analysis wound down. Her old dissatisfaction with her body returned, this time with a tone that indicated a dissatisfaction with the analyst for not making her over completely—again an indication that she was not willing to terminate. On the other hand, she wanted to leave the analysis a week early, once again trying to turn the passive experience into an active one. She showed open sadness and sibling rivalry in saying that other patients she saw would still be here when she was gone and would even be talking about her, thereby indicating her hope that she would be remembered by the analyst. Again using displacement, she said that she had the "worst weekend of my life" because she did not complete a school assignment. She felt that she was not really ready to stop. She hated to think about it because it made her so sad.

In the next hour Amy reported a dream. She was given an

Orange Julius refrigerator. Food kept coming out of it, so much so that it began to smother people around her. So she closed the door and stopped it. The previous day, while visiting her mother who was hospitalized for a hysterectomy, she saw babies in the maternity ward. Amy was interested to see that the nurses carried them around like footballs. She was asked her age and was told to leave because she was too young; this was again like the "rejection" by the analyst. She also agreed to the interpretation that she had a strong wish to have babies, but she added, "I can wait; I just want to do well in high school." The Orange Julius dream indicated to her that she would leave the analysis with many of her strong wishes unfulfilled. She could close the door both on her smothering rage and on her oedipal wishes, yet she still knew what was behind that door.

Not surprisingly, a week before she stopped, Amy regressed from the level of insight and ego functioning reached via this dream by once more turning to animals. Her interest in horses intensified. A teacher she much admired divorced her husband and turned to horseback riding. Amy laughed at this attempt to replace a man with a horse, yet her own equestrian interest helped to diminish the underlying affect of sadness at feeling deserted in the analytic situation. In one hour, during the last week, she both laughed and cried. This helped to demonstrate to her the intensity of feelings about the experience of stopping the analysis, instead of merely "*thinking* about thinking about stopping." Although these affects were accessible during this part of the termination phase, painful events uncovered in her past and intimate details of her transference reactions to the analyst increasingly seemed to undergo repression. Nevertheless, and perhaps even aided by the loosening of the tie to the analyst, her development into adolescence was proceeding satisfactorily. She left with the wish that she could be around when the next patient discovered that she was no longer in treatment. She could therefore project the painful affect from herself onto another patient. Her parting remark, "Have a nice winter," gave the analyst pause and led to the expectation of a visit in the spring.

Follow-up Visits

True to her unconscious intent, Amy called the analyst in March. A ticlike movement of her hands had returned. She was also curious to see the analyst's new office. She talked of her riding lessons and her interest in the riding teacher, whom she regarded almost like a father. She reported that for the past two months she had been going steady with a new boyfriend. Unlike her behavior during the two summer vacations, Amy made no attempt, after her termination, to figure out what might be behind her ticlike movements. In other words, she formed new object relations (riding teacher, horse, myna bird, boyfriend) instead of identifying with the analyst's analyzing ego.[4] However, Amy had had some awareness of missing the analyst and had wondered if he had moved his office into his home. The interpretation was made that the return of the ticlike movements and her not thinking about them were a means of returning to analysis and to see if the analyst still remembered her.

She telephoned the analyst again two months later. This time it was to report that her parents were getting divorced. She denied any need to come in, but said her mother had wished her to call. The analyst told her that she could come in if she wished to and that it was quite understandable that she might want to. She returned for two sessions. The tics had disappeared since the last visit. She seemed much more able to work analytically than she had in the first follow-up hour. She said she felt guilty about leaving her mother to visit her father in his apartment. Amy even believed she might have caused her parents' breakup. She could not analyze this thought further until the analyst reminded her that she had had such wishes when she was younger, to have each parent for herself. Amy was then able to express tearful feelings of disbelief and anger about the divorce, and connected a recent accident with her anger toward her parents. "But I think I can work it out by myself," she said. It was quite obvious that this assertion served defensive purposes because her ability to analyze herself in the postanalytic phase was limited.

---

[4] We agree with Samuel Ritvo who, in a discussion of this paper, stressed that the self-analyzing function in children needs the external support of the analyst's contribution in the therapeutic alliance.

Another hour was scheduled with Amy's consent. During most of this second hour her affect had changed radically and she was very cheerful. She saw a younger patient peek at her from the waiting room, just as she had done with patients when she was in analysis. She talked about drinking beer and not liking cigarettes, but soon the analyst was able to get her back to her reactions to her parents' divorce. She returned to the idea of causing it all and apparently had benefited from the interpretation of the previous hour. With some hint of defensive adolescent intellectualization, she spoke of a paper she had written for class, entitled, "Knowing Yourself Is the Beginning of Understanding Others." She reported that she had ended it with the sentence, "If you cannot learn everything about yourself, you can also get help—a third eye." She cried only at the end of that hour, again attributing her feeling of sadness exclusively to her parents' divorce. Yet she seemed to the analyst to be more grown up than before, and her decision not to resume regular visits seemed appropriate.

A follow-up visit eight months later, again arranged by Amy and coinciding with her first menstruation, confirmed the impression that she was progressing satisfactorily into adolescence in spite of the developmental interference of her parents' divorce. We are not unaware of the fact that she may need further analysis at a later date, or perhaps an "intermittent analysis" to borrow a concept from Mahler.

DISCUSSION

This discussion is focused mainly on the technical issues presented by termination, which for the child involves the impending loss of the analyst as a real object. We must first remember, however, that Amy had a precocious capacity for verbalization, including verbalization of affects, and that at the time of termination was a 13-year-old preadolescent. For this reason, a certain amount of the adultlike quality which pervaded the analysis here and there must be taken into consideration when one uses this case as a general illustration of termination in child analysis. Termination differs in each case (Arlow, 1971), depending both on the nature of the pathology and on the phase of development the child is in.

Throughout most analyses, the topic of termination recurs from time to time, as is illustrated in this case. It is dealt with both as defense and as content. However, this must be distinguished clearly from termination as a reality issue. There comes a time in the course of an analysis when both the analyst and the patient become increasingly aware of the many instances in which the patient as the result of analytic work demonstrates an ability to function well even under stress. We call this space of time the pretermination period. In Amy's case, the analyst and the patient could point to such stressful times as Amy's father's illness, the analyst's vacations, her entry into puberty, and note the obvious improvement in her functioning. During this period the analyst had an opportunity to assess the various aspects of Amy's personality by means of all the Profile considerations, as was described in the first half of this paper. He gradually gained the conviction that termination might be considered as a real issue, rather than as defensive content.

Once termination as a realistic issue has been broached by both patient and analyst, the theme of severing the relationship to the real person of the analyst arises in full force. Even more than adults, children from prelatency throughout early adolescence find it difficult to tolerate the painful aspects of this separation. Normally, children do not have the verbal capacity to express their feelings very clearly. Amy, however, put into words what we ordinarily construct from the nonverbal or indirect communications of other children. When the analyst spoke of termination, she responded, "It is okay when I say it, but when you say it, it really scares me." Moments such as this one, when Amy could consciously confront her conflictual attitudes to termination and bear the pain associated with it are soon overshadowed by other events. These may overwhelm the child's ego and give rise to a variety of defenses. First, and we believe this to be quite typical, there is an immediate displacement of object cathexis. Instead of having an analyst, she will buy a myna bird. Then she transferred her attachment to a horse and a male teacher, and so on. This was analyzed partly in terms of her past object losses, with the analyst showing her that she dealt with the present threat as she had in the past by regressing to transitional and need-gratifying objects. Some of Amy's reactions, however, were not necessarily merely a repetition of past patterns of reaction; they were reactions appropriate for children when faced with current object loss. Although some of Amy's reactions may be considered adaptive and progressive for her age, such as the sublimations and the new object ties, many others were defensive. At times she behaved like a woman who had lost her lover and immediately gets married on the rebound. This makes the working through shallow. Somatization reactions, magical thinking, denial, projection, splitting of the ego, displacements, regression in any part of the psychic apparatus, repression, reversal of affects, turning passive into active, and attempts at sublimation are throughout childhood used to cope with the stress of object loss.

The analyst tries to aid the ego as much as possible in the face of this reality situation. He verbalizes the affect, the defensive activities against the awareness of these affects, and the object loss to the child, trusting that, at least for the period of the termination phase, he will strike a responsive cord in the latent and more mature structures of the developing ego. How long the work of the termination should last depends on how well balanced and how mature the ego's defenses are. Other considerations entering into this decision are the degree of conflict over termination in terms of unresolved issues, such as, in this instance, Amy's castration complex, oedipal and preoedipal conflicts, and the nature of the transference situation. In addition, the analyst must consider what termination implies to the child in terms of the child's past experiences with object loss. We see the impact of termination especially clearly in the last few weeks of the termination phase. Then the child realizes that the analyst really means to terminate and that residual magical wishes such as the wish for a (new) penis will not be fulfilled. The positive aspects of termination, such as more time for parties, are of course acknowledged. These do not raise difficult technical issues and therefore are not discussed at length in this paper (Schmideberg, 1938).

To the extent that the age-appropriate but primitive methods of dealing with termination prevail, postanalytic mourning, insight, the formation of new identifications with the analyst, and further self-analysis are interfered with. It is not surprising that so many, although by no means all, children quickly develop an amnesia (Hall, 1946) for what took place in the analysis. If the child analyst is remembered at all, it is most often in demeaning terms, e.g., he is a baby doctor. This is in sharp contrast to the adult patient who has no amnesia for the person of his analyst (Pfeffer, 1963b) and tends toward idealization, although Helene Deutsch (1959) described postanalytic pseudoamnesia in some adult patients. This tendency in children to forget the analyst already was noted by Freud in the case of Little Hans, who, upon reading his case history as a 19-year-old, at first did not recognize himself and remembered nothing of the events described. Freud (1922) concludes: "So the analysis had not preserved the events from amnesia, but had been overtaken by amnesia itself." We would say that this need for amnesia is not confined to prelatency children. Berta Bornstein (1951) described a "relative amnesia" for latency and Anna Freud (1958) one for the affects of adolescence. The relative amnesia, which in part serves to deal with the object loss of the analyst, also furthers a very necessary and positive goal. The child gives up the constant self-analysis and uncovering, and gradually resumes his ordinary childhood pursuits. A relative closure of the analytic process is thereby accomplished. However, some children continue to analyze themselves, possibly due to a special characteristic of their egos. With others, the analyst himself will actively aid the child in bringing the analytic uncovering and preoccupation with the unconscious to a close.

It is our impression that postanalytic development is in fact aided by a properly conducted termination. Proper analytic attention to all of the factors involved in termination aids the ego in integrating as well as defending against the termination experience. Without this analytic attention, the conflicts aroused during termination would be too powerful for the ego to tolerate, and thus prevent closure. Similarly, analytic assistance in loosening the object tie to the analyst may aid the adolescent patient in the developmental task of object removal. It is of interest, in this connection, that by the end of the first postanalytic year, Amy had been able to progress from her interest in a talking myna bird to obtaining a part-time job in a pet shop. At the same time, however, she was still searching in vain for "just the right horse." Yet, on balance, her postanalytic object ties had a definitely progressive quality. We wish to stress again that in children, more so than in adults, we are dealing not merely with a temporary return of symptoms in the termination phase; the very nature of childhood makes the giving up of the analyst as a real person more complex.

Summary

In this paper we attempt to demonstrate the usefulness, in assessing termination, of an evenly distributed attention to all factors determining the child's overall functioning. Attention is given as well to the quantitative and qualitative changes that occurred in the analysis. Instead of a simple formula or set of criteria for termination, we suggest a multiple aspect view of the child during the pretermination period. The termination process is seen not only as a treatment phase in which ongoing conflicts continue to be analyzed, especially in the transference, but also as a period in which the loss of the analyst as a real person has to be dealt with. Setting the termination date evokes case-specific and phase-appropriate defense mechanisms. Here, to use Anna Freud's term, the analyst may have to give "analytic aid" (van Dam, 1971) in what the child's ego cannot yet accomplish by itself to enable the child to cope with termination and bring about closure of the analytic process in the best possible way.

Uncontrollable events occurring around termination, for example, Amy's entrance into puberty, her mother's hysterectomy, and the parents' divorce, are unavoidable in analytic work. They force us to be cautious in making generalizations concerning our own observations, and challenge us to reexamine our conclusions on the basis of careful follow-up studies.

BIBLIOGRAPHY

ANTHONY, E. J. (1970), Two Contrasting Types of Adolescent Depression and Their Treatment. *J. Amer. Psychoanal. Assn.*, 18:841–859.

ARLOW, J. A. (1971), Some Problems in Current Psychoanalytic Thought. In: *The World Biennial of Psychiatry and Psychotherapy*, 1:34–54. New York: Basic Books.

BALINT, M. (1950), On the Termination of Analysis. *Int. J. Psycho-Anal.*, 31:196–199.

BORNSTEIN, B. (1951), On Latency. *This Annual*, 6:279–285.

DEUTSCH, H. (1959), Psychoanalytic Therapy in the Light of Follow-up. *J. Amer. Psychoanal. Assn.*, 7:445–458.
FIRESTEIN, S. K. (1969), Problems of Termination in the Analysis of Adults. *J. Amer. Psychoanal. Assn.*, 17:222–237.
FRANKL, L. (1961), Some Observations on the Development and Disturbances of Integration in Childhood. *This Annual*, 16:146–163.
FREUD, A. (1958), Adolescence. *This Annual*, 13:255–278.
——— (1962), Assessment of Childhood Disturbances. *This Annual*, 17:149–158.
——— (1963), The Concept of Developmental Lines. *This Annual*, 18:245–265.
——— (1970a), Problems of Termination in Child Analysis. *Writings*, 7:3–21.
——— (1970b), The Symptomatology of Childhood. *This Annual*, 25:19–41.
——— (1974), A Psychoanalytic View of Developmental Psychopathology. *J. Philadelphia Assn. Psychoanal.*, 1:7–17.
FREUD, S. (1922), Analysis of a Phobia in a Five-Year-Old Boy: Postscript. *S.E.*, 10:148–149.
——— (1937), Analysis Terminable and Interminable. *S.E.*, 23:209–253.
FURMAN, R. A. (1964), Death of a Six-Year-Old's Mother during His Analysis. *This Annual*, 19:377–397.
HALL, J. W. (1946), The Analysis of a Case of Night Terror. *This Annual*, 2:189–227.
HEINICKE, C. M. (1965), Frequency of Psychotherapeutic Session As a Factor Affecting the Child's Developmental Status. *This Annual*, 20:42–98.
——— (1969), Frequency of Psychotherapeutic Session As a Factor Affecting Outcome. *J. Abnorm. Psychol.*, 74:553–560.
HOFFER, W. (1950), Three Psychological Criteria for the Termination of Treatment. *Int. J. Psycho-Anal.*, 31:194–195.
HURN, H. T. (1971), Toward a Paradigm of the Terminal Phase. *J. Amer. Psychoanal. Assn.*, 19:332–348.
KENNEDY, H. E. (1950), Cover Memories in Formation. *This Annual*, 5:275–284.
KOHRMAN, R. (1969), Panel Report: Problems of Termination in Child Analysis. *J. Amer. Psychoanal. Assn.*, 17:191–205.
KRIS, E. (1956), The Recovery of Childhood Memories in Psychoanalysis. *This Annual*, 11:54–88.
MAHLER, M. S. (1965), On the Significance of the Normal Separation-Individuation Phase. In: *Drives, Affects, Behavior*, Vol. 2, ed. M. Schur. New York: Int. Univ. Press, 1965, pp. 161–169.
MILLER, J. B. M. (1971), Children's Reactions to the Death of a Parent. *J. Amer. Psychoanal. Assn.*, 19:697–719.
NAGERA, H. (1970), Children's Reactions to the Death of Important Objects. *This Annual*, 25:360–400.
PFEFFER, A. Z. (1963a), Panel Report: Analysis Terminable and Interminable—Twenty-Five Years Later. *J. Amer. Psychoanal. Assn.*, 11:131–192.
——— (1963b), The Meaning of the Analyst After Analysis. *J. Amer. Psychoanal. Assn.*, 11:229–244.

Rangell, L. (1966), An Overview of the Ending of an Analysis. In: *Psychoanalysis in the Americas*, ed. R. E. Litman. New York: Int. Univ. Press, 1966, pp. 141–165.

Schmideberg, M. (1938), After the Analysis. *Psychoanal. Quart.*, 7:122–142.

Shambaugh, B. (1961), A Study of Loss Reactions in a Seven-Year-Old. *This Annual*, 16:510–522.

Solnit, A. J. (1960), Hospitalization. *Amer. Med. Assn. J. Dis. Child.*, 99:155–163.

van Dam, H. (1971), Panel Report: Changes in Technique in Child Analysis. *Assn. Child Psychoanal. Newsletter*, p. 8.

Wallach, H. D. (1961), Termination of Treatment As a Loss. *This Annual*, 16:538–548.

Wolfenstein, M. (1966), How Is Mourning Possible? *This Annual*, 21:93–123.

APPLICATIONS OF PSYCHOANALYSIS

A. Clinical Applications

B. Applications to Other Fields

Analyst in the Nursery

Experimental Application of Child Analytic Techniques in a Therapeutic Nursery: The Cornerstone Method

GILBERT W. KLIMAN, M.D.

IN THIS ESSAY, I SHALL DISCUSS ONE OF THE MODALITIES EMPLOYED AT The Center for Preventive Psychiatry. Emphasis will be placed on how in this modality certain child analytic techniques are used right in the nursery classroom, and illustrative case material will be presented.

THE CORNERSTONE METHOD

IMMEDIATE ORIGINS

When the Center was established in 1965, an analytically supervised nursery was developed.[1] Called the Cornerstone School, the nursery provided (1) primary preventive service as a fortifying

---

Medical Director of The Center for Preventive Psychiatry, 340 Mamaroneck Avenue, White Plains, New York 10605.

Support from the following granting organizations is gratefully acknowledged: the Cleveland Foundation, the Foundation for Research in Psychoanalysis, the Grant Foundation, the Estate of Flora E. Hass, the Harrison Foundation, the Esther and Joseph Klingenstein Fund, the Kosh Family Fund, the Lavanburg Corner House Foundation, the Aaron E. Norman Fund, the Pettis-Crowe Foundation, the Scheuer Foundation, the Van Ameringen Foundation, and the Yasseen Foundation.

[1] The original Center staff included Elissa Burian, M.A., Florence Herzog, Ann Kliman, M.A., Doris Ronald, and Myron Stein, M.D.

milieu for highly stressed healthy preschool children, particularly those suffering from recent bereavement; and (2) secondary preventive service through early life treatment of emotionally disturbed preschool children. I extensively evaluated each child and family before admission to the nursery. Thus, each patient and family had some rapport with me from the beginning. In addition, the children regularly saw me in the classroom where I observed for an hour each day.

Within the first few months, each child continued to relate to me intensely. Several children talked regularly to me about their symptoms. Several had marked reactions to my arrival and departure. They spoke of me after I had left, both in school and at home. Some children told me their dreams in the classroom. Soon a marked thematic continuity in each child's communications became evident.

After a few weeks I cautiously began to respond with interpretive comments akin to my usual analytic work with young children. The experiment was then pursued not only for its clinical value, but also for the scientific value of learning what phenomena would occur.[2]

BASIC FEATURES OF THE CORNERSTONE METHOD

The early experiences eventually led to the development of a clinical method which combines child analysis and early childhood education. It provides treatment daily for children, aged 3 to 6 years, in nursery classes of up to eight pupils. It is a technique with precedents in analytic work with residential and hospitalized patients, in life-space interviews on wards, diagnostic observation within nurseries, and in many collaborations between educators and analysts. (See Redl, 1959; Gratton and LaFrontaine, 1966; Speers, 1965; Anna Freud, 1966; Neubauer and Beller, 1958; Foulkes, 1964.) Yet in none of these precedents did an analyst's work with young children evolve into a persistent, daily, systematic effort to use analytic techniques synergistically within the nursery school educational process.

---

[2] This was first discussed with Marianne Kris, M.D., whose continuing discussion and devoted interest in the project have been vital.

In the Cornerstone method, a therapist works about 6 hours per week right in the classroom, 1½ hours a day, 4 or 5 days a week. Treatment is performed only in the class. Two early childhood educators are in charge of the classroom educational activities, which proceed 3 hours a day, 5 days a week. The teachers conduct a full-scale educational program, encouraging learning in all forms appropriate to the children's abilities and developmental level, with a warm socializing process very much in the foreground. Parents are given guidance by the head teacher each week, individually, and the therapist meets with each parent at least once a month.

As in a regular nursery, the teacher makes no interpretations to the child. Whatever insight she may have into the unconscious sources or connections of his behavior, she does not verbally convey it to the child. That role is left strictly to the Cornerstone analyst. The teacher has a clearly defined educational role, channeling impulses into useful activities and creating and maintaining discipline. In the midst of a treatment situation which liberates children's impulses, this is indeed a very demanding role, and one which the analyst is glad to have performed by an expert. The analyst (or analytically oriented therapist) is relieved of the many educational functions he exercises when alone with a young child in his office. The two teachers will immediately, when necessary, find appropriate outlets for or restrict a child's energies. Previously defended-against impulses can be harnessed by peer activities, or channeled into healthy curiosities and ardent desires to acquire skills. The teachers are on hand when a child is ready to learn, to build, to create, to grow emotionally by the numerous routes which good education provides.

The analyst is present in the classroom 90 minutes daily during the 3-hour school session. What goes on after he leaves is in a sense "extra-analytic," but is nevertheless a clear continuation of treatment. As a result of regular conferences with the teachers, the analyst has knowledge of those many hours a week which the child spends with his teachers after the analyst has left. Even when the analyst is in the classroom, there is much that he cannot observe about all the children. But the teachers funnel a great deal of immediate information to the analyst. A particularly "ripe" or "clear" bit of play, or one the teacher believes the analyst will want to know, is conveyed within a few minutes if he is still in the classroom. Such communications often are made after the analyst has worked with a particular child; he can then go back to that child, having this additional information, and deepen the previous work. Thus, nothing which occurs in the classroom is truly "extra-analytic." In addition to the on-the-spot messages, the teachers and analyst confer about each child's behavior several times a week, so each can use the other's observational powers in a very fresh way—often to sharpen thinking rather than for direct use with the child. Cultivation of the teachers' observational and receptive abilities is crucial for the method, which requires close supportive supervision by the analyst, and a deep sense of "teamness."

The teachers have an educational and guiding role with parents as well as with children. As with the children, they multiply the usefulness of the therapist's time in the parental communication and guidance process—by being his eyes and ears, and working under his supervision. Meeting weekly with each parent or family, the teacher gives educator-appropriate guidance, learns about current family events, expands her knowledge of the child's past development, and shares this information with the therapist, who meets only once a month with each family.

Although the time the Cornerstone therapist spends individually with each child may total only 80 minutes a week, the Cornerstone sessions, being daily, are in fact more frequent than most individual child analytic sessions. Fifteen hours a week of carefully observed classroom communicative play and fantasy process, combined with social and educational activities of many dimensions, also enable the Cornerstone therapist to observe and understand unconscious trends over a period of time and in depth. It then becomes feasible to validate or discard lines of interpretation and clinical hypotheses.

What of a child's need for privacy? We have found that a child rarely requires privacy with the therapist in order to convey a fantasy, behavior, or concern. All children understand that each one in the class is in treatment, and they also know that the teachers will bring their observations to the therapist's attention. Occasionally, a child will ask to speak to the therapist privately. This happened, for example, in the case of a child who was soiling, and another little boy who because of his relationship with his younger brother wanted exclusive contact with the therapist. This can be done in a corner of the room. Once the child has seen that privacy can be obtained, it is interesting how rarely he utilizes it. Nor is there much sustained intrusiveness of one child into another's work. Intrusions and interferences are dealt with by education, often by interpretation, and by the children themselves. The fact that all the children are in treatment facilitates tolerance, acceptance, and respect for each other's treatment.

The Cornerstone nursery classroom is set up in a standard form, and regular nursery classroom activities go on constantly. As in other nursery schools, activities are often structured by the child's interest. Play dough is generally available, as are other creative materials. A phonograph record may be playing at one point. Cookies and juice are available when the children want them, but we tend to have regularly scheduled times for cookies and juice. Children who must retreat, withdraw, avoid, or otherwise resist dealing with processes stirred up by the treatment often do so by turning to educational and social activities. These activities, in turn, are not purely resistant by any means as they increase the therapist's understanding of each child. In older Cornerstone children, emerging into latency, the use of educational and social means as retreats from the therapist is seen more frequently.

When children also interact erotically or aggressively with each other, this interaction may promote growth as well as being equivalent to acting out in the regular child analysis situation. On occasion there will be a synchronized similarity of resistances or defenses on the part of several children, especially when there is much separation anxiety, or in response to shared external factors such as the illness of a teacher or classmate, or a vacation. At these times we can interpret to several children almost simultaneously, but still individualize the remarks so as to keep clear to each child the individual nature of the work he is doing with the analyst. Generally, however, there is a clear individuality of communicative styles and themes.

The Cornerstone child resistant to direct, continuous work with the therapist can pursue treatment work alone, internally, or in social play, or with a receptive and noninterpreting educator. Then the child can return for still deeper work at some mutually agreeable time later in the same session. Resistance is interpreted whenever possible—and therefore frequently. But the ready availability of social action and conversation with teachers and peers is developmentally syntonic with the low tension-binding capacity and low frustration tolerance of preschoolers.

Having given a schematic description of this new application of child analytic techniques, I turn first to illustrative moments in a classroom of six children, and later describe in more detail the work with one child.

A CROSS-SECTIONAL VIEW OF THE CORNERSTONE METHOD

The following examples are from 20 minutes of an ordinary day in Cornerstone, in its second year, when the method had already taken on most of its basic current features.

The children, 3 to 5 years of age, belonged to several diagnostic categories. Leon, a 3¾-year-old black child, had been referred because of a behavior disorder manifested by frenetic, negativistic, destructive acts. Charles, 4¼ years old, suffered from leukemia and a variety of recent neurotic manifestations such as clinging, enuresis, transvestite episodes,[3] and separation anxiety. Ted, at 3¾, was a bright, pathologically obstinate, adopted boy. At age 3, Keith was a pseudoretarded mute child of severely unhappy parents. Anthony was a depressed foster child, a 3½-year-old insomniac. Of Jay, an assaultive 4½-year-old with transvestite behavior, we will hear much more later.

As in most preschool programs, Cornerstone "morning group" children arrive at 9:00 A.M. and stay until noon. Each child is usually brought by his mother, and the opening moments are invaluable for ascertaining a child's mood from the way he leaves his mother and greets his teachers, analyst, and fellow patients. Parents often say a brief word to the staff about current events or behavior changes before leaving.

This day Leon was surly. His father brought him and, in the doorway, mentioned to me that Leon had wet his bed that night.

---

[3] For details of Charles's treatment, see Kliman (1968, pp. 26–42).

The information reverberated in my mind with earlier episodes of bed wetting, usually connected with arguments between Leon's strife-ridden parents. Earlier that morning the teacher had had her weekly conference with Leon's parents and learned of a furious quarrel which Leon had witnessed. She had already informed me briefly of these events.

At first Leon refused to enter the classroom, but the teacher coaxed him in. I was, at this point, chatting with Teddy about a birdhouse on which Teddy had worked for the third session in a row. I commented on the care Teddy took to make the house strong, and how Keith, who also had carefully fed some birds outdoors the day before, was like a parent who took very good care of a family of children. Ted and I discussed how much the birdhouse feeding and caring for the birds were related to Ted's father's temporary absence, Ted's previous fantasies of abandonment, and an episode of nightmares Ted had had during another paternal absence. For five minutes Ted glued the roof quietly and did not otherwise spontaneously express his thoughts.

Without leaving Ted's side, I used Ted's quiet moments to remark to Leon: "It's another one of those upset days, Leon, when you can hardly face being with us. Maybe I can help you because now you and I know more about your troubles." Leon interrupted here and told me, "Come to the fireplace, Dr. Kliman."

Because Ted did not appear inclined to further direct communication I said, "Ted, I'll be back soon and talk with you more about what's on your mind. Meanwhile, I'll be with Leon."

Going with Leon to the fireplace, I helped the child light some wooden sticks, and then listened to Leon's story of the "people" (play-dough figures) he was "melting" and "killing" in the fire. Leon imagined how very hot the people must be, and I commented on how horribly filled with hot feelings they must be. After a while, I made a gentle allusion to how somebody might even think of cooling the hot feelings with water, like a fireman, and later also alluded to the fact that the fire might be special for a boy whose father, like Leon's, was a fireman. Leon said the people were arguing, and he hated them. As the people burned, died, and melted, I mentioned the parents' argument of the night before. Leon responded by saying that once his mommy had beat up his daddy, but then Leon could not proceed any further. He wandered about the classroom so restlessly that I suggested the upset feelings and ideas could be talked about some more in a little while or whenever Leon was ready.

While a teacher (summoned by me) came with another child to help Leon continue with the fire, I moved on. Twenty minutes later in the session Leon resumed working with me, picking up the theme of parental fighting. He spontaneously added that the fight he remembered had taken place when the family moved. (I already knew that this move had occurred over a year ago.) Leon then gave an association related to the morning of the day of the session. He had "scared Natalie" (his baby sister) this morning—put a blanket over her head when she was in the crib. That "made her feel lost. She didn't know where she was." I interpreted, "And on the day your parents were fighting a year ago, you felt lost because your family was moving to a strange place. When your parents screamed at each other last night, that made you feel lost again. You wanted to feel like the boss of that lost feeling, so you made Natalie feel lost." Leon listened with rapt attention, and then played at covering a girl doll with a blanket. He offered no further verbalizations. In the next few days, however, he progressed in his intellectual functioning—an important step for this child whose presenting problems were intellectual inhibitions. He questioned his parents probingly about the death of his grandmother, amazing them with his curiosity.

In the early weeks of the group the analyst's transition from one child to another often led to resentful feelings being vented by the child who was left. These responses were interpreted as they arose. The patients began to appreciate the motives for transitions, which generally occurred when a child's ability for further work with the analyst was at a low ebb. In later weeks, the child himself would often realize that he could not pursue a communication further. Still later, it was often possible to interpret resistances and regularly have long periods of deep work with each child. Moreover, as we gained experience in the use of the Cornerstone method, periods of resistance were no longer sufficient cause for turning to another patient, and the analytic work correspondingly profited.

Many transitions were actively induced by the children themselves, as the following episode shows:

Jay, an intellectually precocious boy who verbalized far more elaborately than most 4½-year-olds, announced that he saw a lobster on a recent vacation. The lobster tried to pinch a child's behind. I said, "A child could have many thoughts about what happens if a lobster pinches his behind." Jay responded gravely that he would think the lobster would "pinch off his peenie and then he would have to make a pee-pee from his poo-poo." I reminded Jay that recently his worries about a boy losing his penis had frequently shown up in ideas about dangerous cracks in the floor that "pinch people" and doors that pinch people's fingers. Thereupon Jay walked away from me, apparently feeling a need for distance. He did not abandon the theme, however. He walked to the block corner and began to construct a "lobster" out of blocks, in full view of the analyst.

I took Jay's walking away and the cessation of direct communication as a signal for momentarily easing my direct activity with the patient. I said to Jay, "It must be hard to continue now because the pinching lobster thoughts are upsetting." Jay persisted in constructing a lobster. During this time, I worked some more with Ted; but I could still see Jay, and later returned to hear Jay's remarkable verbalization of the fantasy: Jay pensively wished he "could be a lady, because the lobster would give the boy's penis away to a lady. So then if I was a lady, I would get my own penis back."

This sequence shows that in respecting the child's defenses, but pointing them out to the child, the therapist had opened the way to a further elaboration of the warded-off fantasy.

ONE CHILD'S CORNERSTONE TREATMENT

The purpose of this section on one child's treatment is limited to describing some aspects of Cornerstone work which are like a regular child analysis. Other than those analytic features, many processes also occur—social, educational, supportive, corrective object relations, and the creation of an artificial family, just to mention a few. But these are not the focus of this essay.

The following brief definition of a child's analysis is useful when considering the phenomena to be described in Jay's Cornerstone treatment: if successfully established, a child's analysis will elicit unconscious material; produce insight into major current and past problems or symptoms; produce transference phenomena; produce a transference neurosis; give the child marked increase of behavioral repertoire; and produce symptomatic, behavioral, and characterological improvement in correlation with insight and working through. With this definition in mind I proceed with the special purpose of the case presentation that follows—to describe the child analytic features of the treatment. It will then be possible to discuss what happens when a psychoanalytic process occurs simultaneously with social, educational, and other therapeutic parameters.

Jay's treatment is chosen for several reasons. Jay was one of the first children treated by our method. His father died 6 weeks after Jay entered our school, so that his treatment had both preventive and therapeutic features. Jay had an unusual ability to play in a symbolically expressive way, verbalize his ideas and memories, and collaborate affectively and self-observingly in both a facilitation of his mourning and an exploration of unconscious aspects of his difficulties. Still further weight is given to his treatment because it was successful and because we have been able to follow his development until age 13.

Background

Jay was $4\frac{1}{2}$ years old when his mother first sought help. Jay's regular nursery school teachers reported that he attacked other children wildly, hitting them dangerously with sticks and rocks. In class he persistently costumed himself as a woman, swishing his hips femininely. He also exposed his genitals and tried to undress other children. He had no friends, and often said that other children hated him. Consultation revealed that dressing up in feminine clothes began at home with an intense interest in his mother's high-heeled shoes at age $2\frac{1}{2}$. His father became angry upon seeing Jay in women's shoes, and Jay would caution his more tolerant mother, "Don't tell Daddy." Jay also wore his mother's pearl necklaces. His body movements often took on a feminine quality as, draped in towels or sheets, he pretended to be a queen, princess, or witch.

Jay frequently harmed himself and was often harmed by his mother. He sometimes ran outdoors in cold weather wearing only his pajamas. Once while he had an upper respiratory infection and was warned that he might get much sicker, he ran out in the freezing rain right after a bath. Since early infancy the mother had been unable to restrain herself from hurting Jay, often pinching or squeezing his buttocks so hard that they were black and blue. She would squeal, "Mine, mine!" while pinching. Jay also squeezed his own buttocks emphatically saying, "Mine, mine!"

During his mother's pregnancy with his brother (born when Jay was 3½ years) Jay became notably destructive. He jumped onto a small table, which obviously could not bear his weight, and broke through it. Quite deliberately, he crayoned an entire terrace floor. On one occasion he punched 15 neat holes in a porch screen and 24 in another; and he could be relied upon to destroy household equipment whenever he was left alone with a maid. After his brother's birth, he was at first cuddly and affectionate with the baby, but soon cruelly hit, poked, and threw hard objects at him. He developed difficulty falling asleep, needed a night light, and early each morning would get into the father's side of the parental bed. His speech was marked by a persistent "s" substituting for "th," but otherwise was clear, often pedantic, poetic, and pseudomature—he had an extraordinary vocabulary and syntax. His social skills were contrastingly very poor. He had failed to develop any social play free of pushing, poking, and bullying other children—most of whom he towered over.

Jay was the product of an uneventful pregnancy during his mother's undergraduate years. His delivery interrupted her final examinations, but she quickly returned to them and managed to breast-feed Jay until he was 3 months old. He was then weaned and left in the care of a succession of nurses. During his fourth month, the mother left on a vacation for several weeks. The nurse said that Jay was uncomplaining and smiled when smiled at. The mother recalled no stranger or separation anxiety during his first year. His motor development and other landmarks were unremarkable. Although he quickly was able to climb very well, Jay was kept in a small crib and a small playpen until he was 2½ years old. Family friends pressed the parents to give Jay a youth bed and let him have free run of the house.

A wrestler in college, Jay's father ran an enterprise relating to feminine fashions. He was alternately gentle and rough with his boy. Sometimes coy with social friends, according to his wife, he nevertheless impressed me as an overtly masculine, serious, friendly, genuinely concerned father.

Early in Jay's treatment the father decided that Jay was too excited by their bedtime ritual of wrestling and kissing bouts. He recalled that Jay once begged, "Please, let's not wrestle before I go to bed, because then I have bad dreams." Except for wrestling and vigorous morning cuddling in bed, father and son shared mostly quiet activities. Jay frequently asked his father to read *Swiss Family Robinson*. The two would go over a chapter and then tirelessly add stories of their own. Jay loved to use his father's carpentry tools, often assisting in house repairs and projects.

The father was filled with realistic plans for business expansions and personal growth. Shortly after Jay's treatment began, he undertook a psychotherapy of his own, seeking to improve his relationship to the boy. He felt he had become too impatient with Jay, and that his anger was making the transvestite problem worse. The weekend before his death he told his wife that he had succeeded in thoroughly enjoying his two children's company even though they fought each other noisily. He began to speak gently to Jay, urging him to talk to me about the problem of dressing up as a girl, and impressed the mother with his new freedom from rancor. There was, however, a frightening carelessness on the father's part after one of the first sessions with his own therapist. While lighting a bonfire in the backyard, in view of his wife and Jay, he poured kerosene directly on the flames.

Jay's mother was a bright, attractive, earnest woman who inspired a benevolent, mildly parental feeling in both teachers and myself. Her intermittently harsh treatment and neglect of her first child were partly understood as resulting from preoccupation with her own needs and her identification with an older sibling who had been cruel to her. Her late childhood was marked by her mother's severe illness, aggravating her difficulty in achieving maternal maturity a few years later. She seemed determined to overcome many of her present difficulties, and entered analysis about a year after her child.

The history of her pinching Jay was not entirely clear. She definitely pinched him black and blue during the first 6 months of his life, causing her husband to be very angry at her. Apparently the pinching continued, with somewhat diminished intensity, right up to the beginning of Jay's treatment. While pinching him, she would grind her teeth so hard that she actually chipped several teeth. At the same time she would exclaim, "I love you! I could eat you up! I eat boys. I think I'll eat your foot first."

Onset of Jay's Treatment

My first session with Jay was an individual one. He was a charming, serious, reflective child with an excellent vocabulary and a high level of information. He easily left his mother in the waiting room, where she was in severe conflict over whether to tell me something. As Jay ran ahead, she whispered to me, "Jay wanted you to know that he touches his penis a lot because it itches. But then he said for me not to tell you."

When we were alone, Jay concentrated on crafts material, especially finger painting. He was quite proud of the multicolored cheerful blots he made by folding the paper over on the thick paint. Although he seemed generally at ease, he was quite concerned about dropping finger paint on my formica table and on his clothes. He claimed that he was going to a party soon and his mother would not like his clothes messed. On the other hand, he went out of his way to drop globs of paint on the floor and did not seem distressed. He did not mention his concern over his penis at all, but told me his trouble was that other children hated him. He thought I might hate him, too, and that his mother hated him because he hit children.

Treatment in the Classroom

After a few days in the classroom, Jay frankly communicated his feminine wishes. He told me he had waked with a "mermaid feeling, . . . wanting to be a mermaid," and also wanting to catch a mermaid and give one to his father. He believed his father would like to have a mermaid, while his mother would like to have a regular fish, a perch. I pointed out to Jay that he felt like the kind of fish he knew would please his father. He was already apparently conveying fantasies symbolically communicative of his sexual problems, and beginning a substantial dialogue with the analyst.

Soon, an intriguing new fear emerged, which I began to suspect was part of the onset of a transference neurosis. Jay took special trouble telling me that he disliked cracks in floors and would like the whole school floor to be smooth. Something about the cracks made him feel upset at school. He clearly understood the analyst's task to help with such a problem. Simultaneously, he was showing me that his block buildings were very tippy. When I pointed out that Jay was talking about tippy buildings just after talking about cracks that upset him, construction of tippy buildings became a long-continuing theme. When I suggested to Jay that perhaps he felt he was kind of tippy himself and not as strong as he would like to be, Jay became more aggressive with other children and adults in school and at home. Within 48 hours he caught two persons' hands in the cracks of doors which he slammed on their fingers. Jay also showed me that he wanted to catch another child's head in a crack between two tables. I interpreted that Jay was trying to make himself feel better by being in charge of this new trouble of frightening cracks, making other people afraid of cracks.

Jay's therapeutic alliance vacillated markedly in its valence at first. He repeatedly told his parents he hoped I would help him stop "itching" his penis, and actually reduced his genital masturbation. This reduction of autoerotic impulse discharge was an early indication that the treatment process could alter Jay's behavior into more frustration-tolerant states at home even while he was increasingly and impulsively discharging aggression in school. At the very least the treatment process was beginning to shift Jay's most turbulent mental processes into the treatment situation and out of his home life. Whether the reduction of masturbation was otherwise desirable is a separate question. At times he would seek me out for long sessions of quiet building and serious talking. At other times the transference was so impulsively hostile or his love for me so defended against that Jay became assaultive. A conspicuous assault followed his discussion of feeling like a mermaid: about 20 minutes later he tried to kick me fiercely.

After a few weeks he showed the treatment team an assortment of ways by which he made other children hate him. He was told that the teachers would help him control himself, while the analyst would try to help him understand himself, so that he could play with other children in a way that made them friendly. It was suggested to him that his way of acting with other children might not yet be completely under his control. For example, he would ask a child, "Do you like me?" and then hit the child with a block a few minutes later. Still later he would complain that the child hated him. He listened attentively when I pointed out that he seemed to be doing just the opposite of what he wanted to do.

Before his father's death both his parents had become regular contributors to Jay's Cornerstone treatment, providing much extra-analytic information during interviews with me and the teachers. They reported that two transvestite episodes had occurred in close connection with seeing his mother undressed. After one observation, he immediately put on her pajamas. On another occasion he dressed in her high-heeled shoes after being kissed by her. Thinly disguised sexual longing for his father was expressed when he asked his father if he could make Jay float to the ceiling.

The day after his father's dangerous behavior with the fire and kerosene, Jay confided somewhat in me about these events, but he was unable to talk about his father's part in the matter. In direct sequence he spoke of his own trouble that night, having pains in his legs and difficulty falling asleep. I was able to point out to him that there was probably some connection between these upsetting things and the upset in his legs, but did not try to interpret further.

It is important to note as a baseline Jay's state of mind and the state of treatment just before his father died. Over a period of several weeks I had interpreted Jay's efforts to make other children afraid of cracks, which he himself feared. Some work had been done on that subject, in terms of a fear of female genitalia, a few hours before his father's fatal crash. When I left the nursery school, Jay seemed to be responding to the interpretation of his classroom violence as a defense against his own dread of cracks. He took several cans of paint and made an awesome mess by spilling them about, then worked very hard helping to clean up, fearing the teacher would be angry and tell his parents. He soon spat a whole mouthful of water on the floor. A while later, Jay abruptly jumped on another child, banging the child's head on the floor. Jay looked very worried, and was told by the teacher that he could not be allowed to hurt other children, and that this was the kind of trouble that Dr. Kliman and she had been trying to help him with.

Jay then took off his sweater very deliberately, hung it carefully in his cubby, walked backward a few steps, then ran hard and fast straight into the far concrete wall, ramming it with his forehead. His teacher was horrified. Jay fell to the floor and sobbed. While being comforted, he allowed himself to be held close. After a long while of perspiring profusely, he calmed down, looked up at his teacher, and said, "I love you, Mrs. Ronald," remaining tranquil for the rest of the morning. This was the first time a furiously self-hurting tendency had been apparent.

The interpretive work concerning his fear of female genitalia had led to many shifts of a rapid turbulent nature. His use of identification with the aggressor changed to an alternation of that defense with aggression turned against the self. Object relations moved to testing of the teacher as a possible transference object for his oedipal love. A shift of symbolic focus regarding cracks had also occurred, with displacement upward from genitalia to the head. From the anxiety-stimulating phallic impulses with regard to cracks he regressed libidinally to the predominantly anal-sadistic impulse level of enraged attacking and messing. From an ego point of view he shifted momentarily to reaction formation against the liberated sadistic impulses, briefly being clean and compliant. He soon returned once more libidinally and symbolically to a phallic concern with heads, but then turned aggression against himself. This was followed by an earlier kind of impulse expression—cuddling the teacher, perhaps taking in the teacher's reading as if it were comforting at an oral level, while also allowing an oedipal gratification.

Jay's Father Dies

Six weeks after Jay entered the Cornerstone School, his father went on a business trip which ended in an instantly fatal plane crash. The loss occurred at a phase of Jay's life when tolerance for painful affects was naturally poor. The work of mourning, aided by therapy though it was, had to go on at a slow pace and low intensity of sadness and yearning for the lost father. After a brief initial phase of overt protest ("I want my Daddy back!"), gross identificatory mechanisms dominated Jay's behavior. He played intently and intricately at being a daddy, far beyond the level and frequency of his prior play. Yet sadness was a definite, conscious, and persistent affect. Rapid, intense expressions also occurred of the need to cathect new objects—including the analyst and teachers—far more quickly than would be expected with an older patient in mourning. The reality-testing aspects of mourning also went on piecemeal and were appropriate to his age.

Other postbereavement trends observed were an increase in the self-directed aggression, which had begun to emerge just prior to the loss. There was increased expression of magical thinking. Sublimatory activities deteriorated. His oedipal strivings became more gross and grandiose. Fantasy themes and play activities became heavily centered about the death, with details about smoke, fire, mystery, and searching. Both instinctual and ego regressive phenomena were evident, with increased greed for supplies, inability to share, and loss of achievements in frustration tolerance and object relations. Although gender identification with the mother had already been in evidence prior to the bereavement, increasing identification with some of her pathological defense mechanisms now emerged, especially in regard to her magical thinking about clairvoyant processes and the power of thoughts.

We wondered whether Jay would develop a permanent split in reality testing and retain a powerful fantasy of father still being alive. The mother's magical thinking and difficulties in impulse control seemed of great importance predictively. They might further restrain the child's already weak functioning in the same areas. At this point it was not possible to say what the short-term and ultimate bereavement effects would be. We could predict, however, that without treatment, a phallic-phase child with transvestite tendencies would do much worse in the absence of his father's protective influence. Further, the partial coming true of his wish to possess his mother exclusively would burden him with extra guilt. Thus the task of assisting this much damaged boy to deal with the new insults to his development was formidable.

Our negative prognostic views were balanced by the vigor with which Jay pursued his therapeutic work. He showed great continuity of themes and a remarkable persistence in working them through despite the intervening bereavement. Continuing work on his girlish thoughts, he expressed a complicated fantasy when he painted a girl with her head cracked open. He then accused me: "You cracked my little girl's head open!" A strange epithet which had rarely been used by him in the past, "Your head!" was now voiced rather frequently, angrily, and energetically. Three weeks after his father's death, angrily objecting to my efforts to interpret his aggressions against other children as a way of mastering his own fears, Jay threatened me: "Mrs. Ronald is going to come and kill you. She'll chop your head off with an axe!"

Following this, Jay stuck a small twig in a crack in the wooden side of the sandbox. He then wondered who was the boss in school, the teacher or the analyst—an exact parallel to his conscious concerns several weeks prebereavement over mother-versus-father dominance at home. His psychological life was increasingly becoming centered on the school, and, as happens often with the Cornerstone method, the child was using the personnel and children in the process of working through his conflicts. His fears of female genitalia and mother were being translated into fears of cracks and fears of what teachers could do to penises and men. As he gained some insight into his fears, a transformation of the related psychological processes became apparent. Instead of raw manifestations of catastrophic anxieties and discharge of impulsive behavior, more structured and more neutral states appeared. There were changes in his relations with people, particularly in the classroom. He began to appreciate them as complicated whole objects rather than need-satisfying or terrifying part objects.

The Treatment Deepens

I shall now skip forward to a time when Jay's relationship to the Cornerstone team was very well established. In the intervening half year much work had been done to reveal to Jay the origins of his intense castration anxiety as well as to facilitate his mourning.

When Jay reentered the Cornerstone School after the summer, his disruptive, poking, and scratching behavior had cleared sufficiently so that he could also attend a regular public kindergarten in the afternoons. At that time, three other children were entering his Cornerstone group—two for the first time.

There was immediate evidence that Jay had elaborate, intense fantasies involving the Cornerstone School. Jay believed he had seen a certain former Cornerstone child in public school, and seriously considered that the former classmate was using a disguise. The disguise theme was already understood by me as part of Jay's transvestite problems. I responded by reminding Jay that being in disguise, like disguising himself as a woman, was a familiar thought in Jay's mind. Then I dealt with the theme of an old friend being in Jay's public school class as a wish, interpreting that having an old Cornerstone friend in public school with him would make Jay feel happier and less lonely.

The next day Jay entered a fierce verbal competition with Charles, claiming, "I'm very smart," and trying to overwhelm Charles with an explanation of what happens "when two chemicals get together." I remarked that Jay had a lot of feelings about being smarter and knowing things about chemicals getting together, which were all very important to him. Jay responded by telling Charles and me that he had a collection of his deceased father's valuables, and in a few minutes added that he wished to "be" a certain uncle. This was Jay's first expression of desire to be a particular grown man, and represented significant progress.

After I left the classroom the teachers (as usual) continued working with the children for an additional hour. They served as recipients, elicitors, and observers of a fantasy which apparently continued and deepened the masculine identification theme Jay had expressed earlier. He lay down on the floor, saying, "I am dead." Although the teachers were aware of the connection of this play to the earlier talk Jay had had with me about his father, in keeping with the Cornerstone method, they made no interpretation. They encouraged the expression of his concern in dramatic play and reported it to me before the next session. They also took note of the fact that Jay again lay on the floor and claimed to be "dead" when his mother arrived to pick him up and go home.

The next day Jay told me that he was not feeling well; he had a stomachache which had started on his way to school. Asked if he thought it could be because there was something on his mind which came up when he "thought about school and the things we work on together here," Jay said, "That's right, there are a lot of things on my mind all night and I don't want to talk about them, but they bother me." Jay soon revealed that last night he had heard a loud noise when falling asleep, and gradually unfolded the fantasy that creatures from outer space had come into his backyard. Perhaps they had come from Venus. If he could have gone out to see, maybe he would have found them, and they would have "antennae on their heads and be mean."

I commented, "Although they were scary creatures and you thought they were mean, too, a boy who is lonely at night and even lonely in public school in the day, and a boy who thinks his father is in outer space [confirmed by Jay at this point—"like in heaven"]—a boy like that might sort of hope and sort of fear that a man from outer space would visit his backyard." In response, Jay expressed considerable interest in a male classmate's behind, which he tried to smear with play dough, and kicked a lady teacher in the behind (rather tentatively). He then wondered whether a certain toy rhinoceros would break easily.

I spoke to Jay about the rhinoceros thoughts and the thoughts about the boy's behind, saying that Jay was worried about the boy getting hurt in his behind and the rhinoceros getting hurt in front. Perhaps Jay was "worried about a boy who wanted to stop being lonely and wanted to do things closer to other people by putting fronts and behinds together, and who worried about what would happen then, and whether fronts and behinds could get hurt that way." This interpretation also used knowledge gained in the prior nine months of treatment during which Jay's poking of other children in the anal region had in part been understood as a wish for and fear of penile penetration of his anus. Apparently in response to the interpretation concerning the rhinoceros front and the boy's behind, Jay made an entirely new kind of block construction which differed essentially from his earlier block play in Cornerstone. He made a building which was sturdy, instead of shaky, solid instead of slender and easily toppled. He insisted that it must be "very strong and very tall" and wanted help whenever he felt uncertain that he could accomplish these goals. Giving Jay a minimal amount of help, and keeping up a "patter" of discourse with him, I commented on how this building was the opposite of a rhinoceros which could break easily. The building then became a kind of garage to which a truck brought cement. The matter of the right-size opening for the truck absorbed Jay for several reflective minutes. He called a teacher to admire the building, "See how big it is. It's taller than the chair."

On the next day, Jay drew what appeared to be a man with a large penis, but he could neither talk about the drawing, nor even acknowledge that what he had drawn looked like a person. He soon became involved in breaking a felt-tipped marking pen, and had to be restrained by one teacher from a rather vigorous attempt to smash it. I observed, but did not physically intervene in, this action, having the advantage of the teacher's availability. I could thus preserve my purely analytic, nondisciplinary function. I commented that Jay was trying to tell us something about his troubles and that these must be connected with what he told us yesterday: things which break. I then remarked sympathetically to Jay about a walkie-talkie antenna which upon entering the classroom he had told the teacher his young brother had broken. I hoped Jay could talk more about problems that were really very hard to talk about.

Jay then used a crocheting needle which was in the classroom, demonstrating some crocheting tricks to other children, who were duly impressed. He complained that his mother did not permit him to crochet because she said only girls should do it. Jay's competitiveness with Charles was now less evident than it had been the previous few days, and he confined himself to disputing one of Charles's remarks. It was a remark of considerable significance to Jay, for Charles had said, "People don't go away forever." Jay said, "People can go away forever." He not only insisted that Charles admit the error, but he was also upset to the point that he became unable to tolerate his own failure in gluing together a three-sided wooden structure whose purpose and nature he had not yet verbalized.

I now engaged Jay in a discussion of how nice it would be if people did not go away forever, acknowledging that Jay knew sometimes people did not come back. I mentioned a maid—one of a string of "missing maids"—who had most recently departed from the home. Jay agitatedly expressed his belief that this particular maid would come back, taking the same view about another maid who had been gone even longer. I wondered "if sometimes a child whose father had died might hope that the father would come back somehow." Jay replied with sadness, "No, that can't happen . . . once he's dead." He seemed relaxed at this point, although an agitated state immediately preceded these remarks. The agitation was absent during the remainder of the hour and a half.

On the following day, Jay played a game of "killing" his closest companion in class, Charles. Then he made up a story that Charles's ghost and his own ghost were playing together. His own ghost was "a very angry and scary ghost." I left the classroom, but the teachers were able to observe the continuation of Jay's expressive fantasy. Jay went outside to join a teacher and Mary, who were playing in the yard while other children were having juice indoors. Jay played in a deep hole for about ten minutes by himself when he called to the teacher, "Please stay here." She sat a short distance from him, while he lined up some flexible dolls which he draped with colored straws. Having established the identities of the dolls as members of a family, Jay described the father as a very kindly man. The boy child would say to him, "May I go horseback riding, Daddy?" "Certainly," was the reply. "Oh, thank you." "May I fly a plane?" "Yes, certainly." "Oh, thank you." "May I drive an automobile?" "Yes, certainly." "Oh, thank you." Suddenly the straws became atomic rays. The father doll came forth to save other dolls, who were being "attacked by atomic monsters." Jay then found a worm, which seemed to be dead. He shrieked, "It's a cobra! Mommy, look, it's a cobra!" The two figures next to the mother doll were now designated as "a nurse" and "a magical sister." The nurse also had a "little girl." Jay exhorted the father doll, "Daddy, Daddy, it's a cobra! Save us!" Daddy was able to kill the cobra, even though it bit him. Several dolls were bitten by the cobra, and buried one by one—all except the father. The father then had sticks attached to each leg and became an airplane which flew around trying to slay atomic monsters. The atomic monsters were dropping dust on the figures below, and also attacked the father-plane. He was wounded, fell to the ground, but was all right and got up again. He flew around attacking atomic monsters and managed to kill them all, although he was struck and fell crashing to the ground several times. Finally, the father went over and unburied every one of the dolls. As he unburied the last one, he pulled the dirt off it with an announcement: "EVEN YOU [are saved], YOU WITCH MOTHER!"

By the end of five days after his return it became clear—with the help of teacher observations—that Jay regarded his mother as a witch, magically responsible for the father's death. He seemed ready to "go deeper," and I would not have expected more of a 5½-year-old child's therapeutic work in a comparable period in the ninth month of intensive treatment. I also had the impression that some of the above material might not have been so readily available in analysis conducted in a traditional playroom setting, especially the poking and smearing of other persons' anal regions, the discussion with Charles of people who do not come back, the visible display of competitiveness with a peer, and the intense creative reactions to my departures. The frequency with which interpretations could be made and had useful consequences suggested to me that an effective analytic process was indeed in progress. The patient had verbalized a fantasy (a child in disguise) which enabled me to interpret his defended-against affect (transference-related loneliness). He responded to interpretation by further elaborating the dominant theme (in terms of an unidentified flying object fantasy), thus enabling me to link the associated affect of loneliness to the death of father and the child's wish for father's return. Some connections between his classroom play activities and his sexual identity concerns were also clarified for him (the fear of breaking the toy rhino's horn was connected with the fear of what happens to boys' fronts and backs), and there was an associated change in ego functions toward improved executive skills and sublimative activity (building sturdier buildings).

I shall now describe a few weeks of the later middle phase, early in the second year of treatment. The material illustrates the continuing thrust of the child's fantasy themes, and their ready emergence in the Cornerstone setting. It also demonstrates some of the special split quality of transference in that situation, and the regularity with which major communications are made to Cornerstone teachers.

As an apparent reaction to my walking to another part of the room, Jay started talking to a teacher about fantasied visitors from outer space. I observed to Jay that the monster-visitors idea was connected with wanting me to stay nearby. Jay then asked me to pretend to be afraid while he pretended to be a monster who followed me. A further aspect of the loneliness theme emerged when Jay mentioned that his mother had been ill for two days, and shortly thereafter put his head down to rest in a teacher's lap. I interpreted to him that a child whose loneliness gets bigger when his mother is not well enough to take care of him could get so lonely that he could even want a monster for company.

A few sessions later frantic needy behavior appeared, with panicky demands for food and crafts equipment. The teachers helped Jay with his wild behavior while I watched from a short distance. Soon he invited me to use some carpenter's tools with him, especially one. I reminded Jay that this particular tool was one he and his father had used together, and his thought about it was connected with loneliness for father and the good feeling he had had when he did tool things together with father. Jay then asked Mrs. Ronald, "Are you smarter than my mommy?"

When Jay's mother once forgot to give him a lunch to take to school, Jay gradually brought this problem to our attention so that a lunch was provided. Jay then pretended to be a robot-monster, and frightened some of the other patients. He then asked other children to bury him in leaves, outdoors, and they cooperated. His identification with his longed-for father was not interpreted by the teachers, and I had already left.

The next day Jay brought in a tool kit belonging to his father and some of his father's coins. He had begged his mother for permission to do so. Again, he buried himself in leaves. He was very anxious, and furtively tried to look under a teacher's skirt. Then he unexpectedly urinated on the classroom floor, under an easel.

We soon learned one reason for Jay's newly heightened anxiety. He was threatened by a tonsillectomy because of tonsillar and associated middle-ear infection. His mother was determined to proceed with the operation, and announced the plan in the classroom, although the entire matter was news to the staff. Jay then wildly wielded a knife which had been used for cutting a face from a Halloween pumpkin. I interpreted to him that he was once more turning his own fear around by making other people afraid. The surgeon scaring Jay was now Jay frightening us with a knife. Simultaneously, the dangerous action was stopped by Mrs. Herzog, our assistant teacher, before Jay came near anyone else.

Jay settled down with Mrs. Herzog, and after I left he told her how to make a genie by a secret formula of flour, salt, and chemicals. It would last a long time. He had a genie of his own, he told her, and would use it to get the teacher all sorts of things—especially a wood-burning set. For himself, he would like lots of money to buy a private plane.

My understanding was that the genie was a magic helper-father, creatively evolved from the child's wishes like the visitors from outer space. It appeared when I left the classroom, at a time of extra need. Jay felt threatened by his mother's recent inattentiveness due to her illness, a threat much aggravated by the planned tonsillectomy. It was powerfully overdetermined because the time of the first anniversary of his father's death was now only a week away. A report from his public kindergarten, which he attended half days, confirmed the ascendancy of thoughts about his father. He cried in the other school, the same day, telling the teacher his father was dead, adding in the same breath that he was going to have his tonsils out.

Another bit of work with Mrs. Herzog further indicated that Jay's mourning was now transference-linked. He mistakenly believed her purse was "made of cobra skin." I told him that perhaps it was the same cobra who inhabited a dream magic mountain. Shortly after his father's death Jay had dreamed that he would have a reunion with his father and a maid in this cobra-inhabited magic mountain.

Two days later the tonsillectomy had been averted by my guidance of the mother and pediatrician. Jay told a story about a bad robot and a bad plane. Both characters had begun their development in my presence. There was a hospital, an overt reference to the preoccupation with current medical matters, which Jay had discussed an hour earlier with me. The hospital was under threat from the bad plane. Apparently the father-plane had returned, angrily, to wreak vengeance on the hospital.

Again, the classroom situation had provided means for continuing and elaborating themes in Jay's analytic work after I left. I had the advantage of the additional material, as usual, in time for inclusion in my thinking before the next day's session.

I told Jay that his wish for an outerspace robot was connected to the hospital bombing because he wanted his outerspace dead father to protect him from the tonsil operation. Jay listened very seriously. I added that it was like the way he wanted me to protect him from his mother's anger. Jay responded elaborately:

"I wish there could be a machine that would make all the other children bad at Christmastime. There would be a bad man who would make that machine and all the children would get into trouble because of that machine. Then Santa Claus would find out about it and he would get a special dart gun and he would shoot that bad man in the behind with the darts." He then detailed the story further while sitting down on the ground next to me and later on the outdoor climber. "The darts would be very sharp and there would be lots of them going into the man's behind." Santa Claus would shoot at the bad man's penis and the darts would go right in the man's penis. He would holler. There would be a special dye in the needle. It would be helium. It would make the man go high in the air. I interpreted that this idea was connected with feelings boys and men have in their penis, which does go up in the air sometimes, by pointing upward. In later days, the theme of building airplanes occupied Jay profoundly. He spent weeks constructing a huge model glider from sheets of balsa wood, making an excellent original design. He believed this might be the largest model airplane I had ever seen, and the largest a child had ever built. It actually was able to fly. Of considerable concern to Jay was whether it would survive crashes, which I related to his wish to have saved his father.

Once, when entering the classroom, he commented both about a minor leg injury he had just suffered and his father's death a year ago. He spontaneously noted he was finding it hard to remember what was going on in school then, showing a remarkable degree of self-observation and interest in his mental processes.

I interpreted both his leg injury and his efforts to remember as connected with his father's death. After I left he apparently responded by composing the following song "for Mrs. Ronald":

> Oh the planet Mars,
> Where the people smoke cigars,
> Each puff they make is enough to
> Kill a snake.
> When the snakes are dead
> They put roses in their heads.
> When the roses die,
> They put tulips in their eyes.
> When the tulips die it is 1965.
>
> Oh, this land is my land,
> It's only my land.
> If you don't get off,
> I'll blow your head off.
> I had a shotgun
> And it is loaded.
> This land is made only for me.

After this song, with its message of guilt and triumph, of anal-sadistic and phallic-oedipal dreads, his further work was marked by an increased mourning through remembering as much as he could of previous work with teachers and me. Often this went in counterpoint with sadly remembering bits of play with his father. It seemed there was a blurring and linking between father-memories and treatment-memories. The reality-testing and affect-discharging work of mourning was facilitated by the transference. He was able to think a good deal about how people's bodies were after burial, and made up songs about "worms eating your bones." In association with thoughts about decomposition of a body, he begged his mother to allow him to visit the attic where his father had kept tools. Other children assisted Jay at times by saying in a matter-of-fact way, "Your daddy is dead, Jay." Jay would reply, also matter-of-factly, "Yes," or "Yes, my daddy is certainly dead."

Contiguous to Jay's increasingly testing the reality of his father's death was his increasingly verbalized insistence that his mother had a penis inside her vagina, and Mrs. Ronald had a bucketful of penises in the school basement. He often put phallic-shaped objects inside vaginal-shaped ones, shouting, "Penis!" as an epithet to the lady teachers. Much work was done with related fantasies of women having a penis inside the vagina. Jay worked through several memories of observations he had made about female relatives. For example, he had seen one woman give herself an enema and described the procedure in some detail. Jay recalled the idea that she had retained the nozzle and was now able to correct this misunderstanding spontaneously.

Fantasies of immortality and rescue by supernatural means occurred intermittently, particularly one of an "eternal lighthouse" which "keeps young people from dying in planes and boats." The link between his longing for his father and the anxiety about his own anatomy became very clear on the anniversary of his father's death, when the eternal lighthouse fantasy merged with a suggestion Jay made to another child that they both go into the bathroom and take their pants off. He soon made remarks about Mrs. Ronald's penis having been taken off, and Dr. Kliman's head having been chopped off. Although he was still working with me on a model of exactly the same airplane in which his father had died, he whispered to Mrs. Ronald, "I want to tell you a secret, but I don't want you to tell Dr. Kliman or anybody. My secret is I believe in God." He soon confided further in Mrs. Ronald that he did not really want to have a penis.

By the 16th month Jay became more relaxed and comfortably warm with the teachers and me. He often joked in a husbandly way with Mrs. Ronald, telling her that she looked funny. Once he amused her and said, "I wish I had a camera so I could take a picture of you laughing like that." At the same time he was able to speak sadly and seriously with his mother about her feelings toward his dead father, "Mommy, you didn't always love daddy. You wanted him to die." Jay seemed relieved to be able to express these ideas, and other children began responding to him with greater friendliness.

Shortly after Jay was able to let his mother know that he blamed her for his father's death, thoughts that his father himself was to blame emerged. Jay began calling me stupid in connection with his wish to spray paint near the school furnace. I was able to point out to Jay that his father had been killed in a burning plane and that his father had been using a dangerous fluid near a fire a few days before the plane crashed. Calling me stupid was a way of criticizing his father for dying. In response, Jay complained that he might die himself from choking on wet crackers, and seriously urged Mrs. Ronald to be good to him.

The Cornerstone Work Ends Successfully

While much could be learned about transvestite behavior and about childhood mourning from a further delineation of Jay's Cornerstone treatment, these are not the focus of my presentation. I am also aware of the fact that the evaluation of the Cornerstone experiment would require the narration of a full treatment record, but this so far exceeds all practical limitations that I can only make a few additional points.

Elaborating on much of the work that had preceded, one day Jay, playing a game in which he pretended to be a crab, told me, "Dr. Kliman, the reason I pretend to be a lady is that the lady and the pinching crab are connected in my mind. If the crab pinches off the boy's penis, then I want to be a lady because the crab gives the penis to the lady. And if I am the lady, I would have my own penis. And I don't have to go without a penis."

This intricate, spontaneously verbalized insight followed many earlier dialogues and interpretations concerning his feminine and transvestite behavior. He had begun to understand his intense fear of cracks in the floor as originating in his fear of and identification with the female aggressor and her genitalia. He had become clearly conscious of current and past fears of his mother, including the specific fear that she would pinch off his penis. This fear had been interpreted to him as being in part a product of his mother's former custom of pinching his behind black and blue.

Interpretations produced several lines of historical material that were highly relevent to Jay's current problems. When I noticed that Jay was making increasing demands for more and more supplies from the teachers, I told him that he was acting "hungry" to get supplies in a big hurry; that he seemed "hungrier" than at other times; and that seeing other children get supplies from the teachers made him "even hungrier." I then added that it must also be hard for him to watch his mother being nice to Eric (who was then 2 years old).

In response, Jay became reflective, and said he could remember when Eric was born, and that Mommy was very nice to Eric. He had a faraway look in his eyes, and I surmised that a process of reminiscence had been set in motion. Encouraging Jay to communicate, I learned that Eric had been breast-fed and Jay now recalled watching his mother breast feeding Eric. "I always wished she would let me do that. But you know what my Mommy would do if I tried? She would have killed me!"

Jay was gradually helped to understand the naturalness of his desire to try the breast, and simultaneously to work through and moderate both his classroom competitiveness for attention and his dread of his mother's ferocity at home. I also acknowledged that his mother did at times act fiercely. As an apparent result of these endeavors, his aggressive acts toward his younger brother diminished further and he showed increasingly tranquil behavior in the classroom.

Jay's aggressive, destructive behavior had begun in the months before the birth of his baby brother. The reconstruction of the historical bases for his animosity in the classroom gave vital impetus to his treatment. Interpretations connecting his classroom behavior to those jealousies were not only helpful in showing Jay the continuity of his emotional life between school and home and past and present. They also helped him correct and work through his tendency to project envy and rage and to perceive others as hating him.

An encouraging development throughout the second year of treatment had been Jay's attachment to the school staff and children. We became a second family, for whom he cared deeply, and of whom he spoke often at home. His mother shared this positive attitude, which helped her immensely in the difficult task of controlling her verbal and physical onslaughts, and developing an identification with our attitudes toward her son. Caring for Jay many hours each week made the teachers particularly important real objects, a force magnified by Mrs. Ronald's weekly meeting with Jay's mother. Although I met with her only once a month, she knew I was available in any emergency and responded well to my confidence in her ability to grow into successful motherhood with our team's help. The rich reality of the Cornerstone School had made this mother's participation and growth possible, and a thinner diet of realistic help, as a less supportive nursery and a more emotionally isolated analysis would have provided, could not have sufficed. Thus when school ended, so did our opportunity for intense work with Jay.

After graduation from Cornerstone, Jay remained in treatment with me on an individual basis. He was seen several times a week for a few months, but then only once a week for a few more months, and finally every few months for several years. My wish to analyze him further was not realizable. The results satisfied his mother and Jay for the most part. His dangerous assaults on brother and other children had ceased. His transvestite behavior had not returned. He was no longer shunned or complained about by other families, and he developed friendships. The disruptive school behavior of prior years and in Cornerstone itself was not present during his first grade in public school. We could judge that major treatment goals had been fulfilled: favorable, progressive alterations of character had emerged with improved flexibility of adaptation to existing social tasks, frustrations, and discharge opportunities. On the other hand, at age 7, he retained a mild phobia of darkness and moderately excessive magical thinking, together with a diffident attitude toward formal learning.

Follow-ups to age 13 showed Jay comfortably masculine, although occasionally "catty" toward mother and adult relatives. He was not interested in being analyzed further, regarding it as a financial extravagance; but in situational crises, usually involving his mother's discipline, he returned for occasional sessions. Although he retained a critic's interest in women's fashions, his transvestite behavior did not recur. He never again injured another child, despite a history of near-murderous assaults. Far from intellectually diffident as he had been in first grade, he now vigorously employed his intelligence in school, where his reading, math, and artwork were outstanding. He was quite logical, and free of floridly magical ideas, using primary process thinking only in well-sublimated storywriting, poetry, and gifted painting. He survived several further life strains of major proportions, with sparing use of my help. His mild phobic tendency was gone, and he appeared ready to enter puberty in good condition. Mourning for his father proceeded quietly, with frequent small doses of sad remembering, and shifting of paternal attachment toward his grandfather and mother's men friends. His transferences to and conscious memory of the teachers and Cornerstone children gradually receded, as did his memory of the analytic work.

At a recent community meeting where I saw him functioning with warmth and poise among his friends and family he took me aside and said with the seriousness and clarity which had characterized much of his early childhood treatment: "I don't know what you did for me. I can't even remember what we did. But I'm sure that without you I wouldn't be here today."

Discussion

It is my contention that Jay's treatment, as well as that of over 100 children conducted along similar lines, is not only based on psychoanalytic thinking. It also showed many of the essential features that are characteristic of the processes occurring in a regular child analysis.

In considering the question whether or not a method of treatment is analytic, I developed a set of criteria as guidelines for judging the existence of a psychoanalytic process. They underlie the definition of child analysis which I stated at the beginning of my presentation of Jay's treatment, and the remarks that follow are based on them.[4]

There was evidence that Jay understood the analyst's work. He collaborated in exploration of, and communicated about, his inner life. He brought fantasies, dreams, and problem-related mental contents; there was marked thematic continuity, and considerable dialogue about psychological functions; and he clearly manifested transference phenomena, which were subject to systematic interpretation. He responded to interpretations with elaborations and new,

---

[4] An extensive list of these criteria is available at The Center for Preventive Psychiatry, where we have attempted to apply them to several cases on a session-by-session basis.

illuminating themes. Often, interpretation of a conflict led on the one hand to oscillation in the psychosexual level of Jay's behavior, and on the other to increased awareness of the relationship between his current anxieties and defenses against impulses. Symbolic representations of his present and past conflicts were understood by him. Progressive growth of character was evident, with increasing flexibility in social tasks and increasing maturity of object relationships as well as insight into and working through of the transference neurosis.

An interesting feature of the Cornerstone treatment is the regularity with which not only profound transference phenomena occur, but with which certain features of transference neuroses are manifested. These correlate closely with the favorable outcome of many of our cases. In Jay's case, there was no doubt he loved and hated the teachers and analyst intensely, and this was not surprising. He also progressed from his perverse, primitive, impulsive state to a more advanced condition in which he created new symptoms—an artificial neurosis in the treatment situation. He expressed many anxious fantasies which crystallized around the Cornerstone personnel. Some of these fantasies were neither currently nor previously experienced consciously as concerning his own family. For example, he not only wished to marry the teacher; he feared her and fantasied she had a bucketful of cut-off penises in the basement, collected from many Cornerstone boys. Further, she would "slip" off Jay's penis or chop off the analyst's head with an axe. He tried to involve other children in sadistic sexual acts, while his behavior was sedate and free of erotic assaults at home and in public school. Meeting one operational criterion of transference neurosis, his neurotic behavior, actions, fantasies, and accompanying distress were largely confined for long periods to the treatment situation.

The ultimate establishment of harmonious relations between Jay and his Cornerstone "family" was accompanied by many positive oedipal fantasies. These in turn permitted working through of his transference neurosis, with its castration anxieties and underlying separation anxieties. As insights developed, their broadening was wrought in a vivid, real-life situation, syntonic with the child's developmental needs and capacities. The analyst then became primarily a benevolent, accepting father-in-transference and the teachers accepting, nurturing, educating, and safe mothers-in-transference.

Because of the techniques used and the phenomena observed, I call the Cornerstone method child analysis conducted within a synergistic educational process.

BIBLIOGRAPHY

CENTER FOR PREVENTIVE PSYCHIATRY (1971), Annual Report, White Plains, N.Y.
FREUD, A. (1936), *The Ego and the Mechanisms of Defense.* New York: Int. Univ. Press, rev. ed., 1966.
——— (1946), *The Psychoanalytical Treatment of Children.* New York: Int. Univ. Press, 1955.
——— (1966), A Short History of Child Analysis. *This Annual*, 21:7–14.
FOULKES, S. H. (1964), *Therapeutic Group Analysis.* New York: Int. Univ. Press.
GRATTON, L. & LAFRONTAINE, C. (1966), Group Psychoanalytic Work with Children. *Canad. Psychiat. Assn. J.*, 11:432–442.
KLIMAN, A. S. (1972), Psychological First Aid in a Natural Disaster. Center for Preventive Psychiatry, White Plains, N.Y.
KLIMAN, G. W. (1965), Oedipal Themes in Children's Reactions to the Assassination. In: *Children and the Death of a President.*, ed. M. Wolfenstein & G. W. Kliman. New York: Doubleday, pp. 107–134.
——— (1968), *Psychological Emergencies of Childhood.* New York: Grune & Stratton.
LURIE, O. (1970), Emotional Health of Children in Family Setting. *Commun. Ment. Hlth J.*, 6:229–235.
NEUBAUER, P. B. & BELLER, E. K. (1958), Differential Contributions of the Educator and Clinician to Diagnosis of the Prelatency Child. In: *Orthopsychiatry and the School*, ed. M. Krugman. New York: American Orthopsychiatry Association, pp. 36–45.
REDL, F. (1959), Strategy and Techniques of Life-Space Interview. *Amer. J. Orthopsychiat.*, 29:1–18.
SLAVSON, S. R. (1943), *An Introduction to Group Therapy.* New York: Int. Univ. Press.
SPEERS, R. (1965), *Group Therapy in Childhood Psychosis.* Durham, N.C.: Univ. North Carolina.
TARNOWER, W. (1966), Extra-Analytic Contacts between the Psychoanalyst and the Patient. *Psychoanal. Quart.*, 35:399–413.
TURKEL, R. A. (1969), Study of New York City Clinics for Children. *N.Y. State District Branch Bull.*, Jan., p. 4.
WAELDER, R. (1932), The Psychoanalytic Theory of Play. *Psychoanal. Quart.*, 2:208–224, 1933.

Preventive Intervention in Adolescence

MOSES LAUFER, PH.D.

PREVENTIVE INTERVENTION IN ADOLESCENCE IS AN AREA OF WORK about which we still know very little, and about which there exist various and contradictory views. Some people believe that the most that should be done during adolescence is to support and counsel. Others believe that intervention should, when necessary, include intensive treatment. Some people state categorically that the process of adolescence and the tasks facing every adolescent are such that it might actually be harmful to intervene before the person has reached adulthood. Others seem less sure about this; they believe that a short period of intervention revolving around specific problems may be useful.

My own views are that, even though the process of adolescence is not well understood, psychoanalytic theory and practice has made available to us important guides which can be used to help many adolescents whose problems may range from transitory disturbances to acute mental breakdowns. However, my own experience, as well as that of colleagues who work with adolescents, indicates that it is not only our limited knowledge which hinders us in this work, but that the somewhat haphazard application of what we do know about mental functioning and about adolescence *to the problem of assessment* adds to our difficulties. Many of the new and the so-called

---

Director, Brent Consultation Centre/Centre for the Study of Adolescence, London; part-time staff member, Hampstead Child-Therapy Clinic.

This paper was presented at the Hampstead Child-Therapy Clinic, October 1974.

more modern ways of helping adolescents are based on the belief that technical changes have hidden in them the cure, and that we only need to go on developing ways of getting to people—a belief based on the implied assumption that everything else will follow from there. I do not, with these remarks, wish to dismiss the outstanding work being done by a whole range of professional people who, through a variety of services in the community, work with and help many very disturbed and vulnerable adolescents. I do think, however, that it falls upon those of us who are psychoanalytically trained or psychodynamically oriented to provide the leadership in understanding, and in the application of this understanding, to work with the disturbed, the vulnerable, or the ill adolescent.

When we set up the Brent Consultation Centre and the Centre for the Study of Adolescence, we were aware that the service and the research we were planning would be expensive and would very likely, for a variety of reasons ranging from lack of staff to lack of money, be difficult to duplicate. Nevertheless, we felt that there was an important place for an organization such as ours. The interrelationship between service and research would enable us to apply what we do know to helping many different adolescents who were experiencing a crisis in their lives, and at the same time would make it possible for us to study, in depth, a number of adolescents who present a type of psychopathology that is often associated with this period of development.

The experiences in preventive intervention which are described in this paper come from the work at the Brent Consultation Centre and the Centre for the Study of Adolescence which has been going on for just over six years. The Brent Consultation Centre is a walk-in service which is supported by the Education Department of the London Borough of Brent. This means that the London Borough of Brent votes us an annual budget—a budget which is used almost totally for the employment of a part-time staff of psychoanalysts and child therapists who carry out interviewing for assessment and who undertake the psychological treatment of adolescents. In effect, the way our service is set up means that any person (but hopefully mainly adolescents) can walk in and be assured of being seen by a member of our professional staff. During the period that we have been open, we have seen somewhat over a thousand adolescents and young adults.

Related to, but actually separate from, the Brent Consultation Centre is the Centre for the Study of Adolescence, a research organization which was set up by us at the same time as the Brent Consultation Centre. The main function of the Centre for the Study of Adolescence is the study of mental breakdown in adolescence. The data for this study are obtained from the analysis or intensive psychotherapy of a limited number of adolescent patients.[1] Until now, our funds for this research have come from foundations and private contributors, but recently we received an award from the Department of Health and Social Security to undertake a broader, statistical study of those adolescents who come to us for help. The Centre for the Study of Adolescence is staffed by the same people who work at the Brent Consultation Centre, which means that each member of the staff has some responsibility for the service and for the research.

When we set up the Brent Consultation Centre as a walk-in service for adolescents, we began with the assumption that there must be a large number of young people who are in immediate need of help, but who, for a variety of reasons, do not make use of the existing services. We also assumed that if we could get them to seek help, we could intervene at a time in their lives when the interferences in development may not yet have seriously disrupted their lives. We assumed that people's fears of mental illness, their guilt about their own thoughts or actions, or their beliefs that they may be irreversibly damaged, would keep many of them away from the more formal agencies, and that very likely they would seek help only following, *rather than before*, a severe and obvious crisis. Our day-to-day work takes such factors and anxieties into account: for example, we have no formal procedure of intake; all information is obtained in the course of the interview (the information about an adolescent's life will vary enormously, depending completely on what the interviewer considers appropriate to discuss, to ask about, or to investigate). We have no waiting list; an adolescent is seen

---

[1] The ideas underlying this research have been described more fully elsewhere (Laufer, 1973).

within a matter of days, or immediately if he requests this or if he or we feel that it is urgent. Our assessment procedure varies; we may see an adolescent for assessment once or twice or fifteen times, if necessary; the interviewer himself decides at what point he has enough information about the adolescent's present and past functioning to make an assessment and to suggest the most appropriate help. Adolescents are discussed at regular weekly staff meetings, which are attended by all the interviewing and assessment staff, who make a final decision about intervention.

Before describing further what we actually do at the walk-in Centre, I shall give more details of how we function from a staff point of view, because there is an important relationship between the people we see, the kind of work we do, and the expectations which the staff members have of themselves. With the numbers of adolescents who come for help, clearly one of the facts is that we see many very disturbed young people who are either experiencing an acute crisis which may include their families, their friends, their future plans, and so on—crises in which we may be able to help, even though we may feel that our intervention is very limited and perhaps only of temporary benefit. At the same time, we see quite a large number of young people who are obviously at risk, and for whom something may have to be done carefully and quickly. I do not want to give the impression that we are a "crisis service"—we are not—it is simply a fact that by being a walk-in service which is available to anybody, we inevitably will see people who are at risk. This means that a member of the interviewing staff may, in one week, see adolescents who are doing quite well but want some help for an acute problem, without there being too much demand on that staff person; during another week, he may be faced with a need to try to do something about a number of adolescents who are seriously at risk.

In such circumstances it may easily happen that we begin to feel that everything we do carries with it an air of urgency or, worse still, that what we are going to do will save the adolescent or change his life. While some of this may be true in some cases, such a tendency carries with it the potential danger of creating an air of omnipotence and the accompanying belief that we can do something for everybody. Some work with disturbed adolescents lends itself to such a belief, especially if there are no built-in safeguards. We have guarded against such a development by (1) our weekly staff meeting where members are expected to present their work; (2) the arrangement where all staff is part-time, with the implied expectation that everybody will continue to do work away from the Centre, *including intensive treatment;* (3) the requirement that all staff will, in addition to their work with adolescents, work with or treat children or adults. Contained in these requirements or these limitations which we place on ourselves is the awareness that work with adolescents, and especially continuous or too much work with adolescents, carries very serious dangers which can be detrimental both to one's work and person—I have already mentioned the air of omnipotence which can be created and perpetuated; other dangers are the unconscious demand to be idealized by the adolescent; the living out, via the adolescent's sexual life, of one's own neurotic difficulties; the need to be the perfect parent, or the savior; and the implied denigration of the adolescent's parents. Such dangers also exist in work with children and adults, but I believe that the specific dangers I have mentioned are greater in work with adolescents, mainly because of the adolescent's own developmental needs and conflicts.

The range of problems for which adolescents seek help is very wide. However, I shall concentrate on a few of the things we have learned, and on some of the areas where important questions still need to be answered. I shall discuss some of the problems in assessment with which we are faced repeatedly; our experience with adolescents who present the "hidden/urgent" problems; special practical problems in the assessment of adolescents whose lives are at risk; and our experiences with the nonintensive treatment of a number of adolescents.

Problems and Functions of Assessment

Some of the difficulties we encounter in assessment reflect our uncertainty about the meaning of certain forms of behavior in adolescence; some are more related to the kinds of young people who come to us. Some adolescents who come in appear to be quite sophisticated about themselves and their problems, and are capable of describing their lives in ways which enable us to know what is going on. Others who also may be worried about themselves have little or no ability to tell us what is wrong. They know that they are worried or different, or that they are isolated and unable to stay on a job, but their relation to their own internal life is such that they are surprised and threatened when we say we want to know about this. These adolescents often feel helpless and bewildered by what is going on; we, too, may feel this way because there may be little likelihood of creating an awareness that something is wrong and that it comes from within themselves. Of course, in every assessment, we take into account a whole variety of external factors which may be important, but finally we must try to understand what is or is not going on internally. For some adolescents, such an approach is either foreign or too threatening, and we get nowhere. But there certainly also are adolescents who can tell us about themselves.

From a technical point of view, I believe that the whole procedure of coming to the Centre, of being interviewed and being encouraged to talk about himself, can be a very important experience in the life of that adolescent. For this reason, I will not only want to find out what I must know for assessment, but I will, when appropriate, encourage the adolescent to participate in the assessment procedure. For example, if I ask a question, I will explain why I have asked the question and what I will do with the answer. I will try to show the adolescent how I go about deciding what I think is wrong and what I think can be done to help. This may seem to be a seductive procedure, but it need not be so if the interviewer conveys his awareness of the adolescent's anxiety. It helps to remove the bewilderment and some of the frightening magic of "assessing"; it also enables the adolescent to begin to feel less terrified of being labeled and of being told that nothing can be done. Many of those who seek help have never before talked to anybody else about their problems, nor have they acknowledged consciously the extent to which they have been and are burdened by what they believe is wrong with them. By the interviewer and the adolescent jointly formulating what is wrong, the frightening unknown becomes a little less powerful and at the same time the adolescent can begin to feel hope that somebody understands what is wrong and may be able to help.

If the adolescent allows me, I will scan his whole present life—his social relationships, his schooling or work, the relationship with his parents. But inevitably I want to be able to establish the severity of the structured pathology which may be present and the extent of interference in the developmental process (A. Freud, 1958, 1962; Laufer, 1965). In other words, I will try to establish whether the disturbance is transitory or neurotic, whether I can spot an established psychotic process or the beginnings of what is a break with reality. How do we do this? And what weight do we give to what we find out?

The way in which the adolescent is responding to the developmental tasks (the change in the relationship to his parents, the change in the relationship to his contemporaries, his reactions to his physically mature body) are of primary importance in assessment. My own bias in assessment is to place the greatest importance on learning about and trying to understand what is going on in the adolescent's relationship to his own body, and in knowing about the central sexual identifications which exist. I will, therefore, want to know how the adolescent is responding to the fact that his body is now physically mature (that he can produce semen and impregnate a female; or that she ovulates and menstruates, i.e., that she can become pregnant and grow a child in her own body). In optimal circumstances, I will be able to get such information either from the adolescent's description of his relationships to people of the same or the opposite sex, from a description of his masturbation activity (including his masturbation fantasies), and generally from the way in which he takes care of his body. The intricate details of the adolescent's relationship to his own body not only can be one of the main means of establishing the extent of the interference in the developmental process, but it can be one of *the* means of establishing the severity of the pathology, and especially whether there are the ingredients either for a "breakdown" (which I shall define later) or for psychosis.

As I mentioned earlier, getting the information which we must have for assessment is often difficult. Sometimes we do not get it, and we may then be stuck, not quite knowing how to proceed. But as has already been implied, my method of obtaining information is an active one, where I will carefully ask the adolescent questions related to all aspects of his life. I am aware of the dangers inherent in such a way of working, but I believe that this way of getting information need be neither traumatic nor anxiety-provoking, especially if we keep in mind that there may be times when it is *not* appropriate to ask too much. I will then not only note the content of the person's reaction, but I will also pay attention to the way in which the answer is given.

AWARENESS THAT PROBLEM IS INTERNAL

For example, a young man said that he had been worried about himself for a long time, but he could not make himself seek help because he thought it might be embarrassing and unpleasant, and in any case he was not sure whether it would be of much use. He became very worried, however, when he realized a short time ago that he had walked to a nearby railway station and had thought of killing himself. But he suddenly thought that he should not do it because he had told his parents that he would never do such a thing. He was dressed shabbily, he kept on glancing away from me, he giggled and blushed when he talked of this. My first impression was of a very disturbed young man—when I went to fetch him from the waiting room, I thought he looked like some of the schizophrenic adolescents I had seen in the acute admissions ward of a hospital. I started the interview by saying that he looked quite worried when I came to the waiting room, and I wondered whether he had been worried about what he might want to discuss with me.

His first answer assured me that his pathology might be less severe than I had assumed. He said that he had felt troubled for years; he had nearly given up; but he had been hoping that I might do something. He talked of his loneliness, of his difficulty in having a girlfriend, of his sudden failure at school after having had a long record of being one of the best in the school, and now of working as a clerk (after he and his family and his head teacher had all assumed that he would go on to a leading university). I acknowledged the feeling of failure, the shame and anger with himself, and the hopelessness.

It was when he could tell me about his masturbation activity that I was able to understand why he presented such a disorganized and shabby picture of himself, and then it was also possible for me to decide that the pathological process was not a psychotic one, even though it reflected the presence of severe interference in functioning. He talked of his long-standing inability to touch his penis, of his humiliation when he could masturbate only by using a vibrator, and of his belief that he was irreversibly abnormal. He was able to describe how he worried about himself, but there was no concern about ominous body changes or weird feelings from his body over which he had no control. In telling me all this, he stared at me to see how I responded, and he could say, with some encouragement from me, that he thought I might be disgusted and that I would confirm that he was a pervert.

From the point of view of assessment, I felt that my primary function was to establish the extent of disturbance (and to assure myself that the process was not psychotic in nature), and also to prepare him for the need for long-term intervention (which we could not offer at that time, but which we would try to arrange for him). With this young man, the question of treatment was not a difficult one to discuss, because he was very much in touch with his anxiety and with the extent of his isolation. That the problem was an internal one was easy for him to perceive, as a result of which the idea of a period of treatment was quite acceptable to him. Discussing treatment with him also gave him the hope that he could change.

THE HIDDEN/URGENT PROBLEMS

At the Centre we see a group of adolescents who present special problems in assessment and who may, from a practical point of view, be in urgent need of help of some kind. These adolescents also say that they are worried, but they do not quite know why. In describing their day-to-day lives as well as their immediate past, they create a picture of suffering or despair that contains a pervasive feeling that everything is worthless or hopeless. I am describing not only the severely depressed adolescents, but those who feel that nothing has changed for years and that nothing will ever change. The depression which they present may not be the neurotic or psychotic type of depression; rather, it is characterized by a feeling that the possibilities of something altering in their lives are nonexistent. Nevertheless, they have not given up completely, and often they come to the Centre thinking that this is a last try. The hidden/urgent problems which these adolescents come with are hidden from themselves, and the urgency is something of which they are not at all aware when they first come to us. With these adolescents one can easily miss the severity of the existing pathology or of the impending danger to their lives, and it is an important function of ours to know when to be concerned and why.

Breakdown

The feeling of worthlessness or hopelessness is, I believe, a reaction to something they experienced earlier in adolescence—an experience that bewildered and terrified them. Some of these people, I believe, felt that they either were mad or might go mad; they felt disorganized by their uncontrollable regressive thoughts or actions—thoughts or actions which were directly linked to the feelings coming from their sexually mature bodies. In assessment, some of these adolescents then describe themselves as dead, not caring, feeling hopeless, hating themselves, and not knowing what to do with themselves.

In such instances the assessment serves a function that goes beyond eliciting the information we need to understand the severity of the pathology. The assessment can be used—very effectively, I believe—to enable the adolescent to try again to come into touch with the anxiety which at one time overwhelmed him. More specifically, the mere act of putting into words his despair, his shame, and his wish simply to give up can be a highly significant step forward. In assessment interviews it is very often not possible for us to determine what these thoughts *really* are about, to what extent the interference is of a secondary nature, or whether the existing pathology is reversible or not. Nevertheless, it is of the utmost importance to establish whether earlier in adolescence there took place what I can best describe as a "breakdown"—an overwhelming of the personality, that is, the experience of being overwhelmed by feelings and the accompanying belief of having lost control of the ability to do anything about it. These adolescents recall the "breakdown" as a time when they had temporarily lost the link with reality—*and it is this which terrified them*—but at the same time they had some awareness that what was happening to them was not really true. The behavior, thoughts, or feelings which these adolescents describe often create the diagnostic impression of a psychosis, but I believe it is more appropriate to categorize them under the headings of "breakdown" because such a description contains the idea of the reversibility of the pathological process (despite the many unknowns inherent in it).

It is my conviction that this kind of "breakdown" regularly occurred in adolescents who attempted suicide (assuming they are not psychotic). They present a special problem of assessment and management, to which I shall come back. The other adolescents for whom "breakdown" is an appropriate description are those who suddenly fail badly at their exams, who suddenly seem to be paralyzed by the experience of going to university, who suddenly isolate themselves and refuse to go out with friends. Less obvious and less clear signs of a "breakdown" are seen in the adolescents who slowly withdraw from the outside world, who drift into drug use and then become dependent on drugs and unable to risk giving them up (as one boy said, "Why should I be mad and empty when I can feel that I have friends"), or who adopt beliefs or behavior which make them into total aesthetes. These adolescents may be viewed as making use of normal adolescent defensive maneuvers; they are often described as neurotic or, more colloquially, as eccentric. But such descriptions help deny the severity of the disturbance which may be present and the extent to which nothing has changed in these people's lives from early adolescence on.

Jane, aged 19, explained to me that she could not concentrate. She had been thinking of seeking help for some time, but she decided to do something about her difficulties when she found that she was refusing time after time to accept invitations from boys to go to parties. Instead, on Saturday evenings, she would read, listen to records, and then just go off to sleep. Once, when she did go out with a boy and he tried to kiss her, she felt disgusted and had to spend a long time when she came home washing her face and looking in the mirror to see that there was nothing unusual about her looks. *She was aware that this behavior was ridiculous*, but she *had to* do it. At present she did not have many friends—she preferred to spend her time alone.

In response to my questions, she described how she hated herself when she first began to menstruate, how she cried and felt that her father would never love her again as he used to. Instead of saying anything which might help her to see what the conflict was about, I said that this must have been an awful time for her, and I wondered whether she continued to have trouble about menstruation. With much embarrassment, she told me that her periods had been irregular for four or five years, but now they were alright.

After I explained why I wanted to know about these things, she went on to tell me about her isolation, her thoughts of suicide which had haunted her for some years, and her feeling that something had happened to her which left her with the feeling that part of her mind was detached from the rest of her. She had given me a number of signals in the interview that something had indeed gone wrong earlier in her adolescence, and when I asked her to describe further her feeling of disgust when the boy tried to kiss her, she casually talked about her eating difficulties in the past. These turned out to be anorexia nervosa—at 17 her weight had dropped from 115 to 70 pounds; it was a time when she felt fine because her body was dead and she felt weak and ugly. She had almost no feelings, so there was nothing to be worried about.

I responded by saying, "You were very right to have come to the Centre. You've been very unhappy for a long time, but you couldn't do anything about it because you were too ashamed. But now that you've come for help, you *must* do something about your life." This experience at the Centre was very important for Jane. Not only could we recognize that her past difficulties were, in fact, an illness, but it was possible to convey to her that she could be helped and that some change could take place. It was as if she now had an ally in her fight against something which until then had simply been terrifying.

Adolescents Whose Lives Are at Risk

The other group of adolescents who come to us with hidden/urgent problems are those who have attempted suicide. Very often, the actual suicide attempt may have taken place some time prior to their seeking help, and often we learn about it only in response to our questioning rather than because the adolescent tells us about it. It is also remarkable how frequently such information is not given to us either by the parents or by professional people (if these are the persons who are first in touch with us). We may be told that the adolescent is feeling depressed, or does not want to work, or is behaving in an odd way, but very often there is no reference to a previous suicide attempt.

My own view about adolescents who have made a suicide attempt is that they have, *at the least*, had a "breakdown" (sometimes the attempt may have been part of a psychosis). Even though the adolescent may tell me that now everything is fine, and that what he is really worried about is his job, or not having a girlfriend, or feeling sexually abnormal, and so on, I react to the information of a past suicide attempt as if it were an urgent crisis, *no matter when it was that the actual attempt was made*. I make it quite clear to the adolescent what view I take of the attempt and why, and I always let him know that I think he is still at risk of repeating it.

From a management or practical point of view, I always involve the parents of the adolescent who attempted suicide, conveying to them as well my view of the seriousness of the situation. Of course, some of the adolescents and parents think I am making a fuss about nothing, and they may try to dismiss what I say. But on the basis of my own experience with the psychoanalytic treatment of adolescents who have attempted suicide, as well as that of colleagues who have analyzed such adolescents at the Centre (as part of our research into mental breakdown in adolescence), I am convinced that from an assessment and practical point of view it is correct to consider such an event an urgent crisis and to make it into a family crisis. To do less than this is to deny the power of the omnipotent fantasy which may temporarily be kept under control, but which can, under certain precipitating circumstances, again seriously interfere with the adolescent's reality-testing function and result in another suicide attempt (Friedman et al., 1972; Laufer, 1974).

The Nonintensive Treatment of Adolescents

I mentioned at the beginning of this paper that our funds for the walk-in service come from the London Borough of Brent. When we first started this service, we insisted that adolescents from anywhere should be able to be seen for assessment. This was agreed, but it was decided that treatment would be reserved only for adolescents from the Borough of Brent. This means that the adolescents coming from outside the Borough of Brent who are in need of treatment have to be referred to other services in the community.

Initially, it was our policy to limit nonintensive treatment to once-weekly sessions for up to one year. This was, at the time, determined primarily by the fact that our budget was very limited. Recently, however, we decided to alter this policy, partly because our budget for the service has been increased substantially, but also because our once-weekly treatment for a limited period was not working out well. Our present policy is to offer up to twice-weekly treatment, without any time limit. While I cannot yet say how this will work out, I shall describe how we go about deciding to offer nonintensive treatment, and in which circumstances I think it to be of use.

A decision about treatment is made at our weekly staff meeting. The reports of all the interviews with the adolescent are circulated in advance of the meeting. It is then up to the staff members attending the meeting to formulate the nature and degree of psychopathology and to recommend the most suitable form of treatment. Whenever the question of nonintensive treatment arises, we encounter much uncertainty about its applicability to adolescents as well as real differences of opinion about its aims and its effectiveness. I find it difficult to decide which factors would account for this—whether it is that we do not understand what intervention does during a developmental process, whether it is our assessment which is at fault, whether the uncertainties reflect our ignorance about the period of adolescence itself, or whether the aims of nonintensive treatment are such that we must expect a good deal of failure. These are some of the questions which we are studying at the moment.

Although we still have a long way to go before we can clarify these problems, I would single out as one of the factors that clouds some of our work the description of our intervention as "treatment." As psychoanalytically trained people, we have certain expectations when we undertake "treatment"; the expectation may be that we can bring about structural change or that we may be able to undo the pathological process which is present. The description of nonintensive intervention as "treatment" superimposes expectations which are different from what I believe such intervention should set out to do. I do not wish to give the impression that I believe that nonintensive intervention in adolescence is not worth doing—far from it. Although such intervention cannot undo the pathological process, it can contribute something of much value to the present and future life of the adolescent. What it can contribute—and I do not think that we should expect anything beyond this—is to help prevent the existing pathology from interfering with the ongoing developmental process; that is to say, it can make it easier for the adolescent to confront the specific developmental tasks, thereby enabling the developmental process to proceed. If we can do this, then we have done something important.

The main developmental tasks of adolescence are: the change in the relationship to the parents, the change in the relationship to contemporaries, and the change in the attitude to the body. More specifically, we assume that the period of adolescence (that is, the time from 13 to 21) will normally enable the adolescent to use experiences in the outside world as well as those related to his internal world (I include those which are specifically related to his own body) in ways which help him with these developmental tasks. If, due to internalized conflict, the adolescent is isolated, or is unable to obtain sexual pleasure from his body, or is unable to risk disapproval from his parents, or is convinced that he or she is socially and sexually inadequate, then the danger is that the failures during the adolescent period will strengthen the already-existing interference in development. When this person reaches the end of adolescence, he will have missed his *once-only chance* to change his relationships to his internal objects, a change which normally would result in his acceptance of the fact that he alone is responsible for his sexually mature body (Laufer, 1968). I use the description *once-only chance* because I believe that the period of adolescence has a specific developmental function which, if interfered with through internalized conflict, cannot simply be undone or caught up with in adulthood. On the contrary, the results of developmental interference or damage in adolescence inevitably have repercussions throughout one's adult life.

If my assumptions about the function of nonintensive intervention are correct, then it follows that the role of assessment of psychopathology and the selection for nonintensive intervention are especially important. The dilemma with which we are constantly faced is that a number of those who come to the Centre for help are very disturbed people, and we know that we may be able to do little for them via nonintensive intervention. Nevertheless, the other side of this is that many of these adolescents are only just beginning to be in touch with the reality of their existing disturbance and to sense the impact of their internalized conflicts on their present and future lives. We know, or believe, that if their psychopathology hinders them in involving themselves in age-appropriate experiences, their infantile fantasies will continue to exert a dynamic power because these fantasies will persist unaltered if they are not tested and checked by reality experiences.

A period of nonintensive intervention can sometimes be of great help to some of these people, but at the same time we cannot lose sight of the fact that we work with many limitations. One of the built-in dangers of offering nonintensive intervention is that we may easily lose sight of the presence of these very important limitations; it is as if the urgency of adolescence as a developmental period makes us want to blur the differences between what takes place in nonintensive intervention as compared to intensive treatment. I have in mind the differences between insight on the one hand, and the internal reality of the transference neurosis and working through on the other (Stewart, 1963). But these issues require much more intricate study, and I hope that our work at the Centre will help to clarify further some of these differences.

Implied in my remarks about nonintensive intervention is that we are still quite unsure about what we are doing, whom we can and whom we cannot help. In our staff meetings we are very careful to define the aims of our intervention, and do not offer such help to adolescents who are clearly either too ill for this or who have no relation to their internal lives. Yet, in selecting patients for nonintensive help we have until now relied on such general criteria as: severity of the disturbance (which presupposes our ability to rule out the likelihood of an ongoing psychotic process), the adolescent's awareness (even if this is only slight) that his problems exist within himself, the extent of the adolescent's suffering, and the adolescent's conscious wish to do something about his present life. This means, in fact, that the adolescents whom we have so far selected for nonintensive help vary enormously from the not-too-disturbed to those who are obviously very disturbed and at risk. I can best summarize this aspect of our work by saying that we think that such intervention is an important part of our service and can be of great help to some adolescents, but we do not yet know which criteria in assessment can help us to be more selective, nor do we know which technical procedures work and which do not.

Summary

In this paper I have described mainly the work of our walk-in service for adolescents. I have not described our research into mental breakdown in adolescence which is being carried out through the Centre for the Study of Adolescence. I am aware that I have avoided discussing a number of important issues related to adolescent development and psychopathology, including: the many gaps in our knowledge about adolescence—unknowns which hamper our work severely; the pros and cons of various forms of intervention; the suitability of the various psychopathological categories which are often used to describe what is wrong. Nor have I mentioned our work with parents. Instead I have chosen to describe a few specific areas of our work which are related to assessment and to intervention. By focusing on what I consider to be the main work of the walk-in Centre, I have also tried to describe what we have learned from this kind of work.

BIBLIOGRAPHY

Freud, A. (1958), Adolescence. *This Annual*, 13:255–278.
—— (1962), Assessment of Childhood Disturbances. *This Annual*, 17:149–158.

Freud, S. (1905), Three Essays on the Theory of Sexuality. *S.E.*, 7:125–243.
Friedman, M., Glasser, M., Laufer, E., Laufer, M., & Wohl, M. (1972), Attempted Suicide and Self-Mutilation in Adolescence. *Int. J. Psycho-Anal.*, 53:179–184.
Laufer, M. (1965), Assessment of Adolescent Disturbances. *This Annual*, 20:99–123.
—— (1968), The Body Image, the Function of Masturbation, and Adolescence. *This Annual*, 23:114–137.
—— (1973), Studies of Psychopathology in Adolescence. In: *Adolescent Psychiatry*, ed. S. C. Feinstein & P. L. Giovacchini. New York: Basic Books, Vol. 2, pp. 56–69.
—— (1974), The Analysis of an Adolescent at Risk. In: *The Analyst and the Adolescent at Work*, ed. M. Harley. New York: Quadrangle Books, pp. 269–296.
—— (1975), *Adolescent Disturbance and Breakdown*. London: Penguin Books.
Stewart, W. A. (1963), An Inquiry into the Concept of Working Through. *J. Amer. Psychoanal. Assn.*, 11:474–499.

The Impact of Surgery on Boys

WILLIAM THOMAS MOORE, M.D.

SEVERAL YEARS AGO I HAD THE OPPORTUNITY TO OBTAIN DETAILED observational knowledge about the immediate and long-term effects of surgery on two boys and their friends. The observations were recorded by their parents at a time when the boys' father was in analysis with me. While a separate paper could be written on the effect which the child's testis surgery had on the course of the father's analysis, I shall limit this presentation to relating the story of the two boys because such observations seem to me to have intrinsic value. Moreover, they highlight several areas that are generally neglected when we apply psychoanalytic knowledge of child development to give "mental first aid" (Bergmann and A. Freud, 1965) to children or advise their parents and our pediatric colleagues.

Report of Observations

THE EMERGENCY SURGERY

One evening Ben, who was then 8 years old, complained of general scrotal discomfort and a slight pain in his right testis which had developed earlier that day as he was sitting in music class. When his parents questioned him he was at first vague, but gradually disclosed that he may have been struck by a hardball during recess. Because his physical discomfort was relieved by lying down, Ben

---

Director of the Division of Child Analysis of the Institute of the Philadelphia Association for Psychoanalysis; Associate Professor of Clinical Psychiatry, University of Pennsylvania.

was able to sleep through the night; however, the next morning pain in his scrotum became severe when he walked. Within the hour he was taken to his pediatrician and then to a pediatric surgeon, both of whom made the diagnosis of torsion and strangulation of the epididymal appendix of the right testis. The surgeon explained that the condition was extremely rare and usually resulted from jumping or falling from small heights. He recommended immediate surgical intervention in order to save the testis from gangrene and loss. With diagrams he then demonstrated to Ben and his parents the anatomical relationships of the involved testis and described the surgical removal of the epididymal appendix, at the same time stressing that the testis and scrotum would remain complete and intact.

Ben was then taken immediately to the hospital. While waiting in the emergency admissions room, Ben asked if he could have a gift following the operation. After his parents responded in unison, "Yes, of course. What would you like?" he replied that he wanted a "new" hardball.

After admission the anesthesiologist spent a good deal of time explaining the procedures of a spinal block. (Since Ben had eaten breakfast, he could not be given a general anesthetic.) The anesthesiologist also told Ben not to be frightened if he awakened during the operation; he would not experience any pain because the spinal anesthesia would cause a loss of feeling from his waist down to his feet. He equated the experience with the numbness Ben may have experienced following a novocaine injection at the dentist's. He further cautioned Ben that at first he would not be able to move his legs, but that this condition would soon change. After the anesthesiologist departed, Ben asked his father to review the details of the impending surgery.

During the half-hour operation, Ben remained alert and followed the movements of the operating room personnel as the anesthesiologist periodically reassured him that everything was going well. Ben's father was told that surgery was performed through the abdominal wall just above the right groin and that the skin incision was closed with a plastic seal so that the operative area appeared as a $2\frac{1}{2}$-inch fine dry line that was to remain bandage free.

As soon as Ben returned to his hospital room he looked at the dry incision and commented that it wasn't "bad looking," and then fell into a light and fitful sleep. He awakened occasionally to check his leg movements or to complain about the continuous intravenous needle that was inserted into his immobilized right foot. Later, when fully awake, he commented that he could not see anything except a towel draped over his chest during surgery, and had experienced no pain, but could feel the surgeon's hands "pulling on things inside my stomach."

On the first postoperative morning, Ben's mother asked if he could recall whether he had fallen or jumped from a height prior to his painful scrotum. Ben remembered that he had jumped from a small stone wall while playing follow-the-leader at the neighborhood Memorial Day picnic, then later while sitting on the wall, he fell backward, and somersaulted in the air before landing on his abdomen. He said he wasn't hurt; in fact, it seemed so funny at the time that he and the other boys laughed.

When his father visited, Ben asked whether he had bought him a new hardball. When his father replied that he would get one by the time he was able to play baseball again, Ben was clearly irritated; however, he quickly recovered and asked his father to play chess. During a lull in the game his father asked if he still had pain in his testis. With Ben's reply that "it only hurts when I touch it," his father suspected he had been checking in order to determine whether his testes were intact.

Later that afternoon as Ben wandered around and acquainted himself with the rest of the surgical ward, he became somewhat distressed over the condition of some of the other children, especially those who were in a critical state. Most upsetting was a 12-year-old boy, who had undergone cardiac surgery earlier that day, and now lay unconscious in an oxygen tent that was surrounded by mysterious life-sustaining medical paraphernalia. The children old enough to understand, discussed the possibility of this boy's death. They were alert to any news they could gather by asking questions or eavesdropping on the hospital personnel. By evening the boy's critical condition had somewhat subsided so that the oxygen tent was no longer needed. Ben was relieved and felt very fortunate by comparison. He expressed a growing eagerness to leave the hospital the next day and was grateful that his mother had been able to stay with him.

Several months later, Ben admitted that he had been afraid of being left alone in the hospital, especially after he had noticed that the parents of other children on the pediatric surgical pavilion were not permitted to remain overnight. He also said he had been less frightened as a result of the explanations and reassurance given by his father and the doctors.

On the second postoperative day, as Ben prepared to leave the hospital with his parents, his father again reassured him that he did not have his testis removed, but only a small part that had "become sick." Ben replied in a serious, but defensive tone that he knew this to be so, as though his father's overzealous attempts at comforting him were at the moment more disquieting than settling to his doubts.

Until then Ben had been quite cooperative and his underlying concerns were not so obvious; however, he began to display an increasing impatience over the delayed procurement of a new hardball. He had also displaced some anxiety about the loss of a testis to a concern about the temporary loss of movement and sensation in his legs, long after the effects of the caudal anesthesia had worn off. Ben's mother had in the meantime consulted with another child analyst, who advised that the purchase of a new hardball be postponed. She explained that the immediate "replacement" might unwittingly reinforce the mechanism of displacement and thereby give more substance to Ben's deep fear that he had lost a testis. While the parents followed this advice, one might question its soundness. The child seemed to experience the withholding of the promised and desired gift as an additional deprivation, which itself may have fostered the feared displacement. Moreover, delaying the gift would scarcely prevent or undo the displacement that Ben seemed to need as an interim defense. One could also argue that the ball might have reinforced Ben's sense of intactness. In any event, without analytic material, it is not possible to determine the meaning which the hardball and its withholding had for the boy.

CONVALESCENCE AT HOME

Ben arrived home and, as he was greeted by his younger brother, tears came into his eyes for the first time. Thereafter, he avoided talking about his operation to anyone until his friend, Paul, visited him later that day. As Paul approached the front door, he began to limp, and as he entered, Ben asked what had happened to his leg. Paul was embarrassed and answered that he didn't know, but that his leg began to hurt as he approached the house. Paul turned out to be an eager and sympathetic listener as Ben gave a full account of his hospital experience. As Ben described the details of surgery to his friend, the accuracy and thoroughness of the explanation impressed his mother, who was within hearing distance.

During seven weeks of convalescence that followed, Paul became Ben's constant companion, and had completely identified with him. He rarely permitted Ben to be out of sight, especially when they played baseball. One evening, as Ben was running the bases, he stopped, winced, doubled over, and folded his arms over his abdomen in an attempt to relieve the sharp abdominal pain. Paul immediately stopped his own activity and watched Ben very closely as he moved toward him. Finally as though in pain, he, too, grimaced, bent forward, and placed a hand on his own abdomen. For several more weeks Paul did not relax his vigil over Ben until he was forced to do so because the two families went separate ways for summer vacation. Paul's intense identification with Ben seemed clearly related to fantasies about his own rather large and "ugly" abdominal scar, a reminder of the critical operation he himself had undergone during infancy.

On the second posthospital day, Ben asked if he could telephone his paternal grandfather who lived in another city. When no one answered, he became visibly shaken. After a suspenseful moment of thought, he telephoned his other grandfather. This surprised his parents because Ben had not been particularly close to either one of his grandfathers. When his maternal grandfather answered, Ben, hesitantly, but, as though under some compulsion, blurted into the telephone, "Grampa, this is Ben. I was in the hospital." He became tear-choked and could say nothing more, as he handed the telephone to his mother. This was the second time he had cried since the beginning of his illness, and it seemed as significant as it was puzzling. But then the parents recalled that two months prior to the operation, Ben had lost a hardball given to him by his paternal grandfather. He was fond of it because it had been used during a major league baseball game and because he had been simultaneously told that his grandfather as a young man had been a successful baseball pitcher. Ben's interest in playing the game increased that spring, and he himself became a successful pitcher for his grade school baseball team. Assurance from his father that he would be given a new hardball by the time he was able to play again apparently had not satisfied Ben. The call to his grandfather suggested that Ben hoped to expedite an immediate replacement and that the displacement of postoperative concern over a damaged or lost testis seemed stronger than ever.

Ben's physical recovery was rapid and he was able to play baseball within a week; therefore, as promised, his father gave him a new "major league" hardball. Never was a hardball given such care. It remained safely nested in Ben's baseball glove for the first few days, after which he rarely played "catch" with the new ball and never permitted it to be used for batting practice.

Ben's mother noticed that since the hospitalization his habit of fondling his genitals, as he watched television, had disappeared. Instead, he now held his new hardball and repetitively slammed it into his baseball glove in order to "make a good pocket like big league players do." As weeks passed, Ben's interest in baseball yielded to other activities; however, for some time to come, the new hardball remained highly cathected, and was kept in an especially safe place on Ben's dresser, separated from other baseball equipment and toys so that it would neither be damaged nor lost.

As the day for his final visit to the surgeon approached, Ben exhibited only negative interest in seeing him; yet he asked if he would be able to see the anesthesiologist, "that doctor who was nice to me in the operating room." On this last visit, the surgeon informed Ben that he had "completely recovered and could engage in any activity," and from this point on the new ball became separated from its resting place. In time, both the ball and the glove, when not in use, were thrown in with other toys.

THE YOUNGER BROTHER'S REACTION

A few incidents in Joe's earlier life have some bearing on his reactions to Ben's hospitalization. Several weeks before Ben's illness, Joe's friend, Billy, had undergone a tonsillectomy, Joe's first experience with this childhood phenomenon. He talked a great deal about Billy's operation and related that his friend had his "testicles taken out," even though he knew the difference between tonsils and "testicles." He had, in fact, known for some time about "testicles"; yet he occasionally caught himself using the incorrect word, "No, I don't mean testicle. What's that other word?" Joe had known of Billy's operation, but did not see him until they met at the neighborhood Memorial Day picnic. Billy's tonsillectomy was the subject of avid interest and conversation, as was his new pet lizard that had been a postoperative gift from his parents. He frequently fished the pet from the pocket of his pants to fondle and display it as Joe and the other boys watched with wide-eyed respect. By late afternoon all of the neighborhood children, including Ben, had arrived and were playing together. (It was during a lull in the play that Ben experienced the unfortunate mishap that led to his emergency hospitalization and surgery the following day.)

Another episode that occurred when Joe was $4\frac{1}{2}$ years old foreshadows his reaction to Ben's operation. Within an hour after his first visit to the dentist, he quietly withdrew into his bedroom and arranged a tray of makeshift dental instruments so that he could play dentist with several of his friends as patients. He was known to repeat the play after each visit to the dentist and informed his family that he would become a dentist when he grew up.

On the day of Ben's hospitalization Joe, age 6, was acutely aware of the events that took place in the morning. After he learned that Ben would not be attending school that day, he was reluctant to go, but finally went. He returned with an air of anticipation, then reacted with alarm when he found only Cora, the maid, at home. She added to his concern when she told him that his parents had taken Ben to the hospital for surgery and that his mother would remain with Ben until he came home. Nothing seemed to calm or please him as Joe alternated between playing outdoors with his friends and clinging to Cora as he whined with impatience at having to wait so long for his father to return. To make matters worse, Gale, age 9, the most vociferous child in the neighborhood, claimed that her mother said Ben had had a testis removed that afternoon. On hearing this, Joe was swept up into a wave of excitement that moved across the neighborhood. The rumors, the questions, the exaggerations—Joe was a witness to them all. The persistence of this rumor later contributed to Ben's own lingering uncertainty about the extent of his surgery. In an atmosphere of loneliness and uncertainty a very worried 6-year-old boy remained close to home.

When his father arrived home, Joe was waiting in the driveway with his friends. He ran to his father's car and asked whether Ben was all right and without waiting for an answer exclaimed, "Gale said Ben had his testicle taken out." When his father assured him this was not the case, Joe shouted the good news to his friends. Gale, her position threatened by Joe's news, adamantly insisted that Joe was wrong, "Ben had one testicle taken off." Joe, feeling uncertain, reversed his tracks in order to check with his father, then returned to the children and angrily directed his resolute remark to Gale, "Ben did not *even* have one testicle taken off." With this, he turned and ran after his father into the house.

Once inside Joe followed his father from room to room and barraged him with questions, which the father answered factually. He first asked about the anatomical location of the operative area. "Where did they cut? Did you see the cut? Did Ben bleed a lot? Can you see the stitches where the doctor sewed him up?" Joe did not ask whether his brother was frightened or had cried and for the remainder of the evening exhibited no interest in anything other than surgical details. Joe had identified with his older brother and seemed to need solid reassurance from his father that both of Ben's testes were intact so that he could effectively deal with Gale and other dissenters on their next encounter. After his questions had been answered, Joe went to bed and slept soundly.

The following morning, after helping his father pack Ben's robe, slippers, and games into a suitcase, Joe went off to school without the reluctance he had shown the day before. After school he embarked on a crusade to convince the remaining disbelievers among the neighborhood children that "Ben did not have his whole testicle taken out, but only a tiny piece that was sick. He didn't even have stitches." By evening he was eager to confront his father with another round of questions about Ben's operation. He inquired in disbelief that a surgical incision can be permanently closed without the use of surgical stitches. "How could the doctor cut Ben open and not sew him up?" He listened in dismay when his father told him that Ben's surgical scar was almost invisible because in place of stitches the skin had been sealed with a new type of plastic coating that held the edges together. No amount of reassurance could convince Joe that Ben's incision would not "break open again if it wasn't sewed up." He did not believe that a plastic coating could have produced a firm seal over Ben's incision. He said he could not wait to see the scar and hoped that Ben would show it to him as soon as he got home. That night his sleep was restive.

When Ben came home from the hospital the following day, Joe could hardly contain himself: "Did the operation hurt? Were you scared?" Then he quickly added that he did not want to see Ben's scar. Later that day he gathered an assortment of "operation tools" consisting of some paper, scotch tape, an empty medicine bottle, a needle, some thread, and a nail file which he placed in "Ben's hospital suitcase." Then he quickly donned his bathrobe, announced that he was a doctor, and sat inside the suitcase, which he said was his "hospital." Before going to bed that evening, he placed his "patients" (several toy animals) along with his "operation tools" in his "hospital" and arranged them by the side of his bed for the night.

For the next few days Joe played in his "hospital" as a surgeon operating on his "patients." The procedure was always the same; first he pretended to cut his "patients," then he would sew them back together before bandaging them. The cutting was simulated, but the sewing and bandaging were realistic. The operative area was the mouth or throat, almost as often as it was the abdomen. Occasionally, when he was bored with using toy animals, he recruited new patients from some of his more easily persuaded playmates. After the third day of this activity, Joe mustered enough courage and asked to see Ben's scar. At first Ben resisted, but later agreed when Joe offered to give him several of his most highly valued baseball cards in exchange for one look at the incisional scar, which by that time was no more than a 1½-inch white line. Joe commented later that he thought the scar was "big" and "ugly." During a restless night, he had a nightmare that awakened him as he cried out, "I have to be Ben." The next day brought a feverish return to full-time, vigorous surgery on all of the toy animals. Joe increased the number of makeshift instruments and used larger, more obvious bandaging. One toy in particular, a rubber bear named "Benny," became the object of frequent, multiple operative procedures. During one "operation" Joe lost the needle inside the bear's abdomen and became frantic until he was able to recover it.

By evening he entreated his family to call him "Dr. Joe" because of his decision to become a pediatric surgeon. He thought he might even study under the same surgeon who had operated on Ben so that he could become the "boss" of the whole hospital, because then he, Joe, could decide who was to become the "patient" and he could demand that all incisions be properly sewn together so that they would not "break open again." When he told his brother of his aspirations, Ben asked incredulously and with repugnance, "How could you look at people's insides?" He added that he himself would rather be a nice doctor, like the one who had talked to him during surgery.

It is interesting to note that from the earliest surgical play Joe had placed great stress on stitching his toys. Finally, after he had become courageous enough to look at Ben's scar, his anxiety increased again and he went into a frenzy of activity that placed even greater emphasis on "fixing up" his patients with sutures and bandages. By that time "Benny Bear" had bandages over five different operative areas, none of which was near the groin or lower abdomen. In order to achieve greater mobility of his "hospital" filled with "doctor tools," Joe exchanged his brother's large suitcase for a small box upon which he printed the words, "Doctor Joe," in bold lettering made of adhesive tape.

Joe's interest in playing doctor diminished as Ben's recovery became apparent. After Ben's dismissal by the surgeon, Joe "operated" less often; however, he kept his portable "hospital" ready for use at a moment's notice. Until the time when the family went on their summer vacation, Joe periodically withdrew into his bedroom and played surgeon, especially after an altercation with his parents or brother. He remained steadfast in his decision that he would someday become a pediatric surgeon.

Ben served not only as a strong rival for Joe, but also as an oedipal substitute for his father. At the same time, Joe identified with his brother as a surgical patient just as he had with his friend Billy. For Joe, surgical loss—whether of "tonsils" or "testicles"—unconsciously was castration. Moreover, since the rumor that Ben had had "one testicle cut off" strongly reinforced Joe's fear, the possibility of castration seemed very real to him. "If it can happen to my brother, it could happen to me." Under such pressure of castration anxiety Joe had recourse to an old pattern of defense that he had previously found to be reliable: identification with the aggressor, changing passivity into activity. This was what he had done when he played dentist at the age of 4. And one would predict that he will deal with future adversity by resorting to activity and reparation.

FURTHER REPERCUSSIONS OF THE SURGERY IN BEN

A month after the operation, Ben and Joe were enrolled for the summer day camp which they had attended the previous year. Within a few days Ben appeared generally unhappy and complained about an inability to fall asleep because of night fears that he thought were engendered by "scary stories" he had heard at camp. One particularly frightening story told of a midnight visit by the "Turnpike Phantom" anticipated by the boys during the annual overnight campout. Another was a story about the moving hand of a mummy bound in white. His parents suggested that the fear of the mummy was probably a reminder of a very scary experience that he was trying to forget. Perhaps the operating surgeon, dressed in white, with only his eyes visible and hands covered with rubber gloves, had looked to Ben like a mummy with moving hands. The father also stressed that it was only natural to be upset about his hospitalization because it had been a disturbing experience for all of them. Ben seemed relieved after this discussion and slept well.

The following morning Ben asked his mother whether he had bled very much during the operation and wondered, "What did my opened-up insides look like?" Before going to bed that evening he told his father that he was afraid the "bad dream" from the night before might recur. He dreamed that he was lying on his back while riding in a convertible "with an open top." Ben had in fact lain on the back seat of a closed convertible when he was taken to the hospital; he had also lain supine and awake with an opened abdomen during surgery. Since mirrors were a part of the overhead light positioned above the surgical field, Ben must have, at least subliminally, seen the reflections of his opened abdomen or "insides," the surrounding operative area, and the surgeon's hands covered with blood.

Within a day or two Ben reported a second "bad dream" in which a hand reached toward him from a hole in the bathroom wall directly above the toilet paper receptacle. Actually, recent plumbing repairs to the boys' bathroom had necessitated such an opening in the wall, and Ben was afraid to urinate because he thought a hand might extend from the hole to grab his penis. Ben's father remembered that as part of the diagnostic examination, the surgeon had taken Ben into the bathroom, stood him on the toilet seat, then darkened the room in order to transilluminate his scrotum. He then left him alone in the bathroom with instructions to urinate into a urinalysis specimen bottle. It seemed likely that Ben's phobia resulted from a condensation of his own and the surgeon's hands, his own hand representing masturbatory pleasure, and the surgeon's signifying punishment for masturbation, which Ben had in fact given up after his surgery.

As time approached for the family's summer vacation, Ben began to frequent the bathroom more than seemed physiologically necessary. He said he was apprehensive about traveling in a car because he feared losing control and urinating in his pants before a rest stop could be made. Even when he had to travel only short distances in town, Ben was very concerned about his need to urinate en route. To allay his anxiety, he rushed to the toilet at the last minute and forced urination before leaving home. At other times he felt like urinating, but couldn't when he tried. He had never been enuretic, but out of fear that he might wet the bed, Ben ran to the bathroom a number of times before retiring. He disclosed that he tried to go to the bathroom while his parents were still awake because he was even more afraid that "the hand" would grab him while everyone was asleep.

Ben also expressed the wish that he could fall asleep immediately upon retiring because as long as he lay awake he thought about his fear that someone would creep into his room while he slept. When asked for details, Ben became very vague, and said he could not remember anything else. One evening shortly thereafter, a group of neighborhood children had gathered on the lawn to tell "spooky stories." Ben created one about a robber, which became so indelibly imprinted in his memory that during the following school term he submitted it to fulfill an assignment for an original short story. The opening paragraph read:

> There once was an old man with a long white beard who went from place to place robbing people's money. The police were going to get him, though, because he was leaving a trail behind him. His beard was so long it dragged on the ground and left a trail. It was so heavy when it dragged, because he hid stolen money in his beard.

Meanwhile, Ben had asked his father what he could do about his nightly fears. The father suggested that Ben might still be worried about what had or had not been taken away from him during his operation; he also might be concerned whether or not the surgery or the anesthesia had permanently affected the normal functioning of his penis. Because of the loss of sensation in his penis during the operation, and for a short time thereafter, it probably was difficult for him to determine when urination began and ended. This in turn made him feel uncertain whether he could control urination, and that in fact some uncertainty still remained. Ben did not reply directly, but asked, "How much longer will my scar be red? Will it ever get smaller? I am embarrassed when anyone looks at it."

Later that week Ben told Joe and his mother that "only a very small bad part" of his testis had been removed. He also spoke openly to them about how frightened he had been when the anesthesia had caused a "dead" feeling in his legs and penis. "It felt like my hand did a long time ago when it went to sleep," an incident that had occurred when he was 4. He had awakened one night crying because he could neither move nor feel his right arm and hand because he had "slept" on them. With this recollection Ben linked two disparate but overlapping experiences, from which one may infer a connection between masturbatory pleasure afforded by hand and penis, and punishment in the form of paralysis and loss of sensation in both offending agents. Berta Bornstein (1953) referred to the castration anxiety in latency boys over manual masturbation that is manifested by guilt, displacements, insomnia, and urinary symptoms.

The choice of the hand had another determinant in Ben's conflict about his impulse to strike his brother. Although prior to surgery his father had routinely warned him, "Keep your hands to yourself," Ben had been free and easy with an occasional punch in Joe's direction. He had always been quick to anger and responded physically when he thought Joe had violated his rights, or appropriated his belongings, or invaded his territory. Ben frequently teased and bullied Joe. After the operation, Ben avoided fighting with Joe, even though he appeared impatient and irritated with Joe most of the time. Ben studiously avoided Joe and his hospital play, especially on those occasions when Joe ventured to ask questions about Ben's operation. In every sense his "doctor" brother was an unwelcome reminder to Ben of things better forgotten. Beleaguered on all sides, Ben did not seem to know which way to turn in his distress. Ben's parents responded empathically to the boy's dilemma. They told Ben that Joe's inordinate interest in his operation made him feel angry and frustrated because Joe kept reminding him of his hospitalization, which Ben was trying to forget. All this really made his brother a burden to him. Shortly thereafter Ben's apprehensions about his night fears, phobias, and inability to urinate gradually began to subside.

The operation had produced changes in Ben's personality, the most obvious of which was the way he handled his aggression. Before surgery, he was overtly aggressive in his play relationships with peers, fighting freely and whenever necessary and sometimes with larger boys. After surgery, Ben seemed subdued and avoided physical contact or confrontations with his friends. He even became annoyed when other boys fought each other in his presence. He no longer teased or bullied Joe; in fact, Ben declared that he did not want to hit Joe anymore because he did not want to hurt him. In time Ben's inhibition of aggression diminished and he again began to stand up for himself in altercations with his playmates. He again teased his brother and delivered a few blows when he felt he could get away with it. However, one more permanent character change began to emerge. Ben assumed a new position among his peers; he became a judge and mediator whenever two friends fought or argued with each other, and no conflict seemed beyond his efforts at arbitration.

As Ben's phobias and his concern about urination diminished, his interest in baseball increased. In order to become a good baseball pitcher, he decided to practice each day by throwing a rubber ball against the garage wall; at the same time he played baseball daily with the neighborhood children. One evening after a game he asked his father why he sometimes developed abdominal side pains while running. "It feels like my stomach will bust." He was also puzzled about the frequent and involuntary nature of penile erections. His father assured him that erections were a daily "normal" function of the penis, just as abdominal side pains, during running, were a natural physical manifestation, which gave most boys some concern. He also told Ben that his recent experiences might have made Ben unnecessarily cautious and overly distressed about abdominal sensations. When his father asked whether the abdominal scar was still sensitive, Ben replied that he was worried about its splitting open if he strained himself too much. Reassurance apparently proved ineffectual. Ben was not fully convinced that no risks were involved in physical exertion.

THE STRUCTURE OF BEN'S PHOBIAS

During the spring term preceding Ben's operation, his second grade class did a detailed study of Egyptian civilization. He was fascinated by pyramids, pharaohs, and especially by the mummification of Egyptian kings, and the concept of death and its undoing. Thoughts about ghosts, spirits, mummies, and other representatives of the resurrected dead—a common preoccupation of latency children—were certainly a familiar part of Ben's mental life prior to his operation. When the storytelling at camp included the mummy tale, Ben claimed there were three things about it that had especially frightened him: the mummy was a man wrapped in "white bandages," the hand of the mummy moved, and the mummy could return to life after being dead for thousands of years. The mummified king was wrapped in white cloth and had a moving hand, as had the white-gowned surgeon.

As previously pointed out, the fear of the mummy's moving hand was probably based on a condensation of Ben's own hand, which delivered pleasure, and that of the surgeon, which rendered punishment. The surgeon's hands had appeared in two episodes: he poked around Ben's scrotum during a painful diagnostic examination in his office and in the darkened bathroom; and during the operation Ben saw the hands of the surgeon extend from his white gown, reach into his abdomen, and emerge covered with blood. In addition, he felt a tugging sensation within his abdomen as the surgeon's hands moved around in the operative site. A chilling recollection of these events persisted well into Ben's adolescence. Small wonder that Ben suffered from feelings of anxiety at the mere thought of seeing bloody hands, whether his own or those of others.

The spinal anesthesia had caused a temporary loss of movement and sensation in Ben's legs and a numbness in his penis. In a sense, these parts of his body seemed dead, but nevertheless returned to life in much the same way as he believed a mummy could be revived. The fear that a mummy's hand could be resurrected also seemed to represent to Ben his concern that penile erections and the desire to masturbate would never cease. He feared that the desire would return, accompanied by a messenger of castration, represented by a mummy, an old bearded robber, or a turnpike phantom—all displaced representatives of the surgeon, who had amply demonstrated his ability to relieve Ben of valuable possessions.

Two additional events in Ben's life seem to clarify one aspect of his phobic symptoms. His fear of the old robber seemed directly related to oedipal strivings. When Ben was $3\frac{1}{2}$ he had a nightmare following an incident involving his parents. Attired in boots, dungarees, his holstered cap gun and belt, Ben entered the living room where he found his mother sitting on his father's lap. He ran over, climbed up his father's leg into his mother's lap, removed the cap gun from its holster, and pretended to shoot his father "dead." He then reached into his father's pocket and pretended to take all of his money. That night he awakened crying that a hairy gorilla was pursuing him. As in his story of a bearded old robber, Ben's fear represented a projection of his aggression against his father and the resultant fear of retaliation.

The second event occurred during the family's preceding summer vacation. One night as the family slept, a "robber" had stealthily entered the summer house and taken money from the father's wallet. The theft remained undiscovered until morning when Ben and Joe observed that the front door screen had been slashed. When in the following year (prior to the hospitalization) Ben learned that his parents were making arrangements to return to the same summer house, he reminded his father of the robbery. Then, at the time of hospitalization, it seemed that Ben made an association between the robber and the surgeon when he overheard his parents discuss the surgeon's fee, amounting to the same sum stolen by the robber.

Concluding Remarks

Latency children often appear to accept surgery with a deceptive stoicism that is likely to be misconstrued as evidence of ego maturity or as an indication that medical procedures produce little, if any, adverse effects on their psychological development. Hospital personnel repeatedly refer to the calmness, detachment, and unemotional attitudes which these children display during hospitalization, without realizing that what they are actually observing are common defensive attitudes employed by children confronted with an imminent physical assault. However, without exception, surgical procedures disrupt the course of a child's development, until the ego has succeeded in reestablishing psychic equilibrium. In many instances, defense mechanisms, once successfully utilized, are again called upon to cope with the anxiety which, though realistic, easily reactivates older anxieties associated with the infantile neurosis. That this link occurs despite the most detailed factual explanations and unusually empathic support by the parents merely underscores the need to reduce the traumatic effects of surgery by applying principles and procedures based on psychoanalytic knowledge about the development of children.

The observations reported here also indicate clearly that the help needs to be extended not only to the child who is undergoing surgery but also to his immediate family, especially his siblings, who generally are doubly neglected because the parents are preoccupied with coping with the immediate emergency and with their own fears which such events arouse. The measures taken in order to help Ben and Joe were successful in reducing the traumatic effects of Ben's surgery on both boys. Detailed explanations about what had already happened and what could be anticipated during hospitalization and surgery unquestionably were helpful to Ben and Joe. It is generally recognized that the presence of the mother or father during hospitalization is helpful to the child in that it diminishes his fear of abandonment and enhances his feelings of being protected. Unfortunately, many present-day hospital administrative expediences exclude the possibility of employing methods that would be psychologically advantageous, and even provide conditions that are psychoanalytically contraindicated. Although preventive pediatric concepts have been understood for a long time, the need for change, based on psychoanalytic knowledge of child development, in most pediatric hospital facilities throughout the United States, is almost as great today as it was at the time of Ben's surgery over 15 years ago.

While realistic explanations of hospital and medical procedures help the child separate fact and fantasy (A. Freud; see Robertson, 1956), they clearly must not be limited to the immediate period of hospitalization. The child's fears persist, reviving archaic anxieties and older fantasies. The child, too, copes at first with the immediate situation, which overwhelms him and makes him helpless. (The "calmness" of hospitalized children may be ascribed to this fact rather than viewed as an expression of psychic balance.) Only as he gradually relives and works over the experience will some of his fears and fantasies come to the fore. While the analytic literature contains many papers stressing the need for preparing children for surgery, there are very few papers (Robertson, 1956) emphasizing the need for continuing the help and guidance for a prolonged period thereafter.

Yet we know from another area that single explanations do not suffice. Child analysts are familiar with the fact that attempts at sexual education fall far short of the good intentions of the educators because children can only understand and assimilate sexual knowledge imparted to them in terms that are appropriate or coincident to their level of development. A 5-year-old girl, after hearing a detailed explanation from her mother about conception and birth, sat silent for a moment, then asked, "But how does the mommy get the baby seed into her mouth?"

Regardless of the psychological help we give to children, each will finally have to rely on his own resources to establish or restore psychic balance. In the case of the two brothers described here, Joe relied mainly on the defense of identification with the aggressor. Ben, however, underwent a much more complicated process of restoration and adaptation. As an outcome of testis surgery, elements of his aggression and his fear of castration seemed to merge as a cluster of events and memories that in effect amounted to a return of his infantile neurosis. To make his situation more bearable he first displaced the reason for his heightened castration anxiety from a concern over the surgical assault on his testis to a concern about the replacement of the lost hardball. When this adaptive attempt failed to provide adequate defense, the same regressive mechanisms, once prevalent during his oedipal conflict, were again called into service.

The revival of the infantile neurosis, following medical trauma, evokes inquiry into its consequences on the character formation of the developing child. The outcome of childhood trauma depends on qualitative and quantitative elements of sublimated pregenitality and effective oedipal resolution; however, longitudinal observations have demonstrated that traumatic events have a tendency to reinforce past developmental dilemmas and to direct the course of future developmental conflicts.

Since I lack analytic material on these two boys and since my detailed knowledge about them was confined to the period when their father was in analysis with me, I can say little about the long-term effect on their development.[1] It is of interest, however, to mention that although Ben has not settled on a specific profession, he has pursued an educational career pointed toward helping children, particularly those who might be in psychological distress. Joe, however, has followed a direct course toward becoming a surgeon.

BIBLIOGRAPHY

BERGMANN, T. & FREUD, A. (1965), *Children in the Hospital*, New York: Int. Univ. Press.
BORNSTEIN, B. (1951), On Latency. *This Annual*, 6:279–285.
——— (1953), Masturbation in the Latency Period. *This Annual*, 8:65–78.
FREUD, A. (1945), Indications for Child Analysis. *This Annual*, 1:127–149.
——— (1952), The Role of Bodily Illness in the Mental Life of Children. *This Annual*, 7:69–81.
——— (1962), Assessment of Childhood Disturbances. *This Annual*, 17:149–158.
——— (1963), The Concept of Developmental Lines. *This Annual*, 18:245–265.
——— (1965), *Normality and Pathology in Childhood*, New York: Int. Univ. Press.
LIPTON, S. D. (1962), On the Psychology of Childhood Tonsillectomy. *This Annual*, 17:363–417.
NAGERA, H. (1966), *Early Childhood Disturbances, the Infantile Neurosis, and the Adult Disturbances*. New York: Int. Univ. Press.
ROBERTSON, J. (1965), A Mother's Observations on the Tonsillectomy of Her Four-year-old Daughter. With Comments by Anna Freud. *This Annual*, 11:410–433.

---

[1] The detailed study by Lipton (1962) demonstrates the complex effects of a childhood tonsillectomy on the character structure of a woman.

Psychological Reactions to Facial and Hand Burns in Young Men

Can I See Myself Through Your Eyes?

ALBERT J. SOLNIT, M.D. AND
BEATRICE PRIEL, M.A.

DURING THE 1973 YOM KIPPUR WAR IN ISRAEL MANY YOUNG MEN incurred moderate to severe burns of the face and hands, especially during tank warfare. At the outbreak of the hostilities on October 6, 1973, the Plastic Surgery Ward of the Soroka Medical Center in Beer-Sheva was one of several such wards in Israeli general hospitals that were expanded and reorganized to take care of wounded soldiers, mainly patients who were injured in tank warfare. More than 50 soldiers were admitted for this injury at the Soroka Medical Center during the first two weeks of the war.

One week after the war began Professor Nahum Ben Hur requested a mental health team to provide psychological services and to record to the extent it was feasible systematic observations

---

Dr. Solnit, Director of the Yale Child Study Center, was attached to the Soroka Medical Center and the Ben Gurion University of the Negev from August 1973 to July 1974. Mrs. Priel is on the faculty of the Department of Psychiatry and Human Development and the Department of Behavioral Sciences, Ben Gurion University of the Negev, Beer-Sheva, Israel. Since Dr. Solnit did not speak Hebrew, Mrs. Priel concentrated on patients who did not speak or understand English and Dr. Solnit concentrated on those, approximately half of them, who did have a working knowledge of English.

that would be useful to others.[1] Our observations and this paper are limited to the soldier's reactions immediately after the injury and for several months thereafter. We do not include the long-term rehabilitation in which some of the patients are still involved.

The burned person suffers from generalized physical stress and discomfort, is subject to long-standing pain and passivity, and faces the fear of death and the possibility of a socially disfiguring handicap. The care of the burns includes a broad spectrum of multidisciplinary personnel and techniques, requiring the integration of specialized therapies with the risk that technicalities may tend to dehumanize the care.

The influence of emotional reactions on the healing of burned patients is widely acknowledged in studies of burned adults (Hamburg et al., 1953), children with burns (Bernstein et al., 1969; Galdston, 1972; Long and Cope, 1961), and in the reactions of hospital staff to the stress of their work (Quinby and Bernstein, 1971). Although all studies agree that psychological care of the burned person is a necessary part of the treatment, there is no consensus about how and when the psychological care should be provided.

Assumptions

The mental health team decided to concentrate on establishing a psychologically therapeutic environment, rather than on case finding and psychotherapy of individual patients. Of course, diagnostic and therapeutic services were provided when indicated in individual cases.

Our assumptions, guided by psychoanalytic theory, were:

1. Injuries of the face and hands that will lead to scarring are

---

[1] Professor Ben Hur's able collaborators included Drs. Sylvia Frohlich and Morris Russo, the chief nurse Ahuva Fishground, as well as an administrative coordinator, Rina Navot. Later, Professor Ben Hur was replaced by Professor Harry Soroff who enthusiastically supported and utilized the mental health team. This team was constituted mainly by the authors, well supported by part-time colleagues Helen Antonovsky, Adina Doron, Esther Horn, and other colleagues from the fields of nursing, social work, and clinical psychology.

among the most psychologically disabling, narcissistically depleting, and competence-threatening risks to human psychological development and functioning. Many psychological studies, including those of Darwin (1872), established that the face is the surface expression of affect and personality. The study of the smile as the first specific social response of the child indicates the maturational and developmental importance of facial expressions as the most basic, unique, and extraordinary repertoire of nonverbal human social communications (Spitz, 1965). One of our patients whose face was massively injured by a burn explosion intuitively gave vent to his understanding when he said, "What identification permit will you give me before I'm allowed to appear in public?" Similarly, the appearance and competence of the hands are crucial for a sense of intactness, for full tactile experience, and for the ability to use the written and printed symbols as forms of expression and communication. Just as the face is an essential expression of personality and emotionality, the hands are an essential expression of competence, skill, and tactile experience. For these men, the hands represented a prominent aspect of their masculinity.

2. A second assumption, based on other studies of patients with severe burns (Hamburg et al., 1953; Galdston, 1972) and on psychoanalytic theory, was that psychological recovery in these patients would tend to follow physical recovery. Ordinarily, psychological difficulties can inhibit or block physical recovery, just as physical injuries can evoke or cause psychological illness. However, because the burns were extensive and concentrated on the face and hands, the psychoanalytic theory of narcissism clearly implied that psychological understanding and assistance should be in the service of improving the effectiveness of the physical care of the patient. In addition to the lifesaving replacements of blood and fluids and the prevention and cure of infection, the physical care had as its end goals the restoration of a covered, socially acceptable, well-structured, mobile face; and hands that were competent and not too disfigured.

In this second assumption we were guided by Freud's statement (1914): "Narcissism in this sense would not be a perversion, but the libidinal complement to the egoism of the instinct of self-preservation, a measure of which may justifiably be attributed to every living creature" (p. 73f.). As Freud pointed out, we may obtain a better knowledge of narcissism through the study of organic disease, as well as through the study of hypochondria and of the erotic life of the sexes. Freud wrote that "a person who is tormented by organic pain and discomfort gives up his interest in the things of the external world, in so far as they do not concern his suffering" (p. 82). These formulations led to three further assumptions.

3. The return of an interest in the external world is a sign of recovery. This returning interest in the outside world is often ushered in by demands, irritability, and what is usually experienced as a lack of gratitude for the care provided by nurses and doctors, especially the former. At times, this tentative return of an irritable attachment to family members and to the nurses and doctors was also misperceived as hostility and poor morale rather than appreciated as the awakening of libidinal ties to these important persons. Before this early evidence of recovery was understood, the staff often reported that the patient was losing ground, was being spoiled, or was too difficult to care for. Ironically, there was a tendency to put the patient into coventry at a time when he most needed encouragement to remain attached and help in becoming socially and emotionally active.

4. This line of thinking, in turn, sharpened our focus on the patient's psychological trauma. These soldiers were suddenly and massively overwhelmed by an explosion and fire, usually when their tank suffered a direct hit by a missile. As one patient said, "I burned like a little piece of wood in a fire." In applying the theory of trauma to the development of a psychologically therapeutic environment, we strongly emphasized that there be opportunities for patients to become active mentally and later physically in planning and implementing their medical and nursing care. This was particularly important for these young men with severe face and hand burns because for weeks they were incapable of caring for their bodies and physical functions. Nurses had to feed them, turn them, and hold them so they could urinate and defecate.

Accordingly, we set as one of our main efforts the goal that patients have the option to hear and ask about the plans for their treatment. The treatment regime included an energetic program of transfusions, antibiotics, debridement, temporary and permanent grafts, physiotherapy, and a high level of nutritional intake. If a patient indicated directly or indirectly that he did not wish to hear about his treatment or participate in its planning, we did not insist that he do so. Each patient's tolerances and preferences were respected. Most of our patients wanted to know what to expect, how the doctors and nurses had planned their treatment, and asked about details or larger issues they did not understand. Where it was feasible we advised, often effectively, that the patient be encouraged to express a preference for alternate treatments or times of treatment. Selecting the day or time of day for graft was often the most important option that patients requested. About half of the time it was realistic to accommodate the treatment plan to such preferences.

While the responsibility for decisions about treatment was not imposed on the patient, taking each patient's wishes and preferences into account provided opportunities for active participation in the recovery process. For example, one of our patients with severe burns expressed fervent reservations about tube feeding as a way of building up his nutritional status. The external aspects of his nose had been largely destroyed by the burn and he anticipated severe pain from the use of the tube. The patient suggested that he try to eat on his own for a day or two to prove he could achieve hyperalimentation as well as and perhaps even better than with the use of a stomach tube. The surgeon decided to defer the stomach tube, and the patient actively demonstrated that he could do it his way.

Such a psychological approach—enabling the patient to be active in his own behalf, without burdening him with decisions about treatment—is also consistent with our best knowledge about the capacities of adolescents and their limitations. Developmentally, many of our patients were in their late adolescent phase when respect for their wishes might be expected to strengthen their realistic appraisal of the situation and rational reactions to it.

There was a repeated tendency to think the decision was being passed on to the patient. We emphasized that the traditional pattern of having the surgeon decide would be psychologically desirable, as long as it took into account the patient's questions, fears, suggestions, and preferences. We acknowledged that such an untraditional pattern of practice would add to the burdens of the surgeon's, nurses', and allied personnel's daily work, but it would also provide them with a more effective working alliance with their patients. In fact, helping patients find an appropriate middle ground between passivity and activity was perhaps the most crucial aspect of the psychologically therapeutic environment.

5. Another vital assumption taken from psychoanalytic theory—that regression is a necessary concomitant of the healing process—was made explicit. This assumption was often misunderstood as our encouraging regressive behavior, rather than, as we repeatedly made clear in group discussions with nurses and physicians, the acceptance of regressive behavior as a transient, necessary, limited aspect of preparing for the work of healing and recovery. In seeking to implement this understanding, an awareness of regressive, self-preservative, narcissistic reactions as preparation for healing became useful in increasing our capacity to tolerate the regressive behavior of patients and to elaborate the therapeutic alliance with them.

Implementation

We considered two conditions necessary to establish a psychologically therapeutic environment:

1. An individualized treatment policy which implied a personal doctor-patient relationship. For example, each patient knew a team of doctors and nurses were caring for him, but one doctor was his main contact, in that sense *his* doctor. The chief surgeon was accepted as the first authority in the conduct of all ward care and activities.

2. The second condition required that the implications of our five assumptions would be accepted and utilized by all the staff of the ward and not only by specialized professionals.

In utilizing our assumptions and establishing the conditions necessary for a therapeutic environment, we adopted several practical methods.

DAILY ROUNDS

Participation in the daily rounds helped the mental health group to become a formal as well as an organic part of the whole staff in terms of our feelings and those of other members of the staff and of the patients. It should be stressed that the relatively very low anxiety expressed by patients in their contact with us was in part due to the extensive participation of the mental health professionals in the important daily hospital routines. We were familiar figures, consistent members of the medical team who saw them regularly.

DAILY INDIVIDUAL CONTACT WITH PATIENTS

It was our conscious choice to become integral members of the ward staff rather than functioning as a special or separate psychiatric group bent on utilizing our diagnostic and therapeutic skills for the purpose of case finding. Thus, we made rounds twice daily with the surgical and nursing staff and participated fully in all aspects of the staff planning and review meeting, of which there was at least one a day.

One of us also made nightly rounds with the nurses, starting at 10 or 10:30 P.M. These rounds were designed to provide a psychological presence in the late hours of the day when physical and psychological discomforts were often very high. Night rounds were expected to promote contact with families and with the evening shift of nurses. These rounds also provided further opportunities for individual patients to request or engage in additional discussion, and to bring up questions, concerns, and complaints that seemed to surface more regularly at night than during the day.

In the course of these daily contacts there were many opportunities for patients to have a catharsis about their war experiences and injuries. With rare exception each of our patients, alone or in a small group, availed himself of this opportunity at a time and in a situation that he chose. We did not systematically interview and encourage each patient to talk about his war experiences, though we had confidence that as it became appropriate and useful, our patients would take an active role in expressing what they felt and what they remembered. According to our view, young men with severe burns needed to have their initial reactions of numbing denial and of regression accepted while their bodies were cared for. Though we hold for the indivisibility of body-brain-mind, such acute, traumatic injuries require first that the physical injury be attended to while the mind's reactions are supported with concern, warmth, and little or no demands. This narcissistic coping pattern is probably lifesaving, since many individuals cannot tolerate, initially, the full impact of what has happened to them.

PHYSICIANS' MEETINGS

In these meetings general problems and policies of the ward were discussed, such as the importance of giving the patients adequate and accurate information about their treatment, according to the patients' willingness to know. Another important topic referred to was the use of analgesic drugs. The mental health professionals encouraged an awareness of the differentiation and overlapping of physical and psychological pain, with the aim of providing appropriate relief of all sources of pain. Within our competence, we felt it natural and sensible to raise questions about sedatives and analgesics. An awareness that psychic and somatic pain are often intermixed enabled us to individualize the questions about analgesics and to resolve the common fear of doctors and nurses that an overdependency on pain-killing narcotic drugs might develop.

The importance of responding to the real needs of the patient was stressed. A controversial point treated in the staff meetings was the influence of discussing treatment policies at the patients' bedside during rounds. Patients, of course, had different opinions about it. Our view was that such an exchange of opinions, when necessary, as it seemed to be, e.g., when looking at the graft site in considerable detail, could be useful to the patient if one conclusion was reached at the patient's bedside. Also, the risk of this necessary discussion could be minimized if the patient was given an opportunity after the rounds to question, complain, or add his suggestions in a discussion with his doctor or an appropriate member of the team.

A good opportunity to review our policies was provided at these meetings when we began to discuss the time of release of patients. An understanding of the patients' ambivalence about leaving the hospital and returning to active life threw light on some of the psychological processes going on during the healing, like dependency and regression. Some of the patients asked to stay for another day or two, while others paid frequent visits immediately after being released, and even arranged to stay overnight in the ward. The staff's understanding of and tolerance for the patients' needs allowed the patients more time to work through feelings about their returning to normal life with their scars.

NURSES' GROUPS

Burns are frequently complicated by serious infections, usually due to pseudomonas aeruginosas, which require isolation techniques. These also tend to isolate the patients from their families and the outside world. Thus, nurses became most important figures 24 hours a day. The most significant emotional material was obtained in these groups of nurses who met two to three times a week. The cathartic functions of these groups were of the greatest importance.

The nurses were heroic in their devotion and skill. They worked on a 12-hour shift. Many returned to nursing work which they had not done for many years as a result of the national need. After weeks of difficult work they became exhausted and often took personally as undesirable some aspects of the patients' regressive behavior. For example, in one room of three severely burned soldiers, as the healing took place in a setting of pseudomonas infection that required the meticulous use of isolation techniques, one soldier was sarcastically critical of how the nurse fed him. Both hands were swathed in huge clublike bandages, his neck was painfully raw, infected, and gradually healing, and his face was partly bandaged so that only his bright brown eyes were clearly visible. The nurse was offended and went off to have a good cry. How could he talk to her that way after she had slaved away for several weeks at doing her best for him, being an auxiliary ego, the one who bathed, fed, toileted, soothed, tenderly dressed, and medicated him? How could the other two in his room, who also were severely burned and also so well cared for, join in supporting and encouraging the sharp tongue and aggressive outburst against the nurse?

The surgeon considered breaking up the combination of these three soldiers, moving them into different rooms, because he could not allow such threats to nursing staff morale. The chief nurse was also considering this solution. A talk with the three soldiers culminated in a statement by the sarcastic soldier, "She is a bloody fool to cry. I was just trying to help her. Before, I couldn't explain which way it was more comfortable."

One of the first subjects brought up by nurses in the group meetings was the conflicting feelings they had about the regressive behavior of patients. The conflict was between noncritical acceptance of such behavior and overprotectiveness on one side and rejection and intolerance on the other side. The very demanding behavior of several patients was interpreted by some of the nurses as ungrateful, humiliating, and to some extent as a threat to their professional image. The main fear nurses had was that patients would become too infantile and dependent. A better understanding of the dynamics of regression and the curative limitations of nursing care helped to increase the nurses' tolerance of regression and their ability to deal with the grown-up parts of the patients' personality. Additionally, we were able to clarify how frustrating and limiting it feels to a nurse or doctor to see his patient recover so slowly and with so much scarring.

GROUPS OF PATIENTS

The groups patients formed had great influence on the healing process. Because of the severity of the wounds most of them were bedridden for weeks. Then room placement determined the structure of the groups. More natural groups were those constituted by patients who had fought and been wounded together. In such groups, patients felt able from the beginning to exchange experiences and elaborate their recollections of the trauma and their discomfort, pain, and worry about recovery. Similar findings have been reported of burned victims of the same road accident who lay together in the hospital (Hamburg et al., 1953).

We made contact with groups in two types of situations: when a "room" approached us as a group and when in some room there was a group crisis. An example of the first case was a room in which all the soldiers were artillerymen who had been wounded together when an enemy plane which had been shot at fell on them. That group went through the healing process as a strong and cohesive group, preferring to stay together and helping each other during the painful treatments, and in supporting each other in discussions of their psychological ordeals.

An example of the second type of situation was the group crisis in one of the pseudomonas isolation rooms described above. In this "problem room," the patients did not cooperate during changes of dressings and had bitter quarrels with nurses and occupational therapists. When the surgeon and head nurse wanted to separate the three patients, we requested a discussion with the patients about what was going on before such a decision was made. In talking with these patients we found that they had difficulties in regaining activity and had great anxiety about being in isolation. One of the patients could not tolerate the isolation. He became so anxious that he went out in the corridor at night, contrary to the ward's rules. We also observed such claustrophobic reactions in other soldiers who, like this one, were wounded by a direct hit on their enclosed tank.

During our discussion the group decided to stay together until they could leave each other naturally. In our experience, such groups were very responsive to discussions that provided clarification and that gave them a voice in the affairs of the ward.

The Role of the Mental Health Team

Because of our understanding that patients with severe physical injuries need psychologically and physiologically to concentrate on overcoming the physical threat to life, we emphasized the establishment of a psychologically therapeutic environment for all patients. We also provided individual treatment for several soldiers whose depression and negative therapeutic reactions interfered with their physical recovery. In other instances, we prepared the way for referral for psychotherapeutic assistance after they had completed the acute phase of their physical treatments and were embarked on the long-term reconstructive aspects of recovery.

The mental health team served primarily as supporters, facilitators, and interpreters in the creation and maintenance of a physically and psychologically therapeutic environment.

There were inevitable conflicts among the professional staff in regard to planning, treatment, and rehabilitation decisions. These conflicts tended to be a matter of timing or of sequence of treatment and usually were resolved by the surgeon with an emerging consensus after adequate discussion.

Decision making by the surgeon was, of course, a complex process in which observations by nurses, physicians, and the patients' responses during ward rounds played a role. In fact, there seemed to be a desirable increase of assertiveness and expectation of participating in the decision-making process on the part of the ward staff when the treatment of burned patients was involved. This is largely explained by the need for more people to work together on an intensive and sustained basis in the modern technical treatment of severe burns. Thus, decision making on a plastic surgery burn ward may reflect the need for greater activity by the staff—evidence of their competence, when coping with the prospects of permanent scarring (limited recovery) of the face and hands of young men.

The group process, as it developed, added a further complexity to decision making. One could expect crises in which the leader would be challenged and accepted anew, if he was competent. The reaffirmation of the team and the leader should facilitate improved levels of communication, collaboration, and a decrease of negative rivalry at the expense of the patient. Occasionally, the mental health team functioned as a soothing catalyst in this process by tactfully introducing observations that could cool and clarify conflict and that restored perspective, temporarily distorted by the unending pressure of intensive, painstaking, frustrating therapeutic demands.

In our experience and that of others (Quinby and Bernstein, 1971), the care of burn patients is associated with recurrent intrastaff tension and considerable risk to good morale because the recovery from severe burns, at the least, is tedious, painful, and associated with significant scarring. The surgical and nursing personnel, especially the latter, are confronted daily with the limitations of their efforts and competence since fire is such a damaging agent. Moreover, nurses are confronted with the irony that in the case of burned patients, they often have to produce pain in order to promote healing, though every effort is made to minimize the pain.

In the staff meetings and informally during rounds when it could be done discreetly and to the degree it was feasible, we presented a review of each patient's past history of physical and psychological deprivations and trauma. We also presented an inventory of each patient's strengths and an account of his past achievements, i.e., his capacity for mastery. Prior deprivations and traumata tended to shape and explicate the patient's attitudes, fears, and narcissistic reactions to the actual injury for which he had been hospitalized.

For example, a soldier with relatively less severe burns and with a potential for recovery without scarring of his face and hands spoke with resentful sadness of how he had felt when his father died when he was 10 years old. He felt he was different from the other men in his room. He evoked pity and resented it. He complained bitterly about any changes in the timing or arrangements for being fed. He spoke pensively of how family life had declined and how he felt cheated after his father died, when the family no longer had their meals together as regularly and dependably.

Marital status played a significant role in the reactions to injuries that produced what appeared to be lasting scars, without regard to the chronological age. Married soldiers' reactions were more directly proportional to the severity of the injury. Single soldiers' reactions were exaggerated by the apprehension that they would not be able to function socially, to have satisfactory sexual relations and to find a desirable young woman to marry. They seemed to be asking, "How can anyone love me if I don't like myself?" A delicate balance of narcissistic supplies was involved in this concern. One soldier expressed his fear by saying that those who did not know him before his injury would meet a different, less attractive, less desirable person, rather than the previous, more complete person he had been. Our patients often conveyed to us an ordeal or baptism under fire in which the rebirth had been disadvantageous. Elements of mourning for their former selves were noted.

The individual attitude toward injury was affected by what happened to other soldiers in the group in which the patient had fought; the reactions were very different if he was the worst wounded, or the least injured, or the only one to remain alive. Anger, guilt feelings, or great confidence in the magic of past luck, and the fear of what the future would bring were then expressed according to personality dynamics. For example, we found negative or paradoxical therapeutic reactions in a severely wounded soldier who was the commander of his tank. He felt very guilty and incompetent because he, the officer, was the only survivor of his tank. In this case, the reactions to the loss of his crew were heightened by his guilt feelings toward his fiancée and his parents because he felt he was coming back to them as a scarred failure. Working with his fiancée, who saw him daily, facilitated our work with the patient who gradually began to assimilate his physical treatment (grafts, transfusions, antibiotics, and analgesics) in a healing way. Gradually, he permitted contact with his parents which he had avoided in the first weeks of hospitalization. This paralleled the turnaround from a negative to a positive therapeutic reaction. Of course, one cannot be certain that this parallelism was of etiological significance, since the recovery from burns is a very complex and gradual process.

Face injuries have a very unique meaning. Disfigurement or scars in the face have a continuing impact on the person's personality, often expressed by these patients as "nothing will be as it was." The overall meaning of those injuries seemed to be a fear of *loss of identity*—the preinjury identity. One soldier explained that if people knew him before, they could remember how he looked, how he was, who he was, and who he is. These were among the most common fears associated with the fear of leaving the hospital. Patients seemed to feel that the community is less tolerant of facial disfigurement than it is of any other permanent consequence of war injuries, such as an amputation, for example.

The precautionary advice given to most patients that they should be careful not to expose burned or grafted areas to the direct rays of the sun was a confirmation to many of our patients that they had lost strength and had been permanently changed to their own detriment. They were told further that cautiousness about exposure to the sun should be assumed to be on a permanent basis. For many, this confirmed their fear that they might be blighted permanently.

Hand burns generally evoke fears about not being able to *function* as an adult and independent man; difficulties in hand functioning invariably elicited conflicted feelings about dependency.

The skin is an organ of protection and of appearance. Our observational and projective test materials show that severe burns are experienced as a significant disruption of the body boundaries, a loss in the body's integrity, in which the symbolic and real meanings of the skin as an organ are implied. These reactions throw some light on the special needs a burned person has to feel protected and on the important psychological meanings that skin grafts and donor sites may have for the patient.

From our observations[2] and our clinical and theoretical background we helped the staff to distinguish between the psychological reactions to the acute phase of the burn injuries and treatment, and the more gradual psychological reactions to the postacute phases of treatment and rehabilitation. We introduced the concept that we as doctors, nurses, and others who were part of the medical team were being asked to lend a part of ourselves, our vitality, our interests, and skills until our patients were able to be active in their own behalf—until the immediate, numbing, fearful reactions that depleted these young men were overcome. Theoretically, we were trying to explain how to restore narcissistic supplies. At the beginning we referred to a repeated observation that these injured young men tried, when they could, to use us as mirrors—how did they look as reflected by how we looked at them and reacted to them.

We pointed out that there was no contradiction between the assumption that patients should be enabled to have an appropriate active involvement in their care; and the assumption that in the acute phase of a burn injury regressive behavior is often a necessary preparation for recovery and not a threat to long-term healing and rehabilitation. It became clear that the first manifestations of healthy active involvement may be missed because of its regressive features, as was so dramatically demonstrated by the sarcastic patient, who said his outburst was meant to help the nurse.

The mental health team played a vital role in identifying conflicts and in facilitating a sustained level of communication. The communications were designed to process and work through the

---

[2] Observations were logged daily and discussed whenever possible. Also, questionnaires with checklists were filled out by physicians, nurses, and other rehabilitation personnel; these provided some data about attitudes toward the patients and their care.

inevitable difficulties involved in a multidisciplinary team working together in providing the most sophisticated, technical, scientific, and humane care of each patient.

In this way we could minimize and often avoid the fragmentation of care that is the risk of all teamwork in a hospital setting. This fragmentation, when it occurs, is experienced by the patient as doctors and nurses being inconsistent, and as jeopardizing the patient's recovery because several different people are trying to treat him in several different ways. Necessary discussions by the team in front of patients can be helpful if disagreements are resolved and explained to the patient, and if the patient has the opportunity to ask his doctor or nurse to explain any technical aspect of the discussion or decision that troubled him.

Thus, a psychologically therapeutic environment on a plastic surgery ward for acutely burned young men must meet the needs of the patients and the needs of the physicians, nurses, and other personnel that staff such a hospital community. A patient with severe face and hand burns is helpless; he becomes dependent on an external source to meet his most basic bodily needs. The external source (medical staff in general and nursing staff specifically) then acts in a mothering, nursing way to alleviate the patient's pain and distress.

Simultaneously with wound healing, the patient begins to overcome the first regressive reactions. Gradually he becomes more active and able to take care of his own body. That change elicits resonating responses in the nurses' and doctors' expectations in line with recovery. The nurse, especially, is required to accept and encourage activity and assertiveness even when its manifestations are provocative or distorted. Psychologically, the recovery process in those burned patients proceeds along lines that are similar to every human growth process—from passivity to activity, from narcissistic withdrawal to interest in the external world, from helplessness to mastery.

By a psychologically therapeutic environment we mean the optimal conditions to promote this recovery-growth process. In such an atmosphere regression is accepted—not encouraged—and activity is promoted when the patient indicates his interest in and readiness for becoming active.

In the achievement of such a psychologically therapeutic environment, the mental health team has a vital role. In addition to promoting communication among the different professional groups and helping to work through the difficulties that inevitably arise, the mental health team's ability to formulate and make interpretations tactfully is crucial. Such interpretations are useful when all of the staff understands and accepts the principle that the best physical care is not only consistent with sound psychological care but essential for a psychologically therapeutic environment.

Summary and Conclusions

Our work was organized according to the following principles:

1. Psychological care was designed to insure that sound physical care would also be sound psychological care, i.e., to validate the assumption that psychological considerations are not in conflict with excellent physical, medical, surgical, and nursing care.

2. Sound psychological care requires that each patient be enabled to become mentally and physically active, in an appropriate manner, in understanding and planning the treatment of his condition.

3. Regressive reactions usually are in the service of recovery. They should be expected both during the initial acute phase when the patient is overwhelmed and finds himself physically relatively helpless; and during the recovery phase when regressive irritability often ushers in the patient's first effort at being active on his own behalf.

4. Planning and treatment discussions among professional health care groups and between those in the same professional group must be ongoing and capable of achieving a reasonable working consensus as a requirement for maintaining excellence in the care of patients and in supporting the morale of the patients and the staff.

The application of these psychological principles meant in concrete terms for the patients that—

1. They had the opportunity to express their fears, questions, suggestions, and complaints so that they felt understood.

2. They received appropriate relief of pain, insomnia, and physical discomfort.

3. They knew who their doctor was.

4. They were cared for by a team of physicians, nurses, and other hospital personnel who worked harmoniously with effective communication and understanding about the care of the patients.

5. They were helped to cope with the injury and its treatment in a manner appropriate to each patient's age, cultural, educational, and religious background.

6. Finally, each patient received warm humane care with acceptance of and regard for his own uniquely individual needs.

BIBLIOGRAPHY

BERNSTEIN, N. R., SANGER, S., & FRAS, I. (1969), The Functions of the Child Psychiatrist in the Management of Severely Burned Children. *J. Amer. Acad. Child Psychiat.*, 8:620–637.

DARWIN, C. (1872), *Expression of the Emotions in Man and Animals.* New York: Philosophical Library, 1955.

FREUD, S. (1914), On Narcissism: An Introduction. *S.E.*, 14:72–102.

GALDSTON, R. (1972), The Burning and Healing of Children. *Psychiatry*, 35:57–66.

HAMBURG, D. A., HAMBURG, B., & DEGOZA, S. (1953), Adaptive Problems and Mechanism in Severely Burned Patients. *Psychiatry*, 16:1–20.

LONG, R. T. & COPE, O. (1961), Emotional Problems of Burned Children. *N.E. J. Med.*, 264:1121–1127.

QUINBY, S. & BERNSTEIN, N. R. (1971), Identity Problems and the Adaptation of Nurses to Severely Burned Children. *Amer. J. Psychiat.*, 128:58–63.

SPITZ, R. A. (1965), *The First Year of Life.* New York: Int. Univ. Press.

Addiction and Ego Function

NORMAN E. ZINBERG, M.D.

SLOWLY BUT DEFINITELY THERE IS A GROWING ACCEPTANCE OF THE idea that in order to understand what motivates someone to use illicit drugs and what effect these drugs will have on him, one must take drug, set, and setting into account (Brecher, 1972; *Drug Use in America*, 1973; Edwards, 1973; Khantzian et al., 1974; Weil, 1972; Zinberg and Robertson, 1972; Zinberg and DeLong, 1974). That is, for such understanding the pharmacological action of the drug, how a person approaches the experience, which includes an assessment of his entire personality structure, and the physical and social setting in which the use takes place must all be considered and balanced. A not unusual paradox has begun to develop: the concept of drug effect being a product of these three variables is becoming a commonplace among mental health professionals before the implications of the notion for psychoanalytic theory, in particular, and personality theories, in general, have been worked through (Eddy et al., 1963; Jaffe, 1970; Khantzian, 1974; Wurmser, 1973; Yorke, 1970). Thus, existing misconceptions about a one-to-one relationship between personality maladjustment and drug use and addiction continue unabated.

In this essay, building on the work of several psychoanalytic

---

Dr. Zinberg is a Faculty Member of Harvard Medical School at The Cambridge Hospital and of The Boston Psychoanalytic Institute. The material for this paper was gathered as part of a study of the social basis of drug abuse prevention funded by The Drug Abuse Council, Inc., 1828 L Street, N.W., Washington, D.C. The work of Richard C. Jacobson and Wayne M. Harding on that project was invaluable to this essay.

theorists (Gill and Brenman, 1959; Hartmann, 1939; Klein, 1959; Rapaport, 1958; Zinberg, 1963), especially that of David Rapaport, I shall present clinical studies of compulsive drug use, describe how the users' responses to drugs have changed over time, review Rapaport's positions and show how these apply to the clinical states described, and, finally, discuss the implications of all this for dynamic theory and therapy.

The Influence of Social Setting on Drug Use

Before turning to the clinical studies of compulsive drug use and users, I shall briefly consider the belief that such use almost invariably stems from severe personality maladjustment or from the individual's being overwhelmed by a powerful chemical. It is true that people described as oral dependent (Rado, 1958), unable to tolerate anxiety (Goldstein, 1972) or aggression (Khantzian, 1974; Wurmser, 1973), or borderline schizophrenics (Radford et al., 1972), do use various illicit drugs to help them deal with their painful affects. Their histories reveal that following the discovery of their drug or drugs of choice, a quick and insistent dependence develops. But it is my contention that these people make up only a fraction, and probably a small one, of even the addict population, let alone the general drug-using population. The idea that certain personality types seek out drug experience because of a specific, early, unresolved developmental conflict, and that such people predominate in the addict group or in the much larger group of controlled users, is based on retrospective falsification. That is, looking at drug users and especially addicts, after they have become preoccupied with their drug experience, authorities assume that these attitudes and this personality state are similar to those the user had before the drug experience, and thus led to it. Then "evidence" from the user's developmental history and previous object relationships is marshaled to show that the addicted state was the end point of a long-term personality process.

This is *not* to say that internal factors are not involved in the decision to use drugs, in the effects of the drugs on the individual, on the rapidity and extent of the increase in drug use, and on the addiction itself and its psychological and social concomitants. But it is to say that there are no psychological profiles or consistent patterns of internal conflicts or phase-specific developmental sequences that can be put forward as the determining factor in the history of drug use and addiction.

Yet, this reasoning persists despite our cultural historical experience with alcohol (Chafetz and Demone, 1962). In the eighteenth century this powerful drug was used very much as heroin is today (Harrison, 1964): 75 or 80 percent of drinkers were alcoholics. Today while there may be 6 to 8 million alcoholics, there are 100 million controlled drinkers of every personality type. Our relative control over alcohol stems from the inculcation of social maxims and rituals (Zinberg and Jacobson, 1974a). "Don't start until sundown," "Know your limit," "Don't drink alone" all serve to minimize excess consumption. There is no consistent effort to select out susceptible personality types, and growing evidence suggests that not even those who do become alcoholics represent specific personality types (McCord and McCord, 1960; Wilkinson, 1970). Hence, it is surprising that there continues to be so much emphasis on the personality of the drug user when there is growing evidence of the power of the social setting to sustain controlled use of a powerful drug among many different personality types (Chafetz and Demone, 1962; Powell, 1973; Zinberg and Jacobson, 1974b).

While the bulk of the clinical work to be presented here will be concerned with the compulsive use of heroin, the history of LSD use over the last decade makes a nice beginning. From about 1965 to 1969 both professionals and the public were terrified by occasional and compulsive use of LSD (Smith, 1969; Tarshis, 1972). Mental hospitals such as Bellevue and Massachusetts Mental Health Center reported that 25 to 35 percent of their admissions resulted from bad trips (Brecher, 1972). The general feeling at that time was that even a single dose of LSD could tip someone who was either seriously disturbed or at a particularly vulnerable life moment, while continued, heavy use, according to this view, would inevitably wear away an individual's psychological capacity to function. Statistics which cited these frequent admissions to mental hospitals, along with lurid accounts in the media of suicides, homicides, and generally bizarre behavior, seemed to justify the fears.

With the passage of just a few years the situation looks quite different. McGlothlin and Arnold (1971) studied 256 subjects who had taken a psychedelic drug *before* 1962, that is, before the enormous publicity of the "Leary era" with its incredible hopes for enlightenment and insight, and the anxiety that inevitably accompanies an act believed to be so daring and potentially disappointing. Although McGlothlin and Arnold's subjects acknowledged that taking these drugs was a powerful experience—indeed some of the subjects thought it had deeply affected their lives—there were no bad trips reported of the kind that lead to mental hospitalization. And today when, according to the 1973 Report of the President's Commission on Marihuana and Drug Abuse, psychedelic drug use is the fastest growing drug use in the United States (*Drug Use in America*, 1973), mental hospitals no longer report bad trips as a factor in admissions. As of July 1974 the Massachusetts Mental Health Center did not know when they last had such an admission, but they were sure that it had been years rather than months ago (Grinspoon, 1974).

Clearly, the pattern of use has changed. The individual taking 200 to 250 trips in one year in a furious search for mystic enlightenment has given way to the two- or three-times-a-year tripper who closely follows countercultural maxims designed to minimize anxiety. To "only trip in a good place at a good time with good people" makes sense with a drug which increases certain perceptual responses. The fact is that the same strong drug is used today by an increasingly wide variety of personality types. Thus the evidence indicates that it was the social setting that got out of hand; before those wild years of the 60s and since, users in a calmer social setting could adapt to and tolerate the experience.

Another excellent piece of work offers further support for this position. The Barr et al. study (1972), which gave LSD to subjects before 1962, strongly suggests that one cannot assume that those people ordinarily diagnosed as significantly disturbed react more severely to these drugs than those considered "healthier." This work shows that a typology of responses to the drug can be constructed, but that they would not be directly determined by the degree of emotional disturbance. Thus personality is a factor in the drug response, just as the drug itself produces unquestioned strong effects, but without a careful understanding of the powerful, and in the case of LSD, almost determining, influence of social setting, many authorities could and did misinterpret what happened in the 60s.

Another example of the power of the social setting to determine drug use and, in this case, the development of drug dependency and addiction comes from our sad experience in Vietnam. Hundreds of thousands of American youths found themselves among people who hated them, fighting a terrifying war they neither understood nor approved, with illicit drugs readily available (Wilbur, 1972, 1974; *Washington Post*, 1971). The Army's misunderstanding of marihuana use led to an "educational" campaign against that drug and the enforcement of penalties. Enlisted men quickly found in heroin an odorless, far less bulky replacement which had the unique property of making time seem to disappear. As almost every enlisted man in Vietnam desired nothing so ardently as to have the year to DEROS (Date of Expected Return from Overseas) pass, many thousands used great quantities of that pure, cheap white powder (Zinberg, 1971, 1972a, 1972b). Data from the rehabilitation centers and from camps processing men returning from overseas leave no doubt that a great many of those using heroin were physiologically addicted. Also, final Army data make it possible to say assuredly (despite the Army's early claims that only those who were heavy drug users before service became addicted) that these young men displayed a wide variety of personality types, that they came from diverse social, ethnic, geographic, and religious backgrounds, and that few were drug users before they went to Vietnam (Robins, 1974). When authorities and professionals alike realized the extent of heroin use in Vietnam, consternation and surprise were expressed that such a variety of people who did not conform to addict stereotypes could become addicts, and fear about what would happen in the United States when these people returned dominated most discussions (Wilbur, 1974). These concerns rested on the traditional view that heroin was so powerful a drug that once one was in its thrall there was no escape. Also, the underlying suspicion remained that, despite the evidence of a variety of personality types using the drug, the users were potential drug-dependents who would have been saved in the United States by the lack of availability of heroin.

Studies of returned Vietnam veterans have shown that for a

fraction (under 10 percent) of those who had become drug dependent these fears of continued addiction were realized, but that the vast majority (over 90 percent) gave up heroin upon return to the United States. The determining factor in their heroin use had been the intolerable setting of Vietnam, and once they returned to the United States neither the power of the drug nor a susceptible personality proved to be decisive in keeping them drug dependent (Robins, 1974).

Description of Addicts

The sample of U.S. addicts was obtained from a large detoxification center and two psychological-treatment-oriented methadone clinics. Over a period of 16 months 54 addicts were interviewed for approximately two hours each. They ranged in age from 19 to 34; 35 were male and 14 black. Addicts were chosen solely on the basis of their having applied to the methadone clinic or having gone into the fourth day of detoxification on a day when the investigator had time available. Although each of the addicts studied was as sharply different from the next in presentation and general superficial personality as any other members of the population, a psychodynamic formulation showed them to be remarkably alike in their psychological difficulties.

To begin with, junkies look a lot alike: they are usually thin, their clothing shabby, and their person somewhat unkempt. Initial conversations reveal their almost total preoccupation with heroin or its replacements and the life style that surrounds its compulsive use. Drug effect, drug availability, drug necessity—getting off, copping, hustling—and a concern with the legal, physical, and psychological hazards that go with those interests preoccupy them. As a result of their addiction they see themselves as deviants with little sense of relatedness to the straight world. Their sense of themselves seems to derive from their negative social and psychological responses such as antisocial activities, rebellion, expressed aggression against the "bastards," and from their own victimization. In Erikson's (1959) terms, they depend on a negative identity for a measure of self-esteem and self-definition.

In our conversations the subjects revealed a direct belief in magic, often centering around the drug and its use, but extending to other areas as well. Junkies frequently tell of how their lives have been star-crossed, with ordinary events being given the power to save or destroy. In these stories frank primary process thinking seems available to consciousness. These thoughts come out as distorted ideas: "I knew if my parents told my grandfather about my sister's marriage, it would kill him, and I was the only one who could stop them." "I knew the train would be late that day before I got on it. There was an aura around the whole station." Or they show an indistinct differentiation between objective reality and a fantasy or magical view: "All it takes is for me to get my shit together, then I can handle all that." The defenses of projection, introjection, and denial are consistently prominent, as is repression, which will be considered separately. As their associations tend to be loose anyway, the combination gives an almost bizarre flavor to most interactions: "I never give in. I'm always fighting the dope and those bastards in the clinic gave me the wrong dope. I know that it doesn't work on me in liquid form and they won't help me cut down by getting the pills."

It must be remembered that despite this presentation of themselves junkies are rarely schizophrenic. Vaillant's 12-year follow-up (1966a, 1966b) found few addicts in mental hospitals, and the clinical impressions of other investigators since then support his work. Since the growth of heroin use in the late 60s, undoubtedly more borderline or schizophrenic people have used heroin as an effort at self-medication, but they remain a small minority—which strikes me as remarkable every time I finish another interview, for it is hard to believe that all addicts are not crazy after talking with them.

There is a general conscious deterioration of the superego. Junkies will tell you fairly frankly that they do what they have to do to survive and get drugs. They know that they cannot be trusted to follow the usual rules, ethics, and codes of social behavior. Tales of stealing from and lying to friends and family abound. Usually there is little real acceptance of responsibility. Their anger and blame for all sorts of troubles are reserved for those circumstances or people that spoiled the perfect deal, the neat setup—often authorities in some form. But always the drug is the basic preoccupation. Their readiness to blame those who interfere with their using the drug so that it works magically is unending. The hours given over in methadone clinics to discussing dosage and whether they are getting enough of the drug, in the right form, by the right person, at the right time, in the right way are literally uncountable. These expressions, while they seem paranoid in flavor and content and carry bitterness and conviction, are nonetheless not paranoid in a paranoid schizophrenic way. The addicts permit their ideas to be more or less susceptible to reality testing if the tester is willing to be subtle, forceful, and extremely patient.

And, as one might expect, while the junkies accept their own unwillingness to play by the rules, they deeply and passionately feel that others, particularly authorities, must. In a way there is no paradox here because their primitive unconscious superego never rests. Junkies are not only self-destructive in the sense that they are incredibly accident prone and constantly arranging to be hurt, but they also manage almost never to do well for themselves in the simplest life transactions. They do lose laundry slips and money, choose the wrong alternative at each instance, and are invariably being gypped at the very moment they think they are slyest. These experiences ostensibly result in an increase in blame for "them" and a feeling that the big strong ones, the doctors, counselors, probation officers, should be more helpful to and more responsible for the poor addict; but this position is invariably accompanied by rigorous and overwhelming self-loathing.

As a result they are argumentative, particularly in a methadone clinic, about matters affecting their precious substance, but very ineffectually so. This need to be unpleasant and to set up struggles that are doomed to defeat arises directly from their insistence on putting and keeping themselves in a weak position. But often if one pushes further into the arcane thought processes surrounding each instance of trouble, fantasy fears that have developed into phobias become apparent. For example, a methadone clinic regulation requires a physical examination; two appointments in a row were missed by several patients, putting them in jeopardy of dismissal from the clinic. Careful questioning revealed that a baseless rumor was circulating that anyone who didn't "pass" the physical would be hospitalized, and since addicts' response to hospitals is truly phobic, they didn't show up for the exam. The development of similar overwhelming fears among junkies is quite common and somehow exaggerated when juxtaposed against the superficial tough (but done in) guy/gal image they try to project.

The breakdown in logical thinking, the disorganization of the ordinary cognitive process above and beyond the difficulty in reality testing is so severe that the inexperienced interviewer fails to understand their educational and vocational accomplishments. Their memories, for example, are terrible, and there seems to be no psychodynamic rhyme or reason to the lacunae. Thinking of repression simply as a defense and an aid to denial and projection does not help one to achieve a dynamic formulation. Neither can one rely for an explanation on conscious dissembling. Certainly the interviewer knows that there is much overt lying to hide real or fancied transgressions and to protect secret pockets of potential gratification. But the forgetting of both significant and insignificant life events and activities often acts more to the addict's detriment on his own terms. Hard as it is to imagine, some even forget a stash of drugs, and they easily manage not to remember addresses, appointments, relevant history, and so on, which could help get them a welfare check or other disability assistance. Running through all this cognitive deterioration is a disorientation of the time sense, which may well be related to the drug experience. Heroin seems to "make time go away," and compensating for that experience may be difficult.

Taken overall, then, this study of addicts shows people whose everyday psychological state seems compatible with a diagnosis of borderline schizophrenia or worse, but who are not schizophrenic; whose current ego functions and cognitive capacities make past accomplishments inexplicable, but who are at times remarkably capable and intellectually able; and who, from this dynamic perspective, appear a lot alike. It is easy to understand the temptation to use this sort of material to work out formulations that would "explain" their seeking drugs and drug dependency. It must be remembered, however, that compared to psychoanalysis or intensive dynamic therapy, these interviews are brief and superficial. Further and more intensive interviewing might disclose more subtle and pervasive evidence of early gross family and individual psychiatric impairment. However, within the severe limitations of this study, the families of these patients were described as consistently different from each other. Only four cases presented frank early histories of emotional disturbance, early school difficulty, and the general sense of oddness associated with early borderline schizophrenia or early severe character disorders.[1]

Addiction and Relative Ego Autonomy

Rapaport (1958) delineated the factors that maintain relative ego autonomy. He began by observing that nonliving matter cannot escape the impact of the environment and thus the results of the interaction are invariant and statistically predictable. This is not true of living matter. At times psychoanalytic theory has tried to pretend that inner forces are strong enough to develop some sort of predictability despite the uncounted variables acting through the physical and social environment, but this has not worked out. Using the Berkeleyian and Cartesian positions to develop a dialectic, Rapaport points out that in the Berkeleyian view man is totally independent of the environment and totally dependent on inner forces and drives. He need have little concern for the external world since it is "created" by inherent forces. The cartoon psychiatrist who is shown asking someone who has been hit by a car, "How did you cause this to happen to you?" is an exaggerated clinical version of this position.

Descartes, on the other hand, saw man as a clean slate upon which experience writes. He is totally dependent upon and thus in harmony with the outside world, and totally independent of, autonomous from, internal desires. In essence, Cartesians, like behaviorists, view such drives and the unconscious supposedly

---

[1] There is some further preliminary evidence that tends to point in the same direction but stems from interviews that were even more cursory, done by social workers and with a different intent. Within this sample, 30 families were interviewed by a social worker to decide upon admission to a methadone clinic. Although there were great differences in the family structure and the degrees of difficulty within the family, the workers found that only two of the families thought that the principal disturbances between the addict subjects and their significant others began before serious drug use.

containing them as nonexistent. This may well account for the failure of learning machines. Human conflicts over success and failure turned out to be more dominant than the desire for M&Ms.

Rapaport reasons that neither of these totally divergent positions speaks to man's experience: that to understand how the ego, whose functions determine and delineate a sense of self, remains relatively autonomous and copes with the demands of the external environment and of the basic, inborn forces Freud termed "instinctual drives" requires consideration of both and their interactions. The autonomy Rapaport postulated is always relative, and the inside drives and the outside environment carefully balance each other. Drives prevent man from becoming a stimulus-response slave,[2] while the constant stream of stimulus nutriment from the environment mediates and moderates the primitive drives[3] by sustaining primary ego apparatuses such as motor capacity, thinking, memory, perceptual and discharge thresholds, and the capacity for logical communication. In addition, external reality nurtures those secondary ego apparatuses—such as competence, cognitive organization, values, ideals, and a mature conscience, determined by each particular culture as adaptive—and allows these characteristics to become successfully estranged from original drive functions.

Thus the relationship between the ego's relative autonomy from the id and the ego's relative autonomy from the environment is one of interdependence. When drives are at peak tension, as in puberty, the ego's autonomy from the id is in jeopardy. Adolescents try to combat their tendency to subjectivity, seclusiveness, and rebellion by the external reality-related converse of these—intellectualization, distance from primary objects, and efforts at total companionship. But it is an unequal and often painful struggle.

---

[2] Rapaport tells the story of the man who did not march in step to an enthralling military band because he was pondering, and points out how falling in love saved Orwell's Protagonist of *1984*, at least temporarily, from the press of that overwhelming environment.

[3] Here, Rapaport uses the story of Moses and the great king who had been told by his seers and phrenologist that Moses was cruel, vain, and greedy. Upon finding Moses gentle, wise, and compassionate, the king planned to put his wise men to death. Moses demurred, saying, "They saw truly what I am. What they could not see was what I have made of it."

The ego's autonomy from the id can also be disrupted by minimizing the balancing input from external reality. Experiments with stimulus deprivation (Bexton et al., 1954; Heron et al., 1953, 1956; Lilly, 1956) showed how susceptible individuals became autistic and suffered from magical fantasies, disordered thought sequences, disturbed reality testing, primitive defenses, and poor memory under such conditions.

Similarly, conditions which permit only restricted and frightening forms of stimulus nutriment impair the ego's relative autonomy from the external environment. When, as in a concentration camp, external conditions maximize the individual's sense of danger and arouse fears and neediness, the drives no longer act as guarantors of autonomy from the environment but prompt surrender. The deprivation of varied stimulus nutriment and its replacement by insistent streams of instructions in the stimulus-deprivation experiments gave those instructions power and engendered belief. In order to maintain a sense of separate identity, values, ideologies, and orderly thought structures, people require support for existing verbal and memory structures. Not surprisingly, Rapaport used George Orwell's *1984* as a text—one which described in exact and clinical detail how this interdependence functioned under environmental conditions intended to turn the individual into a stimulus-response slave.

Throughout his discussion Rapaport insists that the superego in particular is dependent on consistent stimulus nutriment. The convention, or American Legionnaire, syndrome—when moderate, respectable men and women remove themselves from their usual routines and social relationships and behave in an impulsive and uncontrolled manner—makes it very clear how heavily the strictures of conscience depend on social structure.

The junkies described earlier have lost varied sources of stimulus nutriment. Families have been alienated and previous social relationships severed; or, if contact remains, it consists usually of acrimonious or pleading discussions about giving up drugs. Addicts are declared deviant by the larger society and are referred to as an epidemic, a plague, and the "number one problem" of the country. The social input available to them is thus either a negative view of themselves or the ceaseless patter of their compulsive drug-using groups. Have you copped? When? Where? Was it good? What do I need to cop? What if I can't? Who got busted? Will I get busted? These are conditions, albeit self-arranged, which meet the conditions of stimulus-deprivation experiments. At the same time the addict's desire for gratification from the drug itself, and the memory of the result, a withdrawal syndrome, if the drug is unavailable, keeps drive structures at peak tension.

According to Rapaport's formulation, a regressive state should develop when the ego is unable to maintain its relative autonomy from either the id or the external environment. In such a state the barriers differentiating ego and id processes become fluid. Images, ideas, and fantasies based on primary process thinking rise to consciousness, and there develops a reliance on more and more primitive defenses. The sense of voluntariness and of having inner control of one's actions in relation to oneself and to the external environment disappears. Is that not exactly what I have described as the general clinical picture of the junkie?

The necessity to cop, which excessively increases the addict's dependence on the environment, impairs his ego's autonomy from the id. At the same time, being labeled deviant decreases varied contacts with the usual environmental supports and thus also impairs his ego's autonomy from the id. The addicts' efforts to continue some coherent relationships with whatever objects are left to them make them dependent on external cues. They suffer constantly from doubts about their ability to maintain such relationships, and they cling to stereotyped views of themselves. This clinging to what remains of the external environment maximizes the ego's autonomy from the id, but at the cost of minimizing the conscious input of and trust in affective and ideational signals that usually regulate judgment and decision—that is, at the cost of impairing the ego's autonomy from the environment.

Thus the addicts' relative autonomy from both id and external environment is impaired. They are isolated from their own useful emotions and those views of the world which permit a coherent and integrated sense of self. They are at the mercy of primitive impulses and an overwhelming sense of neediness that invades, or more nearly blocks out, a capacity to perceive and integrate "objective" reality. Filled with doubts, they gullibly respond to those in the external environment who offer schemes or promises that might bring magical succor.

As a result of these impaired autonomies the ego must make do with insufficient or distorted input from both id and external environment. The ego must modify its structures to conform to this new, more restricted, and primitive pattern. It is my clinical impression that the addict's ego fights to retain whatever level of ego functioning can be saved. It is this very struggle to retain some measure of ego functions which is a principal source of the rigidity that therapists working with the addicts, in and out of methadone clinics, find so trying. As long as addicts are classified by the larger culture as deviants, it is hard to imagine that they can see themselves as anything else. And as long as their relationships with the external world continue to supply only restricted stimulus nutriment, the blocking of most affective input not oriented to direct gratification *probably* will continue. Whatever new ego homeostasis the individual has achieved, is likely to be rigid and to have a slow rate of change. When threatened, as these people's egos constantly are, by changeable but insistent demands for gratification from drive structures, the new homeostasis of ego functioning cannot easily integrate fresh stimulus nutriment, not even input that is as neutral and sustaining as a therapeutic relationship. Or perhaps it would be more accurate to say: *particularly* the input of a therapeutic relationship because these interactions are *intended* to be at variance with the addicts' usual interpersonal interactions and to make their usual reliance on selective perception, quick repression, projection, and denial more difficult.

There are two other points which stress the importance of the social setting. In showing how the labeling of the addict as a deviant becomes a key factor in impairing his relative ego autonomy I described the extent to which primary process ideation such as interest in magic, belief in animism, generalized unfounded suspiciousness, and acceptance of extremely childish rhetoric become regressively active in regular ego functioning. Junkies often seem to me to be vaguely aware of their own primitive response. But they cannot integrate such thinking sufficiently to make it part of a conscious way of questioning the world, i.e., secondary process, first because the primitive feelings much of the time seem so real. A second interrelated issue is the unconscious effort to retain existing capacity to function no matter how unsatisfactory. In the 60s users of LSD had a similar problem. They too regarded their "trip" as exceptional and at that point found few points of reference between the trip experience and their previous social and psychological experiences. But by the 70s, as a recent study contends (Zinberg, 1974), occasional psychedelic drug users have the same unusual psychic experiences that their counterparts of the 60s had. However, the accumulated and widely dispersed knowledge about the experience prepared them for it. They think about their experiences and discuss them with friends in order to separate out drug effect from essential and usual self-perspectives. Thus the experience is secondary process oriented.

PROSPECTIVE STUDY OF ADDICTION

In 1967–68 I engaged in a large-scale interviewing process to select candidates for a controlled experiment giving marihuana to human subjects (Zinberg and Weil, 1970). Three of those interviewed but not selected for the experiment, who had not used heroin at that time, have gone on to become compulsive heroin users. One is included in the sample of 54 described above, and I have had some lengthy conversations with the other two. They are reluctant to be followed, so I cannot make a full report. Suffice it to say that although all three had many individual quirks and peculiarities in 1967, none was at all like the prototypical junkie then and all three are now. In 1967 the man included in the present sample was rebellious and active in radical politics, intensely intellectual, harshly self-searching, with high standards for himself and others. He had a wide circle of friends and acquaintances which was beginning to narrow at the time I knew him as a result of political disagreements. Nevertheless, his sense of objective reality was not in doubt, his memory was excellent, and his capacity for logical thinking was of the highest order. At that time he had begun to be estranged from his parents, particularly his father, although they too were committed to the political left, and their disagreement was more on method than principle. Previously, despite a lifetime of arguing and concern about economic instability, their relationship had been an enduring one, and he had been quite close to two of his three siblings.

In 1973, while being detoxified for the third time, he had not seen or heard from a family member in over two years. His thought processes were slow and jumpy, and his associations loose. Although he remembered me, he had difficulty in sticking to the subject of the interview, wandering to questions about my hospital function, his medications, and his chances of recovering. When he returned to the subject, his memory was poor, his recall distorted, and his acceptance of responsibility for himself *nil.* At that moment he was on probation for two offenses and had another charge of possession with intent to sell narcotics pending. He gave every evidence of being an impulsive, poorly controlled person. Physically it was hard to recognize him as the same man, and he too said, "I'm not the same person you talked to then."

Both here and in England I have interviewed (Zinberg and Robertson, 1972) many heroin addicts of up to 30 years' standing who showed no emotional or intellectual deterioration. Hence, I do not believe the drug itself was responsible for this man's deterioration, nor can I, on the basis of my previous knowledge of this man, accept the explanation of preexisting addictive personality. I do not at this writing understand what pushed him into addiction. He claims it was fortuity. Following many severe political disappointments and a marked reduction in his social group, he found himself with people whose regular polydrug use, including heroin, was far heavier than his previous standard. They were heavy users of downers (barbiturates), which he had never liked. When they took downers, he used heroin. After a year and a half of chipping (occasional use), he woke up one morning after not using and recognized that the severe stomach cramps, gooseflesh, and sweating meant that he was strung out. He made many efforts to kick, but after that it was essentially downhill all the way.

No doubt somewhere in his psyche the conflicts concerning responsibility, self-sufficiency, and rebellion existed in 1967. But as Freud (1937) argues so persuasively, latent conflicts of all sorts may exist, but whether they will ever become manifest is determined by the subject's life experiences. It is my impression—and I hope to be able to study these three men more thoroughly—that just as with the Vietnam heroin users, it was the changed social setting that was instrumental in impairing their relative ego autonomy.

Treatment of Addicts

Mental health workers of all sorts in methadone clinics, detoxification centers, and the like, already have discovered that therapy must be oriented around current reality. Basically it is important for the therapist to point out again and again what his job is. He wants to work with addicts in ways that will help them to find out how their heads work and how they consistently manage to do the worst for themselves. The therapist is friendly, but he is not there to love them, and anyway his love has no special magical healing property. Neither is he a boss, a job counselor, a dispenser of drugs, or the arbiter of dose increases; he has no prescriptions for living with or without drugs. What stops the addicts from using him appropriately, from trying to make sense of what is going on in their lives? How is it that they want him to be anything but a therapist and want so much to bamboozle, provoke, or seduce him? These are the sorts of questions the therapists find themselves asking.

They are keenly aware of the disappointments, deprivations, and social and psychological isolation of a junkie's life, just as therapists are aware of the high excitement to be found in hustling, copping, and shooting up, compared with which a straight life is seen as a conscience-oriented gray straitjacket, and they try to convey their ability to understand this conflict. Therapists point out how the longings for authoritarianism and the clear-cut concepts of what's right and wrong, at least for others, are based on the junkies' lost trust in their own controls, judgment, and awareness of their own wishes. In effect, the therapy aims at understanding how those ego functions which operate do so; how those that might don't; and what makes such ego functioning difficult; also, how the primitive unconscious superego is active but not helpful. The therapy further intends to show how the remaining ego capacity which at times attempts realistically to modify and moderate behavior is ignored.

This therapeutic approach is well known and intended to help restore the lost relative ego autonomy by using the therapist, clinic, and hospital as a source of fresh, diverse stimulus nutriment. These significant social relationships also act to help the subject's embattled ego be less fearful of his drives. Usually, the theory of technique lags behind the formation of a general theory even if individual practitioners learn how to use theoretical concepts intuitively. This essay is intended to add an understanding of what happens to the ego as a result of the changed social condition of the addict and of how this theoretical position can be extended into technique. Hence, if this theoretical view of the patient's problems is accepted, a therapist would not often or forcefully interpret projection or confront denial. It would be useless and actually psychonoxious to point out that the junkie's feeling that the staff of a clinic is hostile and wants to degrade and deprecate him stems from his own destructive preoccupations with himself and others. Rather the staff members consistently explain what they are there for and ask what troubles the addict about their function; that is, therapists provide him with constant, gentle reaffirmation of reality and show how unnecessary much of his difficulty with it is. Thus, the need for the projection and denial becomes less urgent.

Although some discussion of the addict's past and of his or her family relationships may have occasional usefulness, generally speaking this area is of less interest when working with the addict group than in more usual dynamic therapies. For one thing, such discussions often turn into an interest in the motives and interrelationships that may have led the addict to drug use and drug dependency, and this, if the formulations derived in this paper are accurate, is a fruitless area. At least, when one considers the complexity of drug, set, and setting interactions, it is not one that can be worked on until the addict is in better psychological condition. Incidentally, a further complication with most of the 54 addicts studied—and this is again part of the social setting—is that they are "treatment wise." Almost all of them have had experiences in concept houses and with confrontation groups of all sorts. Although they have rarely followed through with these programs, they have developed a patter about what they are feeling and why they are the way they are that serves as armor against reasonable conversation. A therapist following the theory of technique offered here, rather than showing interest in the motivation for drug use and being drawn into discussions of dependency, neediness, anxiety, aggression, and aspects of early development and early family life, would allow that the addict might have had to do many things *then* but could *now* stop and recognize that this or that action might not be as necessary as he experiences it.

It is around therapeutic interactions such as these that this theory of technique becomes important. At times, dynamic therapists who know that they must work toward reestablishing relative ego autonomy and relieving the pressure of the archaic superego feel that unless they uncover and help the patients understand the initial motivations for the behavior, they are not doing their job. When therapists have a concern that they must do both, it creates a duality in the therapy. With people as embattled and desperate as the addicts, it is a subtle and difficult therapeutic problem to remain constant in outlining the therapeutic context and the reduced fields of relationship both to drive structures and to the external environment. Bringing in long-term motivational conflicts is seductive. Maintaining the awareness that such clarifications are both too confusing to the addicts and too frustrating for the therapist is very difficult. The therapist should remember that junkies do not do well for themselves, and the higher the therapeutic hopes of the therapist, if they are excessive, the greater the disappointment. It is no accident that from Synanon on many "therapies" for junkies involved punishing, authoritarian regimens. Most addicts are provocative. They ask to be contained in a way that could easily be translated into a wish to be punished. It is my impression that, whether the addict asks for punishment or not, fulfilling such a wish sets up a vicious cycle. Punishment is followed by a sense of entitlement, followed by guilt, followed by a fresh, unconscious desire to be punished. A therapy that questions the current premises of the addict's behavior and indicates that he has choices and has to accept responsibility for them is containing and limit-setting; and if it is carried out with respect for the dignity of the patient and a precise understanding of his premises, it is neither punishing nor gimmicky.

To sustain such a therapy requires an awareness of the crucial role of the social setting in the current ego state of the addict. And for many professionals that means a shift in their assessment of what has happened to the individual who has become drug dependent.

Without that shift the tendency to focus on motivations and unconscious conflicts which could have led to the dependency would be well-nigh irresistible. These factors remain important, as set is as integral a variable as setting, but personality conflict is no longer seen as *the* direct cause of the addict's deterioration.

BIBLIOGRAPHY

Brecher, E. M. & Editors of Consumer Reports (1972), *Licit and Illicit Drugs.* Boston: Little Brown.
Barr, H. L., Langs, R. J., Hall, R. R. et al. (1972), *LSD: Personality and Experience.* New York: Wiley Interscience.
Bexton, W. H., Heron, W., & Scott, T. H. (1954), Effects of Decreased Variation in the Sensory Environment. *Canad. J. Psychol.*, 8:70–76.
Chafetz, M. E. & Demone, H. W., Jr. (1962), *Alcoholism and Society.* New York: Oxford Univ. Press.
Drug Use in America: Problem in Perspective (1973). Second Report of the National Commission on Marihuana and Drug Abuse. Washington, D.C.: U.S. Government Printing Office.
Eddy, N. B., Halbach, H., Isbell, H. et al. (1963), Drug Dependence. *Bull. W.H.O.* 2:721–733.
Edwards, G. (1973), *The Plasticity of Human Response.* London: Maudsley Hospital (mimeograph).
Erikson, E. H. (1959), *Identity and the Life Cycle* [*Psychol. Issues*, Monogr. 1]. New York: Int. Univ. Press.
Freud, S. (1937), Analysis Terminable and Interminable. *S.E.*, 23:209–253.
Gill, M. M. & Brenman, M. (1959), *Hypnosis and Related States.* New York: Int. Univ. Press.
Goldstein, A. 1972), Heroin Addiction and the Role of Methadone in Its Treatment. *Arch. Gen. Psychiat.*, 26:291–298.
Grinspoon, L. (1974), Personal communication.
Harrison, B. (1964), *English Drinking in the Eighteenth Century.* New York/London: Oxford Univ. Press.
Hartmann, H. (1939), *Ego Psychology and the Problem of Adaptation.* New York: Int. Univ. Press, 1958.
Heron, W., Bexton, W. H., & Hebb, D. O. (1953), Cognitive Effects of a Decreased Variation in the Sensory Environment. *Amer. Psychologist*, 8:366–372.
——— Doone, B. K., & Scott, T. H. (1956), Visual Disturbances After Prolonged Perceptual Isolation. *Canad. J. Psychol.*, 10:13–18.
Jaffe, J. H. (1970), Drug Addiction and Drug Abuse. In: *The Pharmacological Bases of Therapeutics*, ed. L. S. Goodman & A. Gilman. New York: Macmillan.
Khantzian, E. J. (1974), Opiate Addiction. *Amer. J. Psychother.*, 28:59–70.

——— Mack, J. E., & Schatzberg, A. F. (1974), Heroin Use as an Attempt to Cope. *Amer. J. Psychiat.*, 131:160–164.

Klein, G. S. (1959), Consciousness in Psychoanalytic Theory. *J. Amer. Psychoanal. Assn.*, 7:5–34.

Lilly, J. C. (1956), Mental Effects of Reduction of Ordinary Levels of Visual Stimuli on Intact Healthy Persons. *Psychiat. Res. Rep.*, 5:1–9.

McCord, J. & McCord, W. (1960), *Origins of Alcoholism*. Stanford: Stanford Univ. Press.

McGlothlin, W. H. & Arnold, D. O. (1971), LSD Revisited. *Arch. Gen. Psychiat.*, 24:35–49.

Orwell, G. (1949), *1984*. New York: Harcourt Brace.

Powell, D. H. (1973), Occasional Heroin Users. *Arch. Gen. Psychiat.*, 28:586–594.

Radford, P., Wiseberg, S., & Yorke, C. (1972), A Study of "Main-Line" Heroin Addiction. *This Annual*, 27:156–180.

Rado, S. (1958), Narcotic Bondage. In: *Problems of Addiction and Habituation*, ed. P. H. Hoch & J. Zubin. New York: Grune & Stratton, pp. 27–36.

Rapaport, D. (1958), The Theory of Ego Autonomy. In: *The Collected Papers of David Rapaport*, ed. M. M. Gill. New York: Basic Books, 1967, pp. 722–744.

Robins, L. (1974), A Followup Study of Vietnam Veterans' Drug Use. *J. Drug Issues*, 4:62–81.

Smith, D. E. (1969), Lysergic Acid Diethylamide. *J. Psychedel. Drugs*, 1:3–7.

Tarshis, M. S. (1972), *The LSD Controversy*. Springfield, Ill.: Thomas.

Vaillant, G. E. (1966a), A 12-Year Follow-up of New York Narcotic Addicts: I. *Amer. J. Psychiat.*, 122:727–737.

——— (1966b), A 12-Year Followup of New York Narcotic Addicts: III. *Arch. Gen. Psychiat.*, 15:599–609.

Washington Post (1971), The U.S. Army: Battle for Survival, 8-part Series, September 12–20.

Weil, A. T. (1972), *The Natural Mind*. New York: Houghton Mifflin.

Wilbur, R. S. (1972), How to Stamp Out a Heroin Epidemic. *Today's Health*, July, pp. 9–13.

——— (1974), The Battle Against Drug Dependency within the Military. *J. Drug Issues*, 4:27–33.

Wilkinson, R. (1970), *The Prevention of Drinking Problems*. New York: Oxford Univ. Press.

Wurmser, L. (1973), Psychoanalytic Considerations of the Etiology of Compulsive Drug Use. Presented at the 60th Annual Meeting of the American Psychoanalytic Association, Honolulu, Hawaii.

Yorke, C. (1970), A Critical Review of Some Psychoanalytic Literature on Drug Addiction. *Brit. J. Med. Psychol.*, 43:141–159.

Zinberg, N. E. (1963), The Relationship of Regressive Phenomena to the Aging Process. In: *The Normal Psychology of the Aging Process*, ed. N. E. Zinberg & I. Kaufman. New York: Int. Univ. Press.

——— (1971), GI's and OJ's in Vietnam. *N.Y. Times Mag.*, December 5.

——— (1972a), Heroin Use in Vietnam and the United States. *Arch. Gen. Psychiat.*, 26:486–488.
——— (1972b), Rehabilitation of Heroin Users in Vietnam. *Contemp. Drug Prob.*, 1:263–294.
——— (1974), *"High" States.* Washington, D.C.: Drug Abuse Council Special Studies Series, SS-3.
——— & DELONG, J. V. (1974), Research and the Drug Issue. *Contemp. Drug Prob.*, 3:71–100.
——— & JACOBSON, R. C. (1974a), The Social Basis of Drug Abuse Prevention (unpublished).
——— ——— (1974b), The Natural History of Chipping (unpublished).
——— & ROBERTSON, J. A. (1972), *Drugs and the Public.* New York: Simon & Schuster.
——— & WEIL, A. T. (1970), A Comparison of Marihuana Users and Non-Users. *Nature*, 226:719–723.

The Fall of Man

K. R. EISSLER, M.D.

ACCORDING TO THE OLD TESTAMENT, MAN WAS DESTINED TO LIVE A happy, carefree life in the Garden of Eden, unencumbered by the need to fight for survival and the fearful prospect of death. His disobedience to the Lord, symbolized by the quest for knowledge, resulted in his forfeiting an existence that would have been regulated by the pleasure principle.

There are few who believe in the accuracy of this myth, but it often happens that a myth contains a kernel of truth that is in harmony with later discoveries of science. I believe that this is the case with regard to the myth of the fall of man. Indeed, there can be hardly any doubt regarding the second part of the myth. Man's history is an unending chain of suffering leading finally to the present, in which the whole of mankind seems threatened with annihilation. An anguished mood of desperation has settled over the whole world, and the most illustrious minds have worked out schemes intended to protect us at the last moment against impending catastrophes of whose existence everyone is aware. Yet the various programs of action that have been submitted in great number deserve to be received with considerable skepticism. Even if one disregards the want of agreement among experts and the not so infrequent incompatibility of measures that seem necessary to combat each single fatal danger confronting mankind, one is compelled to record that the structural changes necessary to carry out even only one of the suggested proposals, not to speak of an entire assemblage of schemes, exceed by far what can be reasonably

---

Extended version of the 1974 Brill Lecture of the New York Psychoanalytic Society, given on November 27, 1974 at the New York Academy of Medicine.

expected from societies as they are. Almost every single suggested plan presupposes a mankind whose actions are directed by reason and not tied down by traditions, a mankind ready to bear sacrifices for the benefit of the next or subsequent generations. One must observe with regret that the projects suggested by experts, even if correct, are hopelessly illusory if judged on the basis of the probability that they can be brought to fruition. Consequently, no course of action has been set forth that would gain general approval and promise to unite mankind in a final effort to dispel the darkness that fills every prospect of the future. It seems that such a scheme is beyond the realm of possibility and that mankind's future is doomed.

The present crisis does not surprise the student of Freud's works. In *Civilization and Its Discontents* Freud raised a warning voice, pointing to what seems to be an incompatibility between man's nature and his culture. Many factors, according to Freud, impede man's development into a reality- and culture-adjusted being who would use culture for mankind's general welfare: his aggression, his feeling of guilt, his prolonged childhood and dependence on parents, the prohibition of incest, and the oedipal conflict. The importance and universality of this assemblage of factors have been confirmed repeatedly. Accordingly, I wish to raise the question of whether a deeper, biological basis underlies it.

It has often been said—and I believe rightly—that in order to map what course mankind's history is to follow, one must take into consideration and thoroughly understand organic evolution, which took its inception probably about two billion years ago, and the biocultural evolution of *Homo sapiens,* which began about 200,000 years ago. In studying the matrix out of which man arose, the inorganic layer is usually taken for granted. A meaningful connection between the structure of the inorganic and the structure of the psyche has not been established. Yet it is most impressive that the universe—and therefore, of course, man's existence as well—is based on the fact that for many billions of years electron clouds have been incessantly swinging around atomic nuclei. Biologists are well aware that life as it is known to us rests on surprisingly subtle details of atomic structure. Thus the polarity of water molecules has a bearing on the functioning of cell membranes; the hydrogen bonds on biological systems; the stability of living things in general is guaranteed by the large energy gap between the lowest energy level and the next highest level in atoms and molecules.

Notwithstanding the scientific, that is, explanatory, value of facts of this order, consideration of them does not seem to be necessary for an understanding of man's psyche, except in relation to one distinctive feature of the inorganic layer, the significance of which can hardly be overrated. I refer to the principle of invariance, which is applicable wherever the inorganic is met. The physicist can be certain that the observation he makes with regard to the behavior of an electron in a Geissler tube is valid for all electrons. He does not need to consider the individual electron. Which particular electron it is of the billions that come to his attention is of no consequence, for what is true of one electron is true of all others. The identity of the elements throughout the physical universe is so strictly enforced that the physicist can be dead sure that the spectral lines of light coming from stars a billion light years away prove the existence of atoms identical to those of this planet.

It is possible that isotopes, that is, elements that are identical in chemical behavior but different in nuclear structure, may in rudimentary fashion reflect another principle, whose full-fledged operation can be observed on the organic level. This principle, of course, is that of variation, or variance. At the risk of stating the obvious, the advent of this principle on the organic level is of fundamental importance in making evolution possible. Indeed, one may view evolution as a gigantic struggle between two opposing principles, that of invariant repetition and that of variance or variation. Fascinating as the intricacy of reproduction and inheritance that follow the principle of invariance may be, the real and quite surprising innovation on the organismic level is, however, variance. Handler (1970, p. 165) writes: "The unique attribute of living matter . . . is its capacity for self-duplication with mutation. . . . Reproduction by itself is not a sufficient criterion of life. Many nonliving systems are self-propagating."

With the origin of life we observe almost identical behavior of the most primitive cells, but the electron microscope reveals that the accumulation of such huge numbers of molecules as are gathered in the most primitive organisms does not lead to an identity of structure as rigid as that observed in chemical elements. The individual differences are small and irrelevant to the resulting behavior, but it is noteworthy that with the origin of life the rigid identity of structure is no longer maintained.

When one compares the electron-microscopic features of two protozoons of the same species or even two cells produced by the division of one parent cell, one finds that some parts of the cells are arranged differently so that the distances between given parts are not necessarily exactly the same from cell to cell. It is, for example, not probable that both cells have the same number of molecules. The differences, however, are not so great that they would have a relevant effect on the behavior of these cells. Thus, one finds approximate identity of behavior despite differences of structure.[1] To be sure, a rigid identity of structure is not incompatible with organismal life, but this rigidity is found on the cellular level. "Rotifers and gastrotrichs are 'cell constant.' Each member of a given species is composed of exactly the same number of cells; even each part of the body is made of a precisely fixed number of cells arranged in a characteristic pattern" (Villee, 1967, p. 268). Sometimes a remarkable uniformity is found in the internal structure of organs. Thus flagella of eucaryotic but not procaryotic cells, whether occurring on unicellular or multicellular organisms or on male reproductive cells, invariably contain eleven groups of tubular fibrils in their matrix, nine of which are arranged peripherally and two in the center (Keeton, 1967, p. 76).

The structure of organisms made possible variation of a kind essentially alien to the inorganic level of existence. This new capability of variance that arose with organic life depends on an evolutionary innovation of fundamental importance. The most primitive organisms possess a structural element that is significant in all later organisms: a separation from the environment. The organism is not open toward the environment; there is a membrane which makes it possible to ascribe an inner life to the cell, even at the earliest stages of organic evolution. This factor of inwardness, internality, or insidedness is a fundamental characteristic of life. To

---

[1] Cf. Portmann (1966, p. 422): "The simplest organisms have no individuality in the strict sense of the word."

be sure, the atom has an inside and an outside. But it is not separated from its surrounding in the same way as the cell is. The atom is self-sufficient and does not need support from the outside to survive, even though it, too, will die one day; its electrons will be separated from the nucleus and it will become part of a dead star.

The other evolutionary innovation was the division of the cell into cytoplasm and nucleus, the latter in turn separated by a membrane in eucaryotic cells. The nucleus adhered to a strictly conservative policy and made the stupendous repetition we recognize in nature possible. "*Limulus,* the King-crab of the seashore, is still identical with its ancestor found in the fossils of the Secondary geological era: during all this time the programme has not varied, each generation punctually fulfilling its task of exactly reproducing the programme for the following generation," writes Jacob (1970, p. 5). And yet variation was possible—despite this basic invariance.

These innovations constitute advances of such magnitude that no subsequent evolutionary changes can be considered comparable. The innovations could not have been predicted from a knowledge of the physics and chemistry of the molecules involved, and to this day we have only the slightest idea of how these evolutionary leaps came about.

This structural differentiation admitted the possibility of a systematic basis for variation, and in turn regulated variance became possible. The resulting arrangement tended to favor invariance: the nucleus, in elaborating a genetic structure in which could be encoded the characteristics of the cell, was conservative in that for the most part it programmed daughter cells to be identical. But mutation, or chance variation in the replicated genetic structure, and sexual reproduction made possible variation in the characteristics of the progeny.

Most mutations give rise to nonviable organisms, and only few mutations lead to a new progress that is conveyed to subsequent generations. What determines whether a mutation will become a permanent enrichment of the biosphere is its fitness. The principle of selection dominates organic evolution: what is unfit to live is eliminated. According to present views, inheritance, mutation, and selection constitute the cornerstone upon which the evolution from the Protozoa to the Mammalia was founded. Thus biological evolution is the result of a gigantic experiment that cannot be repeated in a laboratory. Hundreds, well-nigh thousands of variables are simultaneously at work in this experiment, which monotonously leads to the same result: what is fit survives and propagates, whereas what is unfit perishes.

The use of the standard of quantity of organisms reproduced as the test of evolutionary fitness leads, I must note, to an enigma. According to this definition, bacteria, the most primitive organisms of which we know, are the fittest. There is no species that can compete with the propagative potential and actual performance of procaryotic organisms. Omnipresent throughout the biosphere (Stainer et al., p. 687), they are of incomparable adaptability to the simplest as well as the most extreme environmental conditions. No other group of organisms can compete with them in toughness. Are this incredible resistance to most unfavorable environmental conditions and the prodigious rate of reproduction due to their primitiveness, the absence of a separate nucleus, and the scarceness of membranes in their internal structures (the surface membrane being well protected by a dense wall)?

If primitive organisms have the highest degree of evolutionary fitness, why did evolution lead to the formation of organisms that are vulnerable and less fit to reproduce? There can be hardly any doubt that whatever will be the future of our planet, bacteria will still be propagating at a time when *Homo sapiens* will have been extinguished.

Since the human mind is inclined to ask for purposes, even in areas where no purpose may be extant, the question of the meaning of the circle from bacterium to bacterium can hardly be avoided. From this viewpoint organic evolution may appear like a detour that caused senseless pain and anguish and senselessly wasted efforts.

Be that as it may, organic life, which at the time of its inception had minimal chances of persisting in the face of formidable life-inimical physical forces, was well served by inheritance, mutation, and selection. The biosphere extended, filled all available niches, and became so deeply entrenched on this planet that it seemed almost ineradicable.

The world before the advent of man may be called the best

possible world, even though it was by no means a world of harmony. Each living organism had to die, but no single one ever knew of its impending dissolution. Much anguish and pain pervaded this world; many organisms were killed and devoured, serving as sustenance for other species. But that world was one in which a huge number of species lived and grew together, without ever threatening the biosphere and the evolution of differentiated forms—even though a large number of species, and even eight phyla (Simpson, 1967), were extinguished. It was a cosmos marked not by uniformity but by differentiated forms that promised to develop into still more highly differentiated organisms.

Was the kingdom of animals wiser than man? How was it possible that organisms of entirely different structures and living habits, competing with one another for survival, could get along at all, let alone without causing turmoil and chaos? The answer is that animal behavior is severely limited in its freedom. The behavior of even the highest, most differentiated animals has been governed by built-in mechanisms that reduce possible modes of behavior to a very few. Without considering more archaic regulatory principles, one may say that animal behavior is organized by instincts. The regularity of behavior assigned to each species by its instinctual nature was a necessary condition for the effective operation of behavior; organic evolution, and the relative balance which is observed in the world of organisms, would not have been possible otherwise.

Luria (1973, p. 73) emphasizes that natural selection does not work on genes but on organisms. I suggest that selection works on behavior. If there were not regularity of behavior in animals' conduct, selection would never have been able to attain the stupendous results of differentiation.

When I speak of instincts, I step, as is known, into a hornet's nest, since researchers of animal behavior are divided into two camps. Karl Lorenz is the best representative of a school that ascribes to instinct a major role in vertebrate behavior, whereas Ashley Montagu is the most passionate spokesman of the environmentalist school, to which almost all leading animal psychologists in this country belong. It is superfluous in this context to comment on the ongoing discussion. When I use the term "instinct" here, it is not in the sense in which the environmentalists use it. To my way of thinking, instinct and learning do not exclude each other, although there are instincts that are so deeply rooted that they are not subject to any kind of learning.

We know that the state of regulated variance that dominated organic evolution was rudely ended with anthropogenesis, when organic evolution switched to cultural evolution, which is regulated by essentially different principles. A simple consideration will illustrate this difference: Luria (1973, p. 16) says that "The best educated and most superbly conditioned individual, if he dies childless, is evolutionarily a failure," and yet a childless Socrates had more effect on the human race than a royal Bourbon who allegedly begot 300 children.

Before I delineate the differences between organic and cultural evolution, it is necessary to seek out the fundamental evolutionary innovation which differentiates the structure of the psychic apparatus in man from that in animals. No doubt, of the biological changes that made anthropogenesis possible, the most readily observable were the evolution of the brain toward larger size and higher structuralization of the cortex, the assumption of the upright stance, and the superb differentiation of the hand.

In the structure of the psychic apparatus, however, the fundamental innovation that occurred with anthropogenesis was the breakdown of instincts as the main and, as I think, exclusive, organizers of animal behavior and their degradation to drives. I do not claim originality for this often-stated view, but I believe that the importance of that degradation and its full consequences have not been sufficiently stressed. Animals, at least from a certain evolutionary level on, as well as human beings are motivated by urges that are deeply rooted in the physical matrix. But in animals the urges are riveted almost inseparably to the ways in which they are satisfied. Even though learning of course occurs in animals, animal behavior is more or less one-dimensional. The animal's urges to survive, to reproduce, to use and defend its territory, to protect and nurture its progeny, and whatnot are gratified in a way that is almost rigidly predetermined for each species by its genetic programming. The animal does not have to make decisions; it is born with the wisdom of preceding generations that is incorporated in its genes and manifests itself in the smooth working of its instincts. Without the efficiency of instincts as a means of regulating behavior, if each generation had been given the task of finding its own best way of grappling with the biological necessities of survival and propagation, the organic layer of the world would have been in chaos and selection could never have led to organic evolution.

Man, although born with urges comparable to those of animals, is not riveted to rigidly programmed ways of gratifying them. Animal instinct and human drives have in common the inception represented by the physical urge and the consummatory end pathway; both animal and man are driven by hunger, and both gratify it by swallowing food. But whereas instinct forces the animal in the business of providing food to proceed in certain ways that have remained identical since the inception of each species, man has a high degree of freedom, and his history shows a wide spectrum of techniques, from simple food-gathering to the modern industrial production of artificial foodstuffs (Tannahill, 1973).

I feel entitled to refer to the modification whereby instincts became drives as involving degradation, degeneration, or deterioration for the following reasons: instincts are, let us agree, a configuration of a type that contains two constituents or subdivisions: (1) urge, physical demand, or physical tension; and (2) a technique, procedure, know-how, or facility whose execution or use reduces the tension. The drive, however, is a configuration of a kind that has only one constituent, the urge. The drive's gestalt is reduced as compared with that of the instinct, and one may therefore speak of degradation.

This reduction must have been initially one of the greatest threats to man's survival, since he had to invent his own techniques of grappling with external reality. The use of these techniques must have been quite risky and hazardous by comparison with the application of the almost perfect techniques that animals had acquired through the working of organic evolution. We notice here a process that is parallel to that observed at the beginning of life. The existence of early organic compounds was threatened by ultraviolet light, from which the planet was not shielded. Oxygen, then absent from the atmosphere, would have destroyed these compounds. As it happened, they developed a few inches below the surface of water. Oddly enough, they produced oxygen, which became an element indispensable to the development of life and at the same time shielded the planet against the life-destroying radiation. In a comparable manner the dangerous initial loss of predetermined ways of dealing with reality became the prerequisite of cultural evolution, which made it possible for man to dominate almost all other species. In both instances a threat to evolution was converted into a coadjuvant.

The essential change that occurred within the biological sphere when anthropogenesis degraded instinct to drive can be observed most impressively in man's sexual life. No other species is so well endowed to form variations of sexual gratifications. He is helped therein by the anatomical structure required for his upright stance, which permits a variety of positions in intercourse (this is an evolutionary innovation without precedent that is usually not sufficiently emphasized in the discussion of perversions). A seeming paradox results: a person who habitually engages in normal intercourse behaves like an animal, whereas the person who habitually indulges in the whole spectrum of perversions that is accessible to man behaves in an exquisitely human way.

In the gratification of the sexual drive one observes the conspicuous deformation of the biological apparatus that has been made possible by the replacement of instincts by drives. Not only can stimulation of any part of the body's surface elicit orgasm; merely visual or auditory configurations, or a fantasy or a thought can do so as well. The last pathway of gratification can move away from the genitals and be displaced to the mouth or result in anal orgasm. Orgastic dreams without emissions are no rare occurrence in the male. A patient of mine succeeded in training himself to elicit orgasm without ejaculation. Such an accomplishment is rarely observed clinically, but it well illustrates the extreme to which the deformation of a drive may lead.

To put it into psychoanalytic language: whereas the instinct programmed in the genetic structure of the animal determines not only its urges but also the ways in which these urges will be gratified, in man these ways will be supplied by the ego, that is to say, a spectrum of pathways to gratification.

I shall disregard here, without doing injustice to my conclusions, the fact that ego development and the structuralization of the psychic apparatus are also programmed and therefore subject to certain limitations. But it is the basic finding of psychoanalytic research that, given an average constitution, the events of the first quinquennium will decide whether the child will later become a criminal or a saint, an average citizen or outstanding in his performance, a healthy, well-adjusted person or one torn by neurosis and depressions. The principle of unregulated variance that was introduced by anthropogenesis was made possible by the repeal of instincts that had until then regulated animal life.

Of the many objections to my thesis and the extreme consequences I draw therefrom, there will certainly be the argument that a state more and more closely comparable to that of man can be observed as one ascends the evolutionary scale. Animals, particularly the nonhuman primates, have their "quinquennium," during which formative effects on instincts are discerned.

As far as I know, no one has precisely defined the limits of instinctual modifiability. To be sure, in some avian species the song of the adult bird depends on auditory impressions in the young, and monkeys raised under artificial circumstances may be gravely impaired in social behavior and the ability to perform intercourse. Yet in the instance of the birds the possible range of variation of the adult's song is quite narrow; in that of the monkeys, the possibilities opened up by the modifiability of the instinct are limited to proper and improper development of a function or pattern of functions. In man, however, a drive may be modified to an extent that makes the original urge unrecognizable in the developmental end product. As a general statement, despite the elaborate records of extensive learning in animals, it is valid to speak of the rigidity of instincts and the comparative freedom of drives.

There are many conditions which account for man's state as a being without instincts. According to Bolk (1926), fetalization and retardation of the newborn of the species *Homo sapiens* are the prerequisites thereof. The more regressed an organism is, within optimal limits of course, the wider the range of directions in which it can develop, depending on contingencies. This can be observed even within the human species. Males are born more regressed than females, and indeed, the range of developmental possibilities is larger in the male than in the female sex, as can be seen from the fact that genius is very rare, if not even absent, in the female.

Bolk's theory has been modified by Portmann. According to Portmann (1945, 1964), man's evolutionary position should make him precocial, but he is in fact altricial—not primarily altricial, like the higher birds, but secondarily. For man to be born in a precocial state as other mammalians are, the period of gestation would have to be far longer, 21 months. This can be convincingly demonstrated by the fact that for one year the neonate's growth continues the steep curve of fetal growth. It is because of this "physiological premature birth" *(physiologische Frühgeburt)*, as Portmann calls it, that man has the ability to form a large spectrum of behavior patterns without being subjected to the narrow range observed in animals which are born with firmly established solutions of the problems of how to grapple with the tasks of life. It is as if nature took special precautions to assure for man a relatively long period in which to find solutions for the gratification of his drives; one aspect of this can be seen in the fact of man's relatively late sexual maturation.

At any rate, the absence of instincts in man seems well established. Portmann (1968, p. 205) writes: "If I may proceed for a moment in a schematic way . . . we may call the life form of animals . . . instinct bound or instinct secured, the human life form . . . as rather instinct poor" (my tr.).

Man, though still bound to the purposes of survival and propagation, was released from the shackles that nature imposed on the kingdom of animals. He was given a wide realm of choices—not of minor importance such as whether to build a nest in this tree or that one, but rather choices unforeseen in their consequences that deeply and irrevocably affect his own and other species. From this time on, man had to carry out the responsibility hitherto borne unerringly by evolution through the silent work of heredity, mutation, and selection.

This moment I call the fall of man, because it was at this moment that man stepped out of nature, or was released from it, and was burdened with a task for which he was utterly unprepared and in which he was bound to fail, as I shall attempt to show in the rest of my presentation. The antagonistic harmony of the organic world was abruptly disturbed with anthropogenesis. Although mutations occur, of course, in man as in all other species, such mutations cannot lead to functional improvements, except in one area to be discussed later. Mutation might lead to the formation of eyes that can see further than the visual apparatus that is at man's disposal, but mutation could never produce a visual apparatus that can reach the boundary of the universe as man can almost do with the help of a telescope, or decipher the details made accessible by means of the electron microscope. Even millions of years of organic evolution would not have sufficed to create a species able to reach the moon. Technological innovations are the equivalents of new species, but they occur without a corresponding change in the genetic structure. In man, a species was created that would not through mutation become parent to a new species. Organic evolution was replaced by cultural evolution.

Similarly, selection—that other cornerstone of organic evolution—was thrown out of kilter with the dawn of man. All three levels of evolution, inorganic, organic, and cultural, share one principle, that of expansion: inorganic matter fills space to the maximum of its potentiality, stars at the periphery of space being propelled away from the center of the universe; organic life fills all available niches of the planet and propagates to the maximal potential, organic compounds being found even in interstellar space. This tendency of the biosphere is also observable to a certain extent in the culture sphere. New cultural elements, in general, tend to spread, and there are many examples of cultural diffusion.

In cultural evolution, however, this law of expansion no longer holds fully. Thus, the children of Israel did not pursue a policy of propagating their monotheistic religion, but jealously reserved it to their own tribes. When England formed her Empire, she did not export her system of industrialization to the colonies, but degraded them to sources of raw material and market areas, thus reserving the new civilization for herself. Also within the same cultural community, one observes the dominant group trying to limit new cultural elements to use by its own members and even excluding most of the community from the enjoyment of these elements, a problem about which more will have to be said later.

Furthermore, when we turn to cultural evolution, there are the fundamental questions as to what does and what does not favor it, and what is its real goal. The standards of organic evolution seem to be well established: they are differentiation and increase in quantity. Heredity, mutation, and selection actually led to ever more differentiated forms, culminating at last in anthropogenesis, and a huge variety of propagative techniques impelled the biomass to reach the possible maximum. Do we have a yardstick by which to determine what is culturally favorable? Cultural innovations that are heralded as progress may turn out to be destructive and inimical to cultural evolution, destructive of differentiation, and reductive of the quality and quantity of cultural output. Is Christianity culturally superior to pagan antiquity? The question has not been answered.

Moreover, in organic evolution the free interplay of forces necessarily leads to the survival of the fit. This law is invalidated in cultural evolution: the physically fittest is not necessarily—perhaps not even often—culturally most fit, and vice versa. Indeed, instances can be amply documented which show the survival and dominance of the culturally unfit at the expense of the fit. In each generation an undetermined number of human beings that potentially might have been culturally more productive are annihilated in favor of the culturally unproductive or even culturally destructive. There were times when blood relations decided who would be at the hierarchical apex of government, and thus history records many instances in which most unsuitable persons decided the destinies of huge communities. The principle of fitness, even though still operative in some areas of cultural evolution, lost its exclusive relevance and was replaced by the principle of social contingency, which from the viewpoint of cultural evolution is utterly arbitrary and has led frequently to irreparable damage to the cultural process.

I have discussed earlier the principle of invariance in the inorganic sphere, and the principle of regulated variance in organic evolution that led to a state of relative, even though antagonistic, harmony. In cultural evolution the degree and extent of variance are without precedent. In the early phases of cultural evolution, variance was moderate and might have remained within bounds comparable to those of organic evolution. Yet with the change from nomadic life to permanent settlement and the formation of cities, variance apparently started to run wild, as compared with that of organic evolution. Styles and political institutions mushroomed, class distinctions sharpened, specialization took over, wars broke out, and crime spread. The differences in custom, habits, language, beliefs, and occupations between one locale and another, between one member of the community and another, became considerable. Accompanying this was an acceleration of the rate of change whose like has not been seen in physical and organic evolution.

I do not mean to imply that cultural evolution is totally boundless, but rather to stress the difference in regulation of evolution on the organic and cultural levels. The law of regulated variance in organic evolution had to fight against the law of invariance as represented in the conservative nature of the genes. Nor is the chaotic variance in cultural evolution boundless. Behind the dazzling appearances there is a deep-seated tendency to repeat.

Although many analysts reject it, it was a great achievement of Freud to have discovered the repetition compulsion at work in the lives of individuals as well as in the history of nations. In organic evolution, the principle of invariance is still openly visible and it is highly improbable that a principle that operated throughout all preceding phases of evolution should become inoperative in human existence. Cultural evolution, however, faces a general Scylla and Charybdis. Invariance, the compulsion to repeat, continues to rule so long as the cultural process remains at a standstill. Variance, unchecked by selection, would make the cultural process chaotic, transforming human history into pandemonium. Human history is the resultant of both principles, but it is beyond the realm of human decision whether history veers more to the one or to the other direction.

One of the many consequences is the fateful matter of the missed opportunities. I wonder whether its like exists in organic evolution. The frequency of mutation and the watchful eye of selection have probably never ignored a viable differentiation. But human history teaches that splendid opportunities of healthy cultural growth were left unused. Three of them in modern times may be mentioned.

Napoleon Bonaparte had every chance in the world to be greeted by all the nations he conquered as a liberator and an apostle of freedom, if he had but carried out the implicit message of the French Revolution, which had brought him to the pinnacle of power. According to the principle of variance, he should have destroyed the reigning feudal powers and institutions that prevailed in the countries he entered. He had the opportunity of forming a united confederation of republics, consisting of French-, German-, Spanish-, and Italian-speaking territories. But his own ill-fated ambitions to found a new dynasty together with other countervailing forces made him betray his mission, and thus Europe was thrown again into an assemblage of nations, grievously injuring one another in incessant warfare.

Another such solemn moment arose when England formed her incomparable Empire. If the principle of organic evolution were valid also on the cultural level, an opportunity of this kind would have led to the export of the wisdom and experience of age-old democratic institutions and to the integration of a vast empire through an orderly process of industrialization. But national egotism forced her to treat her colonies as vassals and to exploit them, for which she was severely punished, whereas she still might have been—*prima inter pares*—the center of an industrial combine spread all over the world.

A third opportunity was most regrettably missed by this country after 1945. The United States, the only world power relatively unscathed by World War II, failed to seize the opportunity of establishing under her leadership an integrated world economy.

I now turn to some of the psychological consequences attributable to the replacement of instincts with drives in man. This evolutionary innovation caused a basic change in the economy of the psychic energy. Whereas in the animal psychic energy is rigidly bound to vital functions and is activated only within narrow and predetermined channels, the switch to drives set enormous quantities of psychic energy free. The human psychic apparatus has an abundance of energy at its disposal. This, so to speak, free-floating and freely disposable surplus of drive energy, which can be displaced to almost any goal and function, however remote from original biological functions, makes possible behavior that is no longer necessarily in the service of the optimal welfare of the species. This can be observed best in the study of human aggressiveness and destruction. In what follows, I ask you to accept temporarily my opinion, which is not shared by most analysts, that aggression is a drive that is part and parcel of human equipment and demands gratification under whatever circumstances man may be living.

The role of aggression in cultural evolution is essentially different from that in organic evolution. The latter is based on the principle of aggressive parsimony. Aggression is, of course, abundant in nature, but it is kept to an indispensable minimum. Its reduction below that level, wherever it might occur, would lead to the annihilation of the species. Bees mercilessly kill the drones after the queen bee has disemboweled the highest flying drone and the germinal stuff of the next generation has been obtained. If one generation of bees were to take pity on the drones, or if the Drones' Lib were to be successful in protesting the annual killing, this would spell the end of the species.

The biological basis for man's excessive aggressivity is denied by the environmentalist school, which attributes such aggression, in the instances it recognizes, to faulty upbringing and misguided institutions. No doubt, not every person discharges his store of aggressions. Infantile experiences and environment have their say on whether a person behaves peacefully or destructively, but the following deliberation should warn us against visualizing man as a peaceful being.

If a foundation devoted to psychology and education were interested in techniques that would reliably make of the growing child an adult that is dissocial, selfish, ready to kill and rape when he feels frustrated and incapable of postponing the gratification of his desires, the various schools of depth psychology, which can agree on hardly any relevant issue, would quickly concur regarding the way to reach this goal and would present a project that would not be too expensive and would lead most reliably to the desired outcome. If, however, the same foundation were to requisition a project that would lead the child to become an unselfish, social adult, ready to postpone the pursuit of his own advantage in favor of the community's welfare, these same schools would hardly be able to agree on how one ought to proceed. Whatever project were finally instituted, its success would be highly questionable, aside from the enormous costs it would entail. It is, after all, remarkable how easily the child is corrupted, how quickly institutions have deleterious effects.

Reflections having the same meaning have been expressed by philosophers and poets. A notable example of its symbolic presentation is found in the only scene that has been preserved of G. E. Lessing's (1729–1781) *Faust* play: Faust wants to select from seven demons the one who moves with satisfactory speed; he is dissatisfied with those who can move with the swiftness of the plague, the winds, light, or human thought, but he accepts the one that moves with the speed of transition from good to evil. To be sure, man may change from evil to good, but it is rather an exceptional event and usually takes so long that we are often suspicious of the steadiness of the outcome.

As is well known, man is not necessarily at the mercy of his aggression. He develops a variety of defenses, the most notable of which is the formation of the superego, which is brought about by the internalization of aggression. Yet all too often the superego betrays its origin by making man intolerant and thus frequently cruel. A victim may have some chance of arousing pity in the kidnapper, but an inquisitor would betray his Church if he permitted pity for the heretic to influence his sentence.

Alas, even under optimal conditions, aggressions remain alive, simmering as long as man lives. The Franciscan Pater Girolamo Moretti, an outstanding graphologist, made remarkable comments about some Saints whose handwriting he had analyzed. He discovered in St. Francis signs of vanity and restiveness against appointed authority. The handwriting of Teresa de Lisieux was surprisingly similar to that of the Italian mass murderer Rina Fort; and St. Filippo Neri showed a tendency to psychic sadism and avarice (Meng, 1971, pp. 162–165). Freud, who loved his children so much, regretfully had to register, when as an old man he interpreted one of his dreams, that he desired the death of his oldest son, who was fighting at the front and of whom he had not received news for quite a while (1900, p. 558ff.).

The law of aggressive parsimony is not valid in cultural evolution: one may even be persuaded to speak of maximization of aggression. In 1869, Rokitansky, one of the truly great ones of the

Vienna medical school, read a most remarkable paper on the solidarity of all animal life; by this term he referred to a community of action or purpose that is found throughout the kingdom of animals, including man. The paper is very important because it anticipated part of Freud's theory of the death drive. Freud never attended any of Rokitansky's lectures, and no work by Rokitansky is known to have been contained in his library, but this paper was summarized in a paper by Meynert (1892, p. 78f.), Freud's teacher, and Freud may therefore have been aware of Rokitansky's concept.

Rokitansky finds the solidarity of all animal life in aggression. Aggression is rooted in protoplasmatic hunger, which is based on the labile condition of the organic stuff of which animals consist and which requires the continuous incorporation of suitable material from the outside world. Thus, according to Rokitansky, aggression, consistent in character throughout the animal kingdom, is rooted in life-necessary protoplasmatic processes and is structurally represented from an early evolutionary stage on by the evolution of a mouthlike organ.

I follow Ernst Simmel (1944) when I say: the neonate's orality is the first manifestation of human destructiveness. A meticulous observation of the neonate demonstrates that the proposition is not quite complete. From the beginning the mouth serves both libidinal and aggressive functions. Immediately after the neonate's birth one can observe his spontaneous movements of the tongue along the lips which serve exclusively to gain pleasure. These movements are masturbatory and fulfill the characteristics of a libidinal process. The swallowing reflex, however, has the function of incorporating an object. It leads to complete annihilation of an object and is therefore an act of exquisite destruction. I have understood this act of destruction to be a biological necessity without immediate psychological relevance. Yet St. Augustine may have been right when he wrote that if babies are innocent, it is not for lack of will to do harm, but for lack of strength, and proceeded to describe the jealousy, anger, and bitterness observed by him and others in infants, even when they were in a state of full satiation.

The equation of swallowing and maximal destruction strikes our common sense as preposterous. But I ask you to imagine for a moment how we would react if man had been given the privilege of plants, that is, if man could sustain his organic existence by absorbing inorganic compounds—if, for example, he could inhale nitrogen from the atmosphere in order to build up life-necessary proteins. He would turn away with fright, disgust, and contempt from beings that kill animals and push the food into an opening of their organisms. Sensitive minds are aware of the horror of such a process. The author Karl Kraus wondered why civilization did not lead to the establishment of eating toilets.

From clinical observation of melancholic patients it is known that fixation in the "oral-sadistic phase" endows the act of eating with a cannibalistic meaning. Impressed by this frequent finding, I interpreted once the following address to Man found among Leonardo's *Notes* as a sign of depression:

> King of animals—as thou hast described him—I should rather say King of the beasts, thou being the greatest—because thou dost only help them, in order that they may give thee their children for the benefit of the gullet, of which thou hast attempted to make a sepulchre for all animals [Richter, 1883, Vol. II, p. 103f., No. 844].

I should be more cautious today and leave open the question of whether here an oversensitive mind rather than a depressed one preserved its natural feeling for an act of horror which the so-called normal mind mechanizes and reduces to a physiological action, thus negating the atrocity that objectively lies at its bottom.

The entire sphere of food preparation has preserved destructive qualities. Each single action is exquisitely sadistic: cutting, slicing, boiling, chopping, dicing, hashing, skinning, boning, eviscerating, frying, steaming, grilling, etc. It is beyond doubt that if man were an autotrophic being like the plants which absorb inorganic nutrients, if man could live without having to kill, his entire culture and civilization would be essentially different. But would culture have developed at all? Aggression in its internalized form, as we know beyond doubt, is indispensable for the structuralization of the psychic apparatus. But it is also necessary for the evolvement of culture. There must be a deep meaning embedded in the myth of Cain and Abel, that bodeful event of which Rilke wrote: "Yet prior to the first death came the murder." The first man who turned toward God in piety was killed, freakishly enough, just because of his piety, and the murderer and his posterity were protected by a special act of Divinity against his violent death. To say the least, from the viewpoint of modern genetics, mankind's gene pool was exposed to serious deterioration by this divine intercession. To turn to a historical example: Europe probably would never have been Christianized if Charlemagne had not decimated the Germanic tribes that opposed conversion. It may be apposite here to cite also Johann Gottfried Herder, a German philosopher of the eighteenth century, who pointed out the role of hatred in the differentiation of languages.

At any rate, the record of the species *Homo sapiens* shows a luxurious growth of aggression which, in my opinion, was made possible by the change of the oral instinct in animals to the oral drive of man. Man kills and destroys beyond the necessity of self-preservation because, for one thing, he has at his disposal an abundance of oral energy that is by no means bound to the incorporation of food.

This kind of conceptualization of man is rejected by most researchers in the field. It is a thesis of a type which Montagu (1968) characterized as proclaiming man's "innate depravity" and about which he wrote: "It is an unsound thesis, and it is a dangerous one, because it perpetuates unsound views which justify, and even tend to sanction, the violence which man is capable of learning" (p. 6). However, pragmatic considerations ought not to have a bearing on research. Any philosophy and theory can be abused for purposes of rationalization by those who would carry out their designs anyhow, whatever the scientist's theories may be. In view of the Evangel's not detaining those who believed in their divine origin from nefarious practices, Montagu's warning of the evil effects a scientific theory may have seems to me rather to confirm Lessing's belief in the speed of transition from good to evil in man.

At any rate, from the psychological point of view the entire problem may appear in a different light. For the anthropologist a vegetarian diet is a sign of nonaggressivity. When man hunts to satisfy his and his dependents' hunger, he is not a "killer" in the eyes of many of them, and Montagu even asks who the killer is, "the men who are paid to slaughter the animals we eat, or we who pay the cashier at the supermarket?" If the environmentalist school were correct, the danger mankind is facing would be far less acute than claimed by me. Likewise, when the attempt is made to differentiate types of aggression (Lantos, 1958), such as prey and rival aggressions, the problem may appear less formidable. Physiologists demonstrate that the endocrine and other physiological processes underlying these types of aggression are different. To be sure, rival aggression is a later evolutionary acquisition than prey aggression, but if mankind's task of mastering aggression is to be fathomed fully, it is necessary to view man's aggression in its totality. A study that goes beyond the description and social evaluation of a behavior pattern, aiming at the psychological meaning of actions and their unconscious implications, will reveal that in man these evolutionary acquisitions are by no means separate entities but interdependent.

One feature seems well established: the parsimony of aggression in organic evolution is not present in cultural evolution. The lion who when satiated stalks peacefully among his prospective prey but makes them disperse in terror with the first signs of hunger has become almost a cliché in discussions of aggression. It cannot be overstressed that this lion behaves in a nonhuman way. An equivalent state of satiation in man does not dissolve his aggression.

Furthermore, an adequate assessment of the role of aggression in human society must consider the function of tools, as Anna Freud (1972) has emphasized. If one looks for a phylogenetic pattern that might stand as an exemplar of the use of tools, one may cite a biological peculiarity of flatworms: "For defense some flatworms confiscate intact nematocysts from the hydras they eat, incorporate them in their own epidermis and use them for defense, discharging them when appropriately stimulated" (Villee, 1967, p. 264f.). If one accepts phylogenetic models as meaningful, one may emphasize the exquisite aggressiveness and oral nature of what is perhaps the earliest evolutionary instance of toolmaking. Tools in general serve aggressive purposes. "Some tools," Montagu (1968, p. 5) writes, "may be used as weapons and even manufactured as such, but most tools of prehistoric man . . . were . . . not designed primarily to serve as weapons. Knives were designed to cut, scrapers to scrape, choppers to chop, and hammers to hammer." Here, it is important to stress that cutting, scraping, chopping, and hammering are aggressive activities. One may see in technology in general a huge field of aggressive discharge. The purpose for which tools are used may be of a friendly nature, but the aggressive implications can hardly be overlooked. I cite only one example: a scythe is used for cutting and reaping in the process of food production, but then it appears as a symbol of death, rather clearly betraying its innate destructive quality.

Man may lose control over man-made tools, as modern technology seems to be demonstrating. What was originally a means to an end may come to dominate its creators. Modern technology may provide a single person with a destructive potential that is many times that which not so long ago was possessed by whole armies. Such destructive possibilities may exert an irresistible temptation upon an individual so inclined. Thus in registering the grave dangers modern technology has brought upon mankind, one may be reminded of "the return of the repressed" that is well known from the analysis of symptoms. It seems as if the aggressive impulse that originally initiated technology and carried it to its present peak becomes threateningly apparent.

The modern controversy about whether man is a killer, which rages between Ardrey (the best-known representative of the school which answers the question in the affirmative) and Montagu (the spokesman of the school which replies in the negative) has a long history. A charming example, striking in its naïveté and urbanity, can be found in the concluding paragraph of Immanuel Kant's essay on the impossibility of a theodicy. A Mr. de Lucs, presupposing the original harmlessness or goodwill *(Wohlwollen)* of our species, Kant reported, had started a field trip seeking to confirm this view in places where "urban luxuriousness cannot have such influence as to corrupt the minds." After his belief was somewhat shaken by an experience in the Swiss mountains, he concluded that so far as man's goodwill is concerned, it is "good enough, if only there were not present in him a wicked proclivity toward subtle trickery *[ein schlimmer Hang zur feinen Betrügerei]*." Kant, who knew human nature all too well, added: "A result of inquiry which everyone even without having traveled into mountains would have been able to come across among his fellow citizens, yes still closer to his own heart" (my tr.).

This "wicked proclivity toward subtle trickery"—that is the problem, even though it is a far cry from an "instinct to kill." But it implies that even under optimal conditions traces of an inborn hostility can be observed. If one does not stop at merely registering these traces but undergoes the labor of tracing them to their biopsychological roots, one discovers the regular impulse to destroy that which causes displeasure. Initially displeasure is caused by hunger, which forces man to incorporate, that is, destroy, an object in the service of eliminating the unpleasant sensation. The next step is to do the same with anything that causes displeasure, even though it comes from outside. Flight accomplishes the same *psychological* effect, insofar as it eliminates a perception that causes displeasure, and yet the active annihilation of the object whose perception causes displeasure may have evolutionary priority. Indeed, it may have proved to be the more efficient operational mode. Thus, when Ardrey (1961) speaks of "an instinct to kill," he may have been too specific, for the general "instinct," deeply repressed in some and lamentably close to the surface in others, is to annihilate that which causes displeasure. No doubt, in view of the present state of societal organization, that which causes displeasure includes in most instances our fellow creatures.

The abundance of drive energy observed in the aggressive drives is encountered also in the libidinal group. What is quite manifest in the genital drive is also valid for the pregenital ones. As is known, they are the main store of energy that becomes sublimated. But there is a definite limit to the extent to which sublimation and neutralization are possible, quite aside from the fact that extensive and far-reaching sublimations are infrequent and depend on the coincidence of numerous factors. What can be observed is that the abundance of libidinal energy is used for cathexis of the self and manifests itself clinically as an increase in narcissism.

To be sure, narcissism is a life-necessary force. Little as the psychology of animals has been explored in psychoanalytic terms, one can safely say that animals are exquisitely narcissistic. But there again narcissism enforces the biologically useful. The animal becomes completely absorbed by the biological function per se. Narcissism in the human adult in general has different effects. I limit myself to describing one of these: In patients suffering from simple senile dementia, I have observed fairly good orientation and reality testing within the space bounded by their extended arms, that is, only the space within which they are physically able to grasp and seize objects has realistic psychological relevance. Let me use, for abbreviation's sake, the German word *Greifraum* for that space. There is also a psychological *Greifraum*, characterized by a person's authentic interests. Clinical and practical experience proves over and over again that in the vast majority of subjects the psychological *Greifraum* is comparable to that of the senile demented. It is confined within the bounds of their unequivocally narcissistic interests. A passage in a letter by Freud to Pfister may serve as a humorous illustration: "After I started driving about in a carriage all day long, I became annoyed at the carelessness of the pedestrians, just as earlier when I was a pedestrian [I was annoyed] at the lack of consideration by the drivers."

A tragic aspect of the essentially narcissistic nature of man's psychic *Greifraum* is illustrated in a statement made by Françoise Giraud, the present French Secrétaire d'Etat des Conditions Féminines. "There wasn't 1 percent of the population that joined the resistance, but I swear there were 50 percent who would have risked their necks for a pound or two of butter." Whereas culture demands and requires from a certain point of differentiation on an extension of the *Greifraum* far beyond these bounds, man in general is shackled by his narcissism to a very narrow psychological *Greifraum*.

At the inception of life the probability of its persistence was highly questionable. Likewise, at the time of anthropogenesis and the dawn of culture, man's victory and the entrenchment of culture almost all over the earth's surface were quite unpredictable. At that time—when man seemed to be the species least equipped by nature to become a permanent inhabitant, since he was physically weaker than the predatory animals that hunted him, helplessly exposed in his hairless nakedness to the harshness of the climate, without claws and cutting canine teeth, smaller in number than any other species, more prone to develop anxiety and fear than his competitors, and having at his disposal nothing but crudely hewn flintstones—at that time the narrowness of his psychological *Greifraum* was a prerequisite of his survival and its extension would have jeopardized his existence. At that time love, aggression, and narcissism worked harmoniously for the sole purpose of biological survival. But thousands of years later, Dostoyevsky wrote that man is responsible for whatever happens at any time anywhere in the world, thus demanding the maximal extension of the psychological *Greifraum*.

Indeed, such extension is necessary if man is to survive, but this demand and this necessity exceed his potentiality. Witnessing a car accident may easily have a traumatic effect and the memory may haunt us for days; but reading that in an inundation in a far-off country, hundreds of thousands of people were killed evokes in us not more than the cliché response of "How terrible," and we turn readily to the pursuits dictated by the narrowness of our immediate *Greifraum*. Perception wins over abstraction.

The first consequence of excess in aggression and narcissism is man's heightened ambivalence, which has no counterpart in any other species. Man's ambivalence has been a foremost topic of psychoanalytic research, but I believe that its degree and inescapability are still underestimated. Let me point out two examples. For centuries in the West the faithful have prayed daily to the Lord: "Lead us not into temptation." Theologians have, of course, argued that this cannot be taken as indicating that God is the source and cause of temptation. To prove their point, they quote from the Epistle to James (1:13), "God cannot be tempted with evil, neither tempteth he any man," and the even more reassuring passage from I Corinthians (10:13): "God is faithful, who will not suffer you to be tempted above that ye are able, but will with the temptation also make a way to escape, that ye may be able to bear it," which to the unsophisticated may appear to contradict the disastrous consequences that the serpent—for whose presence in the Garden of Eden God, after all, was responsible—had on the course of mankind according to the Old Testament. The ease and lack of logic with which evidently self-contradictory statements in divine scriptures are given the appearance of veracity presuppose a deep ambivalence.

Yet even if it were possible to accept the theologian's reasoning, the sentence in the Lord's Prayer taken per se asserts the very fact that God may tempt His children, and the believer who is unfamiliar with the theologian's reasoning assumes that God may tempt him, though he will attribute to the Divinity infinite goodness.

An even more frightening manifestation of ambivalence is observed when the faithful ascribes to the Divinity a rather Shylock-like trait, inasmuch as God is believed to have forgiven mankind a sin committed thousands of years earlier only after His son had voluntarily submitted to being killed. Such cultural data persisting over millennia in man's mind and religious sentiments should be taken as indicators of all but ineradicable structural features of the human psychic apparatus, whose manifestations may, of course, vary greatly according to particular cultural settings.

Ambivalence in man is so deeply ingrained in the structure of his psychic apparatus that ethical behavior is made impossible, as I shall try to demonstrate. Benjamin Pasamanick, the New York Health Commissioner, terms the condition in which a wealthy society such as ours does not stave off the hunger of its own members "murderous" (*Psychiatric News*, April 7, 1971). Indeed, as we all know, a large number of children and adults even now are suffering from diseases caused by malnutrition that in many instances lead to premature death. Was Pasamanick right in calling this "murder," or was it merely the rhetoric of the reformer who is enraged by society's lethargy vis-à-vis crying social ills? Murder, after all, presupposes intent and everyone is apt to confess his regret about the sufferings social conditions cause.

In 1972 two Frenchmen, Roger Bontems and Claude Buffet, were guillotined in the Santé Prison in Paris. This was quite unusual, since for three and a half years no such sentence had been carried out. Furthermore, what made the event so remarkable was the fact that Bontems had never committed murder. Pompidou, who was the French president at the time, refused clemency. Bontems suffered capital punishment because he had not *prevented* murder, remaining a passive onlooker while his friend Buffet cut the throats of two hostages. In my opinion, sentence and execution were grave miscarriages of justice. But if one believes in capital punishment at all, it might also have been justified in Bontems's instance in terms of a moral principle. Whoever does not prevent death, despite opportunity to do so, makes himself just as guilty as the perpetrator of a capital crime.

What Pompidou overlooked, however, was the implication of his refusal to grant clemency: according to the principle applied to Bontems, Pompidou himself was guilty of the death of an undetermined number of children and grownups who died prematurely because of noxious social conditions. Here we are at the heart of the problem. The members of the community who are favored by social conditions are living in a kind of ghetto surrounded by social misery, and make themselves guilty in relation to its existence by tacitly condoning it. Here it is no longer a matter of famine and mass death in a far-off country, but of the knowledge of destitution in one's neighborhood, and yet this knowledge does not interfere with the enjoyment of social amenities, the voluntary giving up of which would enable each privileged person to reduce misery, even though in most instances this were achieved only in a small island surrounded by a sea of wretchedness.

Oddly enough, the person for whom this callous attitude becomes intolerable exposes himself to criticism. Peter Rosegger (1843–1918), an Austrian author, recounts a childhood experience when he followed the example of St. Martin, who cut his cloak in two in order to share it with a beggar. The little boy did the same with his shirt but was ridiculed by his parents. As an adult, he himself took a patronizing attitude toward his childhood behavior, thus denying its tragic aspect. When Tolstoy at the end of his life was driven to distribute his wealth among the indigent, this was taken as a sign of a mental disturbance brought about by old age. Yet the behavior of both, the little boy and the old man, was nothing but the irrefutable consequence of the religious tenets which their cultural community claimed to be of divine origin.

No doubt, anyone who takes the Sermon on the Mount seriously risks entanglement in a net of dilemmas and may easily become the victim of rejection, perhaps ostracism, and even commitment into an asylum without having significantly alleviated the condition of the poor. Consequently, social survival requires a grandiose act of denial on the part of those who enjoy the amenities of life; only by reducing the psychological *Greifraum* essentially to narcissistic ego interests, limiting himself to token acts of charity, and reducing the live social misery that surrounds him to an abstraction to be discussed in a theoretical frame of reference—that is, by denying in practice the validity of the supreme ethical dogma, thereby in effect inducing in himself scotomata in the perception of his social surroundings—can man survive. But is this alleged necessity of denial for social survival's sake the whole story?

Keir Hardie, the founder and first chairman of the British Labour Party, reports that at the age of 10, in 1866, he was the only breadwinner in the family, his father having been unemployed for a half year because of a lockout. The young Hardie got employment with a "high-class baker," receiving 3 shillings and 6 pence a week for 12½ hours' work per day.

> It was the last week in the year. Father had been away for two or three days in search of work. Towards the end of the week, having been up most of the night, I got to the shop fifteen minutes late, and was told by the young lady in charge that if that occurred again I would be punished. I made no reply. I couldn't. I felt like crying. Next morning the same thing happened. I could tell why, but that was neither here nor there. It was a very wet morning, and when I reached the shop I was drenched to the skin, barefooted and hungry. There had not been a crust of bread in the house that morning.
>
> But that was pay-day, and I was filled with hope. "You are wanted upstairs by the master," said the girl behind the counter, and my heart almost stopped beating. Outside the dining-room door a servant bade me wait till master had finished prayers. (He was noted for his piety.) At length the girl opened the door, and the sight of that room is fresh in my memory even as I write, nearly fifty years after. Round the great mahogany table sat the members of the family, with the father at the top. In front of him was a very wonderful-looking coffee boiler, in the great glass bowl of which the coffee was bubbling. The table was loaded with dainties. My master looked at me over his glasses and said in quite a pleasant tone of voice: "Boy, this is the second morning you have been late, and my customers leave me if they are kept waiting for their hot breakfast rolls. I therefore dismiss you, and, to make you more careful in the future, I have decided to fine you a week's wages. And now you may go!"

I wanted to speak and explain about my home and muttered out something to explain why I was late, but the servant took me by the arm and led me downstairs. As I passed through the shop the girl in charge gave me a roll and said a kind word. I knew my mother was waiting for my wages. As the afternoon was drawing to a close I ventured home and told her what had happened. It seemed to be the last blow. The roll was still under my vest, but soaked with rain. That night the baby was born, and the sun rose on the first of January, 1867, over a home in which there was neither fire nor food [Hughes, 1956, p. 16f.].

Here is what may be termed a typical instance which manifests willful human arrogance, willful exploitation of the helpless, and willful use of one's fellowman for the aggressive purposes of self-aggrandizement. To be sure, such occurrences are rather rare in our present society, and conspicuous consumption will no longer lead to fountains spouting champagne, as happened on the opening night of John Jacob Astor's private theater in New York. But such excesses cannot be reduced to the pernicious effects of special social conditions, as the environmentalist school maintains. They may overtly reflect a tendency that usually remains covered up. In order to grasp how general "conspicuous consumption" is in all fields of life, the following may be considered.

If all human beings were able to make sculptures like those of Michelangelo, or compose music like Mozart's, or write Shakespearean tragedies, such abilities would have to be considered a peculiarity of the species *Homo sapiens* and would lose all inherent value; we would take them for granted, as we take reading and writing for granted, although these latter abilities were so rare at the time of Charlemagne that they were enough to win a court position for the man who had them. One may speak of a "law of negative enjoyment," since the enjoyment of one's abilities, possessions, and so on that is gained by reason of their not being shared by others is almost generic to human nature, although it does not manifest itself in all individuals and societies and is often covered up by its opposite. In our society, good breeding requires the denial of such motivations, but their manifestation is only too easily observable. Insatiability for narcissistic reasons is rampant. Therefore, I conclude that the monumental differences in wealth in our society are not only caused by the operation of economic forces but are wished for and desired because they offer opportunities for narcissistic differentiation. A truly egalitarian society, which reduced economic differences to the utmost, would block one of the most important pathways of crude unsublimated narcissism. The law of negative enjoyment, I may note, is operative when narcissism travels a sublimated pathway. The humble, even the saint and the martyr, do not escape its pitfalls.

The general conclusion one is forced to draw is therefore that Pasamanick's accusation is correct. It is not the necessity of social survival, a sort of self-defense, that makes us callous and forces us to condone preventable death. The basic structure of man's nature makes most of us share in murder.

I shall now present another typical example which may demonstrate that when one takes into account merely the structure of an ethical problem, disregarding man's narcissism, one is forced to state that man's ethical problems are unsolvable.

In July 1931 the 32-year-old German citizen Semmelmann was shot to death in Vienna by a man who had entered his apartment in the morning hours. He had never met his victim before. The murderer, who was arrested by chance, initially refused to give any testimony and for a while it looked as if it might not be possible to establish his identity. However, at the trial seven months later it turned out that both murderer and victim had been members of the Communist Party. Both had been secret agents of the Russian Cheka. Three months prior to his violent death Semmelmann had been dismissed by the Russian organization because the suspicion arose that he entertained relations with rightist circles in Germany. Having lost his livelihood, Semmelmann tried to obtain funds by using his knowledge of Communist secret organizations. He planned to sue the Russian trade organization, in whose service he had worked; he was ready to publish newspaper articles about the Russian secret service; and he was suspected—rightly, as it turned out—of planning to deliver to the Rumanian government a list of all the members of the underground Communist Party. It was not clear whether the murderer had acted on his own initiative or was carrying out the orders of his organization. After a deliberation of half an hour, seven members of the jury found him guilty and five not guilty, which according to Austrian law meant dismissal of the charges. Henri Barbusse, a leading Communist and publicist, had sent a telegram to the court demanding acquittal.

The immorality of Semmelmann's behavior, actual and threatened, is beyond doubt. One should not betray one's former comrades, an action aggravated when it is carried out for mercenary reasons. But what about the ethics of the murderer? Here is a planned, deliberate act of violent destruction of a human being, which is forbidden by ethics. And yet if the slaying had not occurred, an indeterminate number of human beings would have been killed, and hundreds of people would have had to linger in prison for years, even decades. If the murderer had abided by one principle of human ethics, he would indirectly have caused far greater destruction than that due to his deed.

No doubt millions of people would have praised Hitler's murder, but, depending on when it occurred, millions might have condemned it. Similarly, there are many who were and still are of the opinion that Semmelmann would have done a great service by betraying his erstwhile comrades.

It is evident not only that man is bound to be in conflict in his attempt to establish a synthesis between the demands of id, ego, superego, and reality—a conflict that is at the center of psychoanalytic research—but also that the differentiation which has taken place within his superego with the dawn of Christianity has created complications that defy resolutions. The irreconcilability of values which man is admonished to realize has been put forth repeatedly. Indeed, it is impressive to observe the ease with which philosophers present the ideals they cherish without noticing that their exhortations can hardly have the desired effect because of their contrariety. Thus, when Buber asserts that justice and active love *(tätige Liebe)* are the demands of the hour and the hope of the future (Scholem, 1966, p. 42), he combines two values which cannot, I believe, be brought together. Active love in the forms of mercy and compassion excludes punishment, for the more execrable a crime, the more compassion its perpetrator deserves, if one intends to be truly serious about the application of active love. True justice, however, must never be allowed to be weakened by compassion, for from the standpoint of justice nothing must infringe upon the process of reestablishing ethical equilibrium, once that equilibrium has been upset.

A most striking example of an attempt to impose mutually exclusive values was presented in a pamphlet distributed during World War II in the U.S. Army, which advised soldiers that the Catholic Church permitted the killing of an enemy when it was carried out with love in one's heart and without hatred. It is almost unnecessary to say that this is humanly impossible—unless the killer is a sadist. In this case he will, indeed, love his victims and be free of hatred.

In this one area of contrariety of ethical values, which is of utmost relevance in relation to the regulation of individual behavior and community operations, the species is burdened with irresolvable conflicts and no pathway can be delineated that would be optimal for cultural evolution. The serpent's prophecy: "Ye shall be as gods, knowing good and evil," has not come true.

Yet it is not only the self that becomes a receptacle of excess narcissism. Man's culture itself may serve the same purpose, and therefore one may speak of cultural narcissism, meaning the narcissistic gratification a person derives from cultural institutions and products in which he partakes. The animal's narcissism has been mentioned before, as a prerequisite of organic life. Initially, man's narcissism, so different from that of animals, stood him in good stead. But with the evolution of civilization and culture narcissism shifted to the products of culture, and many a man was ready to sacrifice his life for the preservation of an idea, of his culture, of his religion. The culmination of this attitude is perhaps Horace's famous dictum: *Dulce et decorum est pro patria mori*, discovering even sweetness in death if it is a sacrifice for one's country. It should not be denied that such actions may also contain their share of object-related libido, dependent on objective and subjective circumstances, but it can be safely stated that the narcissistic cathexis of one's community, culture, or generally of values is a precondition of culture in various respects.

The use of tools, which began so early and may have been one of the decisive factors at the dawn of mankind, harbors a problem with regard to narcissism. To use an extension of the arm in the form of a stick, or to let the hammer do the work of the fist, presupposed a shift of body narcissism. The machine, in distinction to the tool, which is only the equivalent of a part of the body, made a shift of the narcissistic cathexis of the whole body necessary. A new phase of technology set in when man had to shift the narcissistic cathexis of thinking to computers, which arouse in the layman a feeling of uncanniness similar to that which Sachs (1933) described with regard to the introduction of machines. In each phase the narcissistic loss was compensated by an increase of power and efficiency—that is, the immediate loss of direct narcissistic gratification was repaid with huge dividends by far greater gratifications.

Furthermore, in periods of accelerated cultural growth, as in the Periclean period or the Renaissance, one observes whole cultural groups in a kind of narcissistic frenzy, each member of the establishment vying with the others for cultural exquisiteness. Such temporary flare-ups in group narcissism undoubtedly had beneficial effects. This is also true of individual instances. The artistically productive mind may elevate his claim to perfection to a pinnacle and wrestle tenaciously for its realization. He might prefer a shortening of his life-span over compromise within his value system.

The genius's narcissism is comparable to the animal's narcissism. As organisms take hold of all accessible niches and evolution fills empty spaces with better-adjusted forms, so the genius fills with like tenacity empty cultural niches with his more differentiated products. But the injuries cultural narcissism inflicts on the cultural process may nullify the positive results brought about by creative achievements. Cultural narcissism obfuscates the reality principle. Reality-adequate judgment is obviated.

An example may illustrate this. The American Constitution is surrounded by a halo and considered—indeed, as a document, in many ways deserves to be considered—the greatest achievement American political wisdom has brought forth, the symbol and actual deed on which American democracy rests. But only a minority of the population was permitted to vote on it; if the right to vote had been universal at that time, the result would have been a rejection of the document; it did not prevent the worst form of slavery history records; it did not prevent a civil war which is regarded as having been the cruelest and most destructive war of the century; it did not prevent the partial extermination of the native population; it did not prevent the expropriation of a minority, such as the Japanese at the beginning of World War II; it did not assure a duly elected president the opportunity to start his period of administration; it did not prevent a president from conducting a war in a foreign country without a declaration of war and permission of Congress; it made it possible for presidents to organize civil wars in foreign countries against the will of the majority of the electorate. Nevertheless, it is considered a kind of ideal institution that is without par and should be imitated by all other countries because of its beneficial effect.

How should one explain the unshakable belief in excellence, when failure actually is in front of one's face, notwithstanding the many beneficial effects which can be attributed to the document? One is reminded of the clinically well-known phenomenon of the overvaluation of the love object. True love ascribes to the beloved an excellence which the object of love cannot possibly harbor, but in the case of the national overestimation of a document and its effect, it is a matter of overestimation that is caused by excessive narcissistic cathexes. It is the pride in something that makes the group of which one is a member superior to all other groups. The document is endowed with a perfection which it does not possess, but the illusion of perfection gratifies a deep-seated longing in the person who is living in the shadow of the symbol, for part of the perfection—perhaps even its entirety—becomes either part of the self or part of the group's representation in the self. At any rate, it contributes to the self's elevation, whereas the lover who overvalues his sweetheart feels in comparison with the beloved object, if anything, depleted of personal value, all of which he finds concentrated in his love. The narcissistic hypercathexis of a document such as the Constitution impedes a realistic evaluation; it infringes on the cultural reality principle. The community, if fixated to a certain set of solutions despite the fact that their inappropriateness should be evident, will prevent the choice and introduction of imaginative and daring measures, even when they are imperative in view of threatening emergencies.

Cultural narcissism occasionally takes on grotesque forms in the absolute trust which the believer puts in the dogmas and canons of his particular faith. Admitting that if he had been raised in a different church, he would believe in a different set of canons, he considers himself fortunate that the divinity let him be raised in his particular community and thus enabled him to recognize divine truth. I wish to present an example that shows how a modern, even enlightened mind, too, can infringe upon the simplest of demands of logic in order to save his religious preferences.

In his sermon "He Who Is the Christ," which focuses on the moment when Peter answered Jesus' question as to whom the Apostles believed Him to be: "Thou art the Christ" (Mark 8:28), Tillich calls this "the most important event of human history . . . not only from the point of view of the believer, but also from that of the *detached observer of world history*" (p. 142, my emphasis). Why? Peter's answer denied, so Tillich says, that Jesus was a forerunner like Elija or Jeremiah but asserted that "the Christ, the bearer of the new, had come in this man Jesus. . . . the word 'Christ' was [at that time] still a vocational title. It designated Him, Who was to bring . . . the establishment of the Messianic reign of peace and justice" (p. 144). Thereupon Jesus forbade the Apostles to tell anyone about Him because "the Messianic character . . . did not mean to Him what it meant to the people." They would have expected a divine figure coming from heaven to be the King of glory and peace. "His mystery is more profound; it cannot be expressed through the traditional names. It can only be revealed by . . . the suffering, death, and rising again" (p. 144f.). Tillich admits that "there have been many pictures of creative suffering and of heroic death in human history. But none of them can be compared with the picture of Jesus' death" (p. 146). The Christ had to suffer, Tillich says, "because whenever the Divine appears in all Its depth, It cannot be endured by men. It must be pushed away by the political powers, the religious authorities, and the bearers of cultural tradition" (p. 147).

Tillich goes so far as to say that "whenever the Divine appears, It is a radical attack on everything that is good in man, and therefore man must repel It, must push It away, must crucify It." The Divine "revolts against the human. . . . the human must defend itself against It, must reject It, and must try to destroy It" (p. 147). The Divine, however, "accepts our refusal to accept, and thus conquers us. That is the centre of the mystery of the Christ." Surprisingly, Tillich claims that "a Christ Who would not die, and Who would come in glory to impose upon us His power . . . would not be able to win our hearts. . . . His power would break our freedom. . . . our very humanity would be swallowed in His Divinity. . . . We should be more like blessed animals than men made in the image of God" (p. 147f.).

I have gone into the details of this sermon because they show an accumulation of non sequiturs, inconsistencies, and unpardonable infringements on logical thinking. Tillich, perhaps correctly, says that the divine mystery is humanly unintelligible. Nevertheless, he continually makes positive statements about it, tries to explain it, and expects us to believe his interpretation. His explanation why Jesus did not want the people to know that he was the Christ simply makes no sense. That they expected peace and justice but would not receive it from Jesus as well as the rest of the argument is no valid explanation, in view of the fact that it was after all revealed to posterity, but this posterity had no chance or means of validating His divinity. It is neither cogent nor evident that man must repel the Divine. After all, the Bible reports incidents that bespeak the very fact, for example, in Abraham's instance. A Divine revolting against the human would exclude man's having been created in the image of God. An Adam who strictly obeys God could well be compared to a blessed animal, but man who is forced by his very nature to fight the Divine because the Divine in turn attacks everything good in man would not, if God at last revealed himself as the King of Peace and Justice, destroy his autonomy or freedom at all. Such a divine power would win our hearts most speedily. How little man would lose his liberty can be seen from the fact that even angels were able to fall from grace.

I am certain that if after Christ's rise justice and peace had reigned on earth, Tillich would not have hesitated to use that state as proof that Christ was a divinity. It is, of course, an embarrassing situation for the faithful that despite Christ's death on the cross not an iota has changed in human affairs and man continues to steal, curse, rape, and kill as ever and even worse than before Christ's appearance. It is further embarrassing that an almighty God permits children to be killed or die from terrible diseases as well as condones the outrageous events history records without ever interfering and protecting the good ones against the evil ones.

The theologian has no trouble in converting these embarrassments into proof of God's greatness: man not overwhelmed by His glory preserves liberty, but what kind of liberty is this? It is the liberty of doing anything human—which includes a large area of evil, but excludes the recognition of the presence of God. That seems to be, according to Tillich, the only thing man cannot accomplish. Since the reign of justice and peace apparently amounts to an infringement on human liberty, the theologian has solved the problem for the future, and the absence of the Kingdom of God on earth becomes a sign of God's respect for the dignity of man. One notices a startling perversion of values.

Such a mode of reasoning which is contrary to all logic is the result of an excessive narcissistic attachment to the beliefs in which one has been raised, or, in the case of conversion, to the one newly discovered. It is evident that a person so intensely prepossessed by a conviction which with some distance and impartiality would be instantly recognized as untenable, must have an unconscious reason for that conviction. From clinical experience with pathological instances, we know that the adherence to wrong beliefs has a lifesaving effect on some patients. If he suddenly became aware of the inappropriateness of his delusional conviction, the self would suffer a narcissistic injury of such magnitude that it would initiate a regression which would harm the psychic apparatus far more than the previous disturbance of the patient's reality testing. An equivalent situation might have arisen for a personality as deeply religious as Tillich must have been. However, it would be a mistake to look at his way of solving the Christian dilemma as being related to a psychosis. Nevertheless, one is entitled to conjecture that if some person or event had been able to affect his certainty or shatter his conviction, he might have been seized, at least temporarily, by a psychotic state. Of course, the way of thinking that is characteristic of the religious person makes it practically impenetrable to any argument, and no event could create a serious doubt in his mind, for both the state of justice and peace as well as the opposite prove the existence of the Divinity. He is protected against all eventualities. Here we encounter typical narcissistic attitudes.

The scientist, too, is in his own way narcissistic, but how different is his way of procedure. When Freud realized that—contrary to what he had been convinced of previously—adult neuroses were not caused by acts of sexual seduction experienced in childhood, he did not suffer a breakdown, although he had invested much time and effort in the elaboration of his theory and was filled with great pride. He enumerated in his letter to his friend Fliess all the nice things he had lost by his failure, but went on in his research and evolved new, more suitable theories. At the end of his life he looked back and calmly perceived that the assured part of the psychoanalytic edifice was rather small. Such attitudes within their area of expertise are unfeasible in personalities like Tillich's, and one must register the existence of vast narcissistic structures within their psychic apparatus that deprive them of the necessary flexibility optimal to the cultural process.

One can hardly overrate the detrimental effect of cultural narcissism. It shows up in an overrating of one's language, national and Church membership, political system, and whatnot. It is a major psychological factor contributing to wars. It is passed on to the next generation and therefore involves a fixity and a tenacity that are incompatible with optimal cultural growth.

A further aspect of the problem becomes visible when one considers the uncanny alliance between aggression and narcissism (Rochlin, 1973). Through the operation of a basic law of psychic economy, aggressive discharges are without exception correlated with an increase in narcissistic cathexes. Contrarily, at the peak of the state of love the self is depleted of narcissistic cathexes; this may be one of the many reasons why man is more inclined toward aggressive than loving behavior. The equation is valid in both directions. Aggressive discharges cause an increase in narcissistic gratification, and narcissism in man favors aggressive discharge. That is, man is prone to be aggressive in order to regain the narcissistic level optimal for him.

In the life of animals nothing of the kind is observable. Their aggression follows biological necessities and does not impede organic evolution. On the contrary, it seems to operate regularly in its service, as earlier mentioned. The correlation of aggression and narcissism in man, however, has disastrous consequences, only one of which I wish to go into. This concerns the selection of leaders. Among nonhuman primates, a hierarchical structure of social life is observed. It is not yet quite clear what laws govern the process by which the leader is selected in those societies, but no instance has been recorded in which the leader has operated against the group's welfare without being more or less swiftly deposed.

In human history, such wisdom is encountered but rarely. For the longer part of man's history blood relation determined who was to be at the apex of the hierarchical pyramid. Insane persons have occasionally wielded the power to decide the fate of vast empires and became the cause of their downfall.

In modern society the principle of consanguinity as a basis for selection of leaders has by and large been abolished, but the quality of leadership has not correspondingly improved as might have been expected. Despite the apparent variety, one finds in leading positions, in democratic societies as in others, more frequently than not personages the core of whose personalities is aggressive-narcissistic.

We face here a fundamental issue of cultural evolution. No technique has yet been found that would guarantee the selection of the best qualified or even make his selection probable. With amazing monotony, in a surprisingly large number of instances, one finds in positions of leadership, whether in a scientific society, a corporation, a city, or the whole nation, persons who are smarter than the average, but not of deep intelligence, somewhat ruthless, gifted in manipulating others, and less devoted to the welfare of the group for which they are responsible than to narcissistic self-aggrandizement. They usually are highly attractive to groups. It turns out that most people, usually unconsciously, harbor strong narcissistic-aggressive wishes from whose realizations they are inhibited but which they gratify instead through identification with a person of this type. Thus there is divided responsibility: the prospective leader's ambivalence and the masochism of those who make his acquisition of power possible.

History seems to suggest that cultural evolution, even though eminently successful in bringing forth great minds called geniuses that have made maximal contributions to progress in special cultural fields, was not as successful with regard to the management of mankind's practical affairs. If one can speak of progress in that area at all, one is inclined to say that it has occurred not so much because of leaders as despite them. This, of course, does not negate the fact that at times of crisis great leaders came to power and proved their mettle.

In discussing the bane of aggressive narcissism in the context of leadership, one is led to a group phenomenon that is close to it: warfare. From early stages of cultural evolution on, though probably not from its very inception, warfare has been an integral part of human history. It is difficult to determine whether it was necessary to cultural evolution, but it is a fact, as mentioned before, that Europe would not have been Christianized without warfare; for that matter, the present civilization on this continent is based on the original ruthless fight against its native population. It will be difficult to find an empire or any large civilization that has arisen in the last five millennia which did not at its inception record a massive act of brutal suppression, if not extinction, of a large number of people.

The view that warfare is avoidable because it is the upshot of modifiable noxious institutions is widespread. Thus Immanuel Kant believed that the replacement of monarchies by the republican form of government would abolish warfare, and one cannot blame that great thinker for that error. In his times there existed scarcely any republic, and warfare was ordered by the decisions of monarchs pursuing at least ostensibly dynastic purposes. Similarly, those of our generation, including myself, who believed in their youth that warfare is the concomitant of the capitalistic form of economic organization, cannot be blamed. It was unthinkable that countries that aspired to the realization of socialism could ever resort to warfare with each other. Nevertheless one perceives on the historical horizon the specter of a Russo-Chinese war.

Warfare may be the result of noxious institutions, but it does not follow necessarily that it is preventable by modifying these institutions; one is obliged to concede that no institutions have yet been invented that would make warfare obsolete. In warfare one observes on the collective level and on a gigantic scale the narcissistic-aggressive combination that is encountered in individual life. The biology of war is far more complicated than I have indicated, but here I wish only to stress the anchoring of war in man's psychobiological matrix, a view which is denied by so many.

Before leaving the subject of the grave dangers the cultural process faces through the alliance of aggression and narcissism, I want to quote once more Immanuel Kant, who found in this alliance the very inducement and initiative toward culture. In his essay on ideas about a cosmopolitan history, he states that *antagonism* is the means by which nature creates order. He defines antagonism as man's unsociable sociality *(ungesellige Geselligkeit)*. Man has the proclivity to enter social relations, but also the proclivity to isolate himself. The latter is caused by his impulse to be unsociable and by his expectation of finding resistance in others to his intentions, as he knows of his own resistance to the intentions of those who surround him. "It is this resistance which awakens all activities in man and gets him to the point of overcoming his inclination to laziness and, driven by ambition, imperiousness, or avarice, of procuring rank for himself among his fellow creatures whose company he cannot tolerate well, but whom to dispense with he is unable" (my tr.). Under such conditions, according to Kant, the first steps from barbarism to culture are taken.

It is striking to find here antagonism and desire for isolation, clear representatives of aggression, as well as ambition, imperiousness, and avarice, clear representatives of narcissism, both of which I have described as dangers to culture, promulgated as the main forces to which cultural development is due. It would not be exceptional, however, when factors promoting a process gradually are converted into those that cause its undoing. Kant did not forget to stress the function of love, the desire to socialize, as one prerequisite of culture, a function I have hardly mentioned but for which I may be excused since I am mainly concerned with those forces that are inimical to culture.

Differences of opinion in discussions of mankind's future are frequently caused by what impresses me as a fundamental error in a general evaluation of man. I shall demonstrate the error by a comparison. I once witnessed at Radio City a charming presentation by trained poodles. They were dressed in Tyrolean costumes and danced, and one of them, I believe, even played a musical instrument. In no book on dogs I have ever read are dogs able to waltz and play musical instruments. In general treatises on man, however, he is almost regularly evaluated on the basis of the maximal realization of his highest potential and not that of average behavior. Of course, to understand man fully we have to study both average behavior and individual structure, as is done in other sciences. Statistical thermodynamics has its counterpart in atomic physics; the statistical treatment of large populations has its counterpart in microbiology. It would be a grave error if, in trying to predict the future course of human history, one considered only the behavior of those who have achieved a high degree of internalization and structuralization, instead of considering the average expectable behavior of man, particularly when his autonomy is greatly reduced through acting within a collective.

After having dwelt upon some of the consequences attached to the conversion of instincts into drives in the species *Homo sapiens*, I shall now turn briefly to a particular problem of ego psychology, namely, the antinomies with which the ego is confronted. Antinomies are opposites that are irreconcilable. This quality of irreconcilability may be caused by subjective or by objective factors. But usually a blend of both is involved, as is the case in the following.

Although the progress of science has made accurate predictions possible in some areas, man is still blind to his own future. Imposing as it is that eclipses and other astronomical events can be predicted, in the one area that is of decisive importance man is still bound to act like an inebriate who has lost his sense of direction and staggers vainly trying to find his way. Oddly enough, if man knew the consequences of his actions, this knowledge would paralyze his initiative in many instances. If the early Christians, who were convinced of the imminent Second Coming of Christ, had known the history of the next two millennia, with their religious wars, Inquisition, and mass misery, this would have not only destroyed their conviction but would have also forced them to desist from their devotion to the spread of the Gospels. Similarly, if the Pilgrim Fathers had known that their landing would lead to the Indian Wars, the development of a materialistic civilization, imperialism, and finally the explosion of the atomic bomb, would they ever have left Europe? Here I have referred to man's utter blindness to broad historical processes covering centuries. But the same is true even in relation to a span of decades. Who in 1810, when French armies conquered Europe, would have thought that a mere sixty years later the Prussians would occupy France? In turn, who would have dared to predict that only fifty years later Germany would lie prostrate or, in turn, that a paltry twenty years later Germany would have her armies in France and close to Egypt and, at that time, that it would be only five years before the partition of Germany would start?

I have often thought how lucky I am not to possess the gift of historical foreknowledge. I would never have found employment and probably would not have the honor of addressing you. In 1938, coming from Europe, one was regularly asked for one's opinion of the political future. I was also asked this question by my future chief in my first interview, which was to decide whether I was to be employed. At that time almost every responsible person in this country was convinced that it was out of the question that an American soldier would ever again cross the Atlantic. If I had predicted the landing in Normandy, he would have questioned my judgment. The prediction of Hiroshima he would have relegated to fantasy. Had I claimed that the United States would transport 500,000 soldiers to Asia to fight to preserve a regime in a country not larger than Oklahoma, he would have worried about my common sense. Had I predicted that an American would walk on the moon in thirty years, would he not have thought that I was schizophrenic? The same might have been the case with regard to predictions of cultural developments: had I told him that thirty years later movies would be offered in Times Square that showed intercourse and all known perversions, he would have denied me employment suspecting that I was a pervert.

The German poet Schiller wrote a poem in which a man dies instantly upon unveiling a divine figure that enables him to see the future. A profound truth is here asserted symbolically. We herald the efficiency of the ego's reality adjustment and we admire the superbness of its functions in grappling with reality, and yet the superficial reading of a history text should convince us that if man knew the fate that awaits his progeny of three or four generations later, he would not propagate. To be sure, in organic evolution, according to Simpson (1967), eight phyla disappeared. The proud dinosaurs, ready to become the kings of the land, the water and the air, vanished. But it took a million years for this to happen, and if the dinosaurs had been endowed with reason and known the future of their species, I do not know if they would have acted differently. Their vanishing was possibly not associated with excessive suffering. Louis XVI and Marie Antoinette, however, approaching the guillotine, made a travesty retroactively out of the splendors of the Bourbons and Habsburgs.

Man is forced to act on the stage of history whether he wishes to do so or not; yet at the same time it is impossible for him—be he at the captain's steering wheel or only a cogwheel—to foresee the effect of his actions, although he almost always acts in full conviction that he can do so. Here man faces one of the most serious of the antinomies that confront him.

The second antinomy I wish to discuss is that of man's relation to death. In the Old Testament death quite rightly is pronounced as a punishment that will embitter man's happiness for the larger part of his existence. In his early years he does not know of it and in old age, when life becomes more of a burden than a source of pleasure, he often does not care about it, but in the intervening years something in him rebels against the certainty that life is contingent. With some justification he experiences life as a mockery since it has to end in his dissolution. Moreover, despite his greatness of mind he cannot imagine the state of his own death and cannot represent the state of unconsciousness despite its regular occurrence in sleep. Indeed, everything in a healthy person rebels against the fact of death, and in the deepest, most vital layers of the psychic apparatus the rational knowledge of his end is not only denied but negated. It is well-nigh an impossibility for it to be represented there at all. But man's self cannot escape its awareness. The attempts at escape from this perplexity are well known.

The price man has to pay for being the only species that knows about death is all too great for the privilege of being the crowning product of the process of differentiation.

Again, as in man's relation to history, we encounter here the ego's basic weakness. In sleep all the proud structures which the ego has evolved are buried and the ego must like an infant accept phantasmagoria as reality. Similarly, in death it has to accept defenselessly the victory of what Freud called the death drive. If death were like a period at the end of a sentence, a solitary event concluding life, it would be tolerable, but it is from an early stage on, probably from the latency period on, constantly with man, the only certainty in a life surrounded by contingencies. And it remains a mysterious event, although in the modern scientific mind it should not be. It remains a perplexity, because the human mind is unable to fathom nothingness.

I further should like to discuss here, cursorily, the one antinomy that is represented by the feeling in man of freedom and by its opposite, that of bondage. The feeling of freedom is thwarted, of course, by many factors, partly rooted in man himself, partly in external reality. Yet it is given to man in a form described in the following two lines:

> So every bondsman in his own hand bears
> To cancel his captivity.
>   (*Julius Caesar*, III, 101)

Shakespeare refers here to the extraordinary privilege possessed by man alone, among all species, namely, the ability to put an end to his suffering, to step out of this world of his own accord, when he feels that his creator has let him down. Nothing of this kind is encountered even among man's closest relatives. Animals are condemned to bear their sufferings to the end. It may sound strange when I call the ability to take one's life a privilege, since suicide is generally considered to be a severe form of psychopathology. Notwithstanding the abuse of that privilege, as usually encountered on the clinical level, the potentiality of suicide is an essential characteristic of man's state. As a matter of fact, the number of human beings able to bear their sufferings only by knowing that they have the freedom of ending their lives at will, although undetermined, is undoubtedly rather large. At times this takes an explicit form and is verbalized; but even if not verbalized, it is present in latent form. We are more inclined to be interested in the question of the effect that the knowledge of death has had on man's psychology and culture, but it seems to me that the question of what is the effect of man's awareness of the possibility of suicide deserves equal consideration.

I believe that certain attitudes which are of great psychological import are derivatives of man's ability to commit suicide. Bettelheim (1943) reports that in extreme situations of danger depersonalization protects the self against anguish and pain, which would be otherwise unbearable. A concentration camp inmate gave me once a vivid report which confirmed Bettelheim's thesis. It is almost incredible to hear what tortures a human being can tolerate, when the attitude "It is not I who is tortured" can be activated. Correspondingly, one can understand and empathize when one hears that a German scholar who had survived a prolonged stay in a concentration camp committed suicide shortly after liberation, because he could not withstand the presence of the memories of the indignities he had had to suffer. The lifesaving depersonalization contains mechanisms of denial and undoing. It is based on man's unique ability to put distance between himself and that which he experiences.

This ability not to succumb to the pressures of emotions that are aroused at a particular moment, not to respond to the pains of the body, to banish to the periphery all that which may prevent man from living up to the contingencies of the present, gives man maximum inner freedom. Hatuey, an Indian chief, while being readied to be burned alive, was urged to embrace Christianity in order that his soul might find admission to heaven. When his inquiry as to whether the white man would also go there was answered affirmatively, he exclaimed: "Then I will not be a Christian, for I would not go again to a place where I must find men so cruel." Prescott (1843, p. 123) calls this reply "more eloquent than a volume of invective." Indeed, here is a moment when man shows himself at his best. Facing excruciating pains on his way to death, the representative of a defeated race defies his conquerors in the last moment of his life and hurls at them a reply that contains the prophetic death knell of their own civilization that will ignobly perish one day, crushed by the inherent basic contradiction exposed by the dying captive in one short sentence. Here, indeed, the self emerges in full autonomy and converts defeat into magnificent victory.

But Shakespeare was also aware of man's thralldom, of the utter lack of freedom, which creates the antinomy under discussion. He says:

> As flies to wanton boys, are we to the gods;
> They kill us for their sport.

Although a Shakespeare scholar as renowned as Peter Alexander wrote that "critics of any discernment have long ago given up treating this as the key to Shakespeare's intention" (1955, p. 94), I firmly believe that these two verses contain the essence of the meaning of the tragedy of *King Lear*. Usually Shakespeare takes a while before putting on the stage the focal action around which the play will revolve. No other tragedy of his starts, if I am not mistaken, with an equally forceful action whose consequences will interpenetrate the whole play, as if he wanted to impress on the audience that here the intrinsic nature of the human deed will be discoursed. Indeed, a royal deed, well thought out and reasonable! The contemporary psychoanalyst and also the behaviorist may easily, in view of the crown prince syndrome and generation gap, have advised the aging king,

> To shake all cares and business from our age,
> Conferring them on younger strength, while we
> Unburdened crawl toward death.

There is an additional point which I may advance that speaks strongly in favor of those who see in the earlier cited lines the key to the tragedy. *King Lear* is, as far as I know, the only play by Shakespeare in which an unsuccessful attempt at suicide occurs. Blind Gloucester (4:6) intends to throw himself from the cliffs of Dover, but his son, pretending to be a peasant, leads him to a point from which he throws himself without harm. As if he wanted to annul the great consolation which he had given man in *Julius Caesar*, Shakespeare lets Gloucester say after his thwarted attempt:

> Is wretchedness depriv'd that benefit,
> To end itself by death? 'Twas yet some comfort,
> When misery could beguile the tyrant's rage,
> And frustrate his proud will.

According to the message of *King Lear*, such a degree of

unfreedom and arbitrariness is imposed on man that he cannot even decide upon his own death when he wishes to depart from life.

Man is unable to calculate the consequences of action, not only of historical action as discussed earlier, but also of personal action, even when it is planned, within the narrowest sphere, because of the terrible truth that the gods kill us for their sport. Consequently, action that appears flawless within our earthbound measure may lead to incalculable tragedy.

It is surprising, but we may find in the two verses under discussion the anticipation of recent conclusions of modern biological research, which are summarized in the title of Monod's book, *Chance and Necessity*. It seems to be undeniable that man is the result of chance and necessity, but if this is so then the much vaunted autonomy of the self is an illusion, and indeed man is at the mercy of superior forces "as flies to wanton boys."

The fourth antinomy I selected, among the many there are, has to do with a fundamental property of man's cognitive capacity. Even though one of man's greatest prides is his faculty of abstract thinking and its accomplishments are stunning, his cognitive apparatus is subjected to limits. Splendidly as the concepts of infinity and zero are handled and used abstractly by the human mind, infinity and true nothingness cannot be visualized: they are not accessible to pictorialization in the human imagination—they defy graphicalness. The human mind is of such construction that it is compelled to insist that there must be somewhere a border as well as that there must be something beyond that border. Equally, man is incapable of thinking true nothing. He may exclude substance in his thinking, but he cannot exclude space. A spaceless state is unthinkable. By the question of the origin and the future of space his thinking is checkmated as well as by the infinity of time.

This is a question remote from any practical consequences, and as a matter of fact it disquiets only a few, whereas hardly anyone escapes the disquieting effect of awareness of personal nothingness, that is, of death. Nevertheless, I am inclined to attribute great consequence to the fact that man's thinking is subjected to iron limitations when he turns to the riddles of the cosmos. It is plain that these limitations are not caused by man's unwillingness to recognize the truth, as so often happens when he is victimized by his need for wish fulfillment, that is, a disturbance of the function of reality testing, but by the organic structure of his thinking instrument, the cortex of his brain. Man's brain is prepared by nature to grapple most successfully with medium sizes. Although he has extended by the use of instruments the range of his inquiry beyond that which his sense organs offer him in their natural working, the difficulties accumulate the closer he comes to the almost infinitely large and the almost infinitely small.

The structure of the brain's cortex is, in fact, the one and only place where mutation still has its rightful place and could improve man's efficiency. It is, indeed, a problem why the evolution of the brain stopped at the point it did. According to Dubois (1930), the explosive evolution of the brain in primates was not a gradual one but occurred in leaps. The mammalian psychencephalon did not grow phylogenetically by a gradual increase in brain volume but by repeated duplication of neurons.[2] The question I am raising here in cursory form is why this progressive duplication stopped in man. It may sound like science fiction, but I think one is justified in asking what human life would be like if one more duplication of neurons had occurred. When Freud writes to Putnam that if he were ever to meet God, he would ask Him why He had not endowed him with better intellectual equipment, he raises a fundamental question of human existence (E. Freud, 1960, p. 308). Neuropsychologists like Rohracher (1939, p. 193) state that mankind finds itself in an intermediate state. Cerebral evolution has not terminated. The direction of cerebral evolution and its psychic concomitants, he does not doubt, goes toward "high culture." In such a high culture based on a vastly improved cerebral power, some of the enumerated antinomies would find a solution, I presume, and some of the abstract concepts which now defy pictorial representation may become palpable and open to man's vision, which should greatly contribute to the deliverance of his mind.

It may appear as if I exaggerated the gravity of the antinomies which man is facing, particularly when their effects are compared

---

[2] Versluys (1939) synthesized Bolk's and Dubois's theories into a plausible theory of the biology of anthropogenesis. See, however, Portmann (1962) for arguments against Dubois's theory of leaps in the cephalization of Mammalia.

with the formidable effects on man's destiny of conflicts of such magnitude as the oedipus conflict. But it ought not be forgotten that antinomies have always been the subject of myths and religion, which alone may prove their importance to the human mind. In these sources mankind found answers to the puzzling problems, but science has proved the incorrectness of mythical solutions. In their stead we find abstractions, mathematical formulas, and hypotheses, but no answer that would explain the arcanum.

The antinomies highlight a basic weakness of the ego. As in the instance of the transformation of instincts into drives, one gains the impression that man was released from his bond to nature prematurely, prior to reaching an evolutionary stage at which it would be possible for him to solve the problems of his existence and accordingly organize his behavior: that is, man is bound to fail as a species.

Freud, in examining forces that might cause or contribute to man's psychopathology, found in some individuals a tendency to conflict (1937, p. 244), that is, rival tendencies that although gratified separately without interfering with one another in some, in these individuals clash, creating irreconcilable conflicts.

I wonder whether this observation cannot be extended to the entire species. Is not *Homo sapiens* as compared with other species characterized by a tendency to conflict? To be sure, clinically one finds the whole gamut of attitudes, from the *carpe diem* and *gaudeamus igitur* with all its successful denial and insistence upon momentary pleasurable releases to Nietzsche's dismal exacting demand of "All joy wants eternity" with its tragic implication of constant sadness and disappointment. But underlying the variety of attitudes is the oedipus conflict, which, whatever the society, culture, and particular environment in which a person may grow up in, the child cannot be spared. It is this feature alone, the necessity of going through the oedipus conflict, that permits one to ascribe to *Homo sapiens* a tragic aspect unshared by any other species.

The needs of other higher species can be gratified with ease. It requires relatively little effort to maintain a constant level of contentment in a dog or a monkey. Mankind's history, however, is marked by more or less constant arousal of discontent. In the lives of individuals this discontent is manifested by conflicts observed in two areas where they would have been least expected from the evolutionary point of view: in man's relationship to his own body and in the relationship of the two genders.

In *Faust* (II, 2), a scholar complains to Mephisto that he feels ashamed because one expects from him answers to problems no one has ever solved, such as why soul and body, which fit together so splendidly and hold each other so tightly, as if never to separate, nevertheless disgust each other continuously all day long. Mephisto surprisingly answers that he would rather ask why do man and woman get along so badly. Goethe was quite right when at another place he praised the idea of the two sexes and he called Adam and Eve God's two most enchanting ideas. Indeed, by providing *Homo sapiens* with constant readiness for sexual pleasure, a privilege withheld from nonhuman Mammalia, by providing a body more differentiated and open to a wider spectrum of pleasures than any other species, the stage seemed set for an existence filled with most delightful and exquisite pleasures. But just the opposite came to pass. Most of the human beings who have ever lived have not even been able to satisfy their hunger, and the satiated are tormented by hypochondriacal psychosomatic symptoms that, if anything, make them even unhappier than those whom social reality denies minimal sustenance. The potential of sexual pleasure was severely curtailed by taboos, and the area of greatest bliss was converted into inhibition and conflict.

The tendency toward discontent is also observable in man's relationship to culture. Cultural structures like monotheism and Christianity, which impress one as reflecting colossal evolutionary progress and possess the potential of enriching human existence, turn against man, and there are only very few left who still put any hope in the Evangels.

A new hope arose with the dawn of science. Indeed, rarely has a cultural innovation held its promise so painstakingly as this one did. Sicknesses that seemed to be ineradicable scourges of mankind vanished, and science taught mankind to produce in abundance and with little physical effort all that is needed to gratify not only the basic urges but also the most refined tastes. And again mankind feels deceived, and there are at present perhaps more people who curse science than who praise it. It looks as if all that mankind creates must turn against it, become tainted and corrupted. The promises of bliss, enchantment, and carefree existence are converted into sources of danger, worry, and anguish. This transmutation from hope to despair is a regular historical sequence.

A new movement starts with great promise. A small group puts itself into the service of its elaboration and propagation. They believe with seeming justification in the essential benefits that the innovation will confer upon mankind. Yet to the degree to which the innovation becomes popular and spreads it is partly misunderstood, partly misapplied, and partly abused. In the end it proves itself, even though on theoretical grounds this should not be so, as insufficient to better the human condition. Usually imperfections and weaknesses in the structure of the innovation are held responsible for the default. I doubt, however, that this is actually the case as often as it is claimed, even that it is so in most instances. Is it not rather that the ensemble of factors under discussion here unite to corrupt the innovation? No remedy has obviously been found that could counteract the excess of aggression and narcissism that is a property of the species *Homo sapiens*. Who would have thought it possible when the Evangels started to spread that they would give cause for the bloodiest war that ever had been fought? It came to pass that vast regions were almost depopulated, only because of a disagreement about what meaning was to be ascribed to certain passages of the very Scriptures that had promised the beginning of peace on earth. When Freud (1926, p. 193) asked his interlocutor, "But have you ever found that men do anything but confuse and distort what they get hold of?" he put his finger on this general inclination in man which, circumstances permitting, perverts that which could be a blessing.

The disappointment that turns up in the course of the development of innovations seems to be the fate also of psychoanalysis. With its creation it looked as if mankind had been given a formidable weapon, at last, to acquire by insight power over forces that threaten culture. Beneficial as it has proved to be in alleviating and even curing many forms of psychopathology, it fails in any attempt to use it to solve the grave problems of the present. To be sure, its creator never had thought that psychoanalysis might have such effects, but some psychoanalysts, including myself, thought that proper use of the new science might provide a technique by means of which mankind could gain power over the course of its history, instead of being buffeted around by it.

The present historical moment, however, demonstrates again that there is no measure of insight that could forestall the wildest outbursts of aggression that have to be expected.

I may be permitted to repeat briefly what has become a cliché. An entirely new situation without precedent has arisen on this planet within the last three decades. When more powerful pieces of artillery were invented in the eighteenth century, Montesquieu (1689–1755) expressed fear lest mankind would be destroyed by such potent weapons. Many other thinkers attributed such effects to the weaponry of their times. Yet it is evident that fears and prophecies of this kind were the products of the fantasy of imaginative authors. The hordes of the Huns and Hitler's war machinery, despite their high destructive potential and menace to wide areas of culture, fell far short of being powerful enough to endanger the survival of mankind.

One of the most remarkable features of our times, however, is that according to absolutely reliable information mankind has obtained the power to exterminate life on this planet. According to these sources, it is not a potential power; the existing stockpiles of nuclear weapons—these are the actual means that could, if used, produce this effect. Monarchs had been given in the past the power to set armies into motion that would cause the death of an untold number of people, but ours is the first time in history that the decision of one man alone or at best the decision of a small group of men has the power to initiate a physical process that harbors the potential of ending the life of every man on earth. Will a man or group of men to whose hands this power is entrusted be able to resist the temptation of using it? As experience has taught over and over, temptations to use and abuse power are always lurking in those who possess it.

The other grave dangers which have arisen pale when compared with this one, even though, if unchecked, they would be dangerous to a substantial part of mankind, perhaps to its majority. But even if five-sixths of mankind perished by these dangers, there is justified hope that after two centuries the continents would be adequately populated and the cultural process in full swing. The danger of nuclear warfare goes beyond that. The experts seem to agree that even if man survived a catastrophe such as nuclear warfare, his genetic constitution would be irreparably damaged and man would gradually disappear from the earth's surface as other species have done before. Since nuclear weaponry is equally distributed between two world powers that face each other in uncompromising hostility, each of them claiming that it and only it is able to provide mankind with all the good things in life, one does not need to be a hypochondriac to suspect that such an accumulation of destructive forces as now exists must lead one day to an explosion.

Yet the idea seems to prevail despite all teachings of history that warfare is avoidable, and that man is innately a social being. I have the impression that the present emphasis on the dangers of pollution, the population explosion, and like factors has the function of distracting mankind from the one true cause it should devote itself to exclusively—the destruction of all nuclear weapons. The prospect of nuclear devastation seems so horrible that it is preferred not to think of it, but to propound instead new schemes that promise peace and well-being of the masses while denying man's inherent inadequacy. Man's superiority over all other species is incessantly heralded, although the history of *Homo sapiens* shows irrefutably that he is incapable of resolving the tasks that confront him. Every other species is better adjusted than he, for adjustment means using one's potential to its maximum in the confrontation with reality.

When scholasticism reaches the conclusion that man is less perfect than other creatures by virtue of the very gift of reason which makes him their superior (Willey, 1934, p. 22), one feels inclined to add that this conclusion may also be confirmed by psychoanalysis.

Robert Heilbroner, in his eminent text, *An Inquiry into the Human Prospect*, has described the problem of our time, as well as what the future course of history may be, in an unusually penetrating and concise manner. His outlook is not necessarily less pessimistic than the one I have submitted to your judgment. To my utter surprise, however, he ends his inquiry as follows:

> At this last moment of reflection, another figure from Greek mythology comes to mind. It is that of Atlas, bearing with endless

perseverance the weight of the heavens on his hands. If mankind is to rescue life, it must preserve the very will to live, and thereby rescue the future from the angry condemnation of the present. . . .
It is the example of Atlas, resolutely bearing his burden, that provides the strength we seek. If, within us, the spirit of Atlas falters, there perishes the determination to preserve humanity at all cost and any cost, forever. . . . We do not know with certainty that humanity will survive, but it is a comfort to know that there exist within us the elements of fortitude and will from which the image of Atlas springs.

It is most surprising to witness the realistic, otherwise illusion-free, sociologist-historian in the end taking refuge in a static ancient myth. Atlas, the leader of the Titans, symbolizing rather evil forces, "was awarded an exemplary punishment, being ordered to carry the sky on his shoulders" (Graves, 1955, p. 41). The Atlas myth does not symbolize endurance and patient work toward a better future; rather it symbolizes the man who is condemned to carry passively and endure the burden of existential horror.

The equivalent of the Atlas myth in the world that followed is the image of Christ expiring on the cross. The latter is a dynamic myth because it represents a phase that symbolizes one moment in the course which the world has to take. It is an eschatological image pointing into the future, not only to Christ's resurrection three days hence, but also to his Second Coming. It is apocalyptic, future-directed imagery and not the static imagery of Atlas that is significant of Western thought and feeling.

Possessed by a sentiment, perhaps amounting to a premonition, that something is basically wrong in human affairs, Christianity has, for almost 2000 years, been waiting for His coming.

Indeed, it is possible that Atlas may be freed of his burden in the foreseeable future.

BIBLIOGRAPHY

ALEXANDER, P. (1955), *Hamlet, Father and Son.* Oxford: Clarendon Press.
ARDREY, R. (1961), *African Genesis.* New York: Atheneum.
BETTELHEIM, B. (1943), Individual and Mass Behavior in Extreme Situations. *J. Abnorm. Soc. Psychol.*, 38:417–452.
BOLK, L. (1926), *Das Problem der Menschwerdung.* Jena: Fischer.

Dubois, E. (1930), Die phylogenetische Grosshirnzunahme. *Biologia generalis*, 6:247–292.
Freud, A. (1972), Comments on Aggression. *Int. J. Psycho-Anal.*, 53:163–171.
Freud, E. L., ed. (1960), *Letters of Sigmund Freud*. New York: Basic Books.
Freud, S. (1900), The Interpretation of Dreams. *S.E.*, 4 & 5.
——— (1926), The Question of Lay Analysis. *S.E.*, 20:183–250.
——— (1930), Civilization and Its Discontents. *S.E.*, 21:64–145.
——— (1937), Analysis Terminable and Interminable. *S.E.*, 23:216–253.
——— & Pfister, O. (1963), *Psycho-Analysis and Faith*. London: Hogarth Press, p. 48.
Graves, R. (1955), *The Greek Myths*, Vol. 1. Baltimore: Penguin Books.
Handler, P., ed. (1970), *Biology and the Future of Man*. New York: Oxford Univ. Press.
Heilbroner, R. L. (1974), *An Inquiry into the Human Prospect*. New York: Norton.
Hughes, E. (1956), *Keir Hardie*. London: Allen & Unwin.
Jacob, F. (1970), *The Logic of Life*. New York: Pantheon Books, 1973.
Keeton, W. T. (1967), *Biological Science*. New York: Norton, 2nd ed., 1972.
Lantos, B. (1958), The Two Genetic Derivations of Aggression. *Int. J. Psycho-Anal.*, 39:117–120.
Luria, S. E. (1973), *Life: The Unfinished Experiment*. New York: Scribner.
Meng, H. (1971), *Leben als Begegnung*. Stuttgart: Hippokrates.
Meynert, T. (1892), *Sammlung von Populär-wissenschaftlichen Vorträgen über den Bau und die Leistungen des Gehirns*. Wien/Leipzig: Braumüller.
Monod, J. (1970), *Chance and Necessity*. New York: Knopf, 1971.
Montagu, A. (1968), The New Litany of "Innate Depravity," or Original Sin Revisited. In: *Man and Aggression*, ed. A. Montagu. London/New York: Oxford Univ. Press, 1973, pp. 3–18.
Portmann, A. (1945), Die Ontogenese des Menschen als Problem der Evolutionsforschung. In: *Zoologie aus vier Jahrzehnten*. München: Piper, 1967, pp. 223–230.
——— (1962), Zerebralisation und Ontogenese. *Ibid.*, pp. 230–297.
——— (1964), Die Bedeutung des ersten Lebensjahres. *Ibid.*, pp. 297–311.
——— (1966), Ursprung und Entwicklung als Problem der Biologie. *Eranos Jb.*, 35:411–437.
——— (1968), Der Mensch ein Mängelwesen? In: *Entlässt die Natur den Menschen?* München: Piper, 1970, pp. 200–209.
Prescott, W. H. (1843), *History of the Conquest of Mexico and History of the Conquest of Peru*. New York: Modern Library, n.d.
Richter, J. P. (1883), *The Literary Works of Leonardo da Vinci*, 2 Vols. London/New York/Toronto. Oxford Univ. Press, rev. ed., I. A. Richter, 1939.
Rochlin, G. (1973), *Man's Aggression*. Boston: Gambit.
Rohracher, H. (1939), *Die Arbeitsweise des Gehirns und die psychischen Vorgänge*. München: Barth, 1967.
Rokitansky, C. (1869), *Die Solidarität alles Tierlebens*. Wien: K. K. Hof- und Staatsdruckerei.

SACHS, H. (1933), The Delay of the Machine Age. *Psychoanal. Quart.*, 2:404–424.
SCHOLEM, G. (1966), Martin Bubers Auffassung des Judentums. *Eranos Jb.*, 35:9–55.
SIMMEL, E. (1944), Self-Preservation and the Death Instinct. *Psychoanal. Quart.*, 13:160–185.
SIMPSON, G. G. (1967), *The Meaning of Evolution.* New Haven: Yale Univ. Press.
STAINER, R. T., DONDOROFF, M., & ADELBERG, E. A. (1957), *The Microbial World.* Englewood Cliffs, N.J.: Prentice-Hall, 3rd ed., 1970.
TANNAHILL, R. (1973), *Food in History.* New York: Stein & Day.
TILLICH, P. (1948), He Who Is the Christ. In: *The Shaking of the Foundations.* New York: Scribner, pp. 141–148.
VERSLUYS, J. (1939), *Hirngrösse und Hormongeschehen bei der Menschwerdung.* Wien: Maudrich.
VILLEE, C. A. (1967), *Biology.* Philadelphia: Saunders, 6th ed., 1972.
WILLEY, B. (1934), *The Seventeenth Century.* Garden City, N.Y.: Doubleday, Anchor Books, 1953.

Why Foster Care—
For Whom for How Long?

JOSEPH GOLDSTEIN, PH.D., LL.B.

THIS ESSAY SEEKS TO CLARIFY THE PURPOSES OF PLACING A CHILD IN foster care. It examines two court decisions which came to opposite conclusions concerning the law and administration of foster placements. Both cases illustrate how foster care law and its administration fail to foster continuity of relationships between child and parents from whom the child is separated and between those parents and their absent child. That continuity is necessary to facilitate the resumption of temporarily interrupted family relationships. Each case, in its own way, demonstrates how "temporary" separations in foster care become permanent without fostering the development of permanent relationships between such children and their caretakers. Further, through multiple placements for a single child, foster care has come to be employed to keep a child "familyless" for the duration of his or her childhood. The two cases will be analyzed in terms of the guidelines for decision set forth in *Beyond the Best Interests of the Child* (Goldstein, A. Freud, and Solnit, 1973). Those guidelines for *contested* child placements provide that all such decisions should (a) safeguard the child's need for continuity of relationships; (b) reflect the child's, not an adult's,

---

Walton Hale Hamilton Professor of Law, Science, and Social Policy, Yale University.

I acknowledge the assistance of Janice Abarbanel, Ronald E. Bard, Anna Freud, Sonja Goldstein, Sara E. Huff, Donn Pickett, Spiros Simitis, John G. Simon, and Albert J. Solnit.

Copyright © 1975 by the author who retains all reprint rights. This essay is taken from material prepared for a book.

sense of time; and (c) take into account the law's incapacity to supervise interpersonal relationships and the limits of knowledge to make long-range predictions.

What I say and what justifies much of what I propose is captured in the following brief conversation between a foster daughter and an adopted son in the family to which she was assigned:

"Am I your sister?"

"Oh no, you won't be my sister, not till you've been adopted."

To be "your sister," to be "adopted" expresses every child's need to be wanted—need for continuity of relationships with people and surroundings. For the little girl it meant:

"Can I stay here?"

"Are your mommy and daddy mine, too?"

"Will they love me—even if I'm naughty—even if I make mistakes?"

"Will we be together—always?"

"Will they keep me with them even if someone wants to take me away?"

For the youngster who replied "not until you're adopted," it meant:

"Don't count on staying here. You're only a foster child."

"Someone can always take you away."

"I'm not going to love you—and my mommy and daddy won't either—because you're not staying here forever or else it will hurt too much."

This little conversation is about the "continuity of relationships, surroundings, and environmental influence essential for a child's normal development." Though disruptions in continuity have different consequences at different ages, children of all ages require at least one—preferably two—psychological parents who represent and provide this crucial continuity. For a child to feel wanted and to become a person in his own right, he needs a psychological parent. Psychological parenthood rests "on day-to-day interaction, companionship, and shared experiences." This highly complex and fragile relationship which comes, it is hoped, with being "adopted" and being "a sister" is beyond the law's power to create, but well within its power either to break or to safeguard. To fill the role of psychological parent, it does not matter whether the parents are labeled in law "biological," "adoptive," or "foster." They need only be continually available caring adults. They cannot be continually absent adults, no matter how "caring" they may be. In that sense, the legal labels make little difference. But they make a real difference if society views and treats, as it does through the administration of its laws, the foster relationships as temporary and the biological and adoptive as permanent.

There hangs over current foster care relationships a dual threat which does violence to the child's need for continuity. There is a threat of discontinuity to prior ties not yet broken with the "temporarily" absent parents, and a continuing threat to new, potentially long-term ties with foster parents. These threats alone, whether realized or not, are sufficiently disruptive to prompt both a redefinition of foster care in order to assure that the reciprocal ties between absent parents and child are kept viable and a redefinition of adoption to include foster children whose prior ties, if there were any, are no longer viable.

Two often misunderstood and sometimes apparently conflicting value preferences underlie this analysis of the place of foster care in the law of child placement. The first is a preference for *minimizing* state intervention in all family relationships. It is a preference for safeguarding family privacy, for honoring and respecting the right of parents, biological and adopted, to raise their families as they think best free of government intrusion, except in cases of neglect or abandonment. This value preference comports with, and to the extent that it is reflected in the administration of law reinforces, each child's need for continuity of family relationships. "So long," Anna Freud (1975) has observed, "as a family is intact, the young child feels parental authority is lodged in a unified body and as such is a safe and reliable guide for later identification." Court or agency intervention without regard to, or over the objection of, parents can serve only to undermine that parental authority which is crucial to a child's sense of well-being and ultimate trust in self. Beyond these reasons for minimum state intervention on psychological parent-child relationships, and for safeguarding each child's entitlement to a permanent family of his own, there is another reason which is that the state as *parens patriae* is too gross an instrument to regulate or monitor the delicately complex relationships between parent and child within a family. The state is not and cannot be a substitute for parents. The administration of our delinquency, child neglect, and abuse statutes which have fallen so far short of doing more good than harm makes manifest that self-evident, but often ignored, truth about the limits of law. Before neglect and abuse laws may be invoked to break up families, the state must first use its resources to assist families at risk to remain together by providing, if the parents are willing, a wide range of supportive services in the form, for example, of health, housing, homemaker, and financial aid.

Recognition of an exception to minimum state intervention must not be read as an acceptance of the vague, imprecise, and subjective language of neglect and abandonment statutes. Nor must it be read as a condonation of the not infrequent use of such statutes to tear the delicate psychological fabric of families, particularly poor and minority families, rather than to assist them to remain together. A policy of minimum state intervention calls for a revision of such statutes so as to safeguard families from state-sponsored interruptions of ongoing family relationships by the "do-gooders" who "know" what is "best" and who wish to impose, as if they could, their child-rearing preferences on others. The law must hold in check the rescue fantasies of those it empowers to intrude.

Once a child's placement appropriately becomes a matter of state intervention, however, a second value preference becomes determinative: it is that the child's needs be considered paramount. In such situations the guidelines of finding the least detrimental available alternative for the child becomes operative. That guideline requires that the specific placement and the procedure for placement maximize "in accord with the child's sense of time and on the basis of short-term predictions given the limitations of knowledge, his or her opportunity for being wanted and for maintaining on a continuous basis a relationship with at least one adult who is or will become his or her psychological parent" (Goldstein et al., 1973, p. 53).

I shall now examine, in the light of this overall guideline, two foster care cases and propose a new meaning for foster care.

I

The opinion of the juvenile court judge in the *Appleton* case began inauspiciously with these words:[1]

> Among the few unpleasant burdens which fall upon a Trial Judge is the responsibility to determine the fate of a young child.

Apparently, the judge felt confronted not with an *opportunity* to protect a child's chances for healthy growth, but with the *burden* of destroying that chance.

The Appletons were foster parents of Tom, a 5-year-old who had lived with them for the last four years of his life. They had asked the court not to return Tom to his biological parents as demanded by the County Child Care Service, but rather to allow him to remain in their custody, and, if possible, to be adopted by them. The judge declared that the County agency had "real custody" of Tom and the authority to determine what was best for him. Yet he acknowledged that: "If . . . the best interests of the child received paramount consideration, this court could readily determine that young Tom would obtain greater advantages and benefits" with the Appletons. But they had only *de facto custody*, even though they were for Tom his psychological parents—from his point of view, his only parents. The court observed:

> [T]he agency to whom the child was awarded . . . is satisfied that the causes which gave rise to the committal no longer exist and the child should be brought back to its natural parents.
>
> ["Just like that," one might add. But the court added:]
>
> The Appletons accepted the child with knowledge of the terms of the agreement and received money compensation for their services. The agreement also provided the Appletons were not to institute any proceedings with a view to adoption or placement. While a child's custody should not rest alone upon a contract and a child regarded as mere chattel, the natural parents have natural rights and obligations and are entitled to their child.

---

[1] The names used are fictitious. Therefore, no citation is given to this 1973 decision.

And finally, in an apparent effort to reinforce his decision, the judge mechanically recited:

> Under the present Juvenile Court Act, Section I, 11 P.S. Section 50-101, it is expressly stated that the unity of the family whenever possible is to be preserved. *The family itself is an institution whose sanctity must be preserved.*

Paying lip service to the state's commitment to minimum intervention and to continuity of family relationships, the court proceeded to *destroy* for Tom the only family he had ever known. The integrity, stability, and sanctity of Tom's family was thus shattered by court order. For Tom, the death of the Appletons in a tragic auto accident ultimately might have been easier to manage. He knows that his foster parents really are alive, but out of his reach and sight by court order. To safeguard child care agency policy, to enforce a contract, and to preserve a nonviable family relationship, the court sacrificed the future of a child. In any other breach of contract case, involving personal services, not chattel, in any other case in which disappointed adults, such as the biological parents, might establish pain and suffering, the court could have awarded no more than money damages. It could have threatened no one who breached the contract with imprisonment. Yet, it ordered Mr. Appleton to be jailed if he continued to refuse to give up his son. Certainly, it could not have imposed upon any adult human being, especially one who had no part in making the original contract, specific performance of personal services as it did upon Tom when it ordered him to leave his home to live with "strangers."

Finally, as if blind to reality, the court with apodictic assurance pronounced another principle of minimum state intervention and continuity in support of a ruling which so violently defied it.

> The state is and should be restrained in removing a child from its parents except under the most unusual conditions.

And *so it should*. But the child's parents in this case were the Appletons, not his long absent progenitors from whom he was removed before the age of 12 months.

But the court was unable to apply its own guidelines. It could not or would not recognize which of the two competing units was Tom's real family and who among the competing adults were Tom's real—that is, psychological—parents. The court took a mechanistic blood tie route to identifying Tom's family and parents. It ignored four years of unusually affectionate care as the determinative factor. It did not ask "Whom does Tom possess," but rather, "Who may possess Tom?" The court, misreading in traditional fashion its guide to decision, allowed the state to intrude massively upon Tom's ongoing family relationships and to shatter for Tom and his foster parents their real family.

Even if his biological parents were ideal, even if they were in all ways superior to the Appletons, and even if the state were in error in its initial decision to place Tom in foster care or to leave him there for more than a temporary period, Tom should never have been *awarded* as damages. What was once intended to be a "temporary" placement had become permanent. The relationship between Tom and the Appletons deserved recognition as a common-law adoption—and deserved to be treated with the same finality as the traditional placement of a child with his biological parents. Only in that way could the court have given credibility to its announced policy in favor of family unity and of "restraint in removing a child from its parents except under the most unusual conditions."

Though they are not and indeed ought not to be relevant to the decision in this case, the unusual facts of Tom's repossession by his biological parents add to the tragedy of the court's decision. What the court knew of them offers little comfort to those who entertain some magical expectation that all will somehow turn out for the best. The record revealed that the biological mother had been responsible for the death of a 1-month-old infant son, who suffered a brain hemorrhage after she struck him on the head in anger; that she broke another son's leg in an outburst of temper and later severely burned the same child as punishment; and that she severely kicked a third 16-month-old child in an angry rage. She had been under medical care most of her adult life, including a two-year commitment to a mental hospital. The biological father had had a drinking problem.

Had Tom been accorded party status and been represented as a person in his own right, the court might have been forced to focus on *his* needs rather than allow itself to be trapped in the law's own fictions which made the Appletons *de facto custodians,* which made the anonymous County Child Care Service *real custodians,* and which made the biological parents Tom's *real family.*

II

At approximately the same time, a similar proceeding but with a different result was taking place in another jurisdiction. The opinion of Family Court Judge Tim Murphy, *In the Matter of N.M.S.,*[2] concerns a 9½-year-old child, called Maggie, who lived all but the first eight days of her life with the Thomases, her foster parents. Maggie had originally been committed to the custody of the District of Columbia's Social Rehabilitation Administration (S.R.A.) for foster home placement. She had been declared a homeless child without adequate parental care. Like the Child Care Agency in the *Appleton* case, the S.R.A. who retained legal custody recommended that her biological mother be allowed to repossess her. Maggie was given an opportunity to describe her feelings to the Judge. She strongly objected to being removed from her home. The Thomases asked the court to terminate the S.R.A. custody and to give them legal custody.

Following four days of hearings in which each party, including Maggie, was represented by independent counsel, Judge Murphy found that it would not be in Maggie's best interest to return her to her biological mother. He noted that the S.R.A.'s recommendation, despite its use of best-interest language, was made "without any serious consideration of the best interests of Maggie." He found that the S.R.A. was primarily acting out of fear of unfavorable publicity for the agency from a lawsuit threatened by the biological mother. Judge Murphy saw his obligation to determine instead what would be least detrimental for Maggie. He declared that she was a "neglected child," even though he found that she had not been abandoned or abused and that her biological mother was "not

---

[2] *In the Matter of N.M.S.,* J-51-806, Family Division of the D.C. Superior Court, 1-28 (Jan. 1974). This case, which I call the *Thomas* case, may be cited since the court does not use the real names of the parties to the dispute.

unable to discharge her responsibilities—that she would be able, in the language of the statute, to 'care or control' Maggie in a physical and material sense to adequately clothe and feed and attend to her medical needs." Yet, the court, Judge Murphy advised, "must consider the emotional and mental needs of the child in reaching a neglect determination. [It] would clearly be disregarding the words of that statute were [it not to weigh] the emotional and mental impact on Maggie of the court's decision." Judge Murphy in effect decided, *not* that Maggie was neglected and without care for her emotional health, *but rather that she would be a "neglected child"* if her membership in the Thomas family were to be terminated.

In making this strained but constructive application of the neglect statute, Judge Murphy treated as determinative a child's need for continuity with her psychological parents, here her foster parents. At the outset, he advised:

> A psychological parent is one to whom the child becomes emotionally attached because of the parent's day-to-day attention to his needs for physical care, nourishment, comfort, affection and stimulation.
>
> [He later found that:] Maggie has known only one home during her 9½ years . . . has thrived extremely well in that home . . . and is very happy with, secure in and well-adjusted to the foster home.
>
> [To this finding, he added this footnote quotation:] Psychoanalytic theory establishes as do developmental studies by students of other orientations the need of every child for *unbroken* continuity of affectionate and stimulating relationships with an adult. *(Beyond the Best Interests of the Child)*

Unlike the judge in the Appleton case, Judge Murphy focused on the needs of the child, not on those of the biological or foster parents or those of the child care agency:

> The Court finds that the best interests of this child would not be served by removing her from this warm and happy home she has known all her life, from her foster parents whom she calls "Mommy and Daddy," from her four foster brothers and sisters, to place her in an environment where she feels uncomfortable and anxious, to live in a place she does not want to live and with a woman more an acquaintance than a mother. In reaching its decision, the Court is not finding [the biological parent] an unfit mother in a material

sense, nor is it finding that the Thomases are more fit than [the biological parent.] The Court is considering the best interests of Maggie and Maggie only.

The court turned down Maggie's adoption. It appeared to be a legally unavailable placement alternative. Judge Murphy also rejected, though he seriously considered, placing Maggie with her biological mother for a six-month trial period to see how Maggie might be affected.

> [But the] Court decided against this alternative because the Court finds it unfair, and potentially very damaging, to experiment with this child in order to satisfy [her biological mother's] desire to have Maggie with her, which at this time in the Court's view would be clearly adverse to the child's interests.
>
> The Court believes in her own way [the biological mother] would try to do what is best for Maggie, but it is a question of too little too late. With the wisdom of hindsight, perhaps if a greater effort had been made years ago to join Maggie and [her biological mother], the reunion now could be done without harm. Time, however, has worked against the reunion because the Thomases are now the child's psychological parents and the child needs continuity of this relationship.

The court, not quite able to go all the way to assure Maggie full membership in the Thomas family, ruled that Maggie's foster parents would have legal custody, conditional, however, on the biological mother's being able to visit Maggie in her foster family's home every six weeks.

Aware that a child's sense of time is different from an adult's, that a relatively short period of uncertainty by adult standards may be a long time for a child and a threat to the continuity of family relationships, Judge Murphy, as soon as he had reached his decision, called the parties to his chambers to tell them what it was. He ignored custom and practice which would have had them wait until his opinion had been written and filed. By thus modifying a procedural practice to accord with the least detrimental alternative standard, Judge Murphy spared Maggie, her foster parents, and the biological mother too, but particularly Maggie, more than a month of long days and nights anxiously wondering what their fates would be.

The skill and flexibility required of Judge Murphy to safeguard Maggie's interest must be used not to obscure, but *rather to highlight,* how inadequate and cruel are the foster care laws and their administration. Even the ingenious escape from the statutory straitjacket which Judge Murphy masterminded for Maggie fell short of giving her the same assurance of a permanent family which generally comes with adoption or the assignment at birth of a child to his natural parents. Maggie is still a foster child subject to court-enforceable conditions of visitation which remain to threaten the continuity of the psychological parent-child relationship which the court struggled so vigorously to protect.

Discussion

The remainder of this essay is devoted to a proposal for reducing the likelihood of these law-made tragedies—whether they occur for the child who is insecurely and indeterminately placed with one foster family, as in the *Appleton* or *Thomas* cases, or for the child who is shuttled from one foster family to another in accord with a not uncommon child care agency policy for discouraging continuous and permanent relationships between child and foster parents.

Foster care must have a new face. It must be redefined in practice, not just theory, to be temporary. So long as foster care is expected to be and is in fact temporary in theory only, it can be, as it has become, a legal fiction for destroying families, especially poor ones. A decision to place a child in foster care must carry with it an expectation for all parties, including the court, that the child will shortly, in accord with the child's sense of time, be restored to his or her family, and that during the period of separation provision can be made for keeping alive the ties that bond both child and absent parents. Disturbance to the continuity of his ties with parental figures and of their ties to him must be kept to an absolute minimum if their reunion—which must be the *goal* of foster care—is to safeguard their mutual interests. What this will mean both in terms of temporariness and in terms of provisions for maintaining reciprocity of affectionate relationships will depend in large measure on the child's age at the time he is placed in foster care and upon the extent and form of accessibility of child and parents to each other during the period of separation. The younger the child the shorter should be the duration of such a placement if it is to be temporary.

What foster care arrangements might be made for 2 to 3 weeks, possibly more, for a child between $1\frac{1}{2}$ and $2\frac{1}{2}$ years of age, is suggested by the work of James and Joyce Robertson (1971). Foster "parents" would be required to discuss, whenever possible, with the infant's natural or adopted parents the child's eating, sleeping, and toilet habits and preferences, as well as the ways in which the child is comforted. The foster parents would have an opportunity to observe how the real parents talk, play, and generally handle their child. Plans might be made for the child to have with him in his foster home his own bedding, toys, even a photograph of his parents and of his own room. Plans would be made, where possible, for either or both of the real parents to visit or be visited by the child. Efforts to do this would be facilitated by trying to arrange foster placements in the neighborhood of the child's real home. For the school-age child, continuity of neighborhood surroundings, for example, would facilitate maintaining ties with school and friends. The variations for trying to meet an individual child's as well as his parents' fundamental needs not to break the ties between them are countless and beyond the scope of this essay.

Clarification that the purpose and the expectation of the new foster care are to preserve the family relationships for child and absent parents and that it must be temporary should prompt at the time of decision a realistic evaluation of the circumstances which suggest consideration of foster care and of the opportunities for its effective implementation. Recognition, for example, that the circumstances which justify foster care are more chronic than acute and that the probability of long-term separation is very high should force renewed consideration of supportive resources for keeping the family intact. Barring the availability of such resources, adoption should be considered as the least detrimental alternative for assuring the child an immediate opportunity for the unfolding of his full potentialities as a regular member of a new but permanent family.

If the circumstances, including provisions for preserving existing ties, justify foster care, the court must determine in advance the maximum length of time for that arrangement to remain temporary. That period would minimally take into account the particular child's sense of time, his capacity and his parents' capacity to sustain their relationship during separation, and the nature of the circumstances leading to the placement. To assure that no such placement extends beyond the maximum without reconsideration by the court, each case would be tagged to resurface for review shortly before the expiration of the maximum. Such an *early warning system* would uncover those cases in which the child had not yet been restored to his family. A new determination would now be required to consider the advisability of restoration, with or without supportive services, and if that is found not to be a reasonable option, to arrange for the adoption of the child—possibly and probably preferably within the foster family with whom new ties have begun to develop.

In the event the early warning system fails to uncover a foster placement which extends beyond the maximum time set for the particular child or in the event no such time is set, a statutory cut-off period might be established. It would provide, for example, that for children from infancy to 6 years of age, after 12 (?) months and for those over 6 after 18 (?) months in foster care, the child is presumed to be adopted by his foster family or, if the foster family does not wish to adopt, that the child may be considered adoptable.

In those situations where foster families do not wish to adopt but may wish to continue indefinitely the now long-term foster relationship, it may be less harmful for the child to continue in that relationship than to break it just to fulfill the state policy which perceives foster care only as a temporary relationship. Such long-term relationships might be reclassified as *foster care with tenure*. That classification would provide a relatively high expectation in the child and his foster parents of the continuity that generally is associated with adoption. The law would insulate tenured foster families from the threat of interruption by the long-absent biological parents or by the child care agency whose policy has been offended.

Whatever the statutory cut-off period—which by definition must be arbitrary—provision would be made for foster parents to petition, not only after, but at any time prior to the expiration of the statutory period for a court to find that the foster relationship is no longer temporary and either that the child be found to be adopted by his foster family or that the child be reclassified as *foster child with tenure*. Finally, just as supportive services to keep families at risk is to be preferred to foster care placement, long-term relationships should be secured by adoption or tenure in the foster family and encouraged by not cutting off, but rather even by enlarging, maintenance payments to foster parents willing to accept a long-term arrangement.

Under a statute which so defined foster care and adoption, both Tom and Maggie would have either automatically, by passage of time, or in a very simple legal proceeding, been held to have been adopted by their real psychological parents or been given the status of *foster child with tenure*. At the time of his placement, it is unlikely that Tom would have been seen as a child for whom ties with his natural parents could be maintained or that it was likely that he could be returned to them within a reasonably short time. He would have been directly placed in adoption.[3] As for Maggie, so far as is known, supportive services for her biological mother might have been the preferred alternative to foster care. In any event, foster placement as a temporary arrangement might have been a reasonable prospect.

The proposal goes to future placements. But what of the thousands of children currently in more than temporary foster care? Except for the fortunate few who come to the attention of a Judge

---

[3] Tom was removed once again from his biological family upon the discovery of severe welts on his back. This—and it is difficult to believe one is talking about a human being—prompted Tom's transfer, not to the Appletons but to a children's orphanage. Thus Tom was left in cruel limbo—placed at risk by his *parens patriae*, the state—while the Appletons sought to restore the already damaged psychological ties between them. More anxious to protect its foster care policy than Tom's well-being, the child care agency opposed Tom's return to the Appletons. Unaware of a child's sense of time and his sense of abandonment, and apparently uncomfortable about acknowledging its part in putting him at risk, the court took 6 months to decide that it would be in Tom's best interests to be returned to the Appletons. But Tom's uncertainty about who, if anyone, will care for him on a permanent basis still seems never-ending. The judge noted that Tom had not been abandoned by his biological parents and that adoption by the Appletons is unlikely under current laws.

Murphy, are they to be kept in limbo during their entire childhood?

A large percentage of the children presently in foster care in this country are not likely to be returned to their absent parents; yet most of them face the continuing threat of being removed from the only real home and family they know. They appear not to be entitled as citizens in their own right to that constitutional protection which makes each of us secure in our own homes from the seizure of our person. The continuity of such threats must be removed from the life of these children by interim legislation which would provide that all children presently in foster care for more than, for example, 18 (?) months are either presumed to be adopted by the family in whose care they have been or else are eligible to become foster children with tenure or adoptable if they are not wanted by their foster family. Payments made to foster parents would, of course, automatically continue so as not to discourage but rather to make more secure these families in their assumption of full and permanent responsibility. Under such legislation, a battery of lawyers, a stack of evaluation reports, days of hearings, and lengthy judicial opinions would no longer be required to justify and secure each child's right to continue to live with his or her real, though not necessarily biological, parents. That right would simply be secured.

Such legislative reinforcement of a child's entitlement to a permanent family and the parents' entitlement, no matter how poor, to their children should in turn force focus on the need for a realistic reappraisal of neglect and abuse statutes. Children as well as parents must be assured that they will not be forcefully separated, except in accord with a policy of minimum state intervention reflected in precisely defined standards for intrusion. Those standards must defer to the human dignity and autonomy of parents to raise their children as they see fit. But there is no magic in changing words. Such standards, no matter how precisely defined, must be administered by persons who understand and accept the underlying philosophical and psychological bases for minimum coercive intervention. Otherwise the law of foster care may continue to be used as it must no longer be, to keep children at risk. Through such legislation—administered with full appreciation of its purposes—the law may then begin to assure for each homeless child a home, and continuing membership in a family where he feels wanted.

BIBLIOGRAPHY

FREUD, A. (1939–45), Infants Without Families. *Writings*, 3.
—— (1975), Beyond the Best Interests of the Child. London: *Times Lit. Suppl.* (in press).
GOLDSTEIN, J., FREUD, A., & SOLNIT, A. J. (1973), *Beyond the Best Interests of the Child*. New York: Free Press.
MNOOKIN, R. H. (1973), Foster Care: In Whose Best Interest? *Harvard Educ. Rev.*, 43:599–638.
ROBERTSON, J. & ROBERTSON, J. (1971), Young Children in Brief Separation. *This Annual*, 26:264–315.

Vicissitudes of Narcissism and Problems of Civilization

JEANNE LAMPL-DE GROOT, M.D.

IN THIS PRESENTATION I SHALL ATTEMPT TO PROCEED ALONG THE PATH indicated by the founder of psychoanalysis. Freud repeatedly said that he had only made beginnings. He encouraged others to continue to extend psychoanalysis theoretically as well as practically and to apply it to other human sciences.

A psychoanalytic contribution to the problem of civilized societies can only be a limited one. Nevertheless, I feel that it might be worthwhile to venture a few ideas on this topic. As a psychoanalyst I shall start with observations made in the psychoanalytic treatment situation. In particular, I shall examine the genetic roots of the working alliance.

This term does not appear in Freud's writings. It is a concept that emerged in the psychoanalytic literature many years after Freud's death (Zetzel, 1956; Stone, 1961; Loewenstein, 1969; Greenacre, 1954, and in Greenson's work from 1965 onward). The term is used interchangeably with "therapeutic alliance." I believe the two terms cover the same phenomenon. A patient who has decided to work in an alliance with the analyst does so in order to obtain a therapeutic result, to be cured from his symptoms and his mental distress. Greenson uses, in addition, the term "real or nontransference relationship" between analyst and patient. This relationship is different from the working alliance. It concerns the analyst's

---

Presented as the Freud Anniversary Lecture of the New York Psychoanalytic Institute on April 10, 1973 at the New York Academy of Medicine.

attitude that in addition to being professional should also be humane—an important issue that has sometimes been neglected.

The Concept of the Working Alliance

Working alliance is an appealing concept that must be studied carefully by every analyst. Yet, in going through the literature, I found that it is used rather loosely and with slightly different meanings.

There seems to be a consensus of opinion on the description of its starting point. Jack Novick (1970) summarizes the common denominators as follows: "The core of the alliance is the patient's conscious, rational willingness to do analytic work. The motivation for such work is the awareness of suffering and the wish for cure. . . . The alliance becomes most apparent at times of heightened resistance and transference" (p. 236).

Even this generally agreed-upon formulation, however, raises questions. Experience has taught us that conscious motivation and rationality are overthrown when during the analytic process instinctual and emotional conflicts enter into the picture. If the *core* of the patient's alliance, his bond with the analyst, were no more than his conscious rational wish to be cured, he certainly would run away from the analysis at the very moment when this rational wish is no longer at his disposal. As a matter of fact, there are patients who stop the analysis at such a point. Every analyst has dealt at one time or another with this problem. However, in most of the cases the patient continues the treatment. We must therefore ask ourselves: what is the nature of the patient's tie to the analyst that enables the patient to stay in treatment notwithstanding strong resistances? What makes the patient continue despite his feeling that the analyst mistreats him, is an incompetent therapist, a bore, an inhuman person, or even a criminal?

In fact, Freud dealt with this problem in his early papers on technique. He believed that the affectionate, aim-inhibited part of the transference kept the analysis going in spite of strong resistances. This affectionate tie is part of the object relationship to the parents after the oedipal conflict (colored, of course, by the preoedipal factors) has passed away. At that time (1911–15) analysis was applied only to the transference neuroses, cases in which the core of symptoms centered on the unsolved conflicts of the oedipus complex. Later, when Freud also analyzed character neuroses and narcissistic personalities, he did not explicitly enlarge on his technical arsenal, though he was aware of the fact that these disorders originated in a much earlier phase of development, in the early mother-child relationship.

Narcissistic Versus Object-Libidinal Relatedness

Today we deal more frequently with analyses of character neuroses and narcissistic disturbances than with transference neuroses proper. This may be one of the reasons why the analyst feels the need for a separate term to distinguish the alliance with the analyst from the transference. The classical meaning of the term "transference" relates to the reemergence of the ambivalent object-libidinal tie to the parents in the analytic situation, while the working alliance is a *narcissistic* manifestation. It starts with a self-directed striving—the decision made by the relatively mature "normal" part of the personality to be freed from mental suffering. In view of the fact that the working alliance disappears at times of heightened resistances (which is convincingly described by Novick in his case presentation) but is nevertheless considered to become most apparent in precisely those situations, one has to wonder how these contradictory statements can be reconciled.

The transference of affectionate, object-directed, libidinal strivings is dynamically not sufficiently powerful to enable the patient to uncover and relive strong narcissistic, self-centered, infantile needs. What bond with the analyst, then, enables the patient to reexperience at least part of his unsolved conflicts of infancy and early childhood? One of the principles of psychoanalysis is the genetic approach to mental phenomena. I think we have to look for the genetic roots of that facet of the patient-analyst relatedness which is covered by the term "working alliance." They will be found, I am sure, in the very early bond of the infant with the mother, a bond that is exclusively narcissistic and self-centered. Its dynamics are dramatically powerful. The energy of impulses, drives, and needs is *relatively* much stronger in little children than in adults, because the ego develops only gradually and is still weak and vulnerable in childhood.

In the symbiotic phase the exclusively narcissistic nature of the mother-child dyad is self-evident. However, when the infant becomes aware that the satisfaction of his needs comes from the outside, his tie to the mother is still of a narcissistic nature. I venture the idea that here lie the genetic roots of the working alliance. I shall later describe the ways in which they may manifest themselves in the analytic situation. I continue with the description of the lines of development of the baby's experiential world.

The infant experiences the mother as an extension of his self. This is still the case in the individuation-separation phase (Mahler, 1968). However, the toddler who starts to crawl, to walk, to explore the world constantly meets with limitations, disappointments, and painful hurts. Even the most loving "good" mother cannot fulfill all of his needs immediately. She cannot prevent her little one from bumping himself against a piece of furniture. The little child feels lost, powerless, helpless. Such narcissistic blows are usually much more catastrophic than the physical pain of a scratch or a wound. The intensity of the injury to his self-assurance is often not understood by his mother, who usually has repressed her own infantile experiences and emotions. The little child then desperately tries to take refuge in his fantasy world. In order to compensate for his injured self-esteem he starts to create fantasies of grandeur and omnipotence.

In addition to a "grandiose self" (Kohut, 1971), he idealizes his mother and his parents, who in fact are less powerless than he is. At the time the little child is able to preserve the inner representations of the parents even in their physical absence—when he has reached object constancy—the cathexis of the object and its representation is still mainly narcissistic. The inner image of the parent serves as an extension of the child's self. Several years pass before the child is able to love his parents and other persons living in his small experiential world as personalities in their own right who have their own personal wishes, feelings, qualities, and peculiarities. In other words, it takes time for the child to invest his objects with object-directed libido. I think this kind of object relationship, which develops gradually alongside the narcissistic relatedness, usually becomes more or less settled in the oedipal situation. The precise point of time at which this happens, however, differs from individual to individual. On the one hand, it is dependent upon the infant's innate endowment in regard to drives and the gradually unfolding ego functions; on the other, it is greatly influenced by the kind of mothering and the emotional responses of the parents and other relevant persons in the little child's world.

In relatively "normal" development the object-directed libidinal ties grow during latency and diminish to some degree in puberty during which a relative increase of narcissism is a regular occurrence. In adulthood we consider as sound a durable love relationship in which both partners respect each other's personalities. However, the developmental line of object-libidinal ties (ambivalent as they may be) proceeds alongside the development of narcissism from its archaic, grandiose state into more realistic feelings of self-esteem, longings for self-satisfying achievements, and attainable ideals. A certain amount of self-love is a precondition for the capacity to love another person with empathy, respect, and appreciation.

I have tried to describe briefly the two lines of development of object-relatedness: the narcissistic one originating from the archaic mother-child dyad in the first years of life, and the object-directed libidinal relationship which grows out of it at a much later date.

This differentiation has a bearing on the understanding of the genetic origins of both the transference and the working alliance. To achieve the ability to invest the object with object-directed libido the child must have reached a certain degree of maturation. On the energetic side, drive development must at least in part have reached the phallic stage. On the side of the ego, a number of functions must have matured; for example, the child's reality sense must have reached the stage at which he is able to perceive the object not only as an instrument for fulfilling his bodily and emotional needs, but as another personality in his (or her) own right.

I see the working alliance as having its genetic roots in the very early narcissistic mother-child bond. Transference in the analytic situation is rooted genetically in the *object-directed libidinal* relationship. This sharp distinction is of course clouded in later stages of development. Then the two kinds of object ties become intermingled. In the preoedipal phase the narcissistic tie is prevalent. In the oedipal phase object-directed strivings acquire more impetus. During latency the aim-inhibited affectionate relationship begins to bloom. These various stages can be observed during the analytic process. The distinction between the genetic roots of working alliance and transference may clarify the statement stressed by most authors: that the working alliance is *not* transference, has to be distinguished from the transference, and is of equal importance. It may also explain the contradictory pronouncements that the working alliance disappears at times of heightened resistance, whereas it is supposed to become most apparent at those times. I believe that the solution is theoretically simple. The conscious rational wish to be cured disappears when overwhelming childhood conflicts are uncovered and relived, but the unconscious archaic root of the alliance, the narcissistic tie to the mother that is relived in the analytic situation, persists and is the "carrying power" for the continuation of the analytic process.

In practice the situation is not simple. It is often laborious and time-consuming for both analysand and analyst to disentangle transference manifestations, e.g., of the oedipal object relations, from the earlier narcissistic object ties.

Narcissism in Psychopathology

With the classical transference neuroses the uncovering of the repressed oedipal conflicts, the object-libidinal love-hate relationships that are transferred onto the analyst, is sufficient to bring the strivings and affects under the matured ego's control. The neurotic symptoms can be cured by working through these conflicts. It is different with character neuroses and narcissistic personality disorders, in which an underlying fixation and/or regression to the archaic narcissistic tie to the object is responsible for the uneven development of ego functions.

In these cases the bond with the analyst is of a different nature. The analyst must therefore empathically enter into the experiential world of the infant and toddler. In the most severe disturbances, for example, with an autistic child or psychotics, this primitive narcissistic tie seems to be absent or too weak to be reached in the analytic situation. Infants who never experienced mothering care, e.g., institutional babies, either die or become very retarded children unable to reach a stage of narcissistic relatedness. I myself have no experience with the therapy of psychotics, but I worked a great deal with narcissistic disturbances. Such individuals generally have a primitive tie to a motherly person, unstable as it may be, because it was formed with a disturbed mother whose inconsistent behavior alternated between spoiling and neglecting the baby.

I have discussed some of the technical difficulties presented by these cases in earlier papers (1965, 1967, 1969). Kohut (1968, 1971, 1972) has devoted several publications to the analytic devices needed in the treatment of narcissistic personality disorders and demonstrated them in several case presentations. Kohut (1971) poses the question whether the therapeutic mobilization of the narcissistic structures (including the grandiose self and the idealized parent images) should be covered by the term transference. In a footnote Kohut mentions a comment of Anna Freud's, in which she points out that in these cases the patient uses the analyst not for the revival of object-directed strivings, but for the inclusion in a libidinal (narcissistic) state to which he has regressed or at which he has become arrested. She suggests to call that a "subspecialty of transference" (p. 205). Kohut himself adheres to the term "narcissistic transference."

From the foregoing it might have become clear that I prefer to reserve the term "transference," in its classical conceptualization, to the revival of object-directed strivings in the analytic situation. The term "subspecialty of transference" does not appeal to me. I would call this kind of relatedness *the narcissistic tie*. One of the reasons for my preference is the observation that this kind of bond differs qualitatively from the transference of object-directed strivings with their accompanying affects of love and hate. (In Europe we speak of a different color of this bond.) At the height of the transference neurosis, the analysand does not show concern with the analyst's personality. He is too much involved in his past conflicts. However, at other times he is able to take a certain distance from his childhood troubles and can perceive the analyst as a "real" person—that is, if the analyst is responsive to it. If he is unresponsive, such an inhuman attitude may disturb the patient and damage the course of the analytic process.

In contrast, when in an analytic treatment the stage of the very early *narcissistic* tie comes to the fore, the patient is completely absorbed in his own inner conflicts and *uses* the analyst merely as part of his grandiose self and omnipotent fantasy world. He feels that the analyst is the real, actual, and exclusive source of his complaints, his distress, his emptiness, his powerlessness, and he makes the analyst responsible for everything that threatens his narcissism. He really tries to use the analyst as an extension of his self, like the baby did with his mother.

In the experiential world of the little child the parent really *is* omnipotent and therefore responsible for every mischief. I agree with Kohut that the analyst should not interfere with the unfolding of the patient's idealized world of his self and of the analyst. Such periods may be prolonged and difficult because of the patient's intense anxiety, which he can overcome only with the assistance of the analyst who temporarily must accept the role of an omnipotent parental figure. This applies especially to cases where the actual mothering and parental understanding was absent or totally insufficient. In such situations the analyst needs a lot of empathy and an ability to put himself into the infant's and toddler's experiential world, which is so different from the adult's world. However, after an uncovering and at least a partial working through of the little child's idealized world, the analyst's task should become once more to represent reality to the patient. He should then point out to his analysand that the feelings and fantasies of grandiosity (of self and parents) are "normal" mental products in the magical world of the little child who in reality is small and powerless, but that they are not appropriate in the realistic adult's world. In adulthood one has learned to accept the realistic limitations of every human being as well as the fact that everyone is powerless in a number of life situations.

The working through of these disillusioning facts may be laborious and time-consuming as the earlier phase of uncovering the grandiose world. The patient often clings tenaciously to the omnipotent image of his analyst, on the one hand because he shares in the analyst's fantasied grandiosity and on the other because he can make the analyst responsible for everything. It is the duty of a godlike, almighty creature to fulfill every need and to undo all distress of the poor patient. This magical fantasy is a *creation* of the patient. The fact that it finally must break down may arouse nearly intolerable narcissistic injuries. It parallels in the *emotional world* the severe offense the little child experiences when the *bodily* performance of "creating" feces as a wonderful and originally admired product meets with its final devaluation by the mother, who throws it away as being dirty and worthless. If the mother has failed to accompany her child in his progressive move from one developmental phase into the next one with emotional understanding of his specific maturational course, abilities, and alternating progressions and regression, the analyst later on must try to serve as a *tool* for the patient in his attempt to catch up with this developmental lack. At this point the analyst has to become aware of the changed *quality* of the patient-analyst bond. It reveals itself in the patient's behavior, attitude, posture, tone of voice, stammering, temporary somatic complaints, body language, and other facets. Whether the final outcome of this working through will be a success or a failure depends upon the tact, empathy, and patience of the analyst and on the patient's endurance and special talents and proclivities.

Narcissism and "Normality"

Following the psychoanalytic tradition of turning from pathology to normal development, I come back again to the fate of the original narcissistic tie to the parents and the object-directed strivings in so-called "normal" individuals. This problem is not only of theoretical interest; we also become involved in it with analysands who seek psychoanalytic treatment for reasons other than wanting to be cured from suffering, i.e., persons whose conscious motivation arises from their professional life. There are some scientists working in other fields of the humanities who do not intend to become psychoanalysts, but who want to know more about the unconscious sources of their own mental makeup. The problem is of course most apparent in the training analysis of psychoanalytic candidates.

A certain amount of "normality" is indispensable for the professional task of an analyst. We consider mental health to be the outcome of inner and outer harmony, a well-balanced interaction between the forces of the drives, those at the disposal of the different ego and superego functions, and an *active* or *passive adaptation* to the outer world. This is only, if ever, acquired by a very few. A number of candidates function relatively well in certain areas—their work, their family relationships, their social contacts. If they are really motivated to become analysts, they gain awareness of the special goal of a training analysis—knowing as much as possible about their particular character structure and their personal peculiarities. Certain neurotic manifestations which are present in nearly every intelligent and sensitive person have to be removed first. Next the residuals of the infantile narcissistic experiential world may come to the fore. The rational part of an adult's personality may encounter great difficulties in recognizing a split in his personality and in accepting the persistence of an unconscious part adhering to the images of a grandiose self and idealized, omnipotent parents. If these unconscious, archaic fantasies are subjected to analytic work, the analysand may discover that they are still active and influence his behavior in many instances. They become apparent in the analytic situation by virtue of the different *quality* of the tie to the analyst, as described above. The analysand's resistances to this part of the analytic process can be extremely strong and sometimes they may become unsurmountable obstacles to a favorable outcome. Several factors account for such failures.

1. I have already mentioned the observation that for many people narcissistic injuries are unbearable and can lead to a breakdown of their self-confidence. They feel at a complete loss, empty, incapable of doing anything. The analyst should be on the alert and use his empathy either to forestall such a threatening situation, or to *help* the analysand to master it.

2. Another outcome may be a *secondarily* heightened feeling of grandiosity and an inaccessible delusional attitude. A vicious circle may come into existence. Many decades ago I spoke of "a personal delusion." By this I meant that a "core" of delusional formations remains present in everybody's unconscious, though its impetus varies individually. Whether this delusion will have a detrimental effect or lead to only minor impairment depends on its relative

strength in relation to the other forces available to the "healthy," rational part of the personality.

3. It is a complicating factor in human development that the infantile grandiosity will at some time or other inevitably clash with reality. We also know that disappointments and frustrations evoke, alongside feelings of being unloved, particularly strong narcissistic injuries. It is especially the impaired self-esteem that mobilizes great amounts of *aggression* and *destructive* feelings.

Narcissism and Aggression

The theme of aggression has been widely discussed in the recent psychoanalytic literature. It was the main theme of the 1971 International Psychoanalytic Congress in Vienna as well as of many individual contributions too numerous to list here. I refer only to the study by Eissler (1971) who attempts to lend support to Freud's theory of the life and death drives. I agree with most of his reasoning, since I came to similar conclusions in 1955 (see Lampl-de Groot, 1965, chap. 18). In regard to the drive theory, however, I prefer to use the term "drive" for the psychological manifestations and speak of *biological forces* steering living organisms from birth to death.

Instead of discussing these highly interesting problems in this paper, I turn to observations of other living beings. It is most striking to observe the difference in the effect of both the libidinal and the aggressive forces in human beings and in other species of the animal kingdom.

I was immensely impressed when I saw large herds of all kinds of antelopes and other herbivores, grazing peacefully a few yards away from a group of lions and lionesses, sleeping under a tree in the East African bush and savannahs. Lions and other beasts of prey do not murder for the sake of murdering. They kill whenever they are hungry, or feel threatened, or if they have to defend themselves against stronger animals.

In contrast, man may murder his fellowmen for very different purposes, not merely for survival. In certain circumstances, e.g., in wartime and especially in concentration camps as we know from the time of the Nazi regime, killing and murder may become sources of various shades of satisfaction. It is remarkable that young soldiers, who in civil life actively opposed the establishment, will obey their superiors with docility and sometimes with lust in murdering a civilian population. There are only a very few who refuse to do so. Millions of intelligent youngsters let themselves be lulled by such slogans as "defense of the fatherland" and the need to eradicate "inferior races." Would this be possible if there were no murderous impulses in every human being? Eissler (1971) explains the difference in behavior between animals and man by pointing out that man's object relations are of an ambivalent nature. Together with narcissism they are the steering wheels for aggression. Eissler ends his essay with the dictum: "aggression, ambivalence, and narcissism become mankind's apocalyptic horsemen, when they ride together, as they always seemed to do" (p. 75).

Yet, is there no ambivalence in the animal world? I think there is, at least in the more highly differentiated animals. In animals lower on the evolutionary ladder, destructiveness manifests itself in different ways and serves dissimilar purposes. I am thinking primarily of higher mammals. Jane van Lawick-Goodall (1971), who lived for many years in the bush of Uganda, has recorded her observations on chimpanzees, the closest relatives of men. Chimps live in family groups and keep very closely together. There is usually a strong bond between the members, "loving" each other as expressed, for example, in grooming activities and in the protection of the young and the weaker against dangers. They live in a hierarchical structure, the strongest male being the leader. Chimps are omnivorous and feed mainly on fruit and plants, only occasionally killing a smaller animal. The leader clearly is the first to feed. He can be very angry if a second-in-command tries to take his share. The others meekly wait for the remains, finally fighting each other to get part of the kill or the other food. There is a real ambivalent relationship between the family members, but they will not murder for any other motive than survival.

What then are the special human qualities that enable man to murder without being hungry or having to defend himself against a life-threatening danger? Is it narcissism? Is narcissism an exclusively human feature? There certainly is a biologically founded "body narcissism" in chimps, not unlike that in human beings. Chimps masturbate and they obviously have pleasant sensations in grooming themselves, but we cannot assume that they have a fantasy life and grandiose fantasies like human beings. Chimps communicate with each other by "shouts" or "screams," but symbolic language occurs only in human beings as far as we know. It is a human acquisition which enables man to shape his fantasy life verbally. The result is that fantasies continue to live on in the mind in word representations, though they may become unconscious. The clash between the archaic grandiose fantasies and reality evokes great amounts of aggression.

Another difference between humans and primates lies in the fact that human children grow through an extremely long period of dependence on their environment for survival. With higher mammals this period stretches over a few years. A chimp baby clings to his mother, first onto her tummy and later on riding on her back for some two years, until he is able to feed himself. It is different with human children. This is especially the case in civilized societies, in which the children's dependence on the adults usually extends far into adolescence or even into adulthood. A latency period in drive development is present in chimpanzees too, although it is of much shorter duration than in men. In some illiterate human societies, where a symbolic language in words *does* exist, children are much earlier able to provide for themselves than in civilized countries. They do not learn in schools, but from their parents, elders, and other children.

Jomo Kenyatta (1938) described this extensively in relation to the Gikuyu tribe in Kenya, East Africa, where he was born. According to Kenyatta, the upbringing of children usually follows a smooth course, with parents and child mutually understanding each other. As a result, the child early acquires work skills and independence. Of course, opposition and deviating behavior are not absent, but they are relatively scarce. Disciplining is taken over by the age group at a very early time. The severest punishment is to be considered as an outcast. Another remark by Kenyatta concerns the tribal wars, which are fought solely for survival, for example, when cattle diseases and drought threaten the population with starvation. Even then no women and as few males as possible are killed.

Murder for the mere pleasure of murdering occurs very rarely. This state of affairs was cruelly disturbed when the Western European countries felt compelled to impose their civilization on what they considered "savages." It led to a disruption of the original society. However, here I wish to stress that the early independence and the emotional understanding between parents and child further a more peaceful life.

There are of course other tribes and differently structured societies which exhibit far more violence, e.g., the Dogon and Agri tribes of Africa studied by Parin et al. (1971). But the authors are "Western foreigners" and the French-speaking tribes already "morbid groups of West Africans," according to some anthropologists. It would indeed be a fascinating topic to study different communities from the special point of view of how they deal with aggression. While there exists much more literature on African tribes and on ancient African culture, I cannot go into this interesting topic in this presentation.

Civilization and Destructiveness

I return to the point concerning the destructive forces at work in civilized societies. We are in need of collaboration with various other disciplines, being concerned with human affairs in order to explain the reverse side of the medal in civilization. I mean we should not only be proud of the human achievements of conquering part of nature by science, art, and technology, but also study the drawbacks, the misuse of our achievements in individual, and largely in the joint acts of inflicting distress, humiliation, and destruction on each other. As a matter of fact, I do not intend to suggest that we abandon civilization and return to "primitive" societies, but I believe that we could learn something from their way of life. The European has robbed the Africans of their land and as Kenyatta (1938) says, "He is taking away not only their livelihood, but the material symbol that holds family and tribe together" (p. 317). The land was robbed to make money—for profit and *power*. The rifles and machine guns of the Europeans were superior and much more destructive than bow and arrow of the inhabitants. The conquerors murdered in order to satisfy their *craving for power* and secure submission.

I feel they were living out their personal fantasies of grandeur and omnipotence, with destructive urges breaking through. Is there not a parallel with the older generation in the civilized countries who, having lost contact with their children's world, try to subdue them to make them obedient, submissive, and tractable mass products? There were indeed periods in the history of civilization during which the ethical standards led to attempts to liberalize and to gain freedom for individual development. However, what has become of these endeavors? Time and again the striving for power and omniscience of some leaders has prevailed. Supported by sophisticated rationalizations, they wielded a new kind of power and acted out their unconscious omnipotent wishes, without shunning suppression, discrimination, torture, violence, murder, and war. At first the less sophisticated were subdued, but gradually they became aware of the injustice imposed upon them. Is one to wonder that with the spreading of knowledge by the mass communication media the younger generation resorts to opposition and violence?

As psychoanalysts, we have acquired knowledge about the period in human life when reason is not yet present. An infant's inner world is governed by needs and passions which are often sufficiently satisfied during the symbiotic phase in the mother-child dyad. As soon as he enters the next developmental phases, he becomes aware of his powerlessness, which disturbs his narcissistic equilibrium. Then, I repeat once more, his grandiose fantasies of self and parents have to compensate for the narcissistic injury. The little child's inner world is steered by his feelings of omnipotence and grandeur. When he has acquired speech and thinking, he has his own specific logic; he may, for example, say, "If I will be big, you mommy will be my child and I will wash your hands." Adults may laugh at him, but they usually do not understand the child's inner evidence and the damaging distress they impose upon him by their reaction. It is one example of the misunderstandings between the experiential worlds of children and adults. Being laughed at is one of the most severe damages to a sensitive child's self-esteem. He feels rejected and unloved and therefore inferior and powerless. This inner distress awakens aggression, destructive impulses, and once more fantasies of grandeur, but the latter now have to be kept secret. The consequence is a new estrangement from the parents, and an urgent impulse to live out aggression and destructive urges. Murderous impulses cannot be acted out by the child and are warded off by different maneuvers; but they live on in the repressed, unconscious part of the mind and are accompanied by anxiety and guilt.

The parents in their own infancy were subjected to similar injuries, which they had to ward off and relegate to oblivion. As a consequence they are incapable of empathizing with the child's experience and react with anger, rejection, and punishment. This alienation of the little child's world from the parents' seems to be most prevalent in the so-called civilized societies, in which the system of upbringing apparently fosters this process by laying stress on the intellectual development and sending the children to schools. It is well known that many children then feel abandoned and unloved by the parents. The school may provide new frustrations. The accumulation of distress may make it difficult for the child to adjust to this kind of education and his emotional life may become crippled or distorted. This educational system differs strikingly from the system of upbringing in some of the illiterate societies, e.g., in the Gikuyu and Masai tribes described by Kenyatta.

The smooth and playful learning from elders and one's own age group, without any pressure for intellectual work, seems to prevent or minimize alienation between children and the older generation to a great extent. The emotional life is allowed to express itself in plays, dances, and all kinds of festivities. In Western civilization, the repressed resentment of the lack of empathy in the parents, who fail to understand their little sons' and daughters' predicament of being powerless, creates hostile, self-centered disappointments and narcissistic injuries. Youngsters then may call for revenge and attempt to overthrow their elders' precepts and ethical norms. The clash between generations, with its recourse to more or less violent opposition, has come to the fore periodically during the history of mankind's social development, though in various forms and with different means.

Conclusion

I started this presentation by trying to uncover the early roots of the working alliance in analytic treatment. When I began to discover how difficult and time-consuming it is to undo the split in an adult's personality between his present and his past experiential world, I gained the impression that psychoanalytically obtained knowledge may eventually contribute to the world's problems of individual and social misery. It is man himself, after all, who through countless generations has created his social world. A change from the outside in hierarchical social structure is necessary in many respects, but the frequently voiced idea that this will solve all problems and remove all distress seems to be an illusion. Without a change of the inner emotional world of human beings the outcome of all social and economic corrections may prove to be short-lived and even provoke a reverse reaction.

It is normal for the little child to feel himself to be the center of the world, to have the right to demand all satisfactions, to expect that his "omnipotent" parents will undo every pain and misery, and to experience the impulse to kill whenever he is infuriated as a result of being confronted with his real limitations by the outside world.

In the inner world of an adult such an attitude is rightly considered to be a pathological delusion. Nevertheless, we meet with the reemergence of these repressed delusions in smaller and larger groups of people. In communities and small societies, competition, striving for power, self-aggrandizement, and destructive inclinations come to the fore time and again. Unfortunately, psychoanalytic societies are no exception. Perhaps, analysts should make a start, by trying to conquer the repressed childhood world and letting the hidden forces mature and add to rational behavior in adulthood. Whether this process will ever be achieved in smaller and larger groups and populations cannot be forecast at the present time. The renouncement of personal power, self-aggrandizement, and aggression seems to be a most difficult task, yet these proclivities are the most powerful enemy of the longing for understanding, unity with fellowmen, and love.

When Freud wrote *Civilization and Its Discontents* (1930), it was necessary for him to prove the universality of aggressive and destructive drives in man. Freud saw the destiny of mankind as dependent upon the question whether and how far civilization will finally be able to master the destructive and the self-destructive impulses. As mentioned above, Eissler (1971) added ambivalence and narcissism to the dangers threatening man's future.

I have tried to underline the alienation between the archaic primitive experiential world and the later sophistication as one other of the many factors involved. Civilization promotes rationality, unfortunately at the expense of empathy with the emotional life. Alienation between generations strengthens the lust for power to compensate for the original helplessness and evokes destructive acting out on both sides. This mutual estrangement often finds its way into society at large, with the disastrous outcomes of suppression, robbery, war, and all kinds of misery.

I close by questioning whether man will finally be capable of mastering the repressed residues of his archaic infantile experiential world, allowing its forces to mature and be utilized for more harmonious and peaceful purposes. Will lust for power and aggrandizement together with aggression and destruction prevail, or will loving empathy be recovered in the long run, tiding over the years of upbringing and the emotional gap between generations, countries, peoples, and the differently shaped communities?

BIBLIOGRAPHY

Eissler, K. R. (1971), Death Drive, Ambivalence, and Narcissism. *This Annual*, 26:25–78.
Freud, S. (1911–15), Papers on Technique. *S.E.*, 12:85–171.
——— (1930), Civilization and Its Discontents. *S.E.*, 21:59–145.
Greenacre, P. (1954), The Role of Transference. *J. Amer. Psychoanal. Assn.*, 2:671–684.
Greenson, R. R. (1965), The Working Alliance and the Transference Neurosis. *Psychoanal. Quart.*, 34:155–181.
——— (1967), *The Technique and Practice of Psychoanalysis.* New York: Int. Univ. Press.
Kenyatta, J. (1938), *Facing Mount Kenya.* London: Secker & Warburg, 1961.
Kohut, H. (1968), The Psychoanalytic Treatment of Narcissistic Personality Disorders. *This Annual*, 23:86–113.

——— (1971), *The Analysis of the Self.* New York: Int. Univ. Press.
——— (1972), Thoughts on Narcissism and Narcissistic Rage. *This Annual,* 27:360–400.
LAMPL-DE GROOT, J. (1965), *The Development of the Mind.* New York: Int. Univ. Press.
——— (1967), On Obstacles Standing in the Way of Psychoanalytic Cure. *This Annual,* 22:20–35.
——— (1969), Reflections on the Development of Psychoanalysis. *Int. J. Psycho-Anal.,* 50:567–572.
LAWICK-GOODALL, J. VAN (1971), *In the Shadow of Man.* New York: Houghton Mifflin.
LOEWENSTEIN, R. M. (1969), Developments in the Theory of Transference in the Last Fifty Years. *Int. J. Psycho-Anal.,* 50:583–588.
MAHLER, M. S. (1968), *On Human Symbiosis and the Vicissitudes of Individuation.* New York: Int. Univ. Press.
NOVICK, J. (1970), The Vicissitudes of the "Working Alliance" in the Analysis of a Latency Girl. *This Annual,* 25:231–256.
PARIN, P., MORGENTHALER, F., & PARIN-MATTHÈY, G. (1971), *Fürchte deinen Nächsten wie dich selbst.* Frankfurt: Suhrkamp.
STONE, L. (1961), *The Psychoanalytic Situation.* New York: Int. Univ. Press.
ZETZEL, E. R. (1956), Current Concepts of Transference. *Int. J. Psycho-Anal.,* 37:369–376.

An Attempt at Soul Murder

Rudyard Kipling's Early Life and Work

LEONARD SHENGOLD, M.D.

THE TERM "SOUL MURDER" APPEARED IN THE PSYCHIATRIC LITERATURE after its use by the psychotic Daniel Paul Schreber whose *Memoirs* (1903) were the subject of extensive study, most notably by Freud (1911).

The term does not originate with Schreber. It was used first by Strindberg in an 1887 article on Ibsen's *Rosmersholm*. Strindberg defined soul murder as depriving a person of his basic reason to live. The concept obsessed Strindberg, who was then writing *The Father* (Jacobs, 1969). Soul murder was a repetitive theme of Ibsen's; he used the term directly in the 1896 play, *John Gabriel Borkman*. There he speaks of it as a "mysterious" sin mentioned in the Bible for which "there is no forgiveness" (Archer tr., p. 246), and says it involves "killing the instinct for love" (Paulson tr., p. 334).

Ibsen and Strindberg wrote mainly about the destruction of the souls of adults, and the arena for that destruction was the family. In this century, soul murder has spread beyond the home to become public and institutionalized in brainwashing techniques of political prisons and concentration camps. The confrontation in soul murder is between the all-powerful and the helpless basically between hostile, cruel, psychotic, or psychopathic parents (or authorities) and the children (prisoners) in their charge.

Schreber's much-censored account defines soul murder as inherently vague but involving an assault on his sexual identity and his

---

Director, Division of Psychoanalytic Education, State University of New York, College of Medicine at New York City, Brooklyn, N.Y.

power of rational thought. Niederland's work (1959a, 1959b, 1960, 1963) on the inhuman, crazy child-rearing ideas and practices of Schreber's father has supplied the environmental genesis for the soul murder. The child Schreber was manipulated as if he were a thing. He was purposely, systematically, and, above all, righteously deprived of his own will, and of his capacity for pleasure and joy. And he was not permitted to register what had happened to him.

I shall illustrate this with a clinical example of soul murder (Shengold, 1975). A father entered the dining room. The round table was set for the family meal. Beside each plate was a fresh banana—the dessert. The man made a complete round of the table, stopping at every chair to reach out and squeeze a banana to pulp, but spared his own. The older children and the intimidated mother, used to such happenings, said nothing. But the youngest, a 5-year-old boy, began to cry when he saw the mangled banana at his plate. The father then turned on him viciously, demanding that he be quiet—how dare he make such a fuss about a banana? We know from Orwell's *1984* (a primer on soul murder) of the confusion and split registration in thinking (he calls it "doublethink") that are both the effect of brainwashing and the means by which the torturer keeps his hold on the victim who must not be able to reason about—to know—what has happened to him. After the squashed banana incident, the boy was left in confusion. What had occurred? Who was to blame? A child cannot adequately contain and master a trauma that he is unable to register properly in his mind. Brainwashing is basic to soul murder.

The righteousness, the religiosity of parents like the elder Schreber can undermine the child's ability to know and to hate what is done to him. If the victim is in the tormentor's absolute power, the child can turn for rescue and relief only to the Godlike tormentor. The child needs to see the torturer as good and right. The parent who claims a divine benevolent rightness "consonant with the Order of the World" (Schreber, 1903, p. 58) is so intensely needed for rescue, that the child must compromise his own identity, take on the parent's view. He submits, identifies, and not only exonerates but even glorifies the persecutor. Overstimulation by torture, and the narcissistic deprivation caused by the absence of anyone who cares, can break down even adults—like Winston

Smith in *1984*. The overwhelming anger and hatred evoked by the torment must be suppressed and turned against the self in the terrible urgency to escape annihilation by "loving" and identifying with the "Big Brother" who brought about the trauma (Shengold, 1963, 1967, 1971).

Soul murder can be overwhelmingly or minimally effected; it can be partial, or attenuated, or chronic, or subtle. Kipling's case involved desertion by good parents and their replacement by bad persecutory guardians.

A child can frequently bear much torment if his parents can share the misery, literally or empathically. To experience trauma alone, with no recourse to parents, means that in addition to external insult and the absence of protection, there is the psychic threat of deprivation of the identity-sustaining sense of narcissistic promise. The feelings of identity and of self-esteem depend on the maintenance in the mind of the child of an image of an omnipotent parent who cares and will rescue. Separation from, and transformation of, this parental imago that starts out as part of the self image are necessary for maturation, but to be tolerable the differentiation should be gradual—and the result is always incomplete. No one ever loses the need for "emotional refueling" (Mahler, 1972) so marked in the separating toddler who must periodically return to his mother.

A sudden, an unprepared-for, loss of parental care is one of the greatest human tragedies, even for adults. This is inherent in brainwashing techniques, which involve an alternation of overstimulation and sensory deprivation that is calculated to increase the need for, and destroy the hope of, loving concern. Even iron-willed old Bolsheviks have been broken to a submission to Big Brother Stalin. It is much easier with children, especially if they are separated from their parents. Children have little ability to contain overwhelming stimulation and intense feelings of destructive anger. Anna Freud (1965) reminds us that for children to be able to tolerate hatred directed toward their also-loved parents, those parents' "reassuring presence" is essential (p. 113).

If the child has experienced a period of good parental care prior to the attempt at soul murder, as Kipling did, there is less destruction. Yet the fall from bliss to torment is especially cruel.

Here is a comment of Kipling's, from an autobiographical story (1888b), about parental desertion:

> When a matured man discovers that he has been deserted by Providence, deprived of his God, and cast, without help, comfort, or sympathy, upon a world which is new and strange to him, his despair, which may find expression in evil-living, *the writing of his experiences,* or the more satisfactory diversion of suicide, is generally supposed to be impressive. A child, under exactly similar conditions *as far as its knowledge goes,* cannot very well curse God and die. It howls till its nose is red, its eyes are sore, and its head aches [p. 290; my italics].

Kipling describes the child's helplessness, made so terrible by his lack of understanding. He also hints at a way toward transcendence for himself—the child may grow up and be able to write of his experiences. This means *knowing* what happened to him, and the more he can know (of what happened to soul as well as to body), the freer he can become. The soul, the identity, can be preserved if the adult can say, like Whitman: "I am the man, I suffered, I was there" (1855, p. 21). Kipling used his mind to fight to preserve his soul.

Rudyard Kipling experienced as a child of 6 the fall from the Eden of an overindulged and privileged childhood to the hell of desertion followed by a hostile stewardship that made for years of persecution. He was born in 1865, in Bombay, to a young and ostensibly loving British couple. He was a wanted first child whose every wish was indulged by a self-effacing pair of substitute parents: his *ayah* (nurse) and his bearer. He was the only son of an important Sahib, the center of a world full of wonder. His domain was the garden of a bungalow in the compound of a school of art presided over by his father. He was treated as a young prince. Meeta, the Hindu bearer, talked to him in the native tongue that was the boy's predominant speech in his early years. Rudyard's first memory is of early morning walks to the Bombay fruit market with his *ayah,* a Roman Catholic from Goa. Death and castration were in the background of his idyllic existence. The house in Bombay was near the Towers of Silence, where the Parsee dead were exposed to be devoured by vultures. "I did not understand my mother's distress when she found 'a child's hand' in our garden, and said I was not to ask questions about it. I wanted to see that child's hand" (1937, p. 356). Some of the boy's questions were answered by his *ayah*. She and Meeta often told stories to the children (a sister was born when Rudyard was 2½) at bedtime or before the afternoon siesta. There is an example at the beginning of the autobiographical short story, "Baa Baa, Black Sheep" (in which the children were given the sadomasochistically charged names of Punch and Judy):

> They were putting Punch to bed—the *ayah* and the *hamal* and Meeta, the big *Surti* boy, with the red and gold turban. Judy, already tucked inside her mosquito-curtains, was nearly asleep. Punch had been allowed to stay up for dinner. . . . He sat on the edge of his bed and swung his bare legs defiantly.
> 'Punch-*baba* going to bye-lo?' said the *ayah* suggestively.
> 'No', said Punch. 'Punch-*baba* wants the story about the *Ranee* [princess] that was turned into a tiger. Meeta must tell it and the *hamal* shall hide behind the door and make tiger-noises at the proper time' [1888b, p. 283].

Mostly the stories of early childhood were told by the *ayah* or his mother. In Kipling's description of his earliest years, there appears a theme which resounds through his fiction and poems: he is rescued from a bad mother figure (like the *Ranee*-tiger) by a good father-figure:

> Meeta unconsciously saved me from any night terrors or dread of the dark. Our *ayah*, with a servant's curious mixture of deep affection and shallow device, had told me that a stuffed leopard's head on the nursery wall was there to see that I went to sleep. But Meeta spoke of it scornfully as 'the head of an animal,' and I took it off my mind as a fetish, good or bad, for it was only some unspecified 'animal' [1937, p. 356].

Another bad early experience with the feminine (followed by consolation by a man) was an attack by a hen when Rudyard was crossing the garden:

> I passed the edge of a huge ravine a foot deep where a winged monster as big as myself attacked me, and I fled and wept. [He was comforted by his father who] drew for me a picture of the tragedy with a rhyme beneath—

> There was a small boy in Bombay
> Who once from a hen ran away
>   When they said: 'You're a baby,'
>   He replied: 'Well, I may be:
>   But I don't like these hens of Bombay.'
> This consoled me. I have thought well of hens ever since [p. 357].

Kipling's light humor here expresses a characteristic minimization of fear and hatred, and he ends with a denial. This may be an important memory—later he could identify with his father who set an example for the transcendence of trauma by "the writing of [one's] experiences."

The parents, like so many others in the Victorian age, were in the background of the nursery life. Rudyard was the favorite and lord of a nursery world dominated by maternal and maternalizing figures. He was strengthened against the threats of his own hostility and of the dangerous fascinating world outside the nursery by the grandiosity that comes with maternal favoritism. "If a man has been his mother's undisputed darling," says Freud (1917) of Goethe, "he retains throughout life the triumphant feeling [*Eroberergefühl:* feeling of a conqueror], the confidence in success, which not seldom brings actual success along with it" (p. 156). One thinks of the marvelous self-confidence of Kim, or the more cloying aplomb of Wee Willie Winkie.

There was a sharp break in Kipling's life when he was 2½ years old. His mother was pregnant and the family returned to England where she would have the baby. In old age Kipling wrote about this journey: "There was a train across a desert (the Suez Canal was not yet opened) and a halt in it, and a small girl wrapped in a shawl on the seat opposite me, whose face stands out still. There was next a *dark* land, and a *darker* room full of cold, in one wall of which a *white* woman made *naked* fire, and I cried aloud with dread, for I had never before seen a grate" (1937, p. 357; my italics). One cannot help wondering if this is a screen memory—the frightening woman again appears. The visual stimulation of the dangerous "naked" fire against the dark background might very well have been, then or later, associated with the child's fantasies of the primal scene and of his mother's pregnancy.

When the Kiplings arrived in England in 1868 they stayed with

Alice Kipling's relatives. The indulged Anglo-Indian child was quite uninhibited and rather aggressive; his behavior was not what was required of an English child of those days. He is remembered as charging down the streets of a country town, yelling: "Out of the way! Out of the way, there's an angry Ruddy coming" (Stewart, 1966, p. 1). After the Kiplings left, Rudyard's Aunt Louisa wrote of the visit: Alice's "children turned the house into such a beargarden, and Ruddy's screaming tempers made Papa so ill, we were thankful to see them on their way. The wretched disturbances one ill-ordered child can make is a lesson for all time to me" (Green, 1965, p. 23).

The family returned to Bombay after the birth of Rudyard's sister Alice (usually called Trix). The mother's labor had been difficult. A third child was born and died in India when Rudyard was 5—shortly before his exile. There is no direct evidence of the effects of these births on Rudyard, but they must have profoundly influenced the child, threatening and perhaps compensatorily increasing his narcissism and adding to his aggressiveness (and his hostility toward the betraying mother). But the boy remembered these first six years of indulgence and magic as overwhelmingly wonderful. The motto to the first chapter of his autobiographical fragment, *Something of Myself*, is a maxim of the Jesuits: "Give me the first six years of a child's life and you can have the rest"—a proper Freudian sentiment.

Paradise was lost when Rudyard was almost 6 and his parents again took him to the "dark land." It was customary for the British ruling class in India to send their children to England to be educated. According to Carrington (1955), Kipling's admiring and "definitive" biographer, the timing of the separation in the Kipling family "came early by customary standards" (p. 14). This would appear to be an understatement—Trix was not yet 3! Mrs. Kipling had a large, distinguished, and seemingly devoted family in England. One sister, a lifelong favorite of Rudyard's, was married to the successful pre-Raphaelite painter Edward Burne-Jones. It is a mystery to Kipling's biographers that the children were not left with anyone in the family. A friend of Alice Kipling said that "she had never thought of leaving her children with her own family, it led to complications" (Green, p. 29).

The children were put in the charge of complete strangers who had attracted attention through a newspaper advertisement. Rudyard and Trix were abandoned suddenly, without any preparation or explanation—the parents simply disappeared and returned to India. Not knowing why they had lost their parents was an agony to the children. Rudyard's mother told him later that she had been advised that it was kindest to spare the children the torment of a good-bye. Whatever her motives, and they cannot really be known, at the least she shared the lack of empathy for the child that seems to have been so prevalent in Victorian times, and that was frequently passed down from one generation to the next as part of a compulsion to repeat the past—sowing misery even in the homes of the wealthy and privileged.

When Kipling was grown up, his mother was a loving and charming person, very devoted to her son. Yet it is a mystery how, even after she knew of Rudyard's suffering and breakdown under the care of the foster guardians, she could have left her daughter Trix, a sensitive and nervous child, for several more years with them after removing her son. Here is a description of Alice by her younger sister Edith:

> The Irish blood which is pretty certainly in our family seemed to take effect in Alice; she had the ready wit and power of repartee, the sentiment, and I may say the *unexpectedness* which one associated with that race. *It was impossible to predict how she would act at any given point. There was a certain fascination in this,* and fascinating she certainly was . . . a cheerful, good-tempered, kindly elder sister in my childhood, and a loving friend my life through [Green, 1965, p. 17f.; my italics].

The unexpectedness was a quality in her puzzling character that fascinated and tormented her son. Secrecy and unpredictability are evident not only in her failure to say good-bye to the children; when she returned to England six years later it was also without a word of warning. Years later she had Rudyard's schoolboy poems privately printed without his knowledge or permission—these included early love poems and Kipling was furious. Her brother Frederick tells of Alice's verbal aggressiveness: "Her wit was for the most part humourous and genial, but on occasion it was a weapon of whose keenness of point there could be no doubt, and foolish or mischievous people were made to feel it" (Stewart, p. 5).

The intensity of the overt loving and dependent later relationship with his mother is implicit in Kipling's editorial comment in his short story, "The Brushwood Boy." When the Brushwood Boy returns from India as a man to his home in England, his mother, curious and fearful that he might have marriage plans, comes up to his bedroom to tuck the grown man in: "And she sat down on the bed, and they talked for a long hour, *as mother and son should, if there is to be any future for our Empire*" (1895b, p. 355). Beneath this cosmically significant mother-son harmony lies all the intense antagonism and distrust of women that is so prevalent in Kipling's poetry and prose (e.g.: "And a woman is only a woman, / But a good Cigar is a Smoke" [1885, p. 99]).

Kipling's father, Lockwood Kipling, was a distinguished artist, artisan, and teacher. His brother-in-law Frederick wrote that he was "gentle and kindly in spirit, and companionship with him was a continual refreshing." Rudyard certainly shared that opinion in his later years. Frederick Macdonald goes on:

> [In comparison with his wife his] mind moved more slowly and cautiously, but covered a wider range. His power of acquiring and retaining knowledge was extraordinary. His memory seemed to let nothing slip from its grasp. On what may be called his own subjects, those connected with the plastic arts . . . craftsmanship . . . industrial processes where they come into the domain of art, he was a great expert . . . his curiosity was alive and active . . . all things interested him. He seemed to know something about everything as well as everything about some things [Green, p. 18f.].

Rudyard's formidable intellectual equipment and memory, as well as his intense curiosity, come from his father—by way of inheritance or identification.

The Kiplings left their children in the care of the Holloways: a retired sea captain (a man Rudyard liked who unfortunately soon died), and his wife, called "Aunty Rosa" by the children, a tyrannical, narrow-minded, religiously obsessed woman. She was the boy's prime persecutor—invariably called "the Woman" in his writings. The children always referred to Lorne Lodge, the

Holloways' home in Sussex, as the "House of Desolation." They stayed there, without seeing their parents again, for six years. Trix describes their lodgings:

> Our lessons were always in the dining-room, the basement 'play-room' being too damp for Aunty: there was a rusty grate there, but never a fire, or any means of heat, even in the depths of winter. This perhaps accounted for the severe broken chilblains that crippled me from December to February every year, until Mamma came home. Aunty had an economical theory that if children played properly they kept beautifully warm, but our mushroom-smelling den, with wall cupboards where even a doll's china dinner-set grew blue mildew in two or three days, was too small for any active game [Fleming, 1937, p. 169].

But it was not the physical discomforts that the children minded most, and they were adequately fed. The atmosphere was full of sadism, disguised as religious righteousness. Kipling says:

> It was an establishment run with the full vigour of the Evangelical as revealed to the Woman. I had never heard of Hell, so I was introduced to it in all its terrors—I and whatever luckless little slavey might be in the house, whom severe rationing had led to steal food. Once I saw the Woman beat such a girl who picked up the kitchen poker and threatened retaliation. Myself I was regularly beaten [1937, p. 358].

As long as the old Captain was alive there was someone to intervene and protect him from the Woman. He occasionally gave Rudyard some kind words and, even more important, rational explanations. (Captain Holloway had served on a whaler and undoubtedly was one of the models for that good substitute father, the whaler Captain Disco Troop in *Captains Courageous*.) He had a fascinating *dark* deformity. The old man had been entangled in a harpoon line while whale-fishing, and had been dragged down, but then almost miraculously had gotten free. "But the line had scarred his ankle for life—a dry, *black* scar, which I used to look at with horrified interest" (1937, p. 358; my italics). The Holloways had a son, Henry, who was 6 years older than Rudyard. "Aunty Rosa" apparently was jealous of the brighter younger boy in relation to her Harry. She appears to have treated Trix well, but Rudyard was rejected as a *Black* sheep (which is what he calls himself in his fictionalized account). Trix writes:

> [Aunty] had long wanted a daughter, therefore she soon made a pet of me, and did her best to weaken the affection between the poor little people marooned on the desert island of her house and heart. From the beginning she took the line that I was always in the right and Ruddy invariably in the wrong: a very alienating position to thrust me into, but he, with his curious insight into human nature, said she was a jealous woman, and of such low caste as not to matter, and he never loved me less for her mischief-making [Fleming, p. 169]. [On another occasion she wrote:] She never struck me or threatened me with bodily punishment, and I am still grateful to her for some of her early teaching. But her cruelty to Ruddy poisoned everything [Green, p. 35].

Harry cooperated with his mother in tyrannizing over and punishing Rudyard: "The Woman had an only son of twelve or thirteen as religious as she. I was a real joy to him, for when his mother had finished with me for the day he (we slept in the same room) took me on and roasted the other side" (Kipling, 1937, p. 358). Harry was a prototype for a Big Brother figure, hated and loved, evoking murderous, and (the implications are in the words above) homosexual feelings. Mother and son combined in trying to brainwash the boy:

> If you cross examine a child of seven or eight on his day's doings (specially when he wants to go to sleep), he will contradict himself very satisfactorily. If each contradiction be set down as a lie and retailed at breakfast, life is not easy. I have known a certain amount of bullying, but this was calculated torture—religious as well as scientific [p. 358f.]. [The cross-examination was regularly followed by] punishments and humiliation—above all humiliation. That alternation was quite regular. I can but admire the internal laborious ingenuity of it all. *Exempli gratia*. Coming out of church once I smiled. The Devil-Boy demanded why. I said I didn't know, which was child's truth. He replied that I *must* know. People didn't laugh for nothing. Heaven knows the explanation I put forward; but it was duly reported to the Woman as a 'lie'. . . . The Son after three or four years went into a Bank and was generally too tired on his return to torture me, unless things had gone wrong with him. I

learned to know what was coming from his step into the house [p. 361f.].

The driven, consuming, persecutory regimen deprived the children not only of joy, but even of the opportunity for simple quiet existence—for the timelessness and contemplative relaxation so needed for the growth of the child's soul. The boy was forced into an *adaptive* paranoid attitude: "Nor was my life an unsuitable preparation for my future, in that it demanded constant wariness, the habit of observation, and attendance on moods and tempers; the noting of discrepancies between speech and action; a certain reserve of demeanour; and automatic suspicion of sudden favours" (p. 365). To ward off the persecution, Kipling had to justify the iterated accusation—he was forced to lie; Kipling describes this as having some creative potential. The torment "made me give attention to the lies I soon found it necessary to tell; and this, I presume, is the foundation of literary effort" (p. 359).

The inculcated need to deceive by divorcing action from feeling is documented by Trix. After their mother came to rescue the children, she: "wrote to my father that the children [had] . . . seemed delighted to see her, but she had been a little disappointed by the way we had both hung round [Aunty Rosa] in the evening. She did not know that well-trained animals watch their tamer's eye, and the familiar danger-signals of Aunty's rising temper had set us both fawning upon her" (Fleming, p. 168).

Kipling felt he had been able to survive because of the month each year he spent with his Aunt Georgina Burne-Jones. There love and affection were not stinted and the boy had an important role in the large family's activities:

> It was a jumble of delights and emotions culminating in being allowed to blow the big organ in the studio for the beloved Aunt, while the Uncle worked . . . and if the organ ran out in squeals the beloved Aunt would be sorry. Never, *never* angry! [p. 363f.].
>
> [This is preceded by a passage that links fear of the dark, seeing and being seen, with the need for what was so lacking in the House of Desolation—protection provided by the presence of men:] At bedtime one hastened along the passages, where unfinished cartoons lay against the walls. The Uncle often painted in their eyes

first, leaving the rest in charcoal—a most effective presentation. Hence our speed to our own top-landing, where we could hang over the stairs and listen to *the loveliest sound in the world—deep-voiced men laughing together over dinner* [p. 363; my italics].[1] But on a certain day—one tried to fend off the thought of it—the delicious dream would end, and one would return to the House of Desolation, and for the next two or three mornings there cry on waking up. Hence more punishments and cross examinations.

[In some ways Aunty Rosa's brainwashing was effective—Rudyard never told on her. Here is his explanation:] Often and often afterwards, the beloved Aunt would ask me why I had never told any one how I was being treated. Children tell little more than animals, *for what comes to them they accept as eternally established.* Also, badly treated children have a clear notion of what they are likely to get if they betray the secrets of a prison-house before they are clear of it [p. 364f.; my italics].

Whether children continue to accept what comes to them as eternally established depends in large part on parental attitudes—and a parent figure claiming to speak for God must inhibit the development of the child's own judgment and identity. But Kipling's deepest motivation for keeping silence probably related more to the parents who had betrayed him to the prison-house than to "Aunty Rosa." He had to distance the anger and torment caused by their desertion. The intense need to keep the memory of *good* parents made silence, minimization, and even denial necessary. How could his parents have done this to him? It was too unbearable to keep that question in mind very long.

In her memoirs, Trix expressed the children's feelings about the desertion:

> Looking back, I think the real tragedy of our early days, apart from Aunty's bad temper and unkindness to my brother, sprang from our inability to understand why our parents had deserted us. We had had no preparation or explanation; it was like a double death, or rather, like an avalanche that had swept away everything happy and familiar. . . . We felt we had been deserted, 'almost as much

---

[1] Kipling's work—especially the stories about children *(The Jungle Books, Kim, Captains Courageous)*—are full of the longing for fathers fulfilled by a multitude of good father figures.

as on a doorstep', and what was the reason? Of course Aunty used to say it was because we were so tiresome, and she had taken us in out of pity, but in a desperate moment Ruddy appealed to Uncle Harrison, and he said it was only Aunty's fun and Papa had left us to be taken care of because India was too hot for little people. But we knew better than that because we had been to Nassick [a cool place in the India Hills], so what was the real reason? Mama was not ill . . . Papa had not had to go to a war. They had not even lost their money . . . there was no excuse; they had gone happily back to our own lovely home, and had not taken us with them. There was no getting out of that, as we often said. Harry, who had all a crow's quickness in finding a wound to pick at, discovered our trouble and teased us unmercifully. He assured us we had been taken in out of charity and must do exactly as he told us . . . we were just like workhouse brats, and none of our toys really belonged to us [Fleming, p. 171].

The suddenness and unexpectedness of the desertion increased its traumatic effect by depriving the children of any chance to prepare for, to work out in thought and with the parents what they were to experience. But Rudyard did fight with his mind to keep Trix with him emotionally, and to preserve the memory of the good parents as a refuge from the persecutors. Trix says he called Mrs. Holloway "a *Kutch-nay*, a nothing-at-all, and that secret name was a great comfort to us when Harry practiced his talent for eavesdropping" (p. 169). "Ruddy remembered our lost kingdom vividly" (p. 171). The 6-year-old provided the details that the younger child had forgotten. Remembering the past was a torment to the children, but it supplied the means for restoring the promise of bliss. In Rudyard's stories he conjured up an idealized world and wonderful parents. This strengthened the children and kept them together— the desertion did not mean complete isolation.[2]

---

[2] Compare Orwell's *1984* where the tormentor is successful in his attempt to break down Winston Smith to the point of dividing him from his beloved companion Julia. The soul murder is consummated (i.e., the capacity for love is destroyed) when Winston screams: " 'Do it to Julia! I don't care what you do to her. Tear her face off, strip her to the bones. Not me! Julia! Not me!' " (1949, p. 289). Sibling rivalry is usually tuned up to this cannibalistic pitch under conditions of soul murder. This is effected by the child's need to displace rage away from the

Yet there was so much confusion—an agony of not knowing why, and whom they belonged to, and what their place was in the order of things. No wonder Rudyard was to become an arch-conservative, a pillar of the established order. One can see how the Law of the Jungle in the *Jungle Books*—assigning a place to everyone, making all relationships clear, enforcing "human" decency—represented a wish fulfillment for Kipling; and so did Mowgli's foster parents—wolves!—but of outstanding decency and dependability, with Mother Wolf ready to fight to the death to keep him.

Another soul-saving factor during this time was the boy's absorption in reading. He could not read or write when left with the Holloways, and it was "Aunty Rosa" who taught him. At first he resisted learning, but then he discovered that books offered a way of getting free in fantasy, of distancing his torment. He called it "a means to everything that would make me happy. So I read all that came within my reach. As soon as my pleasure in this was known, deprivation from reading was added to my punishments. I then read by stealth and the more earnestly" (1937, p. 359). Reading then became a "sin" that involved his eyes, his curiosity, and his fantasies. This is stressed in all the accounts Kipling wrote of this time. The sinning was followed by retribution: "My eyes went wrong, and I could not well see to read. For which reason I read the more and in bad lights. [Here he shows his masochism.] My work at the terrible little dayschool where I had been sent suffered in consequence, and my monthly reports showed it. The loss of 'reading-time' was the worst of my 'home' punishments for bad school-work" (p. 365).

The eye trouble amounted to near blindness. This was discovered only shortly before Rudyard's deliverance from Lorne Lodge. Before that there was a terrible humiliating punishment that resembled that given Dickens's alter ego, the fatherless and then orphaned David Copperfield, by the cruel Murdstones. One school report "was so bad that I threw it away and said that I had never

---

tormenting parent, and identify with the tormentor in relation to the sibling. Fortunately the attempt to divide the siblings failed with the Kipling children. Trix's devoted loyalty probably helped save Rudyard's masculinity as well as his identity.

received it. But this is a hard world for the amateur liar. My web of deceit was swiftly exposed—the Son spared time after banking-hours to help in the auto-da-fé—and I was well beaten and sent to school through the streets of Southsea with the placard 'Liar' between my shoulders" (p. 365f.).

What Kipling calls "some sort of nervous breakdown" followed this. The shadows provided by his failing vision were supplemented by shadowy hallucinations—making for a terrible *darkness:* "I imagined I saw shadows and things that were not there, and they worried me more than the Woman." When a doctor sent down by his Aunt Georgina discovered the boy was half blind, "This, too, was supposed to be 'showing-off' [according to "Aunty Rosa"], and I was segregated from my sister—another punishment—as a sort of moral leper. His mother returned to England shortly after this; there is more than a hint of direct reproach (so rare for Kipling[3]) in his dry statement: "I do not remember that I had any warning." On the first evening of her visit to the children, his mother afterward told Rudyard, "when she first came up to my room to kiss me goodnight, I flung up an arm to guard off the cuff that I had been trained to expect" (p. 366). The children were promptly taken away. They had been six years in the House of Desolation.

For some months Rudyard was tended to by his mother in a small farm house near Epping Forest, where he was allowed to run wild; he felt "completely happy . . . except for my spectacles" (p. 366). Although Rudyard was rescued, Trix was subsequently returned to Mrs. Holloway's care. Her experience had been

---

[3] Compare Dickens, who was sent out by his parents at age 10 to work under terrible conditions at a blacking factory: "It is wonderful to me how I could have been so easily cast away at such an age" (Forster, 1873, p. 25). Even when he was a famous writer Dickens was so affected by his memories that he was unable to pass by the site of the factory. What burned in his memory was that his mother had wanted him to stay on even after his father had arranged for his rescue: "I never afterwards forgot, I never shall forget, I never can forget, that my mother was warm for my being sent back" (p. 38). It is true that Dickens was not able to bear talking about the childhood experiences; he wrote about them to Forster, and his wife and children learned only that Dickens had given David Copperfield his own experiences in the blacking factory when they read of it in Forster's biography. But, unlike Kipling, Dickens *knew* how he felt.

different from her brother's since she had been treated as a favorite and had become

> a little Evangelical herself. At the same time she was obstinately loyal to a brother who was constantly being exhibited to her not merely as the Black Sheep of his family, but veritably as among the damned. The strain upon Trix must have been very great, and leaving her with Mrs. Holloway was, upon any possible reading of the total situation, a grave error of judgement. It comes as no surprise when we learn that in later life Trix was subject to recurrent nervous illness [Stewart, p. 11].

Kipling makes two somewhat contradictory statements about the effect of the stay at Lorne Lodge on his subsequent life. He ends "Baa, Baa, Black Sheep" with Punch telling Judy, three months after they have been taken away from the House of Desolation by their mother:

> Told you so . . . it's all different now, and we are just as much Mother's as if she had never gone. [But the narrator adds:] Not altogether, O Punch, for when young lips have drunk deep of the bitter waters of Hate, Suspicion, and Despair, all the Love in the world will not wholly take away that knowledge; though *it may turn darkened eyes for a while to the light,* and teach Faith where no Faith was [1888b, p. 315; my italics].
>
> [As an old man he says of the torment and humiliation at Lorne Lodge:] In the long run these things, and many more of the like, drained me of any capacity for real, personal hate for the rest of my days. So close must any life-filling passion lie to its opposite. 'Who having known the Diamond will concern himself with glass?' [p. 366].

Both statements show realization of the lifelong effects, but the later one denies that he could subsequently hate in a personal way, as if the hatred had been cathartically discharged once and for all.

Kipling was a most complex man; certainly his creativity was not destroyed by the years in the House of Desolation—it may even have been enhanced. He was not deprived of his ability to love, although it may have been damaged. His capacity for humor and laughter survived. But he denies an intense and often cruel personal hatred that is obvious to the most casual reader. It is the terrible destructive hatred of the tormented child who "cannot curse God and die" that is the hardest burden of soul murder. Where is it to go? After his years in Lorne Lodge the free expression of the "angry Ruddy coming" was no longer possible. Part of the rage was bound by identifying with the tormentor. But the child who hates too much must disclaim and deny it—and so it was with Kipling. Yet many—too many—of his poems and stories are about revenge and sadistic practical jokes (for example, 1890b, p. 256f.). Although he can identify with the underdog in his writings, Kipling often hates with the oppressor against the oppressed. Jarrell (1963) comments that Kipling's "morality is the one-sided, desperately protective, sometimes vindictive morality of someone who has been for some time the occupant of one of God's concentration camps, and has had to spend the rest of his life justifying or explaining out of existence what he cannot forget" (p. 146).

His close friend, Mrs. Edmonia Hill, wrote of Kipling when he was working on "Baa, Baa, Black Sheep" while staying at her home in 1888:

> [Kipling has been writing] a true story of his early life when he was sent with his little sister to England to be educated. . . . It was pitiful to see Kipling living over the experience, pouring out his soul in the story, as the drab life was worse than he could possibly describe it. His eyesight was permanently impaired, and as he had heretofore only known love and tenderness, his faith in people was sorely tried. When he was writing this he was a sorry guest, as he was in a towering rage at the recollection of those days [Green, p. 33].

So much for being deprived of the capacity for personal hatred!

There was a short-lived repetition of the desertion and desolation at Lorne Lodge when the 12-year-old Kipling was sent to a public school nine months after his removal from the Holloways. The school had to be inexpensive, and his parents settled on the United Services Colleges (also called Westward Ho!), a new institution designed mainly to prepare the sons of Army officers for a military career. The headmaster was a friend of the Kiplings', Cormell Price, a man known and liked by Rudyard (who called him "Uncle Crom" outside of school). The school was made famous by Kipling's glorification of it in his "Stalky" stories. But these stories conceal, and their comic tone belies, that Kipling's first months at school meant a return to hell. During this time his mother was still in England. Kipling (1937) calls the school "Brutal enough. . . . My first year and a half was not pleasant. The most persistent bullying comes less from the bigger boys, who merely kick and pass on, than from young *devils* of fourteen acting in concert against one butt" (p. 372; my italics). He had found new versions of that "Devil-Boy" Harry.

In "Stalky and Co." (1899), Beetle (Kipling) describes how the bullies "kick the *souls* out" of the new boys who "blub [and] write home three times a day—yes, you brute, I've done that—askin' to be taken away" (p. 162; my italics). And Kipling actually had. His sister writes: "For the first month or so, he wrote to us, twice or thrice daily (and my mother cried bitterly over the letters) that he could neither eat nor sleep" (Stewart, p. 22). Despite her tears, Alice Kipling left England before the Easter holidays when her son could have been with her to tell her firsthand what he had been experiencing. She may have had reassurances from the headmaster. Eventually things did improve for Rudyard—markedly so after the first year and a half. He was accepted by the others and ceased to be a victim: "After my strength came suddenly to me about my fourteenth year, there was no more bullying; and either my natural sloth or past experience did not tempt me to bully in my turn" (1937, p. 372). He found his special friends Beresford and Dunsterville (M'Turk and Stalky in his stories) and they formed a little group that gave him a feeling of active masculine identity. There was a glorious summer holiday when he was 13 and his father returned from India and took him to Paris for the Exposition of 1878 (this was followed by a lifelong fondness for things French). At school he was under the benevolent eye of "Uncle Crom." In this place the Woman held no sway; he lived with brothers who were mostly good, and the fathers were in power.

But the dark past still threatened. The boy was beaten by the masters—a regular part of English public school education. The aura of brutality comes across in "Stalky and Co.," which, writes Edmund Wilson (1941), "presents a hair-raising picture of the sadism of the English public school system. The older boys have fags to wait on them, and they sometimes torment these younger boys till they have reduced them almost to imbecility; the masters are constantly caning the boys in scenes that seem almost as bloody as the floggings in old English sea stories; and the boys revenge themselves on the masters with practical jokes as catastrophic as the Whams and Zows of the comic strip" (p. 21). Trilling (1943) talks of the book's "callousness, arrogance and brutality" (p. 89).

Kipling demonstrates his being on both sides of the persecutor/victim struggle. He shows contempt for the school's compulsory games. There is a general acceptance of the cruelty that is presented, and cruelty to animals is a matter of course. In one story a cat is shot by the boys in Kipling's group and its corpse left to stink in the rafters above the dormitory of offending enemies. (To paraphrase a well-known saying of Freud's, a cat is also a cat. But like the Cigar in "The Betrothal" [1885, p. 99], its symbolic meaning is significant. Here it expresses the hostility toward the female genital ["pussy"] in the predominant anal-sadistic, male, homosexual context of these stories.) The sadistic masters are exposed and get tricked in successful revenge schemes, yet eventually their authority is justified. This is expressed in the poem with which Kipling prefaces *Stalky & Co.*—"A School Song":

> Western wind and open surge
>   Took us from our mothers;
> Flung us on a naked shore
> (Twelve bleak houses by the shore!
> Seven summers by the shore!)
>   'Mid two hundred brothers.
> There we met with famous men
>   Set in office o'er us;
> And they beat on us with rods—
> Faithfully with many rods—
> Daily beat on us with rods,—
>   For the love they bore us!

This last line is ironic and critical. Kipling certainly does not deny the beatings. In his autobiography he is able to express his anger toward the masters, especially toward his first housemaster, the school chaplain, a ferocious and sanctimonious man whom he saw through even as a schoolboy. But his poem ends characteristically with a glorification of the school system: it prepares the boys to go out and rule the Empire. And he praises Big Brother:

> This we learned from famous men,
>   Knowing not we learned it.
> Only, as the years went by—
> Lonely, as the years went by—
> Far from help as years went by,
>   Plainer we discerned it.
> . . . . . .
>
> Bless and praise we famous men—
>   Men of little showing!
> For their work continueth
> And their work continueth,
> Broad and deep continueth
>   Great beyond their knowing!

Soul murder results in splitting the victim's identity into contradictory fragments that function without effective synthesis. In Kipling's simultaneous portrayal of the authorities as good and bad, the personal hatred he claimed to be drained of keeps breaking through. Kipling describes his beginning to write at Westward Ho!, and his motivation is revenge. He had read about "a man called Dante who, living in a small Italian town at general issue with his neighbors, had invented for most of them lively torments in a nine-ringed Hell [it was from "Aunty Rosa" that Rudyard had first heard of Hell], where he exhibited them to after ages. . . . I bought a fat, American cloth-bound notebook, and set to work on an *Inferno*, into which I put, under appropriate tortures, all my friends and *most* of the masters" (1937, p. 378). The italics are by the wonderful Randall Jarrell (1962) who asks: "Why only *most?* Two were spared, one for the Father and one for the Mother" (p. 144).

There is a most important part of the young boy's experience about which Kipling wrote nothing and about which nothing is known—his sexual life. Was the memory of the intense wish to see the child's severed hand a screen for masturbation? It is not hard to imagine the evangelical "Aunty Rosa's" attitude toward masturbation. Did anything sexual happen in the House of Desolation? One infers from his autobiography that puberty came with Rudyard's spurt of physical growth at 14. He developed a precocious mustache and at 17, though short, looked like a man.

The conventions of Victorian literature dictated avoiding sexual details, but Kipling, in contrast to most of his contemporaries, was aware of the existence and power of sexuality and showed it in his fiction. This is implicit in many of the *Plain Tales From the Hills* (1888a), which are full of predatory women. *The Light That Failed*, clearly though discreetly, pictures a sexual liaison between Torpenhow and the streetwalker Bessie Broke, and suggests the lesbian potential of the red-haired girl.

Kipling's first direct reference to sex in his autobiography (1937) concerns his years at school—and it is a disclaimer:

> Naturally, Westward Ho! was brutal enough, but, setting aside the foul speech that a boy ought to learn early and put behind him by his seventeenth year, it was clean with a cleanliness that I have never heard of in any other school. I remember no case of even suspected perversion, and am inclined to the theory that if masters did not suspect them, and show that they suspected, there would not be quite so many elsewhere [p. 370].

Apparently it was Cormell Price's policy to exhaust the boys through sports, but the purported absence of sexuality would make Westward Ho! singular indeed. Kipling's denial is different from the ignoring of sex in the school life by other Victorian memoirists. Minimization of homosexuality goes with minimization of anger for Kipling. Of his being beaten by the Prefect of Games at school he says: "One of the most difficult things to explain to some people is that a boy of seventeen or eighteen can thus beat a boy barely a year his junior, and on the heels of the punishment go for a walk with him; neither party bearing malice or pride" (p. 375). But, do the parties *know,* can they know what feeling they are bearing underneath?

Women in Kipling's early writings are depicted as sexually attractive, but destructive; or cold and asexual. The only real affection in his first novel, *The Light That Failed*, is between men. Kipling's ideal girl at this time of his life seems to have been the "regular fellow," like Miss Martyn (first name Bill or William) of *William the Conqueror* (1895a), who looks like a boy with her cropped hair, is "clever as a man . . . likes men who do things . . . doesn't understand poetry very much—it made her head ache" (p. 172).

Kipling gives Miss Martyn his own feelings toward the literary men of London when he returned there in 1889 (age 24) after his years as a journalist in India:

> But I consort with long-haired things
>   In velvet collar-rolls,
> Who talk about the Aims of Art,
>   And "theories" and "goals",
> And moo and coo with womenfolk
>   About their blessed souls.
>   . . . . . .
>
> It's Oh to meet an Army man,
>   Set up, and trimmed and taut,
> Who does not spout hashed libraries
>   Or think the next man's thought
> And walks as though he owned himself,
>   And hogs his bristles short
>
> [1889, p. 173].

One velvet-collar wearer, Max Beerbohm, whose somewhat feminine sensibilities perhaps helped him sense (and motivated him to ridicule) Kipling's, appreciated that Kipling was a genius; but he loathed his work. He wickedly pretended to believe that *Rudyard Kipling* was the pseudonym of a female author—who else would say "Oh to meet an Army man"?

The Light That Failed was published in 1891. Kipling at 26 would seem to have shared the belief expressed by the friend of the hero of his novel who prophesies his finish as an artist and a man if Dick Heldar falls in love. (This is expressed in dialogue that would fit into the American Western film with its preadolescent unconscious homosexuality. One can almost hear it in the voice of John Wayne:) "She'll spoil his hand. She'll waste his time, and she'll marry him, and ruin his work for ever. He'll be a respectable married man before we can stop him, and—he'll never go on the long trail again" (1890a, p. 78).

I have skipped ahead in time, and now return to the adolescent Kipling. Maisie, the frigid and selfish heroine of *The Light That Failed*, had a direct prototype in Kipling's life—a girl he fell in love with when he was $14\frac{1}{2}$; and she was associated with the House of Desolation. Rudyard met Florence Garrard when he went down to Mrs. Holloway's to take Trix away for a holiday in 1880. Florence was a little older than Rudyard. She was a paying guest at Lorne Lodge; her parents were abroad. Like Maisie, Florence kept a pet goat, and her character, too, was "self-centred and elusive, lacking in sympathy and affection" (Carrington, p. 42). Rudyard felt he was in love with her for five or six years. When he was 16 and about to go back to India, he begged her to become engaged to him. His Aunt Edith "was to recall 'how impressed she had been by the alarming force of his feelings as he gave her an account of his love for Flo Garrard, the girl who took his heart when he was still a schoolboy and did it no good before she tossed it back to him'" (Stewart, p. 32). Kipling met her again in England just before he wrote his novel whose heroine, Maisie, is studying to be an art student, as Flo was. Florence made him recall Lorne Lodge; and, substituting her for Trix, he wrote a first chapter about the two children's stay with an "Aunty Rosa." The boy and girl are described playing with a forbidden loaded pistol; Maisie temporarily blinds Dick by shooting it off. Since Maisie is an amalgam of Florence and Trix, the incident (which prefigures the theme of the castrating and blinding woman) might refer to heterosexual (but incestuous) masturbatory play between Trix and Rudyard. If this occurred, ironically enough, it might well have helped save the boy's masculinity.

Rudyard was nearly 17 when he left England after graduating from Westward Ho! to rejoin his parents in India:

> That was a joyous homecoming. For—consider!—I had returned to a Father and Mother of whom I had seen but little since my sixth year. . . . The Mother proved more delightful than all my imaginings or memories. My father was not only a mine of knowledge and help, but a humorous, tolerant and expert fellow-craftsman. . . . I do not remember the smallest friction in any detail of our lives. We delighted more in each other's society than in that of strangers; and when my sister came out, a little later, our cup was filled to the brim. Not only were we happy, but we knew it [1937, p. 382].

It was paradise regained. Rudyard's mother began the habit, adopted by them all, of calling the four contented Kiplings "The Family Square." (It is in a *square* formed defensively by British soldiers that Dick Heldar gets the wound which eventually blinds him in *The Light That Failed.*)

The period he spent in India Kipling called in his autobiography "Seven Years Hard." During this time he worked as a journalist and began to write the poems and stories of India that made him famous as a young man. He learned about Indian life from the inside, getting to know the Indians, but especially the Anglo-Indians. As a reporter he traveled all over the subcontinent, exploring the levels of the rigid castes of both cultures—from the native underworld of Lahore, and the barracks of Tommy Atkins, to the generals and political leaders of Delhi and Simla. He quizzed and looked and listened, picking up characters for his stories and verses. Kipling's parents became personal friends of the viceroy, Lord Dufferin, providing Rudyard with a view from the top of governmental politics which he made good use of in his newspaper fiction. These stories are told in a tone which implies secret knowledge, that "knowing," grown-up tone so frequent (and sometimes so annoying) in Kipling's writings; it denies the child within who must not know. One expects this from adolescents, but it stayed on with Kipling. Perhaps in part because of this tone, Kipling's stories were eagerly read, and the young man found himself famous in his provincial world. He had the gratification of being asked about the opinions of the enlisted men in the barracks by the Commander-in-Chief himself, General Roberts.

I want to mention some of the nonneurotic aspects of Kipling's personality during these years. Kay Robinson, an editor for whom Kipling worked, describes the young man's unprepossessing appearance, and adds: "The charm of his manner, however, made you forget what he looked like in half a minute. . . . Kipling, shaking all over with laughter and wiping his spectacles at the same time with his handkerchief, always comes to mind as most characteristic of him in the old days when even our hardest work on 'The Rag'—for fate soon took me to Lahore to be his editor—was as full of jokes as a pomegranate of pips" (Green, p. 81). Contemporaries also noted Kipling's intense love for children, and his extraordinary ability to communicate with them. Above all, these years in India brought forth creative work that, despite mixed quality and jejune defects, is marvelous in its variety, quantity, brilliance, and force; several short stories are masterpieces.

His work meant loneliness at times, and even solitude. For years the young man was left in charge of the newspaper during the sweltering hot season when his family and most of the British community left for the cooler hill country. One year, during this abandonment, Kipling had what he calls a "pivot experience." He was 20, the only Englishman left to do all the editorial and supervisory work—it was too much: "It happened one hot-weather evening, in '86 or thereabouts, when I felt that I had come to the edge of all endurance. As I entered my empty house in the dusk there was no more in me except *the horror of a great darkness,* that I must have been fighting for some days. I came through that darkness alive, but how I do not know" (1937, p. 400; my italics). The desertion and darkness must have meant a return to the House of Desolation, with its threat of the hallucinated "shadows and things that were not there," and the incipient blindness. Being alone at night may have brought with it forbidden masturbatory temptation.

We know from the imagery of his writings that darkness meant for Kipling the desolation of spirit of soul murder, the blackness of depression, of hatred and self-hatred mixed with fear of death and castration of the abandoned and tormented child. Kipling's first memories of England were of a dreadful place of darkness. Meeta had not saved the child "from any night terrors or dread of the dark." Dobrée (1967) illustrates the horror of darkness and desolation as a recurrent theme in Kipling's work—usually associated with what Kipling calls "breaking strain"—the unbearable overstimulation that is the essence of trauma. It connects with what he suffered in the intolerable heat at age 20 as well as in the House of Desolation. One of Kipling's last poems is called "Hymn of Breaking Strain":

> But, in our daily dealing
> With stone and steel, we find
> The Gods have no such feeling
> Of justice toward mankind.
> To no set gauge they make us,—
> For no laid course *prepare*—

>   And presently o'ertake us
>   With loads we cannot bear:
>   Too merciless to bear   [1935, p. 298; my italics].

Kipling charges the Gods with responsibility for the "too muchness"—with the specific accusation, so relevant to his parents, that they do not *prepare* human beings for the unbearable strain. Predictably, the condemnation turns to justification—the Gods are needed:

>   Oh veiled and secret Power
>   Whose paths we seek in vain,
>   Be with us in our hour
>   Of overthrow and pain:
>   That we—by which sure token
>   We know Thy ways are true—
>   In spite of being broken,
>   *Because of being broken,*
>   May rise and build anew.
>   Stand up and build anew!   [p. 299; my italics].

In 1907 Kipling told a group of students at McGill University about the blackness of depression:

> Some of you here know—*and I remember*—that youth can be a season of great depression, despondencies, doubts, waverings. The worse because they seem to be peculiar to ourselves and incommunicable to our fellows. There is a certain *darkness* into which the *soul* of the young man sometimes descends—*a horror of desolation, abandonment and realized worthlessness,* which is one of the most real of hells in which we are compelled to walk [1907, p. 21; my italics].

In one of his last stories, a fable called "Uncovenanted Mercies" (1929), Kipling makes Satan, the Prince of Darkness, afraid of the dark: "The glare of the halo he wore in His Own Place fought against the Horror of Great Darkness" (p. 331). For Kipling, Hell was a dark place, blindness a constant threat, and light a promise of salvation—but in a vicious cycle, a promise that leads, by way of the hellfires of sexuality and anger, back to Hell.

Eighteen months after the 17-year-old Kipling returned to India, Florence Garrard wrote him putting an end to their engagement. He commented on this in his verse. The (not very good) poem of

1884 anticipates the novel he was to write in 1890 (*The Light That Failed*). It is called "Failure." The poet brings a girl—called "She"—a gift of "Fire from a distant place." She does not understand the gift "brought . . . of my best" of the "fierce burning stuff" that "gathereth in strength," and she extinguishes the light:

> 'Strange fires! Take them hence with you, O sir!
> Presage of coming woe we dimly feel.'
> Sudden She crushed the embers 'neath her heel,—
> And all light went with Her [p. 101].

The capitalized She's show Kipling is still dealing with the Woman.

Toward the end of his Indian seven years, Kipling broke away from the "Family Square" by taking a job on a newspaper in Allahabad. He transferred some of his familial dependence onto the Edgar Hills, a couple with whom he stayed for some time. He was especially devoted to Mrs. Edmonia ("Ted") Hill who was 30; Kipling was 23. The relationship does not seem to have been sexual or romantic. As had happened previously with "Mrs. Hauksbee," the "wittiest woman in India" to whom he had dedicated *Plain Tales From the Hills*, Kipling was in thrall to an older, forceful, and managing woman. Significantly, Kipling left India and his family with the Hills shortly after Trix became engaged to an "Army man"—one of those doers Kipling so admired. The Hills were going to visit "Ted's" family in America. Kipling decided to go along for a roundabout journey on his way to London where he wanted to further his literary career. He spent several months with Mrs. Hill's family, and was attracted to her younger sister, Caroline Taylor. Then he went with the Hills to London. His Indian stories and poems had attracted some critical attention in England. Kipling's first year in London (1890) was to be a year of marvelous success, very like the success of Dick Heldar, the hero of the 1890 novel, *The Light That Failed*. Each took London by storm with his art (Dick as a painter).

When the Hills left for India, Kipling was again alone. Although his aunts and uncles were nearby, as they had been during the years at Lorne Lodge, Kipling at first deliberately stayed away. He was working intensely—most of the famous Barrack-Room Ballads (published in 1892) were written in London. It must have helped to banish the painful past that he was experiencing once again those feelings of a conqueror of his first six years; like Goethe and Freud, he was conquering with his pen.

Stewart calls *The Light That Failed* a work of genius, but "a very young sick man's book. Its power comes from the irruption, for a time, of something always latent in Kipling: an almost magical fear and hatred of women—of women who are not good chaps, answering to nicknames like William and Ted" (p. 93f.). The women in the novel desert the hero in his need. Most ironic—and it is surely completely unconscious irony—is the dedication poem of the book. On the surface it is a tribute to a loving mother, a mother who would never abandon her son:

> If I were hanged on the highest hill,
>   *Mother o'mine, O mother o'mine!*
> I know whose love would follow me still,
>   *Mother o'mine, O mother o'mine!*
> If I were drowned in the deepest sea,
>   *Mother o'mine, O mother o'mine!*
> I know whose tears would come down to me,
>   *Mother o'mine, O mother o'mine!*
> If I were damned of body and soul,
> I know whose prayers would make me whole,
>   *Mother o'mine, O Mother o'mine!*

The poem presents the fantasy from childhood that the son will die, and the mother will be sorry, love him, and follow him. Despite this tribute to his mother, Kipling portrays himself in the book as an orphan. Perhaps he makes Dick an orphan to keep from writing a direct attack on his mother (no doubt Dickens orphaned David Copperfield for the same reason). Eugene O'Neill makes use of this poem in his autobiographical play, *Long Day's Journey into Night*, but with full awareness of its irony and concealed hatred.

Dick Heldar's blindness begins, as Kipling's had, with the appearance of a grey haze at the periphery of his vision. The theme is introduced in the first chapter based on the stay at Lorne Lodge, where the child Maisie (the transformed Flo Garrard) almost blinds Dick by accidentally shooting a revolver past his face. Heldar's eyes are especially precious since he is a painter. Heldar's masterpiece which he frantically finishes as he begins to go blind is called "Melancolia"—evoking black depression. It represents the head of a woman who has suffered terribly but who insolently laughs at Fate. Dick fears and admires the woman who defies melancholia; the novel covertly shows his identification with her. The portrait's features are taken from cold, selfish Maisie and the model-prostitute Bessie Broke. Bessie destroys the painting to get revenge for the scornful way Dick has treated her (as if she were a *thing* with no feeling) when he broke up her affair with Torpenhow. The female head is apparently malign; Torpenhow says, "Dick, there's a sort of murderous, viperine suggestion in the pose of the head that I don't understand" (p. 154). It is the Dark Woman as Soul Murderer. The novel portrays women as vampires who cannot love and who destroy men and their art. Only masculine love sustains and can be relied on.

The intensity of Kipling's sadism shows in the novel's brutality. Kinkead-Weeks (1964) makes a distinction between Kipling's treating a brutal subject or situation objectively, "and a brutal attitude of satisfaction felt towards it" (p. 198). He gives as example the fine description of the brutal attack of three thousand Sudanese on a square of British soldiers, in contrast to an incident at the end of the attack that shows Kipling's sadism—the description of Torpenhow gouging out an Arab's eye (the oedipal punishment, first visited on an enemy, that is to be the hero's fate). Later, when blind, Dick asks Torpenhow (presumably the irony is to show his ability to laugh at Fate, like his *Melancolia*): "D'you remember that nigger you gouged in the square? Pity you didn't keep the odd eye. It would have been useful" (p. 160).

At the end of the novel, the blind Dick (abandoned by his friends who think Maisie is caring for him) leaves England (and women) to seek out his beloved Big Brother, Torpenhow, the eye-gouger. Earlier, when Dick's blindness became manifest, there was a scene between the two men that conveys homosexual contact, although it is obvious that Kipling does not know it. Dick "made as if to leap from the bed, but Torpenhow's arms were round him, and Torpenhow's chin was on his shoulder, and his breath was squeezed out of him . . . the grip could draw no closer. Both men were breathing heavily. Dick threw his head from side to side and groaned." Dick falls asleep after asking to hold Torpenhow's hand; the scene ends with Torpenhow kissing "him lightly on the forehead, as men do sometimes kiss a wounded comrade in the hour of death, to ease his departure" (p. 157f.). Torpenhow's attentions to Dick (as Meeta's had been to Ruddy) were maternal, protecting from the terror of the dark.

Dick returns to Egypt to die. He has an ecstatic response to getting there in time to take part in, or at least to hear, the battle. Just before finding Torpenhow, Dick again invokes mother: " 'What luck! What stupendous and imperial luck!' said Dick. 'It's just before the battle, *mother*. Oh god has been most good to me!' " (p. 240; my italics). The blinded child can share in the primal scene. Dick then meets Torpenhow and dies in his arms—a *Liebestod*.

In contrast to his hero's death in Egypt, Kipling's success in London made him feel a conqueror of Egypt. After *The Light That Failed* was finished, he sent his parents a telegram that read "Genesis XLV:9." The Old Testament passage referred to reads: "Make haste to go up to my father and say to him, 'Thus says your son Joseph, God has made me lord of all Egypt; come down to me; do not tarry.' " Kipling, whose full name was *Joseph* Rudyard, was identifying with his namesake, the biblical prototype of parental favorites. His ambition and confidence had taken him far from the "depression and realized worthlessness" that he recalled to his student audience at McGill in 1907.

In addition to his presumably platonic ties to two older, domineering, married women, "Mrs. Hauksbee" and "Ted" Hill, Kipling had emotional involvements (and these included marriage plans) with two women prior to 1891: Caroline Taylor, Mrs. Hill's sister, and Flo Garrard whom he merged with his own sister in his novel. He went on to marry another sister, the sister of a man for whom he developed the deepest friendship of his life: Wolcott Balestier. Like Mrs. Hill, Balestier was an American; he came from patrician New England stock. He was 29 years old and with his charm and considerable talent had made himself very influential in literary London. The middle-aged Henry James was "captivated" (Edel, 1962, p. 283) by his young compatriot. Balestier was in

London as the agent of an American publisher, trying to sign up English writers. Despite Kipling's great distrust of publishers and their agents, he immediately became a close friend of the American, and they soon embarked on the project of a mutual novel, set in America and India—*The Naulahka*. Kipling must have been impressed by Balestier's ability to get what he was after, a quality that always attracted him. (Alice James characterized Balestier after his death as "the effective and the indispensable" [Edel, p. 299].) According to Carrington, "No other man ever exercised so dominating an influence over Rudyard Kipling as did Wolcott Balestier during the eighteen months of their intimacy" (p. 178). Kipling soon met the whole Balestier family. Some sort of understanding was quickly arrived at between him and the elder of Wolcott's two sisters, Caroline. Caroline, like Flo Garrard, was older than Rudyard—3 years older. She had taken over a leading role in the family following her father's death and was looking after her beloved brother Wolcott and managing his household.

It is said that when Kipling's mother first saw the rather aggressive Carrie Balestier, she declared (with scant enthusiasm): "That woman is going to marry our Ruddy"; Kipling's father's comment was, "Carrie Balestier [is] a good man spoiled" (Carrington, p. 183). Little is recorded about the progress of the love affair. Partly motivated by poor health, Kipling set off by himself to travel, going to America, South Africa, and the Far East. At this time he wrote some of his first imperialist poems, identifying with and becoming the spokesman for the Empire. In December 1891, Kipling heard that Wolcott had come down with typhoid fever in Germany. When Wolcott died, Carrie cabled Rudyard asking him to come home. Henry James was also summoned, and he arrived to find Carrie in charge of things. He wrote: "The three [Balestier] ladies came insistently to the grave . . . by far the most interesting is poor little concentrated Carrie . . . remarkable in her force, acuteness, capacity and courage—and in the intense, *almost manly nature* of her emotion. . . . She can do and face . . . for all three of them anything and everything that they will have to meet now" (Carrington, p. 191; my italics).

Rudyard married Carrie eight days after he joined the family in London. Henry James gave the bride away, and wrote that Carrie was "a hard devoted capable little person whom I don't in the least understand [Kipling] marrying." Carrington comments: "The reason why Rudyard hurried half-way round the world to marry Wolcott's sister is bound up with his devotion to Wolcott. There is little doubt that Wolcott himself fostered the match, that Wolcott on his death bed commended the care of his family to his friend Rudyard, that Wolcott's wishes were accepted as obligations" (p. 193). Wolcott's death was one of the great blows of Kipling's life. The feeling for the beloved brother figure, shared with Carrie, was part of Kipling's motivation to marry; it was connected with his love for (and identification with) his own sister, Trix. Also, the "manly" Carrie would seem to have had some of the significance for Rudyard of both "Aunty Rosa" and Harry, with their mother and big brother qualities changed from bad to good. Carrie laid down the law in the family, kept Kipling's accounts, watched over his every move; she protected him and kept him from distractions and intruders. She had looked after her brother with her "concentrated" devotion, and she transferred her care to Kipling: "Until Rudyard's death, forty-four years later, the two were inseparable and her services to him were indispensable. . . . [She] gave Rudyard her life's endeavour and grudged him, perhaps, his faculty for withdrawing into a world of the imagination where she could not follow him" (Carrington, p. 194). Here was someone "whose love would follow me still . . . if I were hanged on the highest hill."

After the wedding, the couple traveled to Vermont where they stayed with Carrie's younger brother Beatty. Their first child, Josephine, was born in Vermont, and Kipling having fallen in love with Brattleboro, they decided to settle there. They built a house, called Naulahka (and so evoking Wolcott), which "had one notable feature, to be reduplicated in essentials wherever the Kiplings subsequently lived. Kipling's study had only one entrance, through a room occupied by his wife. There Carrie would sit at a desk, ordering her domestic affairs, and guarding her husband against all possibility of intrusion. He could remain undisturbed for as long as he liked: sometimes, perhaps, for rather longer" (Stewart, p. 104).

I will break off the narrative of Kipling's life at this point; I intend to continue in another paper. The years as the official poet of imperialism, of political conservatism, of hatred against the Boers and the Boches, of becoming the patron saint of engineers and builders, of friendship with Cecil Rhodes and King George V—all lie ahead. So do many years of intense creative work—his masterpiece, *Kim*, and the wonderful short stories written late in his life that some consider his finest work.

Summary and Conclusions

During the time of the attempt at soul murder (ages 6 to 12), Kipling had to face three terrible psychological dangers: the loss of his parents; the soul murder itself (the overstimulation and overwhelming rage); and castration anxiety, since Rudyard, at 6, was at the height of his oedipal development. At Lorne Lodge there was the situation (perhaps true of his first years in India too) of domination by an all-powerful woman, with the much-needed protective father at a distance.

The trauma of the desertion was made more terrible by the boy's being completely unprepared for it. *Suddenly,* the children were in hell. Their fate resembles that of children who were suddenly separated from their parents during the emergency evacuations from London in the blitz of World War II. Anna Freud (1939–45), who cared for and studied these children, concludes:

> In the case of evacuation the danger is represented by the sudden disappearance of all the people whom he knows and loves. Unsatisfied longing produces in him a state of tension which is felt as shock. . . . In reality it is the very quickness of the child's break with the mother which contains all the dangers of abnormal consequences. Long-drawn-out separation may bring more visible pain, but it is less harmful because it gives the child time to accompany the events with his reactions, to work through his own feelings over and over again, to find outward expressions for his state of mind, i.e., to abreact slowly [p. 208f.].

Rudyard, at 6, was more able than the 3-year-old Trix to face the loss, since the images of both parents and the predominantly loving servants were firmly established as part of the structure of his mind. He had achieved object constancy; as long as he could remember and *think,* his parents could not be completely lost. He could use his mind and his creative imagination to fight against that part of himself that turned toward, gave in to, and identified with "Aunty Rosa" and Harry. Yet his power to know and to remember was specifically attacked by them. Reading and writing were crucial skills, and reading (tied to the forbidden *seeing*) became the subject of conflict and symptoms. (Apparently, there were occasional letters from his parents which helped reinforce the children's memories.) Rudyard could fight his passive entrapment with an active ordering of, and playing with, the bad reality in fantasies and memories (with Trix as his eager listener-participant). When Rudyard was very small, his father had written a nursery rhyme that had consoled him after the attack by a hen. In Lorne Lodge, he could identify with his protective father's humor and creativity, to try to ward off the attacks by the Woman. There was, after the near-blindness and the breakdown, a flowering of Kipling's creative writing in the predominantly male atmosphere of school. He emerged as a writer and poet (specifically as a master of *rhyme*). The ambition to become a writer crystallized in adolescence—at a time when there must have been a renewal of conflict over masturbation. He was using the writer's hand to keep away (to use the metaphor from his childhood memories) the severed child's hand. In his struggle with his fear of and fascination with castration, he needed to identify with his father to try to conquer the bad Woman—to conquer her in himself, and outside himself.

The 6-year-old boy in the midst of his oedipal development was subject to intense shifting ambivalence toward both parents. The desertion and subsequent sadomasochistic overstimulation made for libidinal regression and a terrifying access of rage—enhancing parentocidal (and probably especially parricidal) impulses at a time when the boy needed good parents desperately to fight off his inner imagos of the bad parents. Anna Freud (1965) is describing children of about 6 when she speaks of the causes underlying homesickness and school phobias:

> The distress experienced at separation from mother, parents, or home is due to an excessive ambivalence toward them. The conflict between love and hate of the parents can be tolerated by the child only in their reassuring presence. In their absence, the hostile side

of the ambivalence assumes frightening proportions, and the ambivalently loved figures of the parents are clung to so as to save them from the child's own death wishes, aggressive fantasies, etc. [p. 113].

This need to save the internal images of good parents, intense enough for the wartime evacuees at the Hampstead Nurseries where the parental substitutes were good and understanding, becomes desperate under conditions of soul murder, where hatred is deliberately cultivated. Devastation is perpetuated if the parental substitutes, with the fanaticism of the religiously righteous, and the power of concentration camp commandants, can prevent the child from registering the feeling of what has happened to him.

The subjection to "Aunty Rosa" as the Woman—with Harry as her phallic extension—threatened Rudyard's masculinity. He needed a strong father to take her away. Kipling continued to seek for fathers and older brothers in his work and in his life. The fear of the Woman, the need to submit to the phallic parent, the need to deny his parricidal urges, made homosexuality a continuing danger. The ongoing good external relationship with his father in later life must have helped him stave off his strong latent homosexuality. (One can see in his life and work a conflict-ridden range of wishes involving wanting to be, and to have, a man, a phallic woman—the ranee-tiger from childhood—and a woman.) Kipling did manage a heterosexual life with a loving relationship to a masculine, domineering woman. He was a loving father to his children, and suffered terribly when two of them died. His capacity for love was not destroyed. But he had a definite aversion to the sexual woman who is never treated as loving in his early fiction. Sex is not depicted as joyous; at best it is guilt-ridden pleasure followed by punishment.

I have speculated that there may have been sexual play between Trix and Rudyard which had some saving effect on his manhood; certainly her presence at Lorne Lodge helped preserve his sense of identity. Toward her he was able to feel and act like the protective parent that both so needed. Trix was grateful for and craved his care. She was the living link to his home, his parents, and the past. His memory and his gift for storytelling allowed him to become the author of, and Trix his primal audience for, a family romance based on real events. Trix's devotion continued the love from and for a female that was not swept away by the hatred for the Woman. Together the two children could retreat from the desolation and persecution of their daily life to the sanctuary created by the boy's imagination. (In *Puck of Pook's Hill* [1906] and *Rewards and Fairies* [1910], Kipling shows a brother and sister, Dan and Una, meeting people from the past who have observed and participated in historical events; the two travel through history together—and master the primal scene together.) Kipling was able to create a wonderful and sometimes a terrible world for abandoned children, to reward the deserving and punish the wicked. What began with Trix continued in his books.

The effects of the attempted soul murder on Kipling's life after Lorne Lodge were intermittently present and complicated by a struggle against them. There was a need to repeat the sadomasochistic experiences in the House of Desolation. Kipling's predominant position as victim had enforced an identification with the persecutors—out of the child's need for rescue. The destructive hatred had to be turned toward others; he required and found enemies: strangers, Boers, Boches, "the lesser breeds outside the law." But he could also remember what it was to have been the victim, and in some of his best work his empathy for the underdog catches the reader's emotions. He is successful in bringing to sympathetic life the Indians and the Lama in *Kim*; the natives in many of the early stories; the British enlisted men in his prose and verse; above all, the abandoned and neglected children.

But the persecutor part raged against the victim part of himself so that he was subject to attacks of depression. Just as he split the images of himself, he needed to split the mental pictures of his parents into good and bad. With the intolerable rage aimed against those he loved and needed, he was forced to deny his hatred. The denial—the need not to know—existed alongside his driving curiosity. The denial made the split registration possible: contradictory images and ideas could exist side by side in his mind without any blending, as with Orwell's *doublethink*. This kind of compartmentalization is a way of dealing with overwhelming feeling, but it is paid for by sacrificing the power of synthesis that is needed for joy, love, and the feeling of identity. The capacity for mental splitting is not entirely explainable by the defensive need to ward off hatred and fear from the mental images of Kipling's good parents. Even before the assumption of parental roles by the bad Holloways, Kipling had lived through the intense experiences involved in having two sets of parents—white and black, light and dark—as a child in India. It was common in the British colonies for the servants in the family to be closer to the children than the natural parents. The mere existence of the complicated, split mental representations of self and parents does not involve pathology. That depends on how the splits are used. The crucial questions are—can the contradictory mental representations be synthesized; can they be brought together and taken apart again so that they can be worked with in a flow of thought and feeling? Or, must they exist for most or all of the time isolated and beyond criticism, as with Kipling (Shengold, 1974)? Beneath the fragile, seeming clarity of the bad "Aunty Rosa" and Harry, and the good mother and the good father, was a terrible ambivalent fragmentation and confusion. This is beautifully described by Jarrell (1962): "As it was, his world had been torn in two and he himself torn in two: for under the part of him that extenuated everything, blamed for nothing, there was certainly a part that extenuated nothing, blamed for everything—a part he never admitted, most especially not to himself" (p. 144).

Kipling was most comfortable when the separation of the split representations operated to suppress hatred. This could happen when he was active and in control, at one with his "Daemon" (his name, implying dissociation, for his creative powers perhaps unconsciously linked with "that Devil-Boy," Harry) with creative energies flowing. It was necessary above all to achieve *discipline* in his work and in his life—that perfect ordering of things that ruled out sudden desolation so that the good could not suddenly become the bad. Here is the image with which he ends the *Jungle Books* (he had begun them with Mowgli abandoned to the mercy of the tiger): animals and men take part in a magnificent review before the Viceroy, and a native officer responds to a stranger's asking how it was done. The animals "obey, as the men do. Mule, horse, elephant, or bullock, he obeys his driver, and the driver his sergeant, and the sergeant his lieutenant, and the lieutenant his captain, and the captain his major, and the major his colonel, and the colonel his brigadier commanding three regiments, and the brigadier his general, who obeys the Viceroy, who is the servant of the Empress. Thus it is done" (1894, p. 421). In such a well-regulated world, the Empress, the Great Mother, watches over all. The Jungle has lost its terror.

The psychoanalyst who is only a reader has no special source of insight. His view of an author's childhood has to be superficial. From the surface, Kipling's childhood is portrayed as six years of bliss followed by six years of hell. The crucial first six years of life must have provided the strengths that enabled Kipling to survive the efforts to kill his soul in the House of Desolation; he says so himself. How much did these early years also provide the seeds of his undoing? The reader can only speculate, reconstructing from what Kipling wrote, and basing his shaky structure on a general knowledge of human development. In his memoirs and stories, Kipling depicts the narcissistic vulnerability that can accompany the grandiosity of the overindulged child. It would be important to know more about the early relationship with his parents, especially with his mysterious mother. It must be meaningful that Trix writes of herself in Lorne Lodge as having had "no least recollection of" her mother, while "remembering that dear ayah known and loved all my short life in India" (1937, pp. 168, 170). Fears about his anger and his sexual feelings must have been evoked in Rudyard by the births of his sister and the stillborn sibling. These births were probably linked to fantasies about parental intercourse and the first trip to the "dark land," England. The lifelong obsessive metaphors of light and darkness, vision and blindness, show the importance of primal scene fantasies for Kipling, fantasies that had exciting and terrifying connotations. Another evidence is Kipling's intense curiosity and need to know how everything works and is related; this fixation on curiosity is mysteriously transmuted into his creative gifts as an observer and describer and an evoker of realistic detail.

More is known about the second six years, the years of the attempt at soul murder, the effects of which continued to inhibit Kipling's ability to feel joy and to love and sometimes flawed his art. The soul murder was far from completely effected: Kipling preserved his identity, and he became a great artist. Paradoxically the struggle to fight off the soul murder (and its aftereffects) strengthened him, and gave him motive, subject matter, and perhaps even creative powers for his writing. I have connected those terrible years of his childhood to his flaws and to his greatness. Kipling's story touches on the mysteries of the origin of mental illness and of creativity; the explorer must be prepared for contradiction and complexity.

BIBLIOGRAPHY

CARRINGTON, C. E. (1955), *Rudyard Kipling*. London: Macmillan.
DOBRÉE, B. (1967), *Rudyard Kipling*. London: Oxford Univ. Press.
EDEL, L. (1962), *Henry James*, 3. New York: Lippincott.
FLEMING, A. (1937), Some Childhood Memories of Rudyard Kipling. *Chambers J.*, March, pp. 168–173.
FORSTER, J. (1873), *The Life of Charles Dickens*. London: Cecil Palmer, 1928.
FREUD, A. (1939–45), Infants Without Families. *Writings*, 3.
―――― (1965), *Normality and Pathology in Childhood*. New York: Int. Univ. Press.
FREUD, S. (1911), Psycho-Analytic Notes on an Autobiographical Account of a Case of Paranoia (Dementia Paranoides). *S.E.*, 12:3–86.
―――― (1917), A Childhood Recollection from *Dichtung und Wahrheit*. *S.E.*, 17:145–156.
GREEN, R. L. (1965), *Kipling and the Children*. London: Elek Books.
IBSEN, H. (1896), John Gabriel Borkman, tr. W. Archer. In: *Collected Works*, 11:179–353. New York: Scribners, 1926; tr. A. Paulson. In: *Last Plays of Henrik Ibsen*. New York: Bantam Books, 1962, pp. 293–374.
JACOBS, B. (1969), 'Psychic Murder' and Characterization in Strindberg's 'The Father.' *Scandinavica*, pp. 19–34.
JARRELL, R. (1962), On Preparing to Read Kipling. In: *Kipling and the Critics*, ed. E. Gilbert. New York: New York Univ. Press, 1965, pp. 133–149.
―――― (1963), The English in England. In: *The Third Book of Criticism*. New York: Farrar, Straus & Giroux, 1969, pp. 279–294.
KINKEAD-WEEKS, R. (1964), Vision in Kipling's Novels. In: *Kipling's Mind and Art*, ed. A. Rutherford. London: Oliver & Boyd, pp. 197–234.
KIPLING, R. (1884–1935), *Complete Works of Rudyard Kipling*. New York: Doubleday & Doran, 1941.
―――― (1884), Failure. 28:101–102.
―――― (1885), The Betrothal. 25:97–99.
―――― (1888a), Plain Tales From the Hills. 1.
―――― (1888b), Baa Baa, Black Sheep. 3:281–316.
―――― (1889), In Partibus. 28:171–174.
―――― (1890a), The Light That Failed. 15:1–244.

——— (1890b), The Rhyme of the Three Captains. 25:255–260.
——— (1892), Barrack Room Ballads. 25:163–214.
——— (1894), The Jungle Books. 11.
——— (1895a), William the Conqueror. 6:165–206.
——— (1895b), The Brushwood Boy. 6:329–370.
——— (1897), Captains Courageous. 16:1–175.
——— (1899), Stalky & Co. 14:1–377.
——— (1901), Kim. 16:181–525.
——— (1906), Puck of Pook's Hill. 13:1–238.
——— (1907), Values in Life. 24:17–22.
——— (1910), Rewards and Fairies. 13:239–544.
——— (1929), Uncovenanted Mercies. 10:325–348.
——— (1935), Hymn of Breaking Strain. 28:298–299.
——— (1937), Something of Myself. 24:349–518.
MAHLER, M. S. (1972), On the First Three Subphases of the Separation-Individuation Process. *Int. J. Psycho-Anal.*, 53:333–338.
NIEDERLAND, W. G. (1959a), The "Miracled-Up" World of Schreber's Childhood. *This Annual*, 14:383–413.
——— (1959b), Schreber: Father and Son. *Psychoanal. Quart.*, 28:151–169.
——— (1960), Schreber's Father. *J. Amer. Psychoanal. Assn.*, 8:492–499.
——— (1963), Further Data and Memorabilia Pertaining to the Schreber Case. *Int. J. Psycho-Anal.*, 44:201–207.
O'NEILL, E. (1956), *A Long Day's Journey Into Night.* New Haven: Yale Univ. Press.
ORWELL, G. (1949), *1984.* New York: Harcourt & Brace.
SCHREBER, D. P. (1903), *Memoirs of My Nervous Illness.* London: Dawson, 1955.
SHENGOLD, L. (1963), The Parent As Sphinx. *J. Amer. Psychoanal.*, 11:725–751.
——— (1967), The Effects of Overstimulation: Rat People. *Int. J. Psycho-Anal.*, 48:403–415.
——— (1971), More About Rats and Rat People. *Int. J. Psycho-Anal.*, 52:277–288.
——— (1974), The Metaphor of the Mirror. *J. Amer. Psychoanal.*, 22:97–115.
——— (1975), Soul Murder. *Int. J. Psychoanal. Psychother.*, 3:366–373.
STEWART, J. I. M. (1966), *Rudyard Kipling.* New York: Dodd & Mead.
STRINDBERG, A. (1887), Soul Murder. *Drama Rev.*, 13:113–118, 1968.
TRILLING, L. (1943), Kipling. In: *Kipling's Mind and Art,* ed. A. Rutherford. London: Oliver & Boyd, 1964, pp. 85–96.
WHITMAN, W. (1855), *Leaves of Grass.* New York: Modern Library, 1921.
WILSON, E. (1941), The Kipling That Nobody Read. In: *Kipling's Mind and Art,* ed. A. Rutherford. London: Oliver & Boyd, 1964, pp. 17–69.

Acknowledgments

The author is grateful to the following publishers for permission to quote material from their books: Dodd, Mead & Company, Inc., New York (*Rudyard Kipling,* by J. I. M. Stewart, 1966); Doubleday and Co., Inc., New York (*Complete Works of*

Rudyard Kipling, 1941); Elek Books Ltd., London (*Kipling and the Children*, by R. L. Green, 1965); and Mrs. George Bambridge, Macmillan of London and Basingstoke and Doubleday Inc. (*Rudyard Kipling: His Life and Work*, by Charles E. Carrington, 1955).

Frederick Douglass, Portrait of a Black Militant

A Study in the Family Romance

STEPHEN M. WEISSMAN, M.D.

ONE OF THE MOST CHARACTERISTIC ASPECTS OF THE SLAVERY EXPERIence, for the slave, was its disruptive and destructive impact on the traditional family unit. In this paper I shall focus on a single individual, Frederick Douglass, and study the effect of this aspect of slavery on his personality development and identity formation. Douglass grew up, after the age of 5, as an essentially parentless slave child and, after escaping from slavery as a young man, went on to become a major nineteenth-century social reformer.

Although he was deeply affected by this lack of enduring, reliable traditional parental figures, he was nonetheless able to make a remarkably resourceful, creative adaptation to this traumatic experience. By studying Douglass's three autobiographies I hope to trace how this adaptation was in part achieved by the extremely imaginative, active use of childhood fantasy, in particular the family romance. I think that Freud (1908) regarded childhood fantasy from an adaptational point of view when he wrote:

> The liberation of an individual, as he grows up, from the authority of his parents is one of the most necessary though one of the most painful results brought about by the course of his development. It is

---

The author is an Assistant Clinical Professor of Psychiatry at George Washington University Medical School and a Faculty member of the Washington School of Psychiatry. Acknowledgments are due to Drs. Robert A. Cohen and Edward M. Podvoll for their invaluable help, criticism, and friendship.

quite essential that that liberation should occur and it may be presumed that it has been to some extent achieved by everyone who has reached a normal state. Indeed, the whole progress of society rests upon the opposition between successive generations [p. 237].

Freud describes the role these early fantasies play in fostering the child's gradual independence from his parents. The child is able to turn his attention away from his personal parents to his own internal imagery, by means of which he is able to create idealized "good" and depreciated "bad" sets of imaginary parental figures of his own fiction. He is the author of the intricate dramatic plots of these fantasies, and this affords him a degree of control and mastery which he does not have over the actual circumstances in his daily life. The frequency and manner in which aspects of the family romance and its derivatives emerge in the personal analyses of children and adults leave little doubt about its universality and its tendency to persist throughout adult life. In this sense, the romance is a type of mental novel of early childhood which is capable of being mentally revised and rewritten at different stages of life. Douglass's autobiographies are an example of this process of revision and re-remembering.

Otto Rank (1909), writing in close collaboration with Freud, was the first person to point to the role of the family romance in the plot structure of ancient mythological stories of the birth of the hero and his subsequent heroic deeds. By comparing the heroes of ancient myths to the hero of the typical childhood family romance, he pinpointed the features they had in common. In both cases, the hero was the secret, unacknowledged issue of parents of high station. He is separated from them at birth or shortly thereafter either because of fate per se or because of some omen or prophecy. This element of fate or prophecy is taken to signify a sense of specialness and of being destined for great deeds. These prophesied deeds usually portend a threat either to the father in particular or to the status quo of society in general. The hero then finds himself being raised by lowly surrogate parents and only gradually are his true identity and mission revealed to him through incidents which are experienced as signs of destiny and evidence of a personal sense of specialness.

This need to create fictional versions of imaginary parents is more intense in children who have actually lost their parents at an early age. The child protects himself from being overwhelmed by intense feelings of grief and bereavement by reassuring himself that somewhere he has an ideal set of parents and that he is destined for great deeds and happier days. Phyllis Greenacre (1958) described this phenomenon in orphaned children and demonstrated its operation in the lives of several creative individuals. She was able to show a pattern of early childhood loss in the lives of these creative people and to demonstrate how they coped with this loss at the time by creating imagery of their own in the form of vivid, elaborate family romance fantasies. Furthermore, she was able to trace the ways in which they retained this highly developed imaginative capacity as adults and how it became a major resource in their creative activities in later life.

Writing more directly from a clinical point of view, Ernst Kris (1956) made a valuable contribution to understanding the role played by the family romance in the construction of autobiographies.[1] In his analytic work with a number of gifted patients he was able to discover a characteristic pattern of personal myth making in their organization of their biographical pasts. These people began their analyses with consciously available, tightly constructed, historically continuous versions of their pasts. Despite a surface quality of factualness and historical accuracy to these autobiographical narratives, they turned out to contain important distortions. The distortions consisted of explicit factual errors and subtler shifts through emphasis and omission of certain facts. The pattern of these distortions was remarkably uniform. In all cases the autobiographies contained the specific unconscious family romance subtly woven into the fabric of their life stories. Each person had created a personal myth of his past in the form of an autobiographical self image. This mythological self image in turn exerted a major influence on the person's adult life.

Kris's contribution is particularly important to understanding the psychology of autobiographies in general. His work is extremely

---

[1] Kris (1935) had earlier investigated the role of the family romance in the old biographies of artists.

relevant to the subject of this study, Frederick Douglass, since the major source material we have is autobiographical. Douglass was a man who wrote his autobiography at three different points in his life, at the ages of 28, 38, and 64. In each case, the new autobiography did not consist of a mere updating of the previous one by adding the experiences of the intervening years. Each new book included revisions in his accounts of early childhood and adolescent memories. The changes were most marked between the first and second books, and it is the shifts between these accounts on which this paper will focus.

The Life of Frederick Douglass

Before progressing into a psychological exploration of the autobiographies, I shall introduce Douglass himself, identify his significance as a historical figure, and clarify the historical importance of his autobiographies as social documents for the times in which he lived. He was one of a comparatively small number out of a total of three million slaves who escaped from slavery before the general emancipation. After escaping at the age of 21, he actively continued his protest at a public level, agitating for repeal of slavery. After emancipation, he continued as a Negro leader to press for economic, social, and political equality. His voice was heard as a newspaper editor, a political figure, and a government official, but he was best known as an orator.

Douglass was a reformer who brought the case against slavery before the public in a powerfully persuasive manner. He told his personal childhood history as a slave and he told it well. In an age of evangelical fervor and an almost religious spirit of reform, he was among the most eloquent speakers to stand up and personally bear witness to the evils of slavery. Benjamin Quarles (1970), his major biographer, summed up his speaking abilities:

> People simply liked to see him on the platform. There was a dramatic presence about his very appearance—his superb physique, his thick, black hair, and his well formed nose. . . . His voice was created for public address in a pre-microphone America. In speaking he sounded every degree of light and shade. His powerful tones hinted at a readiness to defy faulty acoustics. His rich

baritone gave an emotional vitality to every sentence. With cascading vehemence he could emit invective and denunciation in the best tradition of the Garrisonian school. Added to his earnestness was an impetuous and stirring eloquence [p. 60].

There must have been a heightened sense of dramatic contrast as he told of his transformation from a frightened, parentless slave child to a fiery, angry protester against the injustices of the white slave owners, including his own biological father. As he told his story it was as if the metamorphosis was occurring before the audience itself and they were witnessing the transformation. He was simply narrating the "facts" of his life, but buried within those facts was an ageless story of the struggle between father and son. This second, hidden story, woven into the first, gave fiery passion to his speech and resonated with the unconscious of his audience. It was a tale that had stood the test of time spreading over the centuries from the ancient patriarchal Euro-Asiatic societies to the Oceanic peoples; a story captivating enough that 34 ancient versions of it had been found in the Mediterranean basin and western Asia alone. It was the myth of the birth of the hero.

Douglass was a mulatto child, born in 1817. His biological parents were a black, field-hand, slave mother and an unknown white man. He was separated from his mother at birth and reared by his maternal grandparents until the age of 5. It was his grandmother's job to raise all of the slave children on the small plantation on the eastern shore of Maryland until they were approximately 5 or 6. Then they were customarily sent to live in their owner's home several miles away. Douglass was neither the first nor the only personal grandchild she raised.

At their master's home they lived as part of a kitchen brood of slave children and were supervised by the slave cook. They did a few light household and farm chores but were otherwise left to their own devices until they were old enough to go to work in the fields as quarter hands, half hands, and finally full hands as they approached their physical adulthood. This was generally around the age of 16.

Douglass grew up as part of this kitchen brood until the age of 8 when he was selected as a "loan" to be a body servant and part-time companion for a younger white boy who was a distant relative of his owner. He left the plantation and was sent to Baltimore where he lived with this white family from the ages of 8 to 16. Initially he was affectionately "adopted" by the boy's mother who had never owned slaves before. She responded to him maternally and even began to teach him the alphabet and how to read and write. Later her husband discovered this and forbade it. He warned her of the illegality of literacy for slaves and cautioned her of the danger of intensifying the slave's discontent with his status through literacy. She complied with her husband's wishes both in deed and, gradually, in spirit. Douglass's relations with this "adopted" white mother grew progressively less cordial and more distant.

This attempted ban on literacy served to crystallize Douglass's awareness of the futile social dead end that awaited him as an adult slave. Having overheard the discussions between his master and mistress, he privately vowed to become literate. He was gradually successful between the ages of 10 and 16 in getting his white playmates secretly to teach him how to spell, read, and write. He began to read the Baltimore newspapers whose columns gave him a broad overview of the slavery controversy that was raging in the land. Literacy had allowed him to escape from the intellectual quarantine that was so widely and systematically enforced on illiterate, rural slaves.

He secretly obtained a slim book of speeches of great orators which included several antislavery tracts. He endlessly read and reread this one book during his early adolescence. Later, he was to credit it with helping to kindle his hopes and maintain his dreams of freedom and to have served as the first stimulus for his interest in public speaking.

At the age of 16 Douglass experienced another reversal in his fortunes. His original owner died, the previous "loan" of him to the Baltimore family was canceled, and he was returned to the eastern shore by his new master. Here an attempt was made to reintroduce him into rural chattel slavery as a field hand. He was soon recognized to be temperamentally unsuited to this work by dint of his education, intelligence, and, most importantly, his surly uncooperativeness which was passively expressed in the moody, sullen negativism of the underdog adolescent slave.

He was considered arrogant and was promptly sent to work under a professional "nigger-breaker" whose skill lay in his ability to "break" difficult slaves into passive obedience and compliant cooperativeness. The first six months of this one-year program were highly effective. Douglass became a clinically depressed, suicidally preoccupied automaton that did his master's bidding. A turning point came at the end of six months during an unusually severe and unwarranted physical beating. Douglass physically stood up to the man, successfully fought back, and refused to allow himself to be whipped. His spirits lifted immediately as he began to regain his dwindling sense of his own manhood and to shed the oppressive psychological sense of slavishness that had been growing.

Douglass considered this incident the major turning point in his life as a slave, although he remained a slave for several years more before he successfully escaped. During this period he made one unsuccessful attempt at escaping, after which he was quite fortunately sent back to the family in Baltimore rather than being sold into the deep South, as was the custom with unmanageable slaves. In Baltimore he was taught a semiskilled trade as a ship caulker and was allowed to hire himself out, although his owner kept his earnings. Eventually he was able to secure a set of merchant seaman's identity papers belonging to a black freeman and handily escaped to New York City by train at the age of 21.

He settled in New Bedford, Massachusetts, where he married a black freewoman from Baltimore, began to raise a family, and supported himself as a physical laborer. Here he started to develop an interest in the growing New England abolitionist movement which was headed by his hero William Lloyd Garrison. After several years the two men finally met at an abolitionist meeting in Nantucket at which Douglass was persuaded publicly to tell the story of his slavery experiences for the first time. He spoke with an unrehearsed and moving simplicity. Garrison then rose and, using Douglass as his text, eloquently launched into an electrifying denunciation of slavery that left the audience spellbound.

A strong bond of friendship gradually developed between these two men as an aftermath of their dramatic encounter. Although each man was himself a father in his own right, I imagine that the emotional tone of this union was not unlike the meeting of Stephen Daedelus and Leopold Bloom in Joyce's *Ulysses* where the childless father and fatherless son meet during the course of their respective quests and symbolically unite. Douglass and Garrison developed a highly idealized but productive working relationship, which was to end bitterly 14 years later. During this period of friendship Douglass described himself as studying under the tutelage of Garrison, learning about life, the rhetoric of protest, and the fine points of oratory. Often they barnstormed the abolitionist circuit lecturing as far south as Pennsylvania and as far west as Ohio. First Douglass, the former slave, would tell his story and then Garrison would use Douglass as his text. It was a piece of evangelical vaudeville that drew large crowds and was immensely popular.

The Autobiographies

In 1845 Douglass wrote and published his first autobiography, *Narrative of the Life of Frederick Douglass*. He wrote it himself and it was a summary of his story. His writing it was in part prompted by the growing disbelief on the part of his audiences that this articulate, charismatic black man had ever been a slave. The *Narrative* was well reviewed and was an immediate success. It was translated into several foreign languages and sold over 30,000 copies. There are several reasons for choosing to make a study of the *Narrative* a principal focus in this paper: Of the three autobiographies, it is the one of the greatest enduring literary merit. It also offers the greatest insight into the psychological process of identity formation. Finally, it was the most important of the three books as a historical document. The *Narrative* was perhaps second only to Harriet Beecher Stowe's *Uncle Tom's Cabin* as a major influential piece of abolitionist literature. Its publication won Douglass international recognition and its moving story had an incendiary impact on its audience. It remains a major piece of nineteenth-century American literature and is a passionate indictment of the slavery system by one of its victims.

Even in my attempt to give a neutral summary of the "facts" of

Douglass's early life, the crux of the psychological problem of this study comes clearly into focus. Stated simply, there is no way in which the facts of a person's experience can be told without some degree of interpretive emphasis being placed on one or another aspect of the experience or the personality of the individual. Douglass's story can be told in tragic, heroic, prosaic, pathetic, ironic, and conceivably even comic fashion by either the biographer or the autobiographer. The same is true of a personal analysis in which an individual's life story is remembered and retold from many different emotional points of view. Each of these points of view reflects an organized constellation of memory experiences, fantasies, and corresponding personality traits. The notion of such an organization is reflected in our everyday clinical language when we talk, for instance, of analyzing the depressive or hysterical aspects of someone's personality. In this study I am attempting to analyze the heroic aspects of Douglass's character. I purposely avoid the choice of more clinical terms such as phallic or narcissistic since we lack the corroborative associations from the living patient which lend real meaning and richness to such terms. Instead we will have to content ourselves with derivatives which have been filtered through the secondary process of conscious thought. Through inference these derivatives afford us fragmentary glimpses of aspects of a man and permit us to conjecture about his inner workings. Douglass begins his *Narrative*:[2]

> I was born in Tuckahoe, near Hillsborough, and about twelve miles from Easton, in Talbot County, Maryland. I have no accurate knowledge of my age, never having seen any authentic record containing it. By far the larger part of the slaves know as little of their age as horses know of theirs, and it is the wish of most masters within my knowledge to keep their slaves thus ignorant. I do not remember to have ever met a slave who could tell of his birthday. They seldom come nearer to it than planting-time, harvest-time, cherry-time, spring-time, or fall time. A want of information

[2] The entire chapter 1 and other excerpts from *Narrative of the Life of Frederick Douglass, An American Slave, Written by Himself* are reprinted by permission of the publishers from the Benjamin Quarles edition, Cambridge, Mass.: The Belknap Press of Harvard University Press, copyright 1960 by the President and Fellows of Harvard College.

concerning my own was a source of unhappiness to me even during childhood. The white children could tell their ages. I could not tell why I ought to be deprived of the same privilege. I was not allowed to make any inquiries of my master concerning it. He deemed all such inquiries on the part of a slave improper and impertinent, and evidence of a restless spirit. The nearest estimate I can give makes me now between twenty-seven and twenty-eight years of age. I come to this, from hearing my master say, some time during 1835, I was about seventeen years old.

My mother was Harriet Bailey. She was the daughter of Isaac and Betsey Bailey, both colored, and quite dark. My mother was of a darker complexion than either my grandmother or grandfather.

My father was a white man. He was admitted to be such by all I ever heard speak of my parentage. The opinion was also whispered that my master was my father; but of the correctness of this opinion, I know nothing; the means of knowing was withheld from me. My mother and I were separated when I was but an infant—before I knew her as my mother. It is a common custom, in the part of Maryland from which I ran away, to part children from their mothers at a very early age. Frequently, before the child has reached its twelfth month, its mother is taken from it, and hired out on some farm a considerable distance off, and the child is placed under the care of an old woman, too old for field labor. For what this separation is done, I do not know, unless it be to hinder the development of the child's affection toward its mother, and to blunt and destroy the natural affection of the mother for the child. This is the inevitable result.

I never saw my mother, to know her as such, more than four or five times in my life; and each of these times was very short in duration, and at night. She was hired by a Mr. Stewart, who lived about twelve miles from my home. She made her journeys to see me in the night, travelling the whole distance on foot, after the performance of her day's work. She was a field hand, and a whipping is the penalty of not being in the field at sunrise, unless a slave has special permission from his or her master to the contrary—a permission which they seldom get, and one that gives to him that gives it the proud name of being a kind master. I do not recollect of ever seeing my mother by the light of day. She was with me in the night. She would lie down with me, and get me to sleep, but long before I waked she was gone. Very little communication ever took place between us. Death soon ended what little we could have while she lived, and with it her hardships and suffering. She died when I was about seven years old, on one of my master's farms, near Lee's Mill. I was not allowed to be present during her illness, at her death, or burial. She was gone long before I knew any thing about it. Never having enjoyed, to any considerable extent, her soothing presence, her tender and watchful care, I received the tidings of her death with much the same emotions I should have probably felt at the death of a stranger.

Called thus suddenly away, she left me without the slightest intimation of who my father was. The whisper that my master was my father, may or may not be true; and, true or false, it is of but little consequence to my purpose whilst the fact remains, in all its glaring odiousness, that slaveholders have ordained, and by law established, that the children of slave women shall in all cases follow the condition of their mothers; and this is done too obviously to administer to their own lusts, and make a gratification of their wicked desires profitable as well as pleasurable; for by this cunning arrangement, the slaveholder, in cases not a few, sustains to his slaves the double relation of master and father.

I know of such cases; and it is worthy of remark that such slaves invariably suffer greater hardships, and have more to contend with, than others. They are, in the first place, a constant offence to their mistress. She is ever disposed to find fault with them; they can seldom do anything to please her; she is never better pleased than when she sees them under the lash, especially when she suspects her husband of showing to his mulatto children favors which he withholds from his black slaves. The master is frequently compelled to sell this class of his slaves, out of deference to the feelings of his white wife; and, cruel as the deed may strike any one to be, for a man to sell his own children to human flesh-mongers, it is often the dictate of humanity for him to do so; for, unless he does this, he must not only whip them himself, but must stand by and see one white son tie up his brother, of but few shades darker complexion than himself, and ply the gory lash to his naked back; and if he lisp one word of disapproval, it is set down to his parental partiality, and only makes a bad matter worse, both for himself and the slave whom he would protect and defend.

Every year brings with it multitudes of this class of slaves. It was doubtless in consequence of a knowledge of this fact, that one great statesman of the south predicted the downfall of slavery by the inevitable laws of population. Whether this prophecy is ever fulfilled or not, it is nevertheless plain that a very different-looking class of people are springing up at the south, and are now held in slavery, from those originally brought to this country from Africa; and if their increase will do no other good, it will do away the force of argument, that God cursed Ham, and therefore American slavery is right. If the lineal descendants of Ham are alone to be scripturally enslaved, it is certain that slavery at the south must soon become unscriptural; for thousands are ushered into the world, annually, who, like myself, owe their existence to white fathers, and those fathers most frequently their own masters.

I have had two masters. My first master's name was Anthony. I do not remember his first name. He was generally called Captain Anthony—a title which, I presume, he acquired by sailing a craft on the Chesapeake Bay. He was not considered a rich slaveholder. He owned two or three farms, and about thirty slaves. His farms and slaves were under the care of an overseer. The overseer's name was Plummer. Mr. Plummer was a miserable drunkard, a profane swearer, and a savage monster. He always went armed with a cowskin and a heavy cudgel. I have known him to cut and slash the women's heads so horribly, that even master would be enraged at his cruelty, and would threaten to whip him if he did not mind himself. Master, however, was not a humane slaveholder. It required extraordinary barbarity on the part of an overseer to affect him. He was a cruel man, hardened by a long life of slaveholding. He would at times seem to take great pleasure in whipping a slave. I have often been awakened at the dawn of day by the most heart-rendering shrieks of an own aunt of mine, whom he used to tie up to a joist, and whip upon her naked back till she was literally covered with blood. No words, no tears, no prayers, from his gory victim, seemed to move his iron heart from its bloody purpose. The louder she screamed, the harder he whipped; and where the blood ran fastest, there he whipped longest. He would whip her to make her scream, and whip her to make her hush; and not until overcome by fatigue, would he cease to swing the blood-clotted cowskin. I remember the first time I ever witnessed this horrible exhibition. I was quite a child, but I well remember it. I never will forget it whilst I remember any thing. It was the first of a long series of such outrages, of which I was doomed to be a witness and a participant. It struck me with awful force. It was the blood-stained gate, the entrance to the hell of slavery, through which I was about to pass. It was a most terrible spectacle. I wish I could commit to paper the feelings with which I beheld it.

This occurrence took place very soon after I went to live with my old master, and under the following circumstances. Aunt Hester went out one night,—where or for what I do not know,—and happened to be absent when my master desired her presence. He had ordered her not to go out evenings, and warned her that she must never let him catch her in company with a young man, who was paying attention to her belonging to Colonel Lloyd. The young man's name was Ned Roberts, generally called Lloyd's Ned. Why master was so careful of her, may be safely left to conjecture. She was a woman of noble form, and of graceful proportions, having very few equals, and fewer superiors, in personal appearance, among the colored or white women of our neighborhood.

Aunt Hester had not only disobeyed his orders in going out, but had been found in company with Lloyd's Ned; which circumstance, I found, from what he said while whipping her, was the chief offence. Had he been a man of pure morals himself, he might have been thought interested in protecting the innocence of my aunt; but those who knew him will not suspect him of any such virtue. Before he commenced whipping Aunt Hester, he took her into the kitchen, and stripped her from neck to waist, leaving her neck, shoulders, and back, entirely naked. He then told her to cross her hands, calling her at the same time a d—d b—h. After crossing her hands, he tied them with a strong rope, and led her to a stool under a large hook in the joist, put in for the purpose. He made her get upon the stool, and tied her hands to the hook. She now stood fair for his infernal purpose. Her arms were stretched up at their full length, so that she stood upon the ends of her toes. He then said to her, "Now, you d—d b—h, I'll learn you how to disobey my orders!" and after rolling up his sleeves, he commenced to lay on the heavy cowskin, and soon the warm, red blood (amid heart-rendering shrieks from her, and horrid oaths from him) came dripping to the floor. I was so terrified and horror-stricken at the sight, that I hid myself in a closet, and dared not venture out till long after the bloody transaction was over. I expected it would be my turn next. It was all new to me. I had never seen any thing like it before. I had always lived with my grandmother on the outskirts of the plantation, where she was put to raise the children of the younger women. I had therefore been, until now, out of the way of the bloody scenes that often occurred on the plantation.

The powerful emotional tone of the book is swiftly established.

Douglass writes in the first person talking to his reader in a personal, emotional, and at times imploringly evocative way. He tells the scantily remembered facts of his earliest years and shares the feelings that he had in response to these early experiences. Almost no attempt is made throughout the book to distinguish clearly between what he felt as a child and what he felt looking back as an adult. Regression in the service of the ego has taken place, leading to a powerful piece of writing in which he does not distance himself from his experiences by explicitly adding and sustaining the perspective of an adult remembering aspects of his childhood. Instead things are told from the ambiguous perspective of a half-innocent, half-knowing man-child. This perspective helps to create the image of the omnipotent and omniscient child hero who possesses extraordinary perceptive faculties far beyond his years.

There is also a subtle use of imagery which is sustained throughout the book. We are immediately led into the child's world of darkness, nighttime, ignorance, mystery, whispered secrets, and nightmarish awakening. Douglass tells us that mother left him in the dark and father kept him in the dark. We relive the dreaded childhood experience of being abandoned and left in the dark only to wake up in terror at dawn to a scene of thinly disguised sexual brutality in the form of a passionately jealous whipping of his aunt by his father. The unconscious organizing themes in the imagery are a mixture of separation anxiety and primal scene terror. At the same time there are no concrete memories of the first five years of life. Ten years later, in the second autobiography, this perspective will shift dramatically, but at this point in time Douglass has only this fantasy memory of early childhood. This screen memory substitutes for a factual recollection of the first five years of life and is based on the childhood nightmare which also serves as a prototype in the rest of the autobiography. A dominant unconscious point of view in the imagery of the book relates to the bloody, nightmarish aspects of slavery and the small child's heroic attempts to cope with them by waking himself up. The imagery of waking up becomes an extended metaphor throughout the book for his gradually expanding consciousness, his personal struggle for literacy, and ultimately the establishment of his personal sense of reality, which is highly divergent from the culture in which he grew up.

Douglass begins in a disoriented way with a child who is confused and in the dark about even the simplest facts of when he was born or the circumstances of his birth. This birth confusion is fused with a repressive amnesia for the events of the first five years of his life. These two elements are mixed together to convey an almost fuguelike state. The confusion is used to create imagery of a timeless, legendary world of prehistory. In this archaic, naturalistic world of legend, man is just another animal who experiences and measures the passage of time through the rhythmical change of seasons rather than by use of the artificial man-made calendar. When we are told that his birthday ignorance is typical of most slaves' experiences, it is done in the spirit of establishing his credentials as the universal or prototypical black man.

The second story then is of a boy who speaks for all people. He is born in a timeless legendary world, deprived of his birthrights, separated from his mother at birth, raised by a woman "too old for field labor," later to be turned over to a cruel master who is given to sexual violence and brutality toward women. It is hinted that this cruel white master may be his father, but that, even if it is so, he could not acknowledge paternal ties out of fear of his white wife's jealous anger (the archetypal theme of the wicked stepmother). It is only parenthetically mentioned that the old woman who raised him was his grandmother and no richness of detail is provided about their relationship. The master-father also remains dimensionlessly characterized as the classic tyrant father in the first autobiography.

The remainder of the *Narrative* is book length and can only be summarized here. It is a simple, well-written chronicle of Douglass's childhood experiences in slavery, his eventual revolt and escape. Embedded in the account are the other classic features of the unconscious hero myth: the extraordinary perceptiveness of the child hero, the extraordinary feats of the young hero, and the sense of being specially chosen by fate with signs of divine favor.

As already mentioned, the sense of extraordinary perceptiveness is conveyed through the stylistic technique of writing through the consciousness of the man-child. It is also developed by implicitly contrasting himself to the other slaves who are characterized as docile, unassertive, and, most importantly, unaware victims of slavery. He writes, in this version, as if to suggest that he grew up in a world in which no one else saw the inequities of the system or protested against them by either defiance or escape. Thus Douglass psychologically denies any adult models for his own critical experiences of refusing to be whipped or escaping, thereby creating the aura of extraordinary deeds. Ten years later, in his second autobiography, he will recall living examples of courageous defiance and successful escape that he witnessed while growing up and he will acknowledge their influence on his own experiences. He will also recall that his mother could read and that his black grandfather was a freeman.

Douglass is even more explicit in regard to his sense of personal destiny and his being chosen for divine favor. He talks of his being sent to Baltimore as the first sign of being specially chosen for great deeds:

> I have ever regarded it as the first plain manifestation of that kind providence which has ever since attended me, and marked my life with so many favors. I regarded the selection of myself as being somewhat remarkable. . . . There were those younger, those older, and those of the same age. I was chosen from among them all, and was the first, last, and only choice.
>
> I may be deemed superstitious, and even egotistical, in regarding this event as a special interposition of divine Providence in my favor. But I should be false to the earliest sentiments of my soul, if I suppressed the opinion [p. 56].

So far I have been exercising the analyst's privilege of partially ignoring the writer's literal intended surface meanings in order to detect additional unconscious meanings. This approach is based on an analysis of style, imagery, and organization. An underlying assumption is that these aspects of the autobiography reflect the unconscious feelings, fantasies, and attitudes of the narrator. This technique of psychobiography is analogous to the clinical settings where we only half listen to the straightforward logical meanings in the spoken content of a patient's communications while also focusing on his style, imagery, and nonverbal processes. The conclusions reached through this aspect of the psychobiographical method are speculative since they are based on interpretive conjecture, intuition, and clinical inference as to what else might have been going on in the writer's mind and in his life at the time of writing.

In Douglass's case, the interpretive evidence suggests that an unconscious hero fantasy from early childhood is not being explicitly remembered and recalled as a daydream he once had as a child. Instead, I infer that it is being actively relived and reexperienced with all the vividness of the original childhood fantasy and with a hallucinatory intensity as if the fantasy were actually reality. In other words, the unconscious fantasy actively shapes historical memory and colors recollected incident. What is remembered as factual conforms to the structure and content of the unconscious fantasy.[3]

What independent evidence do we have that such a process is taking place? How do we know that things were not exactly as Douglass remembers them? How do we know that he ever had such childhood fantasies? If there were such fantasies, what role did they play in his life? Working in the clinical situation, Kris was able to document the autobiographical phenomenon I am inferring. With Douglass we are limited to the information he provides us in his subsequent autobiographies, particularly *My Bondage and My Freedom* (1855).

In this second book, the events of early childhood are no longer telescopically condensed into a vague memory of an unhappy abandonment followed by a jolting exposure to a whipping scene. The spontaneous recovery of early memories and the shift in feelings about his master-father are remarkable. Experiences are recalled with more richness and complexity as we now hear the story of a small boy who was affectionately raised as a very definite part of a family unit by his slave grandmother until the age of 5.

Grandmother is glowingly remembered as "a woman of power and spirit [who] enjoyed the high privilege of living in a cabin, separate from the quarter, with no other burden than her own support, and the necessary care of the little children." He describes her as "held in high esteem, far higher than is the lot of most

---

[3] Erikson's (1962) discussion of reality and actuality is pertinent to this matter.

colored persons. [She] was, indeed, at that time, all the world to me; and the thought of being separated from her, in any considerable time, was more than an unwelcome intruder. It was intolerable" (p. 39).[4]

The circumstances of the traumatic separation are clearly recalled. He was told as a small child that he would be sent to live with his master when he was 5 years old. He remembers that after being told of this, the thought of being "separated from my grandmother, seldom or never to see her again, haunted me. I dreaded the thought of going to live with that mysterious 'old master' whose name I never heard mentioned with affection, but always with fear. I look back to this as among the heaviest of my childhood sorrows" (p. 40).

He clearly indicates that he had already developed powerful tyrannical fantasies about his master-father before meeting him: "I had been made to fear this somebody above all else on earth. Born for another's benefit, as the *firstling* of the cabin flock I was soon to be selected as a meet offering to the fearful *demigod* whose image on so many occasions haunted my childhood's imagination" (p. 45).

When the time came to separate, his grandmother took him to his master's home without explaining the purpose of the trip or that she would be leaving him there. "I had never been deceived before; and I felt not only grieved at parting—as I supposed forever—with my grandmother, but indignant that a trick had been played upon me in a matter so serious. . . . I suppose I cried myself to sleep. . . . I cannot withhold a circumstance which, at the time affected me so deeply. Besides, this was, in fact, my first introduction to the realities of slavery" (p. 49f.).

He goes on to recall his adjustment to the transition: "even the much dreaded old master, whose merciless fiat brought me from Tuckahoe, gradually, to my mind, parted with his terrors. Strange enough, his reverence seemed to take no particular notice of me, nor of my coming. Instead of leaping out and devouring me, he scarcely seemed conscious of my presence." That master "could be kind, and at times, he even showed an affectionate disposition.

---

[4] Excerpts from *My Bondage and My Freedom* are reprinted by permission of the publisher, Dover Publications, New York.

Could the reader have seen him gently leading me by the hand—as he sometimes did—patting me on the head, speaking to me in soft caressing tones and calling me his 'little Indian boy,' he would have deemed him a kind old man, and really, almost fatherly" (p. 80).

The picture that emerges from this cross-reading of the two autobiographies is of a young child who is, understandably, outraged by the painful separation and loss that he has just experienced. His anger is partly directed at his grandmother both for being powerless to prevent the separation and for deceiving him. The bulk of his anger is reserved for his master-father whose power to cause the separation is experienced as the ultimate form of tyranny.[5] The child's response is to turn inward to his own imagery and to seek consolation in his daydreams.

Douglass's need to minimize his feelings of grief, disappointment, and vulnerability lead to a temporary disavowal of the positive ties to his grandmother and the lesser ones to his master-father. He sees himself as alone and stranded. He becomes the heroic figure of his fantasies who will go it alone and singlehandedly obtain revenge and secure his personal independence. He tells us that "when yet but a child six years old, I imbibed the determination to run away." There is every reason to believe that just as the origins of his discontent lay largely in this early childhood separation, so the seeds of the wish for freedom, the sense of heroic self-dramatization, and the idealistic wish for social reform were first conceived and elaborated in the imagery of his family romance fantasies.

The fantasies served the adaptive function of creating a heroic sense of identity, which in turn provided him with a sense of personal courage and strength. Thus, the creation of a personal fiction becomes an important psychological resource in childhood. The fiction later takes on a motivational quality as the growing individual attempts to shape his life and personality to the imagery

---

[5] I use the word "father" because it expresses an important psychological aspect of the experience. Regardless of whether his master was either biologically his father or fulfilled the traditional social roles of a father, the young child thought of him that way. Thus, he became a personal object for at least part of the range of emotions that a child develops toward his father. Besides, the evidence suggests that the master was in fact his father.

of the fiction. In Douglass's case, he forged a heroic identity for himself and was able to find a universal form (the myth of the birth of the hero) for the creative expression of his personal discontent. In this sense, the creation of a personal fiction has a power to move and affect others and, as it begins to operate socially, develops the strength and virility of a social and personal fact. This is the type of progression Freud had in mind when he hinted at the role of the family romance as a precursor for individual independence and social change.

This element of heroic self-dramatization was not exclusively confined to symbolic expression within Douglass's writing. He was equally absorbed in living out elements of his family romance in his life. In the *Narrative* he daringly revealed his slave name, Frederick Bailey, and identified his former master as well. He was advised by friends to burn the manuscript. Just as the contents of the story were heroic, the act of publishing it became a dramatic act of heroic defiance since by identifying himself he exposed himself to the risk of recapture and return to Maryland as a fugitive slave. He was also fearful that by revealing the family secrets he would incite his master to recapture him. He fled to England for safety. He described the trip as a voyage to "the land of my paternal ancestors." While in England he wrote a letter to his master in which he defiantly expressed these feelings of symbolically turning to his ancestral grandparents for justice and redress. Many of his dramatic speeches in England were filled with the fiery rhetoric of the wronged and mistreated stepson who was reclaiming part of his cultural heritage. This romantic image of the fugitive son excited the imagination of his audiences. He was an overnight success. He remained in England for 22 months, returning to America after he was safely purchased out of slavery by a group of sympathetic English friends.

As he grew older and more self-reflective, Douglass became aware of his tendency toward heroic self-dramatization. By the time he wrote his third autobiography (1881), he finally revealed the prosaic details of his successful escape from slavery. In the earlier books the escape had always been exaggeratedly shrouded in mystery. After finally describing his exodus, he wryly commented that had the escape been more heroic he would no doubt have told the story earlier. In a sense, each autobiography gives us a glimpse of his maturational progress from angry militant to elder statesman and prompts a question as to what motivated him to write these three separate accounts. Douglass offers little in the way of direct statements to explain his reasons; and his unconscious motives were, no doubt, overdetermined. Nonetheless, it is interesting to speculate about the developmental and unconscious sources of his need to create three separate autobiographies.

Discussion

SELF-EMANCIPATION THROUGH SERIAL AUTOBIOGRAPHIES

The *Narrative* was written at a time when he was still going through the painful experiences of grief and culture shock involved in leaving his native land of Maryland. As he put it, the South was the land of his childhood and, apart from slavery, he missed it sorely. At one level, writing the first autobiography was part of his attempt to work through his feelings of loss involved in ending this chapter of his life.

At the time of writing the *Narrative* he was emotionally bolstered by his hero-worshipping relationship with Garrison, his idealized white father. Ten years later, he had become more of his own man and was painfully breaking the deep emotional tie to Garrison and the abolitionists. Once more he turned to the autobiographical form to deal with the transition and unconsciously commemorate this important emotional loss. Even the title of the second book, *My Bondage and My Freedom,* clearly expresses the central emotional issue of subtler, internal self-emancipation. The final book was written shortly before his wife's death and at a time when he was a spectator of his own decline. This book, like many later-life autobiographies, was probably motivated by the sense of incipient loss of his energetic and vital sense of himself.

Looking at Douglass's writing as a general example of the creative process prompts some thoughts about the psychology of the artist. I would like to focus on something implied but not explicitly stated in Greenacre's formulations on the importance of early childhood losses in the lives of creative people. I think that in these gifted children the process of childhood grief and bereavement is resolved in a way that is characteristic of the future artist. Their extraordinary imaginative ability to cope with loss by protectively creating personal imagery constitutes a special case of denial in fantasy. They do not compromise and replace their childhood loss, after grieving, with another human relationship. Their creative product replaces their personal loss. Greenacre points out that they often remain isolated and lonely as children. Their mourning is incompletely worked through, and they retain a lifelong vulnerability to these feelings, although the intensity of these feelings can fluctuate considerably over a lifetime. This vulnerability comes in part from never having relinquished their highly idealized imagery, heightened expectations, and powerful, idealistic strivings. With sufficient psychological and biographical information one can often detect a correlation between events in their personal lives activating these dormant feelings, which in turn serve as a stimulus for creative activity. For Douglass it was the loss of his grandmother, the South of his childhood, his "white" mother in Baltimore, the loss of Garrison, and the loss of his wife and of his youth which in part prompted his writing. In this sense, the creative activity defends against a full-blown depression just as the original imaginative act of creating the family romance consoled and protected the child.

Looking at Douglass from a more clinical point of view, I see him as having conducted a successful self-analysis. Without listing every criteria of a successful analysis, it is clear that Douglass was able meaningfully to recover traumatic memories from early childhood and to work through his feelings associated with these early experiences and relationships. He became more comfortable with his sense of mixed racial identity, he developed a less nightmarishly depressive view of his childhood, and he achieved a greater sense of personal autonomy. He gradually broke his slavishly dependent tie to Garrison, started his own newspaper, and began to assume his role as an important Negro political leader.

Although there had been genuine feelings of love and friendship between Douglass and Garrison, there were also paternalistic and patronizing elements which were inevitably part of such an idealizing relationship. The emotional turning point occurred when Garrison actively opposed and personally discouraged Douglass from starting a newspaper of his own. Garrison argued that it would only compete with his own paper, *The Liberator*; that Douglass was inexperienced and unqualified to be an editor and publisher; and that Douglass could best serve the abolitionist movement by continuing in his role as the former slave telling his story. The painful break in the friendship mobilized the recovery and integration of a more balanced set of feelings toward and memories of Douglass's original parents—primarily his father and grandmother and, to a lesser extent, his mother.

Douglass's internal growth and maturation are reminiscent of Freud's relationship with Wilhelm Fliess and his self-analysis which took place half a century later. Douglass and Freud each formed intense friendships with male colleagues at critical points early in their careers. The friendships were a realistic source of emotional support and in both cases the friend also served as a transference figure. Both Douglass and Freud used the transference aspects of their respective friendships to work out their specific problems. Douglass confined his insights to serving his personal needs, while Freud attempted to extend his personal observations to human psychology in general. From the point of view of technique, each man made use of writing to substitute for an analyst. Writing allowed each man to structure and organize his fleeting mental impressions and to reinforce his observing ego. Freud made use of written notes, while Douglass used the structure of serial autobiographies. Douglass's achievement is impressive since, like Freud's, it illustrates how an unusually gifted person can intuitively conduct a self-analysis.

RACE RELATIONS IN SLAVERY

Given his creative talents, it is difficult to decide which elements of Douglass's personal experience are representative of the common experiences of slaves in general. Traumatic separations, lost and missing parents, and mixed, unacknowledged racial origins were by no means uncommon events in slavery. Many of Douglass's emotional responses to these events are also typical human reactions, but in the end the personal synthesis of these experiences is uniquely Douglass's and no one else's.

One aspect of his childhood experience and later life story is of particular interest as it reflects on some aspects of race relations in slavery. It is noteworthy that as an adult in a free society, Douglass formed a variety of rich, personal relationships with black and white people as friends, colleagues, and lovers. His first wife was black and his second wife was white. There was also at least one other critically important friendship and possible love affair with a white woman. The early models for these adult love experiences no doubt lay in his childhood relations with his grandmother and his white mistresses.

The emotional ties between blacks and whites in slavery were often strong, although they were highly ambivalent with the positive elements usually disguised. Douglass conveys the spirit of this tie in his letter to his old master where he starts by talking of "the long and intimate, though by no means friendly, relation" which existed between them. His early childhood included a confusing mixture of what were at times poignant but fragmented experiences with caretaking adults of both races. Fortunately, he did have a stable relationship with his grandmother for the crucial first five years of life.

This fragmentation of caretaking relationships was often an important experience for white children as well. Douglass irately informs us in the *Narrative* that his master-father had himself been suckled and raised in early childhood by Douglass's black grandmother. In this sense, grandmother was the earliest childhood love object for both father and son. His master's residual positive feelings toward her are suggested in her privileged status of being allowed to live in a cabin apart from the slave quarters.

Later, as a grown man, this master has a sexual liaison with one of her daughters and has a child by her. Douglass is the child who is then taken from his mother and raised by grandmother only to be taken in turn from her and returned to his master's home. Here he is ambivalently raised for several years in a way that does include fragmentary elements of fatherly interactions as well as nurturing experiences with other members of his white family. Shortly after the death of his slave mother, Douglass is given the special privilege and opportunity of going to live in Baltimore. This was both given and received as a disguised and disavowed form of affection and specialness.

I realize that I am emphasizing the inconsistent and often disguised shreds of positive feelings involved in Douglass's relations with his white family. This is done not to deny the more obvious negative aspects in these family relations, but to emphasize that it was a matter of family relations and that these relations were intimate with deep, unconscious, incestuous undercurrents. Douglass was raised as a second-class member of his master's family and received a great deal of special attention and consideration compared to the standard treatment of other slave children.

When, as an adolescent, he committed the socially unpardonable act of unsuccessfully trying to organize and lead an escape by a group of male slaves, there were outraged members of the local white community who demanded that he be killed or sold into the deep South. His master[6] resisted this social pressure and, out of fear for Douglass's life, returned him to Baltimore to learn a trade with the promise that he would be set free at the age of 25. No doubt, his master saw this as an extremely humanitarian gesture, while Douglass, if he even trusted the promise, indignantly saw it as someone paternalistically offering him something that was his rightful due as a human being.

In many ways, this ambivalent form of black-white interaction was common in slavery and had some of its unconscious roots in early childhood experiences. Modern historical observers generally agree that the black male was more severely disenfranchised from his traditional male status than the black woman was from hers. The standard reasons given are that black women were valued for their procreative functions while black men were exaggeratedly feared for their sexuality. Apart from her financial value as a breeder, the black woman was more personally valued since she often played a critical maternal role in the earliest childhood experiences of white children of both sexes. She was often the wetnurse and primary caretaking figure in early childhood. As such she occupied the place of a highly cherished, emotionally valuable

---

[6] This was his second master who had inherited Douglass. He was a member of the family by marriage, but had known and lived with Douglass since childhood.

figure. For the white child the loss of such a treasured relationship of infancy was almost inevitable in the social system of slavery. It occurred through actual physical separations or, more subtly, as the growing white child went through the disillusioning experience of social learning and came to perceive her degraded, lowly status as a powerless black slave.

The childhood experience of this painful loss led to an unconscious love-hate attitude on the part of Southern whites toward their black nurses and blacks in general. In this sense, whites often experienced a fragmentation of their family units in a disguised way since the emotional importance of black people was often consciously disavowed. This type of early childhood loss, and the repressed grief involved, was one of the important underpinnings to race relations in slavery.

Based on my readings of many other slave narratives and available planters' documents I would guess that many of the crueler and more destructive aspects of the ways whites treated blacks were motivated by the same unconscious ambivalence. The frequent disruptions of the black family unit were partially motivated by unconscious retaliatory envy. The white man's need to repress his childhood emotional tie to the blacks often took the extreme form of seeing them as subhuman or nonhuman. Tenderness was replaced by cruelty in what could be described as a cultural reaction formation. The power and intensity of the white man's exaggerated sexual fear of the black man was probably related to the power and intensity of his own unconsciously determined incestuous wishes toward black women and its accompanying retaliatory fears.

These formulations are based on psychological generalizations which require further refinement and documentation before they can be meaningfully applied to a broad psychological study of slavery. I mention them because the details of Douglass's life lend some support to their validity but not to their universality. The research problem is that no single representative family pattern clearly emerges which can typify the "average" childhood experience of master or slave. Some of the future investigative difficulties consist of trying to formulate useful conceptual models to characterize the different types of family structures and experiences and then to localize where they are applicable in the highly varying subcultures of the antebellum South.

Conclusion

It is difficult to find a way to summarize Douglass except to step aside and talk about him in a personal way, much the way an analyst might think about a patient he has worked with. I think that regardless of the conclusions of this study, Douglass probably would have been pleased to know that a white man had spent so much time trying to understand a black man. In the sense of social progress, I think that he was very much responsible for this growing trend in our society today. I realize that even as I say this, I see him as a man of two races, which he was. In the end I am left with the feeling about him that he is someone I would have liked to have known personally, for somehow his writing and his work, passionate and indignant as they were, were more acts of love than acts of hate.

BIBLIOGRAPHY

DOUGLASS, F. (1845), *Narrative of the Life of Frederick Douglass.* Cambridge: Belknap Press of Harvard Univ. Press, 1960.
——— (1855), *My Bondage and My Freedom.* New York: Dover Publications, 1969.
——— (1881), *Life and Times of Frederick Douglass.* New York: Collier Books, 1962.
ERIKSON, E. H. (1962), Reality and Actuality. *J. Amer. Psychoanal. Assn.*, 10:451–474.
FREUD, S. (1909), Family Romances. *S.E.*, 9:235–241.
GREENACRE, P. (1958), The Family Romance of the Artist. *This Annual*, 13:9–36.
KRIS, E. (1935), The Image of the Artist. *Psychoanalytic Explorations in Art.* New York: Int. Univ. Press, 1952, pp. 64–84.
——— (1956), The Personal Myth. *J Amer Psychoanal. Assn.*, 4:653–681.
QUARLES, B. (1970), *Frederick Douglass.* New York: Atheneum.
RANK, O. (1909), The Myth of the Birth of the Hero. *The Myth of the Birth of the Hero and Other Writings.* New York: Vintage, 1964.

Index

Abandonment of child, 649–50, 660; *see also* Fear, Kipling
Abarbanel, J., 647
Abraham, K., 146, 155, 206–07, 219, 261, 273, 305–06
Accident proneness of addicts, 574
Acting out, 112, 207, 481–82
  with parent, as result of analysis, 419
Activity, 41
  defensive: 539; vs. adaptive, 18
  encouraged in burned soldiers, 552–65
  and identification, 39
  and passivity, 201–02; *see also* Conflict
  restriction, 141–42
  see also Hyperactivity, Hypoactivity
Activity pattern, variations, 133–35
Adams, M. J., 102, 126
Adams, P. A., 108, 125
Adaptation, 110, 119
  active and passive, 672
  alloplastic, 44
  assessment of, for termination, 446–72
  of boy with congenital lack of sensation, 50–71
  and reality anchoring, 33, 42–44
Adaptive modes, 147
Addiction, *see* Drug addiction *and sub* specific drugs
Adelberg, E. A., 594, 646
Admiration, need for, 348–51
Adolescence, Adolescent, 91, 173, 177, 189, 191, 347, 349, 396–98, 450–52, 455, 466–68, 472, 544, 553, 577, 667, 675, 701–07, 717
  acute crisis in, 514
  age-appropriate defenses, 427, 431
  amnesia for, 471
  awareness of internal problems, 518–19, 522, 527
  of boy with congenital lack of sensation, 55–71
  breakdown in, 511, 513, 517, 520–23
  bringing material in displaced form, 437
  developmental tasks, 517, 525
  fear of dependence on analyst, 434, 437
  hidden-urgent problems, 515, 519–23
  masturbation in, *see* Masturbation
  and prelatency child, 422
  prepubertal fatness in, 382–84, 397
  preventive intervention in, 511–27
  severing ties to parents, *see* Distancing, Object removal
  transference neurosis in, 429, 434
  treatment of, 218; *see also* Adolescent analysis
  turn to new partnerships, 453, 455–56, 467
  see also Prepuberty, Puberty
Adolescent analysis, 412, 415–16, 418–19, 422, 425–26, 428–29, 431–35, 437–41, 523
Adoption, 648–60
Aesthetics, 182, 184, 193–94
Affect
  balanced availability, 447–48, 470
  in blind, 9
  development in boy with congenital lack of sensation, 64–65
  and dream, 238
  face expressing, 551
  nonverbal expression, 425–26
  primitive, 110–11
  reversal, 463, 470
  related to awe, 181–85
Affective climate, 86
Aggression
  adaptive, 69
  and ambivalence, 204–07, 218–19
  in animals, 607, 673–75
  assessment, 450, 452–53
  and awe, 193–94
  in blind, 9
  in children, 292–93, 298–300, 446
  conflict about, 350–52, 355
  in cultural evolution, 605–44
  defense against, 427, 606
  development, 258
  direct expression, 107, 112
  and ego interests, 260
  fear of, 111
  inability to mobilize, 136, 140–43
  inhibition of, 542–43, 547
  lusty discharge, 20, 43
  of man, 590–644
  to mother, 25–26, 39, 144
  and narcissism, 246, 254–57, 270–71, 614–30, 641, 673–76

753

Aggression *(Cont.)*
  oral, 305
  and tic, 459
  types of, 610
  uncontrolled, 112
  variations in endowment, 132
  vicissitudes, 191
  see also Ambivalence, Instinctual drives, Rage
Ajurriaguerra, J. de, 97, 123
Alcoholism, 377, 379, 381, 383, 395, 569, 653
Alexander, F., 432
Alexander, P., 636, 644
Alienation, 678–80
Alpert, A., 132, 156
Ambivalence, 86, 177, 264, 267, 359, 439–40, 462, 556, 667, 750
  anal, 148
  of child to mother, 290–91, 299
  concept, 197–219
  conflict, 132, 197–206
  emotional, 198–201, 204
  of father, 295
  forms of, 198
  genesis, 199–200, 204–05
  in man, 614–15, 628
  of mother, 288–90, 301
  and narcissism, 251, 674–80
  to parent, 717–19
  temporal splitting, 210–11
  tolerance, 208–12
  in transference, 665
  types in children, 210–12
Ames, L. B., 105, 124
Amnesia, 263
  for child analysis, 470–71
  infantile, 183
Anal concerns (interests), 25, 131, 292
Anal phase, 25, 86, 163, 172, 202, 261, 425, 439
Anal-sadistic phase, 176, 200, 206, 492, 503
"Analytic aid," 472, 529
Animal
  aggression in, 607, 673–75
  compared to man, 595–633
  studies, 49, 86
Annis, R. C., 49, 71
Anorexia nervosa, 522
Anthony, E. J., 81, 92, 445, 458, 472
Anthropogenesis, 596–613
Anthropomorphizing, 354
Anticipation, defensive, 447–48
Antinomy, 630–39

Antonovsky, H., 550
Anxiety, 184, 216
  expression, 65
  and flight, 143
  low threshold, 97
  mastery, 21, 32, 35
  and narcissism, 251
  in prematures, 103–04
  and respiratory distress, 191
  tolerance, 69
  in transference neurosis, 263
  see also Danger situations, Fear
Apfelbaum, B., 252, 273
Aphasia, 112, 225
Apparatus, mental, 596
  defective vs. secondary interferences, 280
  see also Ego apparatus
Appleton case, 651–54, 660
Ardrey, R., 611–12, 644
Arithmetic, 117, 120, 282, 287, 290, 446
Arlow, J. A., 373, 456, 468, 472
Arnold, D. O., 570, 587
Art, 459, 464
Artist, 308, 336, 347–50, 745–46
Assessment
  of adolescents, 511–27
  of blind infants, 3–12
  of children, 150, 152–53
  diagnostic, 309–14, 335
  of language-disturbed children, 95–123
  of mother, 83
  multiple aspect view and termination of child analysis, 445–72
  see also Developmental Profile, Diagnosis
Atkin, S., 109, 123
Atlas myth, 643–44
Attachment behavior, 63
Attention
  disturbances, 97
  free-floating, 77
  see also Listening
Attention cathexis, 246
Auditory sensation, 63
Austen, J., 185
Autism, normal, 254
Autistic child, 112
Autobiography
  family romance in, 727–46
  of R. Kipling, 686–708
  serial, of F. Douglass, 725–51
Autoerotic activity, 137, 253
  in blind, 11
  excessive, 284
  see also Masturbation
Autoerotism and narcissism, 248–54, 262–63

Index

Autonomy
  secondary, 41–42, 47
  striving for, 44–47
  see also sub Ego
Avoidance, 87, 134, 141, 143, 145, 416, 455, 461
Awe
  maternal origins of, 181–94
  phallic, 181–82, 188–89, 194

Baby, *see* Infant
Baby Profile, 80, 83
  for blind, 3–12
Baby talk, 111
Bach, E., 240
Bach-y-Rita, P., 64, 71
Balestier, C. (wife of R. Kipling), 714–15
Balestier, W., 713–15
Balint, M., 245, 247, 253, 273, 444, 472
Balkanyi, C., 109, 123
Barbusse, H., 620
Bard, R. E., 647
Barr, H. L., 570, 586
Basic core, 22, 40, 148–49
Beating fantasy, 118
Beck, A. T., 65, 71
Bed wetting, *see* Enuresis
Behavior
  adaptive vs. defensive, 18
  destructive, 486–507
  fixed pattern, 414–15
  at home and/or in analysis, 417–23, 425
  rational, 46
  reality-oriented, 25–26
  regressed, 430
  surface and underlying meaning, 80, 201
Behavior constancy, 22, 84
Behavior disorder, 482
Beiser, H. R., 76, 92
Beller, E. K., 478, 510
Bender, L., 101, 108, 123, 125
Benedek, T., 87, 92
Ben Hur, N., 549–50
Bentzen, F., 105, 123
Benveniste, E., 222–23, 240
Berger, M., 279–306
Bergmann, T., 529, 548
Berkeley, O., 570
Bernheim, H., 307
Bernstein, I., 268–69, 273
Bernstein, N. R., 550, 560, 566
Bettelheim, B., 635, 644
Bexton, W. H., 578, 586
Bibace, R., 102, 123
Bibring, E., 247, 273

Bick, E., 75, 92
Biermann, G., 93
Bing, J. F., 245, 253, 273, 275
Biography, personal distortions, 727
Biology, 590–605, 627–29, 637
Birch, H. G., 114, 123, 134, 157
Birth trauma, 191
Bisexuality, 22, 205
Biting, 138
Black militant, portrait of, 725–51
Black-white relations, in slavery, 748–51
Blanchard, P., 305–06
Blanck, G. and R., 63, 71
Blank, R. H., 228, 240
Bleuler, E., 197–98, 201, 207, 219
Blind children, 63, 215
  development, 3–12
Blindness, 228
  threat of, 697–99, 707–08, 711–12, 717
Blind spots, *see* Scotomization
Blos, P., 21, 47, 263, 273
Body
  adolescent's relation to, 517–25
  as claustrum, 188
  dissatisfaction with, 458, 464
  of mother and awe, 182–94
  and narcissism, 262, 268, 622; *see also* Hypochondriasis
  preoccupation with, 345–46, 351
  pride in, 462–63
Body boundary, loss, 563
Body ego, 50, 85–86, 183
Body image (schema), 164–65
  changing cathexes, 262–63
  disorders, 97
Body imagery, 108
Body language, 671
Body memory, 85
Body-mind, mysterious leap, 334–35
Body-phallus equation, 187, 261
Body representation, development, 163–66, 173
Body self, 66–67
Bolk, L., 599–600, 638, 644
Bontems, R., 615–16
Borderline patients, 191–92, 243–44, 265, 573, 575–76
Boredom, 313
Borges, J. L., 341, 355
Bornstein, B., 281, 305–06, 471–72, 542, 548
Boy
  development: 164–66, 169–72, 174, 179; normal, 15–47
  educationally unready, 105–08
  transvestite behavior in, 482, 486–507

755

Bradley, N., 185, 194
Brain, evolution, 638
Brain damage, 12
  minimal, 96, 114, 116
Brainwashing, 683–85, 693, 695
Brayn, G. W., 71–72
Breast, 185, 187–88
Breast feeding, 282–83, 288, 296, 301, 311, 487
  observation, 78, 83
Brecher, E. M., 567, 569, 586
Brenman, M., 568, 586
Brenner, C., 373
Brent Consultation Centre, 511–27
Brodey, W. M., 261, 265–67, 270, 273
Bronson, G., 64, 71
Brunswick, R. M., 162, 173, 179
Buber, M., 620
Buffet, C., 615–16
Burgner, M., 161–80
Burian, E., 477
Burlingham, D., 3–13, 63, 71, 88, 93
Burned soldiers, psychological care of, 550–66
Burne-Jones, E., 689
Burne-Jones, G., 694, 698
Burns, P., 148, 156
Buxbaum, E., 281, 306

Call, J. D., 49, 71
Campbell, A. M. G., 50, 71
Campbell, D., 279
Cannaday, C., 63–64, 71
Caplan, H., 102, 123
Carmichael, E. A., 50, 72
Carrington, C. E., 689, 706, 714–15, 722, 724
Carroll, L., 353
Carterette, E. C., 123
Castration anxiety, 21, 37, 144, 401–02, 439, 454, 716
  and circumcision, 297
  in dream, 186
  in girl, 173, 206, 262, 460, 470
  in latency boys, 542, 547
  and narcissism, 261, 263
  phallic and oedipal, 169–72
  preventing masturbation, 189
  and psychosis, 366
  severe, in boy, 485–509
Causality in dream, 225–27
Central nervous system disturbances, 95–98, 109
Central psychic constellation, 127–55
Chafetz, M. E., 569, 586

Character
  and central psychic constellation, 155
  formation of, and surgery, 547–48
  hysterical, 178
  neuroses, 668–69
  obsessive-compulsive, 458
Character disorders, 576
  narcissistic, 45–46; *see also* Narcissistic disorders
Character trait, narcissistic, 44–47
Character transference, 414–17
Chess, S., 134, 157
Child
  abuse, 650, 653, 660; *see also* Kipling
  admired, 17–18, 44–45
  attributing phallus to mother, 354
  "in the best interests of," 651, 654
  cared for by series of people, 292–95
  complying with denigrated role assigned by parent, 281–306
  custody, 651–61
  dependence of, *see* Dependence
  development, and psychoanalytic training, 75–92
  as extension of narcissism, 250
  educationally unready, 100, 104–08
  entitlement to permanent family, 649–61
  experiential world of, 670–71, 677–80
  firstborn, 301
  language deficit in, 95–123
  need for continuity of relationships, 647–50
  need of mother, 203, 215–19
  neglect, 649–50, 654–55
  "organic," 97, 110
  orphaned, 727
  party status in court, 653–54
  passive-dependent, 104
  premature, 100–04, 108, 288, 292, 301
  raised by two mothers, 399–403
  relation to other children, 416, 531–33, 535–37, 542–43
  seduced, 288–89
  seeing: genitals, 189–90; intercourse, 189; mother's body, 183
  sex theories, 167, 172, 176, 547
  sleeping with mother, 461
  treatment of, *see* Child analysis
  validating parents' expectations, 266–67
  see also Infant, Mother-child relationship
Child analysis, 76, 99
  breaking off, 438
  and child's ongoing relation with parent, 412, 415, 428
  definition and criteria, 485–86, 508

fantasy themes, 478–509
follow-up, 452, 455–56, 467–68, 507–08
intermittent, 468
of latency girl, 307–38
missing sessions, 433
in nursery school, 477–510
"permission to express," 418, 431, 435
phase-related material in, 449–52
of pseudobackward children, 284–306
reaction to interruptions, 419, 425–26
real relation to analyst, 440–41, 444–45, 453, 456–57, 469
silence in, 317–18, 425, 464
simultaneous remedial therapy, 118–19
termination, *see* Termination
transference in, 409–41
treatment situation and technique, 409–41
use of plastic media by child, 321–38
Childhood experience and black-white relations, 748–51
Child placement
court decisions, 647–61
guidelines for contested, 647–48
"temporary" or permanent, 647–61
see also Kipling
Child rearing, 605–06
in Africa, 675–78
routine vs. flexibility, 7
Chomsky, N., 221–22, 231–36, 239–40
Christensen, F., 227
Circumcision, 297–300
Civilization
and aggression, 673–80
and narcissism, 676–80
threats to, 590; *see also* Man, survival of
Clark, L. P., 264, 273
Claustrophobic reaction, 559
Clements, S. D., 97, 123
Clinging, 151, 213, 284, 287–88, 459–60
Coenesthetic functioning, 86
Cognition, 229
Cognitive controls, 133, 147
Cognitive development, 25, 33, 35, 40, 43, 50, 113, 137, 147, 279, 637–39
disturbances, 98–122
see also Sensorimotor development
Cognitive disorders, 102
Cognitive style, 149
Cohen, L. D., 50, 71
Cohen, R. A., 725
Colic, 138, 296
Collective alternates, 183, 376
Colodny, D., 104, 108, 125
Colonna, A. B., 13, 63, 72

Communication
and facial expression, 551
modes in child analysis, 336
between mother: and blind infant, 5–6; and child, 98–99, 122–23, 265–67, 271–72
Compensation, 102, 106, 122
Competition, 449–55
avoidance of, 141, 144
Competitiveness, 310
Complementary series, 122
Compliance
unconscious, 286–87, 300–05
see also Somatic compliance
Component drives (instincts), 149, 168–69, 200, 203
Composition of original tunes, 392–93, 399–406
Compromise formation, 207, 211–12, 238
Concentration camp, 578, 635, 673–75
Condensation, 110, 226–28, 237–38, 544
Conflict
activity-passivity, 22–23, 202
age-adequate, 120
ambivalence, 132, 197–206
about ambivalent feeling, 208–15, 219
anal, 297, 444
continuance of early, and child analysis, 434–35
current, 417–23
dominant, 449
dynamic, and structural assessment, 453–54
between ego and sexuality, 247
internal, 434, 440
internalized, 526
latent, 582
neurotic, 305–06
with object, and narcissistic needs, 351–53, 355
obsessive-compulsive, 458
optimal distance from, 42, 47
part of normal and neurotic development, 23–25
pathological vs. "normal," 41–44
patterns, 128
phase-adequate, brought into analysis, 417–22
phase-related, 21–23
predisposition to, 205
preoedipal, 470
present at termination of child analysis, 446
of pseudobackward child, 286–87
psychosexual, 106, 108, 114

Conflict *(Cont.)*
  solution, 128
  superego-ego-id, 620
  tendency to, 639
  types, 208
Congenital sensory neuropathy, 53
Connelly, K., 115, 123
Conrad, K., 115, 123
Conscience development, 113–14; *see also* Superego
Conscious(ness), 112, 198, 204, 222
  altered state, 344–54
Constipation, 117–18, 139, 307–08, 311, 458
Constitution, 106, 109, 114, 205, 264, 280, 599; *see also* Ego, Endowment, Heredity
Constructions, 360–73
Contagion, verbal, 99
Conversion, 85, 334–35
Cope, O., 550, 566
Cornerstone method, 477–510
  cross-sectional view, 482–85
  longitudinal view, 485–508
Cornubert, C., 190, 194
Corrective emotional experience, 432
Counterphobic mechanism, 450
Countertransference, 90
Cragg, B. G., 49, 71
Cramer, B., 15–48, 129
Creativity, 43, 375–76, 398–406, 464, 686–722
  and early losses, 727, 745–46
Crush, 438
Curiosity, 691, 697, 719, 721
  in prephallic phase, 171–72
  sexual, 26, 168–69, 280–81, 294, 304, 437
Curson, A., 3

Danger situation, 366, 371
Darwin, C., 551, 566
Daydream, 34, 45, 223–24, 346, 381, 433, 459, 743
Day residue, 344
Deaf child, 63, 113–14
Deaggressivization, 255, 257
Death, 589, 595, 609, 633–35, 642
  of daughter, 346
  in family, 189–90
  of father, 394–95, 486–508, 561
  of grandmother, 292, 295
Death instinct, 199, 204, 247, 256, 607, 634
Death wishes, 213, 215, 333, 343, 383, 397, 462, 718
Defense, 235
  and adaptation, 33, 35–36, 42–44, 47
  in adolescence, 427, 431
  age-appropriate, 452, 456, 472
  against aggression, 427, 606
  against ambivalence, 132, 212–14, 219
  archaic, 87–88
  balanced availability, 447–48, 455, 470
  against castration anxiety, 170–71
  choice, 151–52, 427
  chronology, 87, 427
  against close relations, 416
  against devalued self image, 302–03
  development, 87–89
  against fantasy, 35–36
  flight into health, 430
  forerunners, 80, 87–88
  habitual, 416
  ignorance as, 281
  in latency, 444
  against loss, 341, 346, 354–55
  and mirror dream, 342–55
  narcissistic-regressive, 353–55
  against object-directed impulses, 414
  obsessional, 213
  against passivity, 18, 22, 25, 28
  phase-appropriate, 39–40
  primitive, 108, 578–79
  reality-syntonic, 35
  self-sufficiency as, 425–26
  against separation, 460–61
  termination material as, 460–61, 469
  see also sub specific mechanisms
Degoza, S., 550–51, 558, 566
de Hirsch, K., 95–126
Déjà phenomena, 182, 193
Delong, J. V., 567, 588
Delusion, 626, 672, 679
  childhood memory as content of, 357–74
  end of world, 369
  persecutory, 368–70
Demandingness, 284, 311–12
Demone, H. W., Jr., 569, 586
Denial, 35, 63, 88, 270, 281, 292, 302, 304, 354, 448, 616–17, 695, 699, 719
  acceptance of, 555
  in addicts, 575, 580, 584
  of affect, 425–26, 464
  of castration, 345, 354
  of death, 341
  of dependence, 463
  in fantasy, 465
  of hate, 699
Dependence, 260, 463, 562
  of blind, 7, 9, 215
  of child: 203, 215–18; prolonged, 590, 675
  on love object, 248–49

oral, 439
wish, 27
Depersonalization, 191, 635
Depression, 184, 187, 337, 342, 345–46, 437, 559
  in adolescence, 519–20, 523
  in child, 299, 448, 451
  defense against, 746
  and narcissism, 243, 251
  see also Mother
Deprivation, 259, 267, 270
  oral, 174, 187
  sensory, 685
Descartes, R., 576
Desexualization, 247, 249, 254, 256–57
Destructiveness, 256
  and civilization, 675–80
Destrudo, 255
Deutsch, H., 162, 174, 179, 262–63, 273, 471, 473
Development
  adaptive approach, 67–69
  arrest, 96, 114, 268
  atypical, 96–123
  of boy with congenital lack of sensation, 55–71
  change of function, 152
  continuity and change in, 22–24, 40–41
  critical: periods, 106, 115; reorganization, 146–52
  disturbances, 153
  earlier phases "coloring" later, 425
  early, 665–67
  equipotentiality of intake channels, 85
  external and internal factors, 279–80
  first five years decisive, 599
  longitudinal study of, 91–92
  normal, 15–47, 667
  objectless stage, 253–54
  organizers, 260
  pathology interfering with, 517–27
  pattern of phase progression, 130–31, 135, 139–40
  phase-adequate, 84–85
  precocious, 30
  prediction of, 10–11, 17
  progressive forces, 446
  role of narcissism in, 252–72
  of self and ego, separate lines, 66, 70–71
  slowed, 283–305
  "style," 15
  symbiotic phase, 254, 666, 677
  undifferentiated phase, 246
  uneven: 95–123, 668; vs. even, 29–31
Developmental lags, 95–123

Developmental lines, 67, 85, 87, 149, 153, 445
  of narcissism and object relatedness, 270, 666–68
  of self and ego, 66, 70–71
Developmental point of view, 151–52, 218
Developmental Profile, 3, 128–29, 153
  applied to termination decisions, 445–72
Diagnosis, 90–92
  differential, autistic and dysphasia, 112
  of language deficit, 95–96
  see also Assessment, Developmental Profile, Labeling
Dickens, C., 697–98, 711
Direct observation, 75–92, 127–29, 155, 259
  interpretation of data, 18–19, 80–82
  in nursery school, 168–69, 175–76
  technique, 81–83, 89–90
Disappointment, 270, 416, 455–56, 673–79
Discharge patterns, 130, 132–33, 140–41
Displacement, 88, 110, 210, 212–13, 218, 228, 249, 261, 298, 463, 465, 469, 532–34
  away from and to analysis, 436–37
  of current conflict and wish to child analyst, 417–24
  from mother to analyst, 438–39
  types, 226, 229, 238–39
  upward, 492
Distancing, 213
  from parent in adolescence, 434, 437, 455–56, 462–63, 577–80; *see also* Object removal
Dobrée, B., 708, 722
Doctor game, 82
Dondoroff, M., 594, 646
Doone, B. K., 586
Doron, A., 550
Dostoyevsky, F., 614
Double, 184, 341, 354–55
Doublethink, 684, 719
Douglass, F., 725–51
  autobiographies of, 725–51
Downie, A. W., 50, 72
Dream
  absurd, 224
  awe experience in, 186–87
  of blind, 228
  body as phallus, 187
  of boy with congenital lack of sensation, 58
  censorship, 222, 227, 236–39
  of child, 238
  coitus, 183
  distortion, 237–39

Dream *(Cont.)*
  fear of, 540
  frightening, 31–33
  influence of mass media on, 229
  interpretation, 193, 223–24, 228
  latent and manifest content, 211–30, 238, 342–43
  of limp trombone, 389–90, 398–99
  and linguistics, 221–40
  logical and causal relations in, 224–30
  mirror in, 341–55
  and narcissism, 243
  orgastic, 598
  and psychosis, 372–73
  as rebus, 211
  representability in, 222, 224, 235, 237–39
  representing castration, 341
  sensorial, 228
  society's influence on, 229
  syntax in, 225–26
  in termination phase, 463, 465–66
  theory, 211–40
  wish to avoid, 34–35
  see also Nightmare
Dream language, generative theory, 230–36
Dream screen, 352
Dreamwork, 223, 233, 236–37
Drivenness, organic, 107, 112
Drug addiction, 376–77, 379–80, 389, 395
  and ego function, 567–86
Drugs, psychedelic, 570, 581
Drug use, 521
  before and after serving in Vietnam, 571–72, 582–83
  influenced by social setting, 568–86
Dual unity, 254, 271
Dubois, E., 638, 645
Dubovsky, S. L., 49–73
Duplication, 350–55
Dynamic viewpoint, 154, 263–65
Dyslexia, 106, 108, 115
Dysnomia, 107, 120
Dysphasic child, 103, 110–13

Easser, R. B., 113, 125
Economic point of view, 251–54
Ecstasy, 182
Eddy, N. B., 567, 586
Edel, L., 713–14, 722
Edelheit, H., 109–10, 113, 124
Edelson, M., 221–22, 224, 230–40
Edgcumbe, R., 161–80, 204, 219
Education, 605
  and child analysis, 478–510

Educational therapy, 116
Edwards, G., 567, 586
Ego
  achievements, 451
  of addicts, 580–81, 585
  in adolescence, 577
  and aggression, 255
  alteration, 248
  archaic states, 191
  autonomous: and addiction, 576–81, 583, 585; function, 28, 42–44, 47, 249, 252, 259, 261, 271, 454
  defect, 264
  deficiencies, 50
  and dream censorship, 237
  of dreamer, 373
  and Eros, 256–57
  and identification, 249
  and mirror dream, 341, 352
  modification by identification, 38–39
  and narcissism, 245–272
  in normal boys, 31–36, 42–44
  and object loss, 267
  organ of adaptation, 62
  pathology, 267
  pathway of gratification, 598
  pattern of response to drives, 131
  primordial, 366–68
  restrictions, 141, 143
  synthesis of ambivalence, 219
  and termination, 445–49, 455, 469
  and transference, 413
  variations in equipment, 130, 133–35, 141, 143, 147–48
  see also Id
Ego apparatus, primary deficits in, 104
Ego boundary
  loss of, 183, 185, 192
  unstable, 110
Ego cathexis, 246, 248, 255, 260–61
Ego development, 38–39, 280, 598–99, 666–68
  advance and regression, 25–29, 47
  arrest, 96, 114
  and body representation, 173
  of boy with congenital lack of sensation, 62–64, 68–71
  defects in, 258
  and hand-mouth integration, 85–86
  lag in, 107–08, 116
  and language, 96, 108–14
  and learning readiness, 106–07
  and libidinal development, 259–63
  precocious, 29–31
  in premature child, 103–04

preobject period, 261, 272
and sensory experiences, 49–51, 63–64, 67–69
Ego energy, 246
Ego feeling, 257
Ego ideal, 21, 28, 35, 38, 47, 136, 152
and narcissism, 249–50, 262–64, 272
Ego instincts, 199–200, 204, 246–47, 255
Ego interests, 246, 260, 262
Ego libido, 246, 248–49, 256, 263
Ego nuclei, 252
Ego psychology, 128, 151, 243, 631
Ego strength, 33, 37, 42–43, 50, 104, 106, 148
Ego weakness, 148, 633, 639
Eidelberg, L., 255
Eisnitz, A., 341–42, 352, 355
Eissler, K. R., 46, 48, 589–646, 673–74, 680
Ekstein, R., 124
Elation, 243
Elkisch, P., 341, 355
Emde, R. N., 49
Emerson, P. E., 63, 73
Emotional refueling, 685
Emotional starvation, 50
Empathy, 70, 86, 145
Encopresis, 303
Endowment, 68, 134–35, 148, 264; *see also* Constitution, Ego, Heredity
Enema, 118, 361
Energy, psychic
discharge, 264–65
and narcissism, 246–72
neutral, 254, 257
transformation, 259; *see also* Neutralization, Sublimation
undifferentiated, 246, 252–55, 257–58
Enuresis, 139, 287, 289, 293, 296, 303, 482–83
Environment, 81
addict's dependence on, 578–79
average expectable, 61
ego's relative autonomy from, 578
and endowment, 134–35, 148
psychologically therapeutic, 550–66
Environmentalists, 595–96, 605, 618
Envy, 145, 187, 190, 209, 315–16, 336–37
Epigenesis, 146–47, 152
Equipment, *see* Constitution, Ego, Endowment, Instinctual drives
Erection
concern about, 543–44
exhibiting of, 24
Erikson, E. H., 22, 146, 156, 165, 179, 376, 406, 572, 586, 741, 751
Eros, 256

Escalona, S. K., 134, 148, 156
Ethics, 614–26
Evans, R., 307–39
Evolution
cultural, 596–610, 628
organic, 590–610, 627, 632–33, 638–40
Exceptions, 44–45
Excitation, spread, 85
Excitement, sexual, 364–71, 461
Exhibitionism, 24, 162, 168–69, 174–75, 179, 251, 385, 391, 393, 397–98, 435
Externalization, 111, 261, 265–66, 302, 304, 412–14, 431, 434, 439
of controls, 447–48
Eye symptoms, 335

Facial burns, psychological reactions to, 549–66
Family
of addicts, 575–76, 578, 584–85
biological, 648–60
blindness in, 4
direct observation of, 75–92
interactions, 129
interrupted relations, 647–61
secret, 281, 289, 291–94, 304
supportive, 309, 337
Family romance, 400–01
of F. Douglass, 725–51
Fantasy
of abandonment, 483
vs. action, 151
aggression and libido in, 141
analyst as superparent, 381
archaic, 672
of being: in mother's body, 187; one with object, 193; parent to parent, 400
of birth, 22, 25
of childhood, 725–26, 741
curtailment, 34–35, 46
enacted, 316–17
of father's infidelity, 385–87
fears, 574
feminine in boy, 22
grandiosity, 670–80; *see also* Grandiosity
of having twin, 354
homosexual, 308
illusory phallus, 136
of incorporation, 259
of intercourse, 167, 438
and learning, 117–18
life, 135, 137, 139–45
magical, 31, 578–80, 671
of mother about child, 289–90, 301
of mother's destructiveness, 189

Fantasy *(Cont.)*
　oedipal, 168, 173, 460, 509
　omnipotence, 111–12, 523
　oral, 144
　oral impregnation, 167
　oral-incorporative, 261, 401
　passive feminine, 387
　phallic, 170
　of phallic phase girls, 174
　primitive, 104, 107, 453–54
　and reality, *see* Reality
　regression confined to, 28
　regressive, 294
　restitution, 145
　retaliative, 35
　sadomasochistic, 300, 329
　self-devaluing, 284–85
　and sexual activity, 166–68
　about surgery, 546–47
　visual media, 212–13
　voyeuristic, 187
Fantasy-reality ratio, 33–36
Father
　absent, 138–41, 144–45, 419, 483
　ambivalent, 293
　attack on child, 449–55
　death wish for child, 215
　deserts family, 287–88, 301
　fear of, 182, 421, 439
　jealousy of, 452–54, 462
　longing for, 144
　loss of, 440; *see also* Death
　obsessional, 293
　oedipal, 450
　primal, 184–85
　punitive, 299
　rejecting, 284–85
　relation to, 486–505
　role in early development, 183
　of Schreber, 358–69
　seductive, 460
　separated from family, 377, 379, 383, 385
　sex play with child, 304
Father-son relationship, ambivalence in, 205
Fear
　of abandonment, 286, 297, 300, 415–16
　of addicts, 574–75
　archaic, 111
　and awe, 187–89
　of death, 37
　of desertion, 461
　of disintegration (dissolution), 108, 192
　of engulfment, 188
　of external reactions, 431
　of failure, 294–95
　of falling, 139
　of father, *see* Father
　of instincts, 36
　of knowing, 294
　of loneliness, 343–44
　of loss: 145; of analyst, 460–61; of object, 216, 343–47, 351–55; of self, 341
　that mother would forget child, 434
　of narcissistic injury, 35, 46
　primal, 191
　of rejection, 216–17, 294
　of retaliation, 21, 170–71, 545
　of therapist, 439
　see also Anxiety, Night fears, Phobia
Feces smearing, 284, 288
Federn, P., 255, 257, 261–62, 273
Feeding, 20, 80, 85–86, 97, 139, 141, 249, 292
　of blind infant, 5–6
　see also Breast feeding
Feigelson, C., 341–55
Feinstein, S. C., 528
Fenichel, O., 305–06
Ferenczi, S., 307–08, 315–16, 334, 336, 338
Fetalization, 599
Figure drawing, 102, 119
Fillmore, C., 233, 240
Firestein, S. K., 445, 473
Fishground, A., 550
Fiske, D. W., 72
Fixation
　anal, 335
　at anal level, 424–25
　and developmental advances, 143
　and narcissism, 270
　to narcissistic tie, 668
　neurotic, 460
　normal, 23
　oral, 171, 305
　in oral-sadistic phase, 608
　in phallic-narcissistic phase, 175, 177–79
　in phallic phase, 131
　in pregenital phase, 268
　prephallic, 147, 171, 175
　and regression, 80, 151, 154, 424
Fixation point, 424–25, 449
　absence of, 20, 23–24, 31, 40
　forerunners in blind, 11
Flapan, O., 16–17, 48
Flavell, J. H., 50, 71
Fliess, R., 179
Fliess, W., 198, 248, 627, 747
Fleming, A. [Trix Kipling], 689–722
Fleming, J., 87, 92
Flechsig, P. E., 357–71

Index

Food
  and aggression, 608–09
  fads, 144
Forrest, T., 108, 125
Forster, J., 722
Foster care, 647–61
Foster parent with tenure, 659–60
Foulkes, S. H., 478, 510
Fraiberg, S., 10, 13, 49, 63–64, 71
Frank, A., 109, 112, 124
Frankl, L., 447, 473
Fras, I., 550, 566
Free association, 79, 82
Freedman, D. A., 50, 63–64, 70–71
Freeman, R. D., 49, 72
Freeman, T., 373–74
French, S. L., 107, 124
Freud, A., 3, 16, 20, 29, 75, 80, 85, 87–88, 91, 107, 116, 128, 148–49, 153, 163, 207, 210, 214, 279–82, 309, 338, 358, 409, 412, 414, 416, 457, 471–72, 478, 517, 529, 546, 610, 649–50, 669
  on adolescent analysis, 438
  bibliographical references to, 13, 48, 92, 124, 156, 219, 339, 441, 473, 510, 527, 548, 645, 662, 722
  on child analysis being determined by external and internal events, 420
  on child's relation to parent, 685
  on chronology of defenses, 427
  on developmental assessment, 150
  on differences between child and adult, 428–29
  on effect of separation from parent, 716–18
  on fixation point and fixation at a level, 424
  on Hampstead Index, 410
  on intact family, 644
  on language and instinct mastery, 112
  on method of direct observation, 77
  on normality, 41
  on precocity in development, 30
  on real relation vs. transference, 440–41
  on regression, 23–24
  on symptoms being drawn into transference, 424
  on technical problems, 415
  on termination of analysis, 443
  on transference neuroses, 429
Freud, E. L., 638, 645
Freud, I., 83, 93
Freud, S., 44, 50, 66, 75, 84, 112, 146, 162–63, 166, 191, 193, 215, 217, 308, 366, 371–73, 417, 444, 471, 577, 582, 590, 606–07, 613, 627, 634, 639, 641, 663–65, 673, 702, 711, 747
  on ambivalence, 198–206
  on awe, 183–84
  bibliographical references to: 48, 71, 93, 124, 156, 179, 194, 219–20, 240, 273–74, 355, 374, 473, 528, 566, 586, 645, 680, 722, 751
  on childhood fantasies, 725–26, 744
  disturbance of memory on the Acropolis, 190
  on double, 341
  on dream, 223–27, 237–39
  on ego, 49
  on experience of unpleasure, 64–65
  on girl's puberty, 262
  on Goethe, 688
  The Interpretation of Dreams, 221–39
  on love, 199–200
  on narcissism, 243–64, 272, 551–52
  on normal development, 23
  on psychoanalytic technique, 77–78, 89
  on religion, 184–85
  on Schreber, 359–60
  on uncanny, 184
Freud, W. E., 3, 13, 75–94
Friedlander, B. Z., 98, 124
Friedman, M., 523, 528
Friedmann, M., 167
Friendship, 731–32, 745–47
Frohlich, S., 550
Fromm-Reichmann, F., 372
Frost, B., 49, 71
Frustration, 203, 211, 218, 256, 259, 272
  and aggression, 673–80
Frustration tolerance, 12, 209, 482, 490
  good, 26, 31
  low, 105
Functional hierarchy, 43
Furman, R. A., 457, 473
Furth, H. G., 113, 124

Galdston, R., 550–51, 566
Galenson, E., 193–94
Games, 448–51, 464
Gardner, H., 229, 240
Garrard, F., 705–06, 709, 711, 713–14
Garrison, W. L., 731–32, 745–47
Geleerd, E., 306
Genetic fallacy, 41, 200
Genetic point of view, 151–52, 154, 258
Genital primacy, 202–03, 452
Genius, 600, 622, 628
Gilbert, E., 722
Gill, M. M., 264, 275, 568, 586

Gilman, A., 586
Giovacchini, P. L., 528
Giraud, F., 613
Girl, development of, 164–66, 169, 173–77, 179, 262
Glasser, M., 523, 528
Gleitman, L., 113, 124
Globus hystericus, 307–08
Glover, E., 305–06
Goethe, J. W., 606, 640, 688, 711
Goldberger, A., 3
Goldblatt, M., 307
Goldstein, A., 568, 586
Goldstein, J., 647–62
Goldstein, S., 647
Goodman, K., 124
Goodman, L. S., 586
Grandiosity, 191, 267, 666, 670–80; *see also* sub Self
Grasping, 85
  in blind, 6, 8
Gratton, L., 478, 510
Graves, R., 644–45
Greed, 217, 283
Green, R. L., 689, 691, 693, 700, 707, 722
Greenacre, P., 103, 124, 181–83, 185, 189, 193–95, 252, 274, 317, 339, 375, 396–98, 400, 402, 405–06, 663, 680, 727, 745–46, 751
Greenson, R. R., 81, 83, 89, 93, 663, 680
Greifraum, 613–17
Grief, *see* Mourning
Grinspoon, L., 570, 586
Grinstein, A., 197, 220
Groban, S. E., 49–71
Grobstein, R., 72
"Ground-language," 361–65
Group psychology, 250–51, 629
Guidance
  of mothers of blind children, 3–4, 12
  see also Parent guidance
Guilt, 113, 118
  and frustration, 351
  and masturbation, 138–39, 329, 349, 542
  in mother: 292–95, 299; of physically handicapped child, 4
  oedipal, 350, 352–53
  relieved by mirror dream, 349–55
  of survivor, 562
  unconscious vs. conscious, 433

Halbach, H., 567, 586
Hall, J. W., 470, 473
Hall, R. R., 570, 586
Hallgren, B., 108, 124

Hallucination
  childhood memory as content of, 357–74
  a discharge phenomenon, 368
Hamburg, B., 550–51, 558, 566
Hamburg, D. A., 550–51, 558, 566
Hampstead Index (treatment situation and technique), 409–41
Hampstead Nursery School, 282, 284; *see also* Nursery school
Hampstead War Nurseries, 77, 718
Hampstead Well-Baby Clinic, 282–83, 286
Hand
  burns, 549–66
  phobic fantasy about, 539–44
  symbolic and real meaning, 551, 562, 687, 703, 717
Handler, P., 591, 645
Hand-mouth coordination, 85–86, 164
  in blind, 8, 10
Hardie, K., 617
Harding, W. M., 567
Harley, M., 528
Harlow, H. F. and M., 49, 71
Harms, R., 240
Harnik, J., 262, 274
Harris, D. B., 126
Harrison, B., 569, 586
Harrison, I. B., 181–95
Hartmann, H., 18, 23–24, 30, 33, 41–43, 46, 48, 61–62, 72, 148, 152, 156, 200, 205, 220, 244, 246–47, 252, 254, 257–58, 275, 366, 568, 586
Hartnup, T., 161, 210
Hate object, 218–19
Hayles, A. B., 50, 73
Hayman, A., 3
Heart rhythm, 402
Hebb, D. O., 65, 72, 578, 586
Heider, G., 134, 156
Heilbroner, R. L., 643–45
Heinicke, C. M., 443–74
Helen of Troy, 45
Hellman, I., 281, 303–06
Helplessness, 64, 114, 138, 675–80
Hendrick, I., 257, 274
Herder, J. G., 609
Heredity, 293, 594; *see also* Constitution, Ego, Endowment
Herman, K., 108, 124
Hero
  birth of, 726
  fantasy, 739–41
Heroin, 569, 571–73, 575, 581–83
Heron, W., 578, 586
Hertzig, M., 134, 157

Herzog, F., 477, 501
Hill, E., 700, 710, 713
Hinde, R. A., 64, 72
History, 589–644
Hitler, A., 620, 642
Hobbies, 295
Hoch, P. H., 123, 587
Hoffer, W., 86, 93, 164, 179, 444, 473
Holder, A., 165, 180, 197–220
Holloway, R., 49, 72
Holt, R. R., 252, 274
Homosexuality, 251, 264, 353, 702–05, 712, 718
 fear of, 366–68
Hopelessness, 519–20
Horace, 621
Horn, E., 550
Hospitalization, repeated, 51–71
Hostility, irritable, and recovery from illness, 552–65
Huff, S. E., 647
Hughes, E., 618, 645
Humor, 120, 251, 448, 688, 699, 717
Hunger, 216, 609–15, 640
 absence of experience of, 52
Hurn, H. T., 444, 473
Hyperactivity, 95, 119–21
Hyperkinesis, 112
Hypnosis, 251
Hypoactivity, 101
Hypochondriasis, 248, 250, 254, 263, 312, 552, 640
Hypotaxis, 229–30
Hysteria, 308–09, 334–35
Hysterical attacks, 430

Ibsen, H., 683, 722
Id, 148, 248–49, 252, 256–57
 ego's relative autonomy from, 577–79
 and object loss, 267
 undifferentiated from ego, 248, 257
Ideal ego, 249
Idealization, 193, 209, 251, 272, 432, 438, 471, 515, 745–46; *see also sub* Object, Parent
Identification, 80
 with absent father, 21, 36–37
 with active party, 38–39
 with aggressor, 33, 39, 492, 539
 with analyst, 470
 with analyst's analyzing ego, 467
 bisexual, 165
 with boy who underwent surgery, 533
 of child with mother's image of child, 286–87
 defensive, 21, 447–48
 and desexualized libido, 256
 exaggerated, with adult, 22–23, 36
 with father, 24–26, 36–39, 171, 256, 261, 299, 450
 feminine, 174, 177
 and libido transformation, 248–49
 masculine, 28, 36–39, 44, 172, 495
 with mongoloid brother, 294
 with mother, 493
 with mother's: narcissistic style, 45; speech mannerisms, 289–91
 and narcissism, 243–44
 with object, 260
 and object loss, 249, 264, 267–68
 with persecutor, 719
 preoedipal: 193; and oedipal, 459
 primary, 253, 261
 primitive, 267
 and regression, 47
 and release of aggression, 193
 role in normal development, 36–40
 and self representation, 163–66, 173
 sexual, 517
 with surgeon, 539
 with tormentor, 684–85, 697
 unconscious, 99
 vicissitudes, 36–39
Identity
 development, 267, 685–722
 disturbance, 190
 and face injury, 562
 formation, 165
 heroic, 743–44
 maintenance, 260–61
 masculine, 136, 701, 706
 mixed racial, 746
 negative, 572
 primary narcissistic, 260
 sexual, 163–66, 170–72, 179, 683
 split, 703, 720
Ilg, F. L., 105, 124
Imagery, use of in: autobiography, 738–40, 743, 746; writing, 708
Imaginary companion, 354
Imitation, 265
Immaturity, physiological, 119–21
Impulse control, 50, 62–63
 lack, 107–08
Impulsivity, 107
Inanimate object, 193, 212
 attack on, 133
Incest prohibition, 590
Incorporation, 201, 206, 259
Independence, 18, 28, 30, 132, 450

Individual differences, 84, 129, 131, 147, 151
Individuation, *see* Separation-individuation
Infant
   blind, 3–12
   placid, 286
   uncuddly, 82–83
   see also Child, Neonate
Infantilization, 104
Infantile neurosis, 148, 151
   and surgery, 545, 547
   vicissitudes, 24–27
Inhibition, 144, 189, 455, 542–43
   in child, 299
   of curiosity, 169, 281, 294, 304
   intellectual, 281, 303–05, 484
   motoric, 459
   of success, 449, 454
Injury, "accidental," 54–69
Insight, 452, 456, 466, 470, 486, 494, 526
   psychological, of child, 31–36
Instinct, 595–604, 631
   of mastery, 257
   oral, 609
   see also Death instinct, Ego instincts, Life instinct, *and sub* Self preservation
Instinctual drives, 597–98, 604–31
   active and passive aims, 199
   assessment of development at termination, 445–46, 450–52
   balance, 130, 132–33, 140–41
   concept, 252, 264
   deformation, 598
   defusion, 205, 247, 254, 256, 258
   energy, 604, 612; *see also* Energy
   and environment, relative autonomy from, 577–81
   fusion, 204–05, 247, 254, 258, 260
   lack of control over, 107–08
   mastery and language, 110–12
   and object relations, development, 161–63, 178–79
   oral, 609
   polarities, 201–02
   theory and narcissism, 245–73
   variations in endowment, 132
   see also Aggression, Libido
Integration difficulties, 96–122
Integrative function, 148, 152, 341; *see also* Organizing function, Synthetic function
Intellectual development, 26, 29–30, 34–35, 280
Intellectualization, 112, 427, 463, 468, 577
Intelligence tests, 16, 34, 52, 100, 105, 117, 282, 284–85, 287, 291, 295, 299–300, 455

Intercourse, 167, 178, 183, 438
   sadistic concept, 439
Internalization, 28–39, 113
   of aggression, 608–09
Interpretation
   in child analysis, 467–68
   of defense, 416, 420
   guided by child's current feelings, 435
   premature, 192
   psychoanalytic, in nursery school, 479–510
   reaction to, 314–17, 332
   of resistance, 437, 444, 481–82
   of transference, 428–29, 432, 437–38
   see also sub Dream
Intervention, brief, 511–27
Interviews, 16–19, 128–29, 155
   of addicts, 581
   of adolescents, 512–27
In the Matter of N. M. S., 654–57
Introjection, 38, 88, 248, 270, 354, 573
Introspection, 113
Isakower phenomenon, 183
Isbell, H., 567, 586
Isolation, 35
   of affect, 462

Jacob, F., 593, 645
Jacobs, B., 683, 722
Jacobson, E., 44–45, 48, 135, 156, 193, 244, 246, 249, 252–54, 257–60, 263, 270, 274, 376, 400, 406
Jacobson, R. C., 567, 569, 588
Jaffe, J. H., 567, 586
Jakobson, R., 225, 240
James, H., 713–14
Jansky, J., 100, 105, 107, 118, 123–24
Jarrell, R., 700, 703, 720, 722
Jazz, 378
   and blues, 383, 398, 405
Jealousy, 251, 298, 343; *see also* Envy, Sibling rivalry
Jelgersma, G., 374
Jessor, R., 50, 72
Jewesbury, E., 50, 72
Joffe, W. G., 164, 173, 179, 251, 272, 274, 336–38
Johnson, A. M., 305–06
Jokes, 113, 464–65
Jones, E., 229, 240, 281, 306
Jones, M. R., 156
Joyce, J., 732
Julia, H., 148, 156
Jung, C., 247
Junkies, 572–76
Justice, 615–25

Kagan, J., 99, 124
Kane, F. J., 50, 72
Kant, I., 611-12, 629-30
Kanzer, M., 157, 190, 195, 246, 253, 274
Kaplan, B., 111, 126
Kaplan, D. M., 104, 124
Kapp, R. O., 262-63, 274
Kardiner, A., 247, 252, 274
Karush, A., 247, 252, 274
Katan, A., 109, 111, 125
Katan, M., 357-74
Katz, J., 233, 240
Kaufman, I., 587
Kaywin, L., 341, 355
Keeton, W. T., 592, 645
Kennedy, H., 3, 75, 93, 279-306, 307, 409-441, 463, 473
Kenyatta, J., 675-76, 678, 680
Kernberg, O. F., 243-44, 265, 270-71, 275
Kernberg, P. F., 243, 275
Khantzian, E. J., 567-68, 586-87
Killing, 608-12
Kinkead-Weeks, R., 712, 722
Kipling, R., 683-724
 early life, 686-720
 relation to: sister [Trix], 696-97, 706, 715, 717-19; women, 703-19
Kipnis, D., 50, 71
Klein, E., 305-06
Klein, G. S., 147, 156, 568, 587
Klein, M., 81, 207, 211, 305-06
Kliman, A. S., 477, 510
Kliman, G. W., 477-510
Koffka, K., 121, 125
Kohrman, R., 444, 456-57, 473
Kohut, H., 50, 63-64, 66-67, 72, 193, 195, 243-45, 251, 254, 257-58, 261, 263-64, 269-70, 275, 350-51, 355, 402, 406, 666, 669-70, 680-81
Kolansky, H., 109, 125
Korn, S., 134, 157
Korner, A. F., 72, 134, 156
Kraus, K., 608
Kris, E., 16, 22, 24, 28, 30, 41, 43, 48, 75, 84, 93, 205, 220, 247, 252, 255, 274, 375, 406, 473, 726, 741, 751
Kris, M., 81, 93, 478
Krugman, M., 510
Kubzansky, P. E., 50, 71
Kunkle, F. C., 50, 71
Kurlander, L. F., 104, 108, 125

Labeling, and choice of therapy, 96, 114-23
LaFrontaine, C., 478, 510
Lakoff, G., 233, 240

Lamarck, C., 228
Lambert, E. H., 50, 73
Lampl-de Groot, J., 18, 48, 162, 179-80, 663-81
Landauer, K., 281, 306
Langford, W. S., 100, 123-24
Langs, R. J., 570, 586
Language
 and cognition, 102, 109
 comprehension: 98; difficulties, 101-03, 106
 deficits, 95-123
 generative theory, 230-36
 and psychic organization, 108-14
 see also Communication, Speech, Verbalization
Language-stimulation program, 116-21
Lantos, B., 610, 645
Laplanche, J., 207, 220
Latency, 20, 24, 37, 91, 116, 121, 205, 303, 307-38, 343, 349, 396-97, 400, 444, 452, 456-58, 471, 481, 634, 667-68, 675
 and central psychic constellation, 129-55
 masturbation in, see Masturbation
 normal, 422
Laterality, 105-06
Laufer, E., 523, 528
Laufer, M., 511-28
Law
 and administration of foster placement, 647-61
 cannot supervise interpersonal relations, 648
Law of aggressive parsimony, 606-10
Lawick-Goodall, J. van, 674, 681
Learning, 609
 capacity, 141, 169
 difficulties (disturbances), 95-123, 280-81, 287, 289, 300, 304-05, 446-55, 518
Legs, use in blind, 9
Leonardo da Vinci, 332, 608
Leshan, L., 103, 125
Lesser, S. R., 113, 125
Lessing, G. E., 606, 609
Levin, D. C., 66-67, 72
Lévi-Strauss, C., 232
Lewin, B. D., 184, 195, 243, 275, 352, 355
Lewis, M. M., 98, 125
Liberman, D., 221, 240
Libidinal types, 251
Libido, 612
 adhesiveness, 219
 and aggression: 254-57; balance, 147-48
 assessment of distribution at termination, 451-52

Libido *(Cont.)*
  development: 146; assessment, 450–52
  and ego development, 30, 259–61
  lusty discharge, 20, 43
  narcissistic: 248–63, nature of, 257–58; vs. object-directed, 621, 665–68
  theory, and narcissism, 245–73
  variations in endowment, 132
  see also Instinctual drives, Sex
Lichtenstein, H., 244, 253, 260, 275
Liendo, E., 221, 240
Life cycle, 146–47
Life instinct, 199, 204, 247
Lilly, J. C., 578, 587
Lindzey, G., 156
Linguistics, 221–40
Lippman, H. S., 267, 275
Lipton, S. D., 547–48
Lisping, 109
Listening, 98–99, 106, 116
  in blind, 5–6, 8, 10–11
Litman, R. E., 474
Little Hans, 166, 198, 471
Loewald, H., 188, 195, 262–63, 275
Loewenstein, R. M., 48, 125, 195, 205, 220, 246–47, 252, 255, 274–75, 339, 663, 681
Long, R. T., 550, 566
Longitudinal study, 127–55
  description, 16–19
  of progressive development, 15–47
Looking, 85
Lorenz, K., 595
Losing and feeling lost, 415
Love
  aggressive, 206
  and hate, 198–219, 247, 256; *see also* Ambivalence
Love object, 218–19
  overvaluation, 250, 623
LSD, 569–71, 581
Lundberg, S., 279
Luria, R. R., 102, 125
Luria, S. E., 595–96, 645
Lurie, O., 510

McCollom, A. T., 134, 146, 156
McCord, J. and W., 569, 587
McDevitt, J. B., 259, 275
Macdonald, F., 691
McDonald, M., 402, 406
McFie, J., 105, 125
McGlothlin, W. H., 570, 587
Machines, 622
Mack, J. E., 567, 587

McLaughlin, F., 245, 253, 273
McLuhan, M., 229
McMurray, G. A., 50, 72
MacNaughton, D., 268–69, 275
Maenchen, A., 193, 195
Magee, K. R., 50, 72
Magic, 189, 226, 470
  belief in, 572–74, 580
  see also Thought processes
Mahler, M. S., 50, 66–67, 110, 125, 135, 148, 156, 165–66, 180, 192, 195, 253–54, 259, 269, 275, 281, 306, 352, 355, 457, 468, 473, 666, 681, 723
Malony, P., 221–41
Man
  fall of, 600
  survival of, 589–644
Marburg, R. O., 245, 253, 273, 275
Marcotte, D. W., 50, 72
Marijuana, 376, 571; *see also* Drug use
Markowitz, R., 279
Martin, M., 228, 240
Masculinity, 41, 454–55
  complex, 251
  discouraged, 292–95
  and femininity, 201
Masochism, 201, 628
  moral, 268–69
  and narcissism, 244, 247, 251–53, 270
Mason, E. A., 104, 124
Mastery, 34–35, 40
  active, 46–47, 65, 279–80
  instinct, 257
  of internal world, 46–47
  language in service of, 111
Masturbation, 140, 284, 303, 490
  in adolescence, 347, 349, 351, 390, 397, 517, 519
  in boy with congenital lack of sensation, 52
  compulsive, 390–91, 398
  conflict: 315, 327–29, 350, 717; of Schreber, 360–66, 369, 373
  fantasy in adolescence, 517
  fight against, 300
  given up following surgery, 534, 540, 542
  inhibition of, 189
  involving mirror, 343–55
  in latency, 343, 351, 542
  in phallic phase, 166–68
  screen for, 703
  and soul murder, 364–65
  without orgasm, 187
  see also Autoerotic activity, Guilt
Materialization, 307–38

Maturation, 10, 228, 249, 259, 261–62, 269, 271
  and central psychic constellation, 130
  and development, 258
  interferences, 95–98
  lags and deficits in, 96–123
Meaning, 232
Medical procedures, explanation to patient, 530, 545, 552–66
Meers, D., 165, 180
Megalomania, 191–92, 263
Melancholia, 243, 264, 267
Memory, 141, 271
  of addicts, 575, 581–82
  of blind, 11
  as content of schizophrenic delusions, 357–74
  disturbances, 190
  historical, 741
  poor, 578
  spontaneous recovery, 746
  traces, 259, 262
Meng, H., 606, 645
Menstruation, 262, 345, 462, 468, 517, 522
"Mental first aid," 472, 529
Mental health team and burned soldiers, 550–66
Merging, 188, 193
Metaphor, 226, 234
  of mirror, 342
Metapsychology, 243, 251, 253, 258, 271
Methadone clinic, 572–76, 583
Metz, C., 228, 240
Meyer, M. M., 447
Meynert, T., 227, 606, 645
Miller, E., 92
Miller, J. B. M., 457, 473
Miller, M. L., 341, 355
Minimization, 704
Mirror dreams, 341–55
Mirroring, 260
Mirror transference, 350
Mistrust, 415
Mitscherlich-Nielsen, M., 76, 93
Mnookin, R. H., 662
Model, E. E., 3
Money, J., 126
Monod, J., 637, 645
Montagu, A., 595, 609–11, 645
Montesquieu, C., 642
Moore, B. E., 243–76
Moore, W. T., 529–48
Morgenthaler, F., 676, 681
Mortido, 255
Moses, 184, 577

Moss, H. A., 99, 124
Mother
  ambivalent, 288–91, 301
  anger at, 25–26, 39, 144
  anxiety in, 104, 138–39, 141
  attitude: and child's backwardness, 279–306; latent and manifest, 83
  as auxiliary ego, 7, 63
  of blind infant, 3–4
  cannot tolerate child's masculinity, 292–95
  childhood theories of, 88–89
  conflict of, 338
  denigrating child, 283, 299, 301–05
  depression in, 19–20, 138–39, 141, 282, 292–96, 449
  devalued self image of, 302
  disappointed in child, 299
  externalizing undesirable self-aspects to child, 302–05
  lack of admiration of child, 280
  looking for damage in child, 292–95, 301
  need to have child repeat own experience, 289–91, 303
  phallic, 20–21, 451
  of physically handicapped child, 3–4, 54–70
  preferring son to daughter, 139, 284, 287, 302
  pregnant, 24–26, 420
  of prematures, 104
  recognition of, by blind infant, 7
  regressive reunion with, 353–55
  as seducer, 299
  staying with hospitalized child, 532, 546
  transference, 206, 213
  unconscious collusion with child's symptom, 293
  unmarried, 287, 301
  use of denial, 281, 292, 304
Mother-child relationship
  ambivalence in, 205–06
  and blindness, 4–6
  early, 265, 271, 385–87, 665–68, 677
  and language development, 98–99, 110, 122–23
  and learning, 303–05
  and mirroring, 260
  observation of, 75–92
  prolonged symbiosis, 67
  sadomasochistic, 213, 300
  see also Communication, Dual unity
Mothering
  and development of boy with congenital lack of sensation, 61–63, 70

Mothering *(Cont.)*
  inadequate, 283, 301–06, 670
  inhibitions, 268–69
  and narcissism, 254
Motility
  in blind, 9–10
  disturbances, 96–122
  global, 96, 101, 107
Motor inactivity, 134–35, 138, 141
Motor instinct, 134–35
Mourning, 65, 248, 452, 457–58, 470, 486, 493–508
  incomplete, 746
Mouth, 607
  as tool of perception, 8
Murder, 615–20, 673–78
Murphy, L. B., 44, 46, 48
Murphy, T., 654–57
Murray, J. M., 263, 275
Murray, T. J., 50, 72
Musician, 459
  analysis of, 375–406
  meaning of trombone for, 381–82, 387–406
Mutations, 593–603
Myers, W. A., 342, 355
Mysteries, 294
Mystic experience, 184
Mythology, 192, 199, 726

Nagera, H., 13, 63, 72, 85, 93–94, 219, 457, 473, 548
Narcissism
  in animal, 612–13, 621–22, 673–75
  clarification of concept, 243–72
  cultural, 620–27
  development, 44–45
  and diagnostic criteria, 44–47
  dynamics, 263–65
  an economic concept, 251–54
  as energy concept, 248, 251–57
  and hand and face injuries, 550–52
  healthy, 46, 244, 264, 451–52
  in man, 612–30
  and mirror dream, 342, 350–55
  normal, 270
  a nuclear organizing concept, 270–72
  and phallic phase, 162–79
  primary, 244, 248, 252–56, 271, 367
  secondary, 244, 249, 252–53, 262, 271
  and self representation, 135–37, 142
  stages, 244
  transformations, 250–51, 270
  vicissitudes: 663–80; early, 191
Narcissistic disorders, 151, 258

  genetic aspects, 265–71
Narcissistic injury, 626, 671–72
Narcissistic mortification, 183, 342
Narcissistic personality, 243, 254, 260, 270, 341, 350, 668–69
Narcissistic tie, 669–71
Narcissus myth, 260–61
Navot, R., 550
Near-sightedness, 311–29
Need, 202–03, 215–18
  defined, 202
Negative therapeutic reaction, 433, 559, 561–62
Negativism, 24–25, 176
Neonate
  lip movements, 607
  male, compared to female, 599–600
  see also Infant
Neubauer, P. B., 15–17, 48, 125, 127–57, 478, 510
Neurology, 51–53, 95–97, 114
Neurophysiology and psychological problems, 116–17
Neurosis
  in adolescence, 517
  and central psychic constellation, 155
  in child, 112; *see also* Infantile neurosis
  and educational difficulties, 112, 116
  and narcissism, 243–44
  and oedipus complex, 149–51
  and preoedipal development, 151
  seduction theory, 627
  underlying conflict, 247
Neutralization, 255, 257–58, 260, 612; *see also* Sublimation
Niederland, W. G., 269, 275, 357, 360, 365, 374, 684, 723
Nietzsche, F., 639
Night fears, 539–41
Nightmare, 37, 117, 190, 238, 483, 544
Night terror, 708
Nitzburg, A. C., 123
Nobel Prize complex, 45–46
Normality, 16–47
  concept, 46–47
  diagnosis of, 41
  and narcissism, 671–73
  and oedipus complex, 151
  and pathology, 16–19, 22–24, 40–47, 209
  variations, 84
Novick, J., 664–65, 681
Noy, P., 402, 405–06
Nunberg, H., 152, 156
Nursery school, 91
  analyst in, 477–510

Index

see also Hampstead Nursery School
Nursing, 552–65

Oberndorf, C. P., 281, 306
Obesity, 382–83, 385, 387
Object
  attachment, 148
  fantasy relation to, 139–43
  good and bad, 206
  idealized, 136, 142–43
  need-satisfying, 212, 218, 264, 469
  need vs. love for, 202–03, 215–19
  real vs. fantasied, 428
Object cathexis, 246, 248–49, 255, 259–62
Object choice, 244
  homosexual, 248, 250
  narcissistic, 264
Object constancy, 148, 203, 211, 666–67, 716
  lack of, 67, 70, 110
Object hunger, 270
Object libido, 248–50, 256–57, 260, 267, 269
Object loss, 136, 249, 470, 727, 745–47, 750
  early, 267–68
  fear of, 216, 343–47, 351–55
  see also Death, Separation
Object love
  development, 200–06
  and narcissism, 243–51, 253, 255, 269
Object relations
  in adolescence, 517–23
  ambivalent, *see* Ambivalence
  anaclitic, 7
  and central psychic constellation, 134–35, 139–41
  development: 42–43, 50; in boy, 168–73; in girl, 173–77
  early, 161–63
  extension of current, to child analyst, 417–23
  immature, 258, 284
  instability of, 115
  levels, 161–63, 178–79
  and narcissism, 243–72
  narcissistic and libidinal, 665–68
  nurturing, 384–85
  on phallic-narcissistic level, 177–79
  preoedipal, 168
  prestages, 7
  and regression, 25
  sadistic, 268
  sadomasochistic, 425, 435
  and termination, 451–56
Object removal, 460, 470; *see also* Distancing
Object representation, 130, 133, 135–37, 142–43, 148, 165, 171, 178–79, 188, 193
  and narcissism, 246, 253, 257, 261, 263, 270–71
Observation, in psychoanalytic situation and direct, 79–80
Observer
  desirable attitude, 82–83
  role of, 77–79
Obsessive-compulsive mechanisms, 108
Obsessive-compulsive neurosis, 30, 43, 184, 226
  and ambivalence, 198–99, 213–14
  in child, 431
Oceanic feeling, 191, 194
Oedipal phase, 188, 212–13, 267–68, 285
  influenced by preoedipal development, 425
  and phallic phase, 161–79
Oedipus complex, 20–22, 24, 37, 39, 114, 152, 399, 590, 716–17
  central feature of development, 149–50, 155
  and central psychic constellation, 127–55
  and circumcision, 297
  in girl, 176–77
  and identity, 166
  and narcissism, 261, 263, 667–68
  negative, 25, 152, 168, 436
  positive, 152, 168, 436
  and preoedipal development, 127–55
  revival, 544–45, 547
  and transference neurosis, 664–65
  variations in solution, 151–52
Ogden, T. E., 50, 72
Old age, 262
Omnipotence, 37, 46, 213, 218, 250, 254, 256, 342, 459–60, 514–15, 670, 674, 677–79
Omwake, E., 134, 146, 156
O'Neill, E., 711, 723
Ontogenesis, 184, 224
Oral-incorporative phase, 201, 206
Orality, 131, 187
  and creativity, 376, 400
Oral phase, 163, 171, 205–07, 248
  and intellectual inhibition, 305
Oral-sadistic phase, 608
Oremland, J., 375–407
Organ inferiority, 248
Organismic immaturity, 108–09, 119, 122
Organizing function, 42–43; *see also* Integrative *and* Synthetic function
Orgasm, 43
  and reality testing, 368
  ushering in psychosis, 361, 371
Orton, S. T., 108, 125

Orwell, G., 577–78, 587, 684, 696, 719, 723
Osteomyelitis, chronic, 50–71
Overeating, 387, 397
Ovesey, L., 247, 252, 274
Owen, F. W., 108, 125

Pain
  congenital absence of, 50–71
  physical and psychological, 565
Painting, during child analysis, 319–21
Panic, 216, 398
Paranoia, 337, 358, 574
Parapraxes, 81, 214–15
Parent
  deserting child, *see* Kipling
  divorced, 138, 467–68, 472
  exhibiting unusual affect, 189
  idealized, 269–70, 669–74, 677, 696, 726
  lack of pleasure and pride in child, 280, 302–06
  narcissism of, 250, 260, 266–69
  overpermissive, 310–11
  preferring one child to other, 139, 284, 287, 298–300, 302
  psychological, 648–51
  quarreling, 458, 483–84
  separated, 19
  severing ties to, *see* Distancing, Object removal
  split image, 695–96, 719
  tolerating uneven development, 31
  unconscious need to denigrate child, 281–306
  see also Father, Foster parent, Mother
Parent-child relationship
  and foster care, 647–61
  and legal decisions, 647–62
  safeguarding, in absence of parent, 658
Parent guidance, 3–4, 12, 479–80, 506, 529
Parin, P., 676, 681
Parin-Matthèy, G., 676, 681
Part object, 254, 259
Pasamanick, B., 615, 619
Passeron, R., 228, 240
Passive experience, turning into active, 39, 88, 269, 470
Passivity
  in boy, 447–56
  and creativity, 404–05
  defense against, 18, 22, 25, 28
  encouraged in child, 292–95
  enforced, 300, 550–65
  see also Activity

Past
  determines health and neurosis, 20–21
  revival of, vs. extension of present concerns, 417–22, 424–25
Pearson, G. H. J., 305–06
Peekaboo, 88
Peller, L. E., 109–10, 125
Penis
  manipulation of, 297
  and narcissism, 261–62
  trombone as, 387–91
Penis awe, 181–94, 317
Penis envy, 87, 168–69, 173–76, 186, 206, 213, 285–87, 311, 315–16, 345, 352, 460, 470
Perception, 270–71
  auditory and visual, 105–06
  in blind, 8, 10–11
  development, 259
  disturbances, 96–121
  and gratification-frustration, 259
  of need satisfaction, 254, 259
  and repression, 263
  selective, 580
  and self, 67
Perceptual sensitivity, 134–35, 141, 313
Perez-Reyes, M., 50, 72
Perlmutter, D., 235–36, 240
Personality
  aggressive-narcissistic, 628
  changes following surgery, 542
  characteristics of prognostic relevance: 80; in blind, 12
  distorted, 306
  nonpsychotic part, 371
  type and drug use, 568–69, 586
  "wrecked by success," 360
  see also Narcissistic personality
Personal myth, 23, 727, 741–42
Perversion, 248, 704
Pettigrew, J. D., 49, 72
Pfeffer, A. Z., 444, 471, 473
Pfister, O., 613, 645
Phallic-narcissistic phase, 161–79
Phallic phase, 20, 24, 37, 186, 189, 212, 261, 285, 492–93, 503, 667
  and central psychic constellation, 130–55
  premature entry, 297
  preoedipal and oedipal aspects, 161–79
Phallus, *see* Penis *and sub* Dream, Fantasy
Phase dominance, 450–51, 455
Phase primacy, 20–22, 40
Phobia, 37, 144, 507, 574–75
  reactive to surgery, 539–45
Phobic response, 106, 114

Phylogenesis, 224, 252, 610
Physical illness
　in childhood, 138, 283, 288, 297
　of father, 462, 469
　of mother, 292–95, 466, 472
　and narcissism, 250, 262, 269
　see also Burned soldiers, Medical procedures, Surgery
Physiology, 252, 610
Piaget, J., 99, 111, 113, 125, 147
Pick, A., 115, 125
Pickett, D., 647
Plank, R., 185, 195
Plasticity, primitive, 101, 106
Play, 137, 168
　regression confined to, 28
Pleasure, congenital absence of, 50–71
Pleasure ego, 255
Pleasure principle, 88, 103–04, 122, 280
Pleasure-unpleasure, 218
　balance, 148
　in blind infant, 7–9
　indications, 80
　see also Pain
Podvoll, E. M., 725
Poe, E. A., 189
Pollock, J., 3
Pontalis, J. B., 207, 220
Portmann, A., 592, 600, 638, 645
Postal, P., 233, 240
Potency disturbances, 346–47, 349
Powell, D. H., 569, 587
Practicing, 67
Preambivalent stage, 206
Preconscious, 79, 83–84, 198, 204
Prediction, 100–01, 105, 631–33
　of development, 90, 134, 338
　inability to make long-term, 648
　short-term, 650
Pregenital phase (drives), 202, 253–54, 267–68, 612; see also Preoedipal phase
Pregnancy, 4, 262, 292, 296, 301; see also Mother, pregnant
Prematurity, see sub Child
Preoedipal phase, 128–55, 189, 263, 439, 668
　and phallic phase, 161–79
　see also Pregenital phase
Prepuberty, 20–21, 41, 205
Prescott, W. H., 635, 645
Prevention, 477–78, 486
Preverbal phase, 80
Price, C., 700–01, 704
Priel, B., 549–66
Prieto, L., 221

Primal scene, 228–29, 315, 460, 719
　and mirror dream, 342, 344, 347, 352, 354
　terror, 738
Primary process, 35, 110–11, 114, 280, 367, 371–72, 572, 579–80
Principle of variance and invariance, 591–603
Professional choice, 548
Progressive drive, 20
Projection, 35, 63, 88, 209, 249, 261, 270, 272, 342, 352, 431, 452, 463, 470
　in addicts, 573–75, 580, 584
　of aggression, 545
　and externalization, 413
　of mother, 266–69
Promiscuity, 380, 387
Protest, 87, 286
Provence, S., 134, 146, 156
Pseudobackwardness, 279–306
Pseudostupidity, 281, 320
Psychiatrist, 95–96
Psychic apparatus, see Apparatus
Psychoanalysis
　applied to pediatrics, 545–46
　fate of, 641–42
Psychoanalytic theory
　applied to management of burned soldiers, 549–66
　concepts, 85–87
　phases, 198–206, 245–47, 264, 271
Psychoanalytic therapy and technique
　of adolescents, see Adolescent analysis
　breaking off, 218
　and central psychic constellation, 154
　of child, see Child analysis
　and direct observation, 77–82, 89–92
　fundamental rule, 78
　obstacles to cure, 672–73
　pseudoamnesia for, 471
　of talented musician, 375–406
　termination, 394–96, 405, 443; see also Termination
　widening scope, 243
Psychoanalytic training
　desirable experiences, 90–92
　role of infant observation in, 75–92
　supervision, 373
　training analysis, 671–72
Psychobiography, 740–41
Psychological tests, 16–18, 25, 34, 52, 107, 117, 119, 129, 447, 454–55, 459
Psychopathology
　assessment of adolescent, 511–27
　and narcissism, 668–71

Psychopathology *(Cont.)*
  transitory, 511, 517
  see also sub Normality and specific syndromes
Psychosis, 151, 244, 248, 251, 265, 341
  in adolescence, 517-27
  transient, 348-50
  see also Schizophrenia, Schreber
Psychosomatic matrix, 148-49
Psychosomatic phenomena, 85, 337
Psychotherapy
  of boy with congenital lack of sensation, 58-61, 69-70
  dynamic, 584-85
  of father, 377, 379
  intensive, with adolescents, 513
  of parent, 447-48, 455
Puberty, 22, 206, 262
  delayed, 382, 397
  see also Adolescence, Prepuberty
Pulver, E., 245, 251, 258, 272, 275
Punchinello, 229
Punishment, 585
Putnam, H., 232, 241
Putnam, J. J., 638
Putzel, R., 161

Quarles, B., 728-29, 733, 751
Quinby, S., 550, 560, 566

Rabinovitch, M. S., 102, 123
Race relations, in slavery, 747-51
Radford, P., 568, 587
Rado, S., 568, 587
Rage, 192, 293, 343, 352, 466, 716-19
  of father, 449-50, 452
  against mother, 450
Rangell, L., 334, 338, 454, 474
Rank, B., 268-69, 275
Rank, O., 341, 355, 726, 751
Rapaport, D., 264, 275, 568, 576-79, 587
Rapoport, J. L., 50, 72
Rappaport, S. R., 109, 125
Rationalization, 32-33, 88, 465, 609
Rat Man, 198
Reaction formation, 18, 21, 25, 63, 302, 492, 750
  in latency boy, 444
  psychotic, 371
Reading, 696, 717
  difficulties, 102-03, 106, 108, 119-21, 282, 305, 448
Reality, 620
  and actuality, 741
  allegiance, 36, 43
  distortions, 259
  and fantasy: lack of differentiation, 573; ratio, 33-36
  and infantile grandiosity, 673, 675
  orientation: 33-36, 42-43; in blind, 10-11
  treatment oriented to current, 583-86
Reality ego, 255, 366-67, 370
Reality principle, 122, 280, 622-23
Reality testing, 28, 44, 47, 62-63, 247, 523
  of addict, 574, 581
  image vs. object mode, 265-66
  impaired, 626, 638
  and language, 111-12
  split, 493
  surrender of, 366-69
Reconstruction, 18, 437
  in child analysis, 449-50
  of development, 152, 154
  and infant observation, 75, 91
Redl, F., 478, 510
Rees, K., 16, 127-57
Regression, 18, 21, 23-24, 87, 135
  anal, 21, 25, 369
  in analysis, 418
  and awe, 185, 188, 193
  and birth of sibling, 87, 284
  and condensation, 238
  and conflict, 151
  controlled, 27-28, 31, 36, 47
  in early adolescence, 520
  of ego, 139
  energetic, 254
  fate of, 24-29
  fear of, 422, 437
  and fixation, see Fixation
  and identification, 37, 264
  language used in service of, 111
  and loss of boundary, 192
  and mirror dream, 352-55
  and narcissism, 248, 270, 626
  to narcissistic tie, 668
  to need-satisfying object, 469
  after nursing, 185
  and object loss, 268
  and oedipal conflict, 352-53
  oral, 26, 420-21
  to oral phase, 248
  and overstimulation, 717
  partial, 25-27
  permitted, 430-31
  to phallic-narcissistic phase, 177-79
  during phallic phase, 171
  to primary process, 114
  and release, 431-32
  resistivity to, 42-44

in service of: ego, 43–44, 738; healing, 554–65
and simultaneous progress, 25–26
structural, 254
and surgery, 547
and symptom formation, 26, 37
and termination, 466, 470
tolerance of, 555–64
and undifferentiated state, 366–68, 370
Regression-progression balance, 27–29, 40, 130, 140, 143, 147, 449–50, 455, 460–61, 671
Regression rate, 84
Reich, A., 193, 195, 263, 276
Reik, T., 83, 94
Reisen, A. H., 49, 72
Rejection
avoidance of, 416
inviting of, 416
Religion, 601, 606, 614–15, 624–26, 631, 640
Religious feeling, 182, 184, 191–92
Remedial therapy, 95, 116–23
Repetition
of anal-sadistic relationship, 423–25
of mother relationship, 436
of past experience, 423–27, 438
Repetition compulsion, 251, 269, 603
Repression, 249, 448, 453, 612
and addiction, 573, 575, 580
and ambivalence, 213–14, 218
lack of, 63
and narcissism, 247, 249
of pleasure, 262–63
return, 611
of sexuality, 262
and symbolic expression, 334–35
and termination, 465–66, 470–71
Research
methodology, 16–19
and service, interrelation, 512–13
Resistance, 79, 294, 444
adolescent crush as, 438
to anal material, 315–16
and defense, 89
interpretation of, 437, 444, 481–82
and narcissism, 247, 251, 672
normality as, 46
and therapeutic alliance, 664–65, 668
and transference, 436–37
Restitution, 145, 263, 267
Retardation, 285
intellectual, 304
see also Pseudobackwardness
Reverie, 344

Reversal, 421, 463, 470; see also Passive experience
Richardson, S., 50, 72
Richter, J. P., 608, 645
Riess, A., 133
Rilke, R. M., 608
Ritvo, S., 134, 146, 156, 467
Robert, F., 50, 72
Robertson, J. A., 567, 582, 588
Robertson, James, 658, 662
Robertson, Joyce, 546, 548, 658, 662
Robins, L., 571–72, 587
Robinson, J. S., 63–64, 71
Rochlin, G., 267–69, 276, 627, 645
Rohracher, H., 638, 645
Roiphe, H., 193–94
Rokitansky, C., 606–07, 645
Rolland, R., 190
Ronald, D., 477, 492, 494, 500, 503–06
Rooney, W., 227, 241
Rosegger, P., 616
Rosen, V. H., 109–10, 125
Rosenblatt, B., 164–65, 180
Rosenzweig, N., 50, 72
Rousey, C. L., 109, 125
Rubinfine, D. L., 180, 267, 276
Ruskin, J., 182
Russo, M., 550
Rutherford, A., 722–23

Sachs, H., 622, 646
Sackett, G. P., 65, 73
Sadism, 247, 264, 267, 692, 712
anal, 201
in English public schools, 701–02, 704
Safety, feeling of, 286, 305
Salk, L., 402, 406
Sander, L. W., 146, 148, 156
Sandler, J. J., 161, 164–65, 179–80, 208, 220, 251, 272, 274, 279, 409–41
Sanger, S., 550, 566
Santostefano, S., 147, 156
Sapir, S., 123
Sarcasm, 144
Schaffer, H. R., 63, 73
Schatzberg, A. F., 567, 587
Schatzman, M., 358, 373–74
Schilder, P., 121, 125, 259
Schiller, F., 632
Schizophrenia, 263, 357–74
and addiction, 573, 575–76
in adolescence, 518
analyzability, 371–372
in child, 101, 110
see also Psychosis

Schmideberg, M., 470, 474
Schneider, S. F., 50, 73
Scholem, G., 620, 646
Scholnick, F. K., 102, 126
School failure, 280–81, 518; *see also* Learning
School phobia and homesickness, 717–18
Schreber case, 357–74, 683–84, 723
Schur, M., 473
Scoptophilia, 162, 168–69, 179, 280–81
Scotomization, 134, 141, 144, 445, 617
Scott, T. H., 578, 586
Screen experience, 463
Screen memory, 190, 461, 738
Secondary elaboration, 227
Secondary gain, 251
Secondary process, 110–11, 280, 366, 368, 373, 580–81, 583
Secret, sexual, 281, 289, 291–94, 304
Seduction
 of child, 288–89; *see also* Father, Mother
 homosexual, 365, 369–70
Séglas, M. J., 362, 374
Selection, 594–601, 628
Self
 absorption with, 351–53
 awareness of, 113
 and breast, differentiation, 188
 cathexis of: 246, 255, 259, 271, 612, 627; changes, 262
 concept, 260
 discovery, 252
 and ego, 246–47, 257
 fragmented, 254
 grandiose, 269–70, 351, 666–67, 669–74, 677
 and ideal self, discrepancies, 336–37
 loss of, 188; *see also sub* Fear
 narcissistic split, 218
 as organizer of ego activity, 67
 sense of: 110, 122; in boy with congenital lack of sensation, 66–68
Self-analysis, 470–71, 746–47
Self-criticism, 26
Self-destructiveness, 255–56, 268, 487, 492–506
 of addicts, 574
Self-dramatization, 744
Self-emancipation through serial autobiography, 745–47
Self-esteem, 21, 45, 173–74, 451–52, 462, 666–67
 impaired, 672–73, 677
 low, 284–306, 315, 332, 336–38
 regulation, 130, 135–37, 142–43, 145, 251, 263, 272, 338

Self image
 devalued in child, 284–306
 development, 253, 259, 265–70
 "dumb shit," 451–55
Self-love, 248, 253, 255, 264, 667; *see also* Narcissism
Self-nuclei, 254
Self-object, archaic, 270
Self-object differentiation, 135, 259–60
 and awe, 183–94
 incomplete, 353
 lack of, 65–67, 272
Self-observation, 28, 31–33, 42, 47, 351, 502
 capacity, 455
 defensive, 32–33
 lack, 113–14
Self-portraits, motives, 350
Self-preservation, 202–03, 249, 551–52, 609
 instinct, 199–200, 246–47
Self-regard, 249, 264
 disturbance, 265
Self representation, 66–67, 130, 135–37, 142, 148
 and identification, 163–66, 171, 178–79
 integration, 404
 of mother imposed on child, 304
 and narcissism, 246, 253, 257, 259–67, 270
 split, 720–21
 and transference, 413
Semiology, 221–40
 cinematic, 222, 228–29
Semmelmann, G., 619–20
Sensation
 congenital absence of, 49–71
 substituting for lacking, 63–64
Sensitivity, *see* Perceptual sensitivity
Sensorimotor development, 50, 80, 110, 115; *see also* Cognitive development
Separation
 child from mother, 288, 290, 292–96, 298, 434, 438
 experience, 738, 742–47
 fear of, 461; *see also* Fear, of loss
 and foster care, 647–61
 legal provisions for period of, 657–61
 from parent, 459, 685–722
 problems, 86, 213
Separation anxiety, 24, 37, 482, 509
 in mother, 266
Separation-individuation, 20, 66–67, 69, 110, 135, 143, 148, 165, 269, 352–53, 450, 457, 666
Settlage, C. F., 375, 401, 406
Sex differences, 164–79, 599
Sex education, 547

Index

Sex instincts, 199–204; *see also* Libido
Sex, Sexuality
  female, 173–77; *see also* Girl, Woman
  gratification possibilities, 598
  phallic, 292
Sexual roles, 167
Shakespeare, W., 618, 634–37
Shambaugh, B., 457, 474
Shane, M., 443–474
Shengold, L., 342, 355, 683–724
Sibling(s)
  aggression to, 446–47, 452–53
  ambivalence to, 210
  birth of, 26, 31, 145, 186–87, 213, 283, 296–98, 311, 325, 417–21, 426, 487, 689, 721
  different vulnerabilities of, 337
  mongoloid, 291–95, 301, 304
  neglect of healthy, 546
  observation, 86
  reaction to brother's surgery, 535–39
  relations, 129, 310–13, 322, 337–38
  sex play, 138–40, 718–19
Sibling rivalry, 87, 120, 174, 298–300, 346–47, 352, 465, 696
Sigel, I. E., 99, 124
Silence, 317–18, 425, 464
Silverman, M. A., 16, 127–57
Similarity, in dream, 225–26
Simitis, S., 647
Simmel, E., 607, 646
Simon, J. G., 647
Simpson, G. G., 595, 633, 646
Singh, R., 221–41
Skin
  contact, 5–6
  symbolic and real meaning, 562–63
Slavery, 725, 729–51
  escape from, 728, 731, 749
Slavson, S. R., 510
Sleep, 80, 84, 88, 97, 188, 633
  in blind infant, 5
  disturbances (difficulties), 287–88, 539–41, 556, 565
  and narcissism, 243, 251
  withdrawal into, 134, 139
Slochower, H., 190, 195
Smell, 52, 64
Smile, 551
Smith, D. E., 569, 587
Society, primitive, 675–78
Soiling, 292–95, 303, 435, 480
Solnit, A. J., 134, 146, 156, 375, 457, 474, 549–66, 647, 650, 662
Somatic compliance, 85, 148

Somatization, 87, 470
Soroff, H., 550
Soul murder, 360, 364–65, 373
  attempt at, 683–722
Space disorientation, 102–03
Speech
  development: 98–99, 102; retarded, 298
  difficulties, 291
  mannerisms, 289–91
  not used for communication, 110–11
  see also Communication, Language, Verbalization
Speers, R., 478, 510
Spelling difficulties, 102, 106, 108, 121
Spiegel, L. A., 66–67, 73, 259–60, 276
Spitz, R. A., 49–50, 63–64, 73, 80, 86, 94, 146, 148, 157, 243, 253, 260, 276, 551, 566
Splitting, 206, 210, 212, 214, 218, 270, 272, 342, 439–40, 470, 719–20
Sprachgefühl, 115
Sprince, M., 281, 304, 306
Stainer, R. T., 594, 646
Staver, N., 281, 304, 307
Stealing of food, 288
Stechler, G., 148, 156
Stein, M., 477
Sternbach, R., 50, 73
Stewart, J. I. M., 689–90, 699, 701, 705, 715, 723
Stewart, W. A., 526, 528
Stimulation
  blind infant's need for, 7, 9, 11
  sadistic over-, 717
Stimulus deprivation experiments, 578–79
Stimulus nutriment, 577–80, 583
Stolz, H. R. and L. M., 382, 407
Stone, L., 191, 195, 276, 663, 681
Stowe, H. B., 732
Strachey, J., 191, 247, 305–06
Strindberg, A., 683, 723
Stross, J., 75
Structuralization, 18, 108–09, 134, 596, 598, 608
Structural theory (viewpoint), 154, 204, 243, 251
  and narcissism, 258–63
Structure
  defined by function, 264–65
  formation and narcissism, 249–50, 258
  identity of, 591–92
  linguistic, deep and surface, 211–12, 231
Stubbornness, 117–19
Style, analysis of, 738–40
Subirana, A., 105, 126

Sublimation, 249–50, 259–60, 470
  deteriorating, 493
  lack of, 63
  potential, 149
  and termination, 457, 464, 470
  see also Narcissism, transformations; Neutralization
Suicide, 634–37
  attempted, 521–23
  tendencies (thoughts), 458, 518, 522
Superego
  of addicts, 573–74, 585
  and aggression, 255
  analyst a representation of, 432
  anxiety, 21
  defect in child, 305
  and denigrated self image, 303
  dependent on stimulus nutriment, 578
  development: 26–27, 37–39, 63, 89, 193, 280, 600; feminine, 145; and identification with father, 256; and language, 113–14; and object loss, 268; precocious, 26, 29–31
  and dream censorship, 237
  identification, 193
  internalization, 28–39
  and mirror dream, 342
  and narcissism, 250, 261, 263–64, 272, 452
  and oedipus complex, 152
  punitive (strict), 22, 352
  sadistic, 297, 300
  and transference, 412–13
Surgery
  explanations to child, 530–32, 546
  impact on latency boys, 529–48
  need for prolonged guidance following, 546–47
  plastic, 549–66
  preparation for, 546
  repeated, 51–71
Swallowing reflex, 607–08
Symbol
  acquisition, 99–100
  comprehension, 229
  unconscious, 239
  verbal, 229
Symbolic function, 231–36
Symbolic system, 221, 231–32
Symbolism
  of bee, 185
  childhood, 229
  in dream, 228–29, 237–39
  phallic, 186–87, 189

Symptom
  anal, 424
  developmental significance, 152–53
  formation: 263–64; in schizophrenia, 357
  narcissistic, 189
  psychosomatic, 640; *see also* Psychosomatic phenomena
  removal and termination, 444
  somatic, 223, 243, 254
Syntax and dream, 222–30
Synthetic function, 152; *see also* Integrative *and* Organizing functions
Szurek, S. A., 305–06

Taboo, 183–84, 186, 226
Tactile sensation, 63–64
Talent, 459
  and creativity, 375–76, 396–406
  masturbatory component, 398
Tannahill, R., 597, 646
Tanner, J. M., 105, 126
Tarnower, R. A., 510
Tarshis, M. S., 569, 587
Tartakoff, H. H., 45–46, 48
Taste, absence of sensation, 52–71
Teacher, 95
Teething, 138, 141
Temper tantrum, 50, 292, 309, 312–13, 453
Tension discharge, 85, 265–67
Tension tolerance
  high, 136
  variations, 133, 136
Termination
  of child analysis: 330–34, 440, 443–72; premature, 443; technical problems, 456–72
  child turning into active experience, 462–66
  experienced as loss, 456–57, 460–61, 469–70
  and parental environment, 454–56
  positive values, 457
  reactions to, 457–72
Terror and awe, 181–94
Testis surgery, 529–48
Therapeutic alliance, 78, 218, 314, 467, 490, 554
  genetic roots, 664–68
  and narcissism, 663–70
Thomas, A., 122, 126, 134, 157
Thought processes, 112
  of addict, 572–76
  distorted, 578
  magic, 111–12, 218, 493, 507

Index

obsessive, 292
omnipotent, 218
Thrush, D. C., 50, 73
Thumb sucking, 284
Tic, 318–19, 326, 446–55, 458–65
Tillich, P., 624–27, 646
Time
   child's sense of, 265, 647–48, 650, 656, 660
   disorientation, 102–03
   loss of sense of, 193
Tizard, E., 125
Toilet training, 20, 41, 117, 139, 172, 283, 288, 292–93, 296–97, 449
Tolstoy, L., 616
Tonsillectomy, 285, 500–01, 535, 548
Tools, 610–11, 621–22
Topographic point of view, 204, 247
Totemism, 232
Touching
   inhibition, 519
   prohibition against, 184
Transference, 79, 207
   in adolescence, 439
   affected by therapist's treatment of father, 379
   clinging, 438
   of current relations, 417–23
   of defense, 426
   differences between child and adult, 428–29
   and dominant conflict, 449, 458, 470
   envy and gratitude, 209
   fantasy, 400–02
   genetic roots, 664–68
   of habitual modes of relating, 413–17, 421
   homosexual, 370, 437
   improvement, 430
   magic, 459–60
   manifest: as derivatives of repressed, 423–27; vs. transference neurosis, 415
   narcissistic: 669–71; vs. object-libidinal, 665–668; to sexual object, 250
   of need to be admired, 350–51
   negative, 199, 218, 315
   of oedipal relationship, 418, 421–22
   of past experience, 418, 423–28
   phallic-oedipal material in, 214
   phenomena, 486, 508–10
   positive, 199, 216–17, 315
   preoedipal factors, 664–65, 668
   of pseudobackward child, 284–85
   and real relationship, 663; *see also sub* Child analysis
   resolution, 439, 452, 456, 470
   of Schreber, 369–71
   and self-analysis, 747
   split, 499
   stages of, 436–41
   and therapeutic alliance, 664–65, 668
Transference neurosis, 263, 415, 490, 509–10, 526, 664
   in adolescence, *see* Adolescence
   apparent, 422
   in child analysis, 427–35
   and mirror dream, 351
Transformation, 259
   in language and dream, 223–36, 238
   see also sub Narcissism, Neutralization, Sublimation
Transitional object, 269–70, 400, 469
Transitional phenomena, 402–05
Transvestite behavior, 482, 486–507
Trauma
   in adolescence, 382–83, 385, 397
   early, and awe experience, 188–91
   effect of, 547
   in phallic phase, 189
   primary genital, 174
   psychological, and war injury, 552–66
   sexual, 297–300
   visual, 315–16
Treatment
   of addicts, 580
   of adolescents: intensive, 511, 515, 519, 526; nonintensive, 515, 524–27
   of preschooler, indications, 153–54
   see also Adolescent analysis, Child analysis, Psychoanalytic therapy and technique, Psychotherapy
Treatment alliance, *see* Therapeutic alliance
Trilling, L., 702, 723
Tunes, as transitional phenomena, 402–05
Turkel, R. A., 510
Tyson, R. L., 409–41

Uncanny, 182, 184, 190
Unconscious, 79, 84, 204, 224
Underachievement, 95–96
Underdog, 22–23, 44–45
Unpleasure, 255–56
   primitive reaction, 87
   see also Pain, Pleasure-unpleasure

Vaillant, G. E., 573, 587
van Dam, H., 443–474
van der Waals, H. G., 253, 264, 276
Variance and invariance, 591–603
Verbal capacity, 63–70

Verbalization, 99, 110–12, 468–69
  advanced, 485
  capacity, 27–33, 42, 47
Versluys, J., 638, 646
Vestibular sensation, 64
Villee, C. A., 592, 610, 646
Vinken, P. J., 71–72
Vision
  disturbances, 190, 247
  and dream, 221–23, 228–29
  prehensile, 183
Visual alertness, 134–35, 140–41
Vomiting, 424
Voyeurism, 178, 342
Vygotsky, L. S., 102, 111, 126

Waddington, C. H., 67–68, 73
Waelder, R., 113, 126, 244–45, 255, 276, 510
Walk-in clinic, 512–15, 524, 527
Wallach, H. D., 457, 474
Walsh, M. N., 191, 195
War, 629–30, 642–43
War neurosis, 251
Weaning, 20, 86, 139, 283, 288, 487
Weil, A. P., 22, 48, 108, 116, 122, 126, 132–34, 148, 156–57
Weil, A. T., 567, 581, 587–88
Weiss, E., 247, 255, 257, 276
Weissman, P., 375, 407
Weissman, S. M., 725–51
Weitzner, L., 447
Welbourn, R. B., 87, 94
Well-Baby Clinic, 75–78, 82, 91; *see also* Hampstead Well-Baby Clinic
Werner, H., 100, 111, 126
White, R. W., 50, 73
Whitman, W., 686, 723
Whorf, B., 230
Wilbur, R. S., 571, 587
Wild analysis, 77
Wilkinson, R., 569, 587
Willey, B., 643, 646
Willick, M., 346
Wills, D., 3, 10, 13
Wilson, C. P., 50, 70, 73
Wilson, E., 701, 723

Winkelmann, R. K., 50, 73
Winnicott, D. W., 193, 195, 404, 407
Wiseberg, S., 568, 587
Wish
  boy's to be girl, 170
  for child, 466
  and dream, 223
  and fear, 416
  girl's to be boy, 285
  oedipal, 466
  oral, 138, 145
  regressive, 27–28, 31, 187, 432
  return to womb, 187
  revival of: 423–27; vs. release in child analysis, 431
  see also Death wishes
Withdrawal, 87–88, 134, 137, 139–43, 284, 287, 344
  in blind child, 11
  of cathexis, 249
  of mother, 5, 7, 9
  narcissistic, 133
Wohl, M., 523, 528
Wolfenstein, M., 457, 474, 510
Wolf Man, 228
Woman
  masculinity complex of, 251
  narcissistic, 250, 262
Word representation, 112
Words, sense and meaning of, 111
Work inhibition, 324
Working alliance, 78; *see also* Therapeutic alliance
Working through, 285, 436, 448–70, 486, 494, 509, 526, 668, 670, 741, 746
Writing, 686, 707–22, 747
  difficulties, 96, 102–03, 106, 115, 119–21
Wurmser, L., 567–68, 587
Wyatt, G. L., 99, 126

Yorke, C., 567–68, 587

Zangwill, O. L., 109, 126
Zetzel, E. R., 309, 338, 663, 681
Zimmerman, R. R., 49, 72
Zinberg, N. E., 567–88
Zubin, J., 123, 587